Handbook of Essential Oils

VOLUME 1

Handbook of
Essential Oils

VOLUME I

W. Gunkel ○ **L.C. Fraser** ○ **S.C. Bhatia**

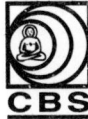

CBS Publishers & Distributors Pvt Ltd
New Delhi • Bengaluru • Pune • Kochi • Chennai

Volume 1

Handbook of
Essential Oils

ISBN: 978-81-239-1820-4

First Edition: 2010

Published by Satish Kumar Jain and produced by Vinod K. Jain for
CBS Publishers & Distributors Pvt Ltd
4819/XI Prahlad Street, 24 Ansari Road, Daryaganj,
New Delhi 110002, India.   Website: www.cbspd.com
Ph: 23289259, 23266861, 23266867   Fax: 011-23243014   e-mail: delhi@cbspd.com

Branches

• Bangalore: Seema House 2975, 17th Cross, K.R. Road,
  Banasankari 2nd Stage, Bangalore 560070, Karnataka
  Ph: 26771678/79   Fax: 080-26771680   e-mail: cbsbng@gmail.com

• Pune: Shaan Brahmha Complex, 631-632 Basement, Appa Balwant Chowk,
  Budhwar Peth, next to Ratan Talkies, Pune 411002, Maharashtra
  Ph: 020-24464057/58   Fax: 020-24464059   e-mail: pune@cbspd.com

• Cochin: 36/14 Kalluvilakam, Lissie Hospital Road,
  Cochin 682018, Kerala
  Ph: 0484-4059061-65   Fax: 0484-4059065   e-mail: cochin@cbspd.com

• Chennai: 20, West Park Road, Shenoy Nagar, Chennai 600030, TN
  Ph: 044-26260666, 26202620   Fax: 044-45530020   email: chennai@cbspd.com

Printed by: Paras Offset Pvt. Ltd.

Preface

Essential oils occur in various parts of the plant anatomy. In some cases, they are found throughout the various organs and in certain cases they are restricted only to one special portion of the plant, such as leaves, bark, roots, and flowers of fruit. Himalayan pine is a type in which the oil is found in most of its parts; rose oil is present only in flowers, cinnamon oil is confined to the bark, leaves and little in the roots. These oils are composed of a number of chemical compounds, such as hydrocarbons, alcohols, esters, aldehydes, lactones, oxides, ketones and occasionally compounds containing nitrogen and sulphur.

Essential oils for all practical purposes may be defined as odoriferous bodies of oily nature obtained almost exclusively from vegetable sources. These are generally liquid (sometimes semi solid or solid) at ordinary temperature and volatile without decomposition. Some of the essential oils are partially decomposed during distillation.

Handbook of Essential Oils is a complete treatise on essential oils and is in five volumes. First Volume deals with chemistry, origin and function of essential oils in plant life; spice essential oils and oleoresing; flavour and and fragrances; production of essential oils; design of equipments for essential oils; Indian attars, determination of physical, chemical and odour properties; detection of adulterants in essential oils; project profiles for manufacture of essential oils and uses and storage of essential oils is the first volume of essential oils.

Second Volume is about the constituents of essential oils—hydrocarbons and their derivatives, alcohols, aldehydes, ketones, phenols, acids, esters, lactones, coumarins and coumarones, furan derivatives and oxides, terpenes, sesquiterpenes and derivatives of unknown constitution. The Volume is divided into two parts: Part A and B. Part A is divided into nine sections (I to IX) and Part B into six sections (X to XV).

Third Volume provides an exposition of genus citrus, lemon, orange, bergament, lime, tangerine, balm, basil, lavender, peppermint, sage, rose, cardamom, pepper, curcuma, sandalwood, ylang ylang, and jasmine.

Fourth Volume deals with essential oil of the palmarosa, gingergrass, lemongrass, citronella, Bois de Rose, cinnamon, cassia, camphor, linaloe, clove, eucalyptus tea tree oils, ajowan, caraway, carro celery, coriander, lovage, geranium, garlic, onion, orris root, calamus, coconut oil, thuja, cypress and cupressus and cedarwood, etc. This Volume is divided into sixteen sections, each one providing useful information.

Fifth Volume is concerned with essential oil of cananga, ylang ylang, concrete and absolute of jasmine and lilac, anise, magnolia, American turpentines, thuja, cedarwood, etc. This Volume also provides an analysis of important essential oils by capillary gas charomatography and carbon-13 NMR spectroscopy. It is divided into eight secions.

Together, all the five volumes constitute a wealth of information for scientists and professionals associated with oil industries. Thus, the *Handbook of Essential Oils* is a complete treatise/manual covering all the aspects related to essential oils and their derivatives along with manufacturing aspects, properties, testing and uses. This reference is essential reading for all students pursuing chemistry and specialisation in aromatic and medicinal plants and persons doing doctorate in these fields. This book will also be helpful for leading industrialists manufacturing essential oils and allied products. Diagrams, figures, tables, and appendices further add to the values of the volumes.

W. Gunkel
L.C. Fraser
S.C. Bhatia

Contents at a Glance

Contents

Chapter 1

Essential Oil and Perfumery Industry: A Review

INTRODUCTION

Essential oils for all practical purposes may be defined as odouriferous bodies of oily nature obtained almost exclusively from vegetable sources. These are generally liquid (sometimes semisolid or solid) at ordinary temperature and volatile without decomposition. Some of the essential oils are partially decomposed during distillation.

Essential oils occur in various parts of the plant anatomy, in some cases found throughout the various organs and in certain cases restricted only to one special portion of the plant such as leaves, bark, roots, flowers or fruit. Himalayan pine is a type in which the oil is found in most of its parts; rose oil is present only in the flowers, cinnamon oil is confined to the bark, leaves and little in the roots. These oils are composed of a number of chemical compounds such as hydrocarbons, alcohols, esters, aldehydes, lactones, oxides, ketones and occasionally compounds containing nitrogen and sulphur.

INDIAN ESSENTIAL OIL INDUSTRY

The Natural Essential Oils and their fragrance are perhaps the most remarkable products of plant metabolism and these products have influenced human thoughts and emotions since the beginning of our civilisation. The art of perfume making was first conceived and employed in the East, especially in India, Egypt, Persia and China. The realisation of their therapeutic values later made use of these materials in medicine as curative, cooling, antibacterial and preservatives including their value in flavouring of foods and drinks. Modern advances in chemistry led to the development of technology for separation of odouriferous constituents from these aromatic plant materials. Thus, large production units have been established which not only isolate their subtle aromas but also blend them for use in aerosols, perfumes and in making of great variety of products ranging from food, medicine, soap, cosmetics, toiletries, paints, varnishes, petroleum products, insecticide, adhesives and host of several others.

The very thought of essential oil and perfumery was first conceived and technically applied in eastern world particularly in Egypt, Persia, China and India. Presence of perfume inside the coffin from the ancient Egyptian monuments is a glowing tribute to Egypt's own technical advancements in perfumery industry in ancient times. The Persians were first to distil rose buds to get natural oil.

The essential oil and perfumery industry has been in existence since the times immemorial in India. Indian perfumes and 'Attars' had been famous for their aroma and flavour throughout the world. Old Hindu literature mentions the use of perfumery materials for pharmaceuticals and religious purposes. There was a time when only the Indian scents had the monopoly and were very much appreciated by the people of foreign countries.

Recent excavation of a copper plate dated 1000 A.D., in Etawah district indicated that there was an organised trade of perfumes in Kannauj and that the kings of Kannauj used to levy tax on the production of 'khus'. Jaishri and Harshvardhan (700 A.D.) were the lovers of perfumes and encouraged their production. Moghul kings were also lovers of perfumes.

Otto of rose was discovered by the queen Nurjahan, wife of Emperor Jehangir in the 17th century. We have also ample references in Vedas and Sutras on the use of different perfumes in religious functions. Sandalwood oil, ambar, 'kasturi' (musk), otto agar and 'kesar' (saffron) have been used since the Vedic age.

Objectives

In view of the interests of the distillation units, farmers and the research organisations—a systematic and thorough survey of this important plant based industry has been conducted. The main objectives of conducting this survey are:

1. To study the organisational, economic and technological aspects of this industry.
2. To develop close rapport with industrialists and thus generate mutual confidence for healthy cooperation to modernise this industry.
3. To study the market trends of this industry.
4. To bring farmers and the distillers close together so as to avoid instability in the trade.
5. To acquaint the growers with the latest techniques of cultivation and utility of aromatic plants.
6. To feed the scientists and the data bank with the latest information on cultivation practices and processing of these plants.
7. To suggest measures that this industry, Central and State Governments and the research organisations might take in order to re-establish the lost image.

Present Status

The most important essential oils produced at present in India are those of sandalwood, palmarosa, mints (*Mentha arvensis, M. piperita and M. citrata*), cedar wood, turpentine and vetiver. The main producing centre of these oils in north India is western U.P. Major quantities of these oils are produced here and rest of the oils are produced in other parts, i.e. Punjab, Jammu and Kashmir, Rajasthan and Himachal Pradesh. Small quantities of oils, i.e. ajowan, rose, dill and camphor, etc. are also produced at Aligarh, Kanpur, Kannauj and Dehradun.

In addition to the oils, a few aromatic products such as scented hair oil, 'Attar' and perfumed waters are also manufactured by the Kannauj based traditional perfumers. Delhi is the main centre in north India where synthetic perfumes are being manufactured by blending different compounds. Other centres where blending is also done are Kannauj, Lucknow, Kanpur and Varanasi.

METHODS OF PRODUCTION

Essential oils and natural perfumes are produced by distilling different vegetable crops. The following methods are adopted in north India for the manufacture of various essential oils and perfumes.

Water Distillation

It is very simple process and has been in use since time immemorial. At present major quantities of 'Khus' oil, natural perfumes and 'Kewda' and rose oils are manufactured by this method. In this process of distillation flowers and roots are mixed with a good quantity of water and put in a copper still called 'Deg'. This still is directly heated at the bottom and the vapours produced are condensed and collected in a copper vessel known as 'Bhapka' connected with 'Deg' through a bamboo condenser called 'Chonga'. Attars are manufactured by absorbing flower distillates either over sandalwood oil or liquid paraffin. There are different sizes of the copper stills used at present which can distil 40 kg to 100 kg of the material Total oil is not extracted by this process of distillation and the quality of the oil depends upon the temperature maintained during distillation. Fuel consumption in this system of distillation is more in comparison to steam distillation.

Water and Steam Distillation

This system of distillation is used by the small farmers for field distillation of fresh crops like *Mentha arvensis, M. piperita, M. citrata* and palmarosa, etc. In this process of distillation, the charge is kept over the false bottom of the still. Fresh water is also fed during every charge at the bottom which is separated from the crop by a perforated grid. This still is heated directly from the bottom and the steam produced extracts the oil from the crop and the vapours produced are condensed and collected in a receiver connected with the charge still through condenser. This type of distillation unit is generally made of steel. This process requires less time and fuel and gives more yield of the oil than water distillation.

Steam Distillation

Major quantities of the essential oils are produced by steam distillation some of the important oils which are distilled by this method are those of sandalwood, cedar wood, camphor, *Mentha arvensis, M. piperita, M. citrata*, 'nagarmotha', 'ajowan' and celery seed, etc.

This process consists in applying steam under pressure to the still containing the charge. These stills are made of steel. Vapours thus produced and condensed are collected in a receiver. These receivers are connected with the charge still through water condensers made of either steel or copper sheet. In sandalwood oil distillation, these condensers are made of copper. Time required for distillation varies from crop to crop. Great care must be taken for temperature control as sometimes high temperature resulting from rise in pressure can decompose the oil produced. Industrialists continue the distillation of a particular charge for the extraction of oil till they find that charge is not running economically. At times distillation is continued for period longer than necessary resulting in off odours in the product.

Expression

This process is employed only for extracting oil from the peels of the citrus fruits. In this process, peels separated from the fruit are dipped or moistened with lime solution to render its cell turbid. These are then separated from the water emulsion by centrifuging.

SIZE AND GEOGRAPHICAL DISTRIBUTION

Total area under aromatic plants has increased considerably since the beginning of seventies. Important plants grown in north India (particularly Uttar Pradesh and Punjab) are *Mentha arvensis, M. piperita, M. citrata*, palmarosa, rose, java citronella and lemon grass. These crops occupy small area in Jammu and Kashmir and Himachal Pradesh also. In U.P., the important centres of cultivation are Moradabad, Rampur, Nainital, Badaun, Bareilly, Dehradun, Saharanpur, Aligarh, Jaunpur and Ghazipur. Although there is no regular agency for collecting and supplying the data on the area under these crops, yet it has been estimated that in 2002 it occupied about 10,000 hectares. This area depends largely on the market trends of the crops.

Besides the regular cultivation of the above mentioned essential oil bearing plants, there are certain plants, i.e. vetiver, 'nagarmotha', camphor, cedarwood, pine trees, etc. which grow wild and are collected for distillation. The important centres of their growth are Bharatpur, Mauranipur, Musanagar, Hardoi, Barabanki, Etah and Himalayan tract.

PRODUCTION OF VARIOUS ESSENTIAL OILS

Essential oil production largely depends upon the crop production, collections from wild sources, imports of the essential oil bearing seeds and spices from other parts of the country, market demand and the market trend. There are about 150 distillation units existing in an organised sector and about one thousand water distillation units (Deg, Bhapka type) for manufacturing of natural perfumes and 'khus' oil.

Sandalwood Oil

In India the sandalwood oil is produced from the east Indian sandalwood botanically known as *Santalum album*. It grows wild in Mysore, Tamil Nadu and Andhra Pradesh. It has also been introduced in Rajasthan, Madhya Pradesh, Maharashtra, Kerala and Uttar Pradesh.

It has been estimated that 6000–7000 tons of the wood is produced annually in the country. Mysore contributes the major portion of it. Other main centres for sandalwood oil in the country are Indore, Ujjain, Bombay and Kannauj. Major quantity of wood produced in Mysore is retained by the state government for oil distillation, a part for export and the rest for carving. Maximum quantity of the wood consumed in Uttar Pradesh is purchased from Tamil Nadu Government auctions. The auction takes place twice in a year in the months of June and December.

Sandalwood oil production of the country depends upon the quantity of the wood available. The main centres of production are Kannauj and Kanpur in U.P. and Karnataka. There are 50 distillation units in all, of which eight are existing in Kannaj and two in Kanpur. Only fifty per cent of the installed capacity of these units is utilised for the distillation of sandalwood which is due to the lesser quantity of the wood auctioned every year. In order to utilise the full capacity of the units, industrialists distil other crops during the non-availability period of the wood.

Sandalwood oil is produced by steam distillation of the wood or roots. It consists of reducing wood by chipping and cutting and then finally converting to fine powder by passing through disintegrator. It is a very important step as it affects the cost of production, influences the distillation and steam consumption, etc. These distillation units are generally made of steel and their capacity is 500 kgs of the wood per charge. Distillation is carried out at low pressure, i.e. 0.7 kg/cm^2 to 2.8 kg/cm^2. It takes about 4–5 days to carry one charge and the distillation of a particular charge is stopped only when it is found that it has become uneconomical to run the batch. The average yield of the oil in north India is 5 to 5.5 per cent of the wood. The oil produced is light pale yellow, optically clear with the characteristic sandalwood odour. Sandalwood oil produced at these places contains 91–92 per cent of santolol.

Sandalwood oil is used mainly as a basic raw material in perfumery and a little quantity also in soaps, face creams, toilet powders, etc.

Rose Oil

Rose plantation in India was introduced several hundred years ago but was restricted only for decorative, ornamental and religious ceremonies. For industrial purposes, the plantation in an organised manner was initiated on commercial scale only during the beginning of nineteenth century.

Uttar Pradesh is the only centre where rose plantations are carried out for industrial purposes. The principal centres in Uttar Pradesh are located at 'Hussain and Barmana' in Aligarh, Kannauj, Ghazipur, Lucknow, Kanpur and 'Sikandpur' in Ballia. About 800–825 hectares of the area is under rose plantations. Rose flowers produced at Aligarh and Barabanki are also consumed for making rose oil. Most of the rose gardens are of small sizes and the bushes growing in them are even 40 to 50 years old. New rose plantations are rarely traceable. It has been found that the rose growers are switching their crops to other profitable crops which promise better returns.

Two types of rose varieties are grown in Uttar Pradesh, namely *Rose damascena* called 'rose fasli' and *Rose edward* known as 'rose cheenia'. Rose 'fasli' variety is planted in Aligarh and Lucknow while that of rose 'cheenia' is planted in the rest of rose growing areas.

The soils where rose is growing are alkaline, light loam and stiff clays majority of the rose growing gardens are dependent on canal waters for irrigation. Planters do not apply proper compost or fertilisers to the plantations. Majority of the farmers use only animal dung and some of the farmers are using 25–30 kg/ha of calcium nitrate mixed with animal dung. 'New plantations are raised from cuttings in the months of July and August planted at a distance of about 60 cms to 100 cms apart in rows. About 5000 plants are planted in one hectare. Pruning is carried out every year either in December or January.

Rose plant flowers are grown twice a year, in March-April and September-October. Major quantity of the flowers are produced in March-April and little quantity in September-October. Plucking of flowers is by hand when the blooming starts and in the case of Rose 'Fasli' it continues for 40–60 days. Maximum yield of the rose flowers is about 2 T/ha in case of Rose 'Fasli' and 1.5 T/ha in case of rose 'cheenia'.

Flowers produced and collected by the farmers are either brought to the mandis for their disposal or are directly sold to the distillers.

Rose oil is produced from flowers of *Rosa damascena* variety. Kannauj has monopoly in this trade. It is produced by water distillation using 'Deg-Bhapka' system. Ten to twelve grams of the oil is produced by using about 200 kg of flowers. It has been observed that the oil is not completely extracted from the flowers by using this method of distillation.

Indian rose oil which was once known in the world market for its quality is now loosing its significance due to the high prices and deterioration in quality.

Mint Oils

Mentha industry accounts for a significant portion of the essential oil trade from the point of view of the capital employed, total value of production, number of people employed and the potentiality for future growth. Several species of this group have been introduced in India for experimental purposes but only three species, i.e. *Mentha arvensis, M. piperita* and *M. citrata* have been used for commercial utilisation. Essential oils of these species are produced by water and steam distillation.

Mentha arvensis oil

The main centres of its cultivation are Moradabad, Rampur, Bareilly, Saharanpur, Badaun in Uttar Pradesh and Ludhiana, Batala and Moga in Punjab.

Japanese mint is grown in North India in loamy and alkaline soils and agroclimatic conditions of U.P. and Punjab are most suitable for this crop. Plantation is generally done in January–February by suckers. Mixed fertiliser containing P_2O_5 and Nitrogen is applied. Weeding in the fields is done annually twice or thrice before flowering. No serious disease has been observed in 'the plants'. When the crop reaches the flowering stage, it is harvested. Two to four (usually three) harvests are obtained depending upon the yield of the oil and the market trends.

First harvesting is carried out in the last week of May to early June, second is taken in August and the third and final harvest is taken in November.

Mint oil is produced by steam, and water and steam distillation of the crop after keeping it for 24 hours. Major quantity of the oil is produced by steam distillation.

Mentha piperita oil

It is a perennial, glabrous, strongly scented herb cultivated in a temperate region of Europe, Asia, North Australia and India. In India, it is presently grown in Uttar Pradesh and Jammu and Kashmir.

It is planted in the months of January or February in deep rich loam soil. It is propagated by cuttings of root stocks. It thrives well in humid and temperate climate of Tarai area. Farm yard manure and artificial fertilisers are applied during cultivation. Care must be taken for its proper irrigation. The crop is harvested when it starts flowering. Generally two or three cuttings of the crop are obtained, first in May-June, second in August-September and the third in October-November. The average yield of the fresh green herb is about 10–12 T/ha. Peppermint oil is produced by steam distillation or water and steam distillation in U.P. from the partially dried herb. Oil produced here is a pale yellow liquid with strong agreeable odour followed by a cooling sensation. This oil is extensively used for flavouring and in pharmacy and offers a good scope for its increased production.

Mentha citrata oil

This perennial herb is a native of Europe largely cultivated in European countries. Cultivation of this crop is of recent origin in India. It is only cultivated on a commercial scale in Uttar Pradesh and that too at Kashipur, Moradabad and Haldwani. Kashipur is the main growing centre of this crop.

Same cultivation practices are adopted for the plantation of this crop as for *M. arvensis* and *M. piperita*. It is planted in the month of January and two to three harvests are obtained in the months of May–June, July–August and October-November. Mostly urea is used as a fertiliser. No serious disease has been observed. Citrata oil is produced by steam distillation of the fresh green crop. An average yield of 100 kg/ha has been observed.

Palmarosa Oil

India is the main producer of palmarosa oil, obtained from Rosha grass botanically known as *Cymbopogon martini*, var. *Motia*. The important centre of production of this oil is Madhya Pradesh. It is a tall, perennial and sweet scented variety of grass which grows wild in the drier localities. In Uttar Pradesh, it is cultivated as a regular crop. The main centres of its plantation are Dehradun, Badaun, Lucknow and Rai Bareilly.

Rosha grass is raised from seeds or nursery plants on a loamy soil or well drained clayey soil in Uttar Pradesh. These are planted just after the break of monsoons. Animal dung is used as a fertiliser. Full care of irrigation is taken. The plants are harvested as soon as the flowers appear. Generally one harvest is taken in the month of October but sometimes two cuttings are also taken, i.e. first in July and second in October. The total yield of the crop is about 125 to 150 quintals per hectare annually.

Palmarosa oil is distilled by steam distillation. A small quantity of the oil is also produced by water distillation. The grass is subjected to distillation soon after the harvest.

Palmarosa oil is used as a base for perfumes and cosmetics especially in soap.

Java Citronella Oil

Java citronella oil is produced by the distillation of *Cymbopogon winter ianus* Jowitt grass. The main producing areas of this oil are Assam, Nagaland, Meghalaya, Mizoram, Tripura, Arunachal Pradesh and Uttar Pradesh.

In north India, it is cultivated on commercial scale, only in Uttar Pradesh. The main growing centres of this crop are Kanpur, Allahabad and Nainital. A little plantation of this crop is also carried at other places in Uttar Pradesh. Plantation in Uttar Pradesh is carried out in the months of April and May by slips in rows giving spacing ranging from 60 to 90 cm in humid soils. The fields are properly irrigated by the growers and majority of them use animal dung mixed with a little quantity of nitrogen as a fertiliser. Generally two harvests are taken in the months of August–September and November–December but at certain places, the farmers even take the third cutting also.

Java citronella oil is produced by steam distillation of fresh green grass. At present Java citronella oil is widely used in perfumes, soaps, cosmetics and pharmaceutical industries.

Costus Root Oil

Costus root oil known as 'Kuth' oil is produced by steam distillation of the roots. Kuth roots are grown in Lahaul-Spiti in Himachal Pradesh and the snowy areas of Jammu and Kashmir. The area under cultivation is showing a downward trend in the country. It has been observed that the yield of 'Kuth' roots/ha and the oil content are decreasing every year. Kuth produced in Jammu and Kathmir is considered to be the best. Farmers are slowly switching their crops to seed potatoes due to fall of the market prices and their inability to find out a customer. Only a part of the roots are consumed in India for their distillation and the rest are exported.

The main production centres of this oil in North India are Kanpur and Kannauj and their production largely depends upon the market demand. Roots used for the oil production are generally brought from Himachal Pradesh.

Khus Oil

'Khus' oil also known as 'ruh khus' is a thick viscid liquid appearing dark greenish or brownish. It is obtained by the distillation of *Vetiveria zizaniodies* roots. These plants grow wild throughout the country in plain, as well as the foothills, particularly Assam, Bihar, Orissa, Hyderabad, Mysore, Uttar Pradesh, Punjab and Rajasthan. It flourishes well in warm damp climate especially on the banks of rivers. Regular plantation of the crop is also carried out in Kerala. There are two varieties of wild grasses one flowering and the other nonflowering.

In North India, vetiver plants are widely distributed in Uttar Pradesh, Punjab and Rajasthan. The important centres of its occurrence are Bharatpur, Musanagar, Lakhimpur, Kheri, Barabanki, Pillibhit, Hardoi, and Etawah. Bharatpur is the main centre where maximum quantity of the roots are dug every year. 'Khus' roots produced here are of yellowish brown to reddish colour and vary in length from 10 to 35 cm. These roots are dug out in North India at the intervals of two years and are harvested in December to beginning of March. It has been observed that the area covered by this wild plant is decreasing day by day due to the conversion of barren lands to cultivated fields. High cost on digging the roots has been noticed.

This industry is managed by a few firms from Kannauj who send oil extraction parties during the season to different place,

Khus oil is produced by water distillation and steam distillation of the roots. Steam distillation of roots is of recent origin and the roots for distillation are brought from different places to Kannauj, Kanpur and Lucknow. Water distillation is carried out in the fields by the traditional method using 'Deg-Bhapka' system. About 0.1–03 per cent of the oil is extracted from the roots by using this method of distillation. There are about 500 units which operate annually at different places. In both these method, the roots are first cleaned, steeped in water for about 12 hours, chopped into small pieces (2–4 inches long) and then distilled. Although steam distillation is more economical and gives yield of oil yet it is not preferred by majority of the distillers. It is because of the fact that the oil produced by steam distillation does not give the same colour and note as produced by water distillation. Khus oil is widely used in perfumes cosmetics and soaps.

Nagarmotha Oil

Nagarmotha oil is produced by the distillation of *Cyperus scariousus* tubers. This plant grows wild in damp places in Madhya Pradesh, Bengal, Southern parts of the country and Uttar Pradesh. The tubers are collected by poor people and are brought to the markets. The main markets in North India are located at Mauranipur and Lalitpur. These tubers are sold to the distillers after removing dust, unwanted grasses and roots and after completely drying.

'Nagarmotha' oil is extracted by steam distillation of the tubers. The main centres for its production are Kanpur, Kannauj and Lucknow.

Turpentine Oil

Turpentine oil is one of the most important essential oils obtained by distillation of oleoresin from *Pinus longifolia* (Chir pine). Whole of the turpentine oil is produced in North India. The main centres of its production are Uttar Pradesh, Punjab, Jammu and Kashmir and Himachal Pradesh.

Pinus longifolia grows abundantly in the sub-mountain regions of the Himalayas upto an altitude of 1600 m. above mean sea level. This forest tree covers an area of about 8–9 lakh hectares in Uttar Pradesh, Jammu and Kahmir and Himachal Pradesh.

Tapping of resin from chir commences in March and continues till November after which the flow of resin practically ceases. The average yield of the resin is about 400 kg/100 blazes. The tapping and selling of the resin in these states is managed almost entirely by the respective government forest departments. Resin produced and collected is auctioned for the manufacture of rosin and turpentine oil.

Turpentine oil is extracted from crude resin by two types of distillation processes namely, by steam distillation and by direct heating of resin. The main centres of its production are Uttar Pradesh, Himachal Pradesh, Punjab and Jammu and Kashmir. The average yield of the oil is 15–17 per cent by weight. The quality of the oil varies considerably depending upon the area and mode of collection, storage and processing.

This clear, limpid and transparent oil with a pungent odour is widely used as a solvent in paint, varnish and boot polish industries. It is also employed in pharmaceutical and perfumery industries. Major quantity of the oil produced is utilised for making synthetic camphor and pine oil.

Cedarwood Oil

Cedarwood oil is produced by steam distillation of roots, stumps and wood of *Cedrus deodara* tree. 'Deodar' trees are widely distributed in the Himalayan forest areas of Jammu and Kashmir, Himachal Pradesh, Uttar Pradesh, Jammu and Kashmir is the biggest producer of cedar wood. Roots contain the maximum quantity of cedarwood oil.

The main centres of cedarwood oil production are Jammu, Kannauj, Dehradun, Kanpur and Mukerian. Major quantity of the oil is produced from the roots and it is more economical. The roots, stumps and the wood are crushed to powder before they are subjected to steam distillation. The maximum quantity of the oil produced is of dark reddish colour which is not being preferred by the users. However, this oil can be improved by alkali wash and redistillation.

Celery Seed Oil

Celery seed oil is produced by distillation of celery seed botanically known as *Apium graveolens*. It is a dried fruit of a herb belonging to the parsley family. It is known locally as 'Karnauli'. Its cultivation in India is done in Punjab, Uttar Pradesh, and Haryana. It is mainly grown in Amritsar, Ladwa and Saharanpur. Other small growing areas are Karnal, Pahawa, Jagadhari, Shamli, Julandhar, and Ludhiana.

Celery seed is sown in the month of December and transplanted in the months of January and February. The vegetable growers transplant it on the ridges in the standing crops of cauliflower and tomato to save it from frost. In Amritsar it is cultivated in those areas which are irrigated by sewage water and in Saharanpur along the beds of Yamuna river. The harvesting is done in the month of May. The average yield of celery seed is 10 to 15 q/ha.

Celery seed is completely freed from dust before it goes to the market. Celery seed oil is extracted by steam distillation of the seeds. The main centres of its production are Kanpur and Kannauj. Oil yield varies from crop to crop and place to place but the seeds obtained from Amritsar contain the maximum oil percentage. The average yield of the oil is 1.80–1.85 per cent by weight. Celery seed oil is used as an antispasmodic and nerve stimulant.

Camphor Oil

Camphor oil is produced in North India by steam distillation of camphor leaves and wood. Camphor trees are distributed in the forest area of Uttar Pradesh. The major concentration of these trees is restricted only to Dehradun district. Regular plantation of these trees have also been introduced in Herbertpur distt. Dehradun.

Cinnamon Oil

Cinnamon oil is produced from the bark and leaf of *Cinnamomum zeylanicum*. The main centres of its distillation are Bangalore, Malabar, South Kanara and Kanpur. The oil in North India is generally produced from the leaves. Kanpur is the only centre in North India where cinnamon oil is produced. Leaves which are pungent and bitter type are brought from Assam for their distillation. Cinnamon oil is produced by steam distillation of leaves. The average yield of the oil produced here is 1.2 per cent. Oil produced in Kanpur is a brown pungent liquid containing 70 to 90 per cent Eugenol. It is used for flavouring confectionery and as an embrocation in rheumatism.

Dill Seed Oil

Dill seed oil in North India is produced by the steam distillation, of *Anethum sowa*. The average yield of this pale yellow oil is 1.5 per cent and contains 44 to 50 per cent of carvone. This oil is used in flatulence, hiccough, colic and abdominal pains.

Ajowan Oil

Ajown oil is obtained from the seeds of *Trachyspermum ammi*. It is cultivated in Madhya Pradesh, Uttar Pradesh, Bihar, Bengal and Punjab. Ajowan oil is mainly produced in Indore but small quantity of it is also manufactured in Uttar Pradesh. Ajowan produced in Madhya Pradesh is considered to be best in the country.

Ajowan seed for extracting its oil is brought from Indore to Uttar Pradesh for its distillation. Ajowan oil is extracted from the seeds by steam distillation. The main centres of production are Kanpur and Kannauj. The average yield of the oil produced in north India is 2–3 per cent by weight. The oil produced contains 44–50 per cent of thymol. Ajowan oil is sold on the basis of its thymol content. Ajowan oil is used in colic, atonic dyspepsia, diarrhoea and spasmodic affections of the bowels.

Other Essential Oils

Besides the above mentioned essential oils, small quantities of other essential oils, i.e. lemongrass, valerian root, ginger, kewda, morpunkhi, eucalyptus, calamus root and jatamanshi root, etc. are also produced in north India. These oils are produced only in Uttar Pradesh. The main centres of their production are Kannauj, Kanpur, Dehradun, and Rampur. It has been observed that these oils are produced either for their experimental trials or the production is not regular and depends only on the market orders.

NATURAL PERFUMES

Natural perfumes are mostly products of plant metabolism and they occur generally in the form of volatile oils. As already mentioned earlier, this industry has been in existence in India since time immemorial. Kannauj, Kumbakonam, Bangalore, Pandharpur, Poona, and Patna have long been famous as centres of perfumery industries in the country. In north India, the important centres producing natural perfumes are Kannauj, Jaunpur, Ghazipur and Ballia. Of all these centres Kannauj is the biggest producing centre and a few industrialists from Kannauj have monopoly in this trade. Small quantities of perfumes are also manufactured at other places in North India.

There are about 50 large scale units and 800 small scale units engaged in the manufacture of different perfumes. There are about 500 old type distillation units (Deg-Bhapka system) of different capacity consuming 40 to 100 kg of the raw material per charge. Out of these about 800 units are mobile and sent out to the fields for extraction of oils.

Natural perfumes are produced by collecting flower distillates over sandalwood oil or liquid paraffin. Some of the producers also use mobil oil as a base oil. Paraffin liquid and mobil oil as base are used to manufacture low grade perfumes.

The proportion of flower oil in the product determines the quality of perfume). The process used for the production of these perfumes is water distillation of the flowers or aromatic plant materials. The vapours from the still are condensed and absorbed on a base oil. Keeping base oil as same in 'Bhapka' a few more distillation batches are run with fresh flowers till the desired concentration of natural oil in the base oil is built up. The resulting product is remarkably stable and resembles the natural fragrance.

Attar Rose

Rose attar is prepared by collecting distillate of rose 'Fasli' and rose 'Cheenia' over sandalwood oil or liquid paraffin. Kannauj, Aligarh, and Sikanderpur are the main rose growing centres. Rose flowers produced are sold to the distillers by the farmers either directly or through the dealers. Major quantity of the rose 'Fasli' variety of flowers produced are consumed for making Rose attar. The main centres of rose attar production are Kannauj, Aligarh, and Sikanderpur.

Jasmine Attars

Jasmine attars are produced by absorbing distillates of different varieties of Jasmines, e.g. 'bela', 'chameli' and 'juhi' over sandalwood oil. Aligarh, Kannauj, Jaunpur, Sikanderpur and Ghazipur are the main Jasmine growing centres. Flowers are sold to the distillers either directly or through the dealers. It has been found that the area under these plantations is decreasing year by year due to the low flower prices and the development of cheaper synthetic perfumes.

The main centres of oil production are Kannauj, Jaunpur and Ballia. (Maximum quantity of 'bela attar' is produced in Kannauj. Only a limited quantity of the flowers produced are used for making 'attars' and the rest being used for making perfumed hair oils. Rates of Jasmine 'attars' largely depend upon sandalwood oil and the flower prices.

Hina Attar

'Hina attar' is produced by distillation of large number of aromatic ingredients, i.e. vetiver, patchouli, saffron, musk, 'mehndi' flowers, ambergus, agarwood, nagarmotha, etc. The main centres of its production are Kannauj, Delhi and Lucknow. 'Hina attar' is produced by absorbing the distillate of aromatic ingredients over sandalwood oil, mobil oil or liquid paraffin. The types and quantities of the ingredients used vary from industry to industry and are kept as confidential.

Attar Gulhina

Attar gulhina is produced by absorbing distillate of 'Mehndi' flowers over sandalwood oil. Hina trees are wildly distributed throughout north India but Uttar Pradesh is the main centre from where the flowers are plucked for its commercial utilisation. In Uttar Pradesh the plants are widely grown on the road sides and the outer ridges of the agricultural fields.

Kewda Attar

Kewda attar is produced by absorbing distillate of kewda flowers over sandalwood oil and liquid paraffin. A few firms from Kannauj have monopoly in this trade. They send their representatives to Ganjam in Orissa, which is the main flower growing area for the extraction of attar.

Perfumed Hair Oils

Perfumed hair oils are produced by absorbing the perfume of different flowers over sesame. The main types of flowers used in hair oils are 'bela', 'chameli', rose and 'juhi'. The important centres of hair oil production are Kannauj, Ghazipur, Jaunpur, and Sikanderpur in Uttar Pradesh. Cleaned and husked sesame seeds absorb the flowers fragrance. Exhausted flowers are removed after about 24 hours and are replaced by fresh flowers. This process is repeated again and again till the seeds are highly saturated with perfume. The seeds are then crushed in 'Ghanis' producing perfumed hair oils.

Agarbatties

Agarbatti making in north India is only a cottage industry. The main centres of its production are Kannauj, Agra and Delhi. The basic raw materials used in this industry are the Perfumery wastes, i.e. sandalwood residue, cedarwood residue, etc. Agarbatties are generally made manually by poor women or children belonging to the labour class families. These are prepared by giving a thin layer coating of a mixture of different perfumery residues and other spices and resinoids, i.e. gum benzoin, gugul, gum acacia, etc. over bamboo sticks of different sizes. These agarbatties are sold to the persons who after giving their own scented dip to these agarbatties sell in the market under their own trade name.

Rose Water

Rose water is produced by distillation of rose flowers with water. Major quantity of the rose water is produced from 'rose edward' variety of flowers. The main centres of its production are Kannauj, Sikanderpur, and Aligarh. The maximum quantity of the rose oil is produced at Kannauj.

Kewda Water

Kewda water is produced by distillation of 'Kewda' flowers with water. The main centres of its production are Chhatarpur, Berhampur, Jagannathpur and Gopalpur. Perfumery firms from Kannauj and other places in North India send their representatives to different flower growing centres during the season for carrying out distillations. Kannauj people have the monopoly in this trade.

SYNTHETIC PERFUMES

The important centres for the production of synthetic perfumes in north India are Delhi, Kannauj and Lucknow. Small quantities of these perfumes are also produced at other important perfumery centres. Delhi is the main producing centre of synthetic perfumes. These perfumes are produced by the blending of different organic compounds in order to provide the suitable fragrance resembling to the natural one. Synthetic perfumes produced sold at much lower prices than the natural perfumes. This factor is responsible for the down fall of the natural perfumery industry in India. It has been noticed that the aromatic compounds used in this industry are either brought from other parts of the country or are imported from the foreign markets.

Essential oils and perfumes are consumed in soaps, cosmetics, pharmaceuticals, confectionery and aerated water, attars, scented tobacco, agarbatti, incense, paints and varnishes.

ROLE OF ESSENTIAL OILS IN PERFUMERY BLENDING

Perfumery blending is a very unique art wherein there are no fixed principles, or restrictions while composing a perfumery blend. It may be very complex formulation or a good perfume can be created with simple and few odouriferous materials consisting of aromatic chemicals, essential oils and resinoids. Ultimate result should be appealing and homogenous.

Essential oils are oils derived from naturals sources of various plant materials. These materials are grass, leaves, barks, roots, flowers, and fruits, etc. These materials are collected at right stages and are distilled or pressed and distilled to obtain essential oils. Every oil has its own characteristics like odour and colour so also viscosity. These essential oil bearing plants are grown in various climatic conditions in different altitudes all over the world. India having bestowed with all major climatic conditions of the world is capable of growing many such essential oil bearing plants.

Essential oils in perfumery play a dual role. Oils can be used in neat form or they are processed and the resultant products are used in blending.

Let us take for granted that all essential oils are available to work with, whether imported oils or indigenous oils. We think of using the same in blending with other odouriferous materials like aromatics chemicals and resinoids.

Major Routes of Essential Oils in Perfume Compounds

There are four major routes while using the essential oils in perfume compounds:
1. Using the oils in neat form.
2. Using terpineless oils.

3. Processing oils to make isolates and derivatives.

4. Using isolates and derivatives there off.

In addition to types mentioned above, there are few more oil varieties like colourless oils, iron free oils and few captive oils from different manufacturers.

While recollecting the use of fragrant liquids as perfumes by stone age humans, history reveals that the essential oils attracted men and women to each other by applying oils on their body as 'perfume'. In primitive period it may not be even oils, but just juices of citrus or apple, strawberry like fruits having strong aldehydic odour. In addition to this they must have used some fragrant powder of barks and other dried natural materials. Thus preparing blends of natural odours. Shall we call it a first natural perfume? As the science and technology advanced, the quality and availability of odouriferous materials also improved. Art of blending also became a science. In this scientific art of blending the natural essential oils play a most important role.

Essential oils in perfumery blends

In well crafted perfumery compound essential oils play a major role of contributing all 'feel good' factors. These important qualities can be described in perfumery terms as follows:

1. To get new shades of odour.
2. To achieve homogeneity.
3. To get substantivity.
4. To get richness.
5. To achieve natural freshness.
6. Overall perfumistic effect.

Perfumer has at his disposal about two hundred or more commonly used essential oils. Some of these oils are used liberally, some of them are used sparingly, and some are used in small proportions to get exotic effects. Selection of oils required in a perfume while its conception depends fully upon perfumer's artistic imagination, consistent availability of oil and in industry the cost of natural products. Rest depends upon final fineness of perfumery compound.

CONCLUSION AND RECOMMENDATIONS

No doubt, the industry has progressed well during the last five years but in the production of certain essential oils and perfumes the industry has gone considerably down. India lost its dominant position as a supplier of high grade perfumes and aromatics due to its failure in keeping pace with technological developments in western countries. A further set back was due to poor quality control. This lost image can be achieved if proper coordination between the producers, users and the research organisations is made. It is, therefore, expected from all concerned with this industry to consider the following factors for its development:

1. Majority of the farmers are illiterate and are not aware of the latest developments taking place in cultivation practices. With the result they are unable to produce the crops giving them better returns. Therefore, it is expected from the research organisations to send regularly a team of scientists in these plant growing areas so as to provide them research and development facilities for the introduction of latest cultivation practices. It is also expected from the farmers to adopt the latest developments without hesitation.

2. Research organisations should work for the development of new strains which should be disease resistant, give better yield and quality of oil.

3. Farmers are ignorant of the exact utility of their produce and they are not offered exact prices, with the result there are great fluctuations in the market. This creates uncertainty regarding the cultivation and production of essential oils. It is, therefore, suggested that an association of the farmers and the users of these oils may be formed which should fix up the prices at the time of cultivation.

4. There is considerable scope for the development of essential oil industry. In addition to the materials which are now being exploited for the production of essential oils, a number of other essential oils, such as caraway, cananga, lavender, clove, nutmeg, patchouli, spearmint, cassia and coriander, etc. are imported in large quantities. Research laboratories should give more emphasis on the development, of these aromatic plants in the country.

5. Training courses for the farmers and the distillers should be arranged to educate them with regard to the latest techniques of cultivation practices and distillation methods.

6. There should be a thorough techno-economic survey of the flora to discover new indigenous aromatic plants and introduction of exotics for cultivation on semi-commercial and commercial scale.

7. Regional research laboratory, Jammu should strengthen data bank system so as to provide the latest information to those concerned with the development of this industry. For this, the farmers and the industrialists should contribute not only financially but also by supplying the exact figures whenever required.

8. There should be a coordination between the research organisations, farmers and the perfumers to develop and cultivate new perfume bearing plants.

9. It has been observed that the yield and quality of the oil vary from batch to batch and industry to industry. Moreover in certain cases, the oil yield is far below the expected level. It is due to the lack of knowledge on the distillation techniques. It is, therefore, suggested that the distillers should not hesitate in approaching the research organisations for adoption of modern distillation techniques.

10. Research organisations should provide testing facilities for the essential oils sent by the industry at concessional rates.

11. Research should be initiated to design and produce presentable containers for attars and other essential oils meant for export.

12. Steps must be taken to boost the export of essential oils and perfumes and there should be adequate arrangements to know the market demands in foreign countries.

13. There should be adequate arrangement for the identification of synthetic and natural essential oils. This lack of knowledge creates great hindrance during the import of essential oils.

14. There should be coordination between the various research laboratories, so that they can jointly contribute their services for the development of this industry.

15. Quality improvement of synthetic perfumes is very much required in north Indian perfumery industry. For this purpose, research laboratories should develop new organic compounds and new techniques of blending so as to provide the required fragrance to blend the perfume.

16. A high power advisory council be set up to facilitate development of essential oil industry, help in fixing prices for raw materials, to boost export of essential oils and to rationalise imposition of sale tax and excise tax structures.

17. It is suggested that authoritative information with regard to this important growing industry should be collected and published from one central source. Maintenance of such information on a up-to-date basis is vital to a further study of the problems and progress of the essential oil and perfumery industry.

18. Except in a few cases, the industry is technologically backward, organisationally weak and not in a position to take full advantage of technological developments that are available. Industrialists should not hesitate in approaching the research organisations through their associations in pin-pointing their problems. It is also expected from the research organisations to concentrate sincerely in solving the problems mentioned to them.

19. There is a great and urgent need for expanding educational and technical facilities available to the industry.

20. Standardisation of the quality of essential oils and perfumes and production of high quality goods are the major factors that should contribute to a rapid expansion of their exports.

21. This industry seems to be one of the most labour intensive industries which can also be highly machanised. Therefore, a rapid expansion of this industry would lead to the creation of employment potential.

22. In view of the importance of this industry, the industrialists should make special efforts to produce quality products. These iudustrialists should also keep close contact with the users of their products, find out their quality problem and attempt to solve them.

23. In view of the widespread distribution of the industry in north and because of its growing importance and in view of the paucity of technically trained men in this industry, there should be an adequate arrangement to institute full time training courses in essential oils and perfumes. Further, for the sake of the small entrepreneurs in this trade who may not be in a position to employ qualified staff, part time training courses should also be available in the research organisations or in the big industrial houses. Such part time training will be an important factor in raising the general level of technology and efficiency in the industry.

24. The essential oil association of India and perfumes and flavours association of India should create and maintain technical services and make these services available to their members in order to improve their productivity.

25. It is in the long-term interests of the essential oil and perfumery industry to produce uniform quality products. Standardisation of the quality on a state and national basis so that all industries should adopt them. Standardisation within the factory and inspection procedures to ensure that these standards are observed would go a long way in improving quality ensuring customer satisfaction, giving boost to exports and in creating a good public image for the industry.

Besides above, our country's biodiversity coupled with competent scientific force, make our country as the best choice to become a foremost leader in fragrance and flavour business. We have to review our strength and weaknesses and plan a joint strategy with growers, scientific community and users.

Our strength is:
1. Biodiversity.
2. Forest resources.
3. Infrastructure.
4. Scientific force.
5. Farming community.
6. Trading community.
7. Processing industry.

Our weaknesses are:
1. Agriculture policy.
2. Role of R & D institutes and facilities.
3. Marketing support.
4. Interaction.
5. Commodity boards.

Chapter 2

Chemistry, Origin and Function of Essential Oils in Plant Life

INTRODUCTION

Early in his history, man evinced a great deal of interest in the preservation of the fragrant exhalation of plants and those who were later to be called chemists occupied themselves with separating the essence of the perishable plants. It was probably observed that heating of the plant caused the odoriferous principle to evaporate and that upon condensation and subsequent cooling, droplets united and formed a liquid consisting of two layers—water and oil. While, in such primitive experiments, the water from the plant is used to carry over the oils, additional water or steam was later introduced in 'stills' to obtain better yields and quality. In early work, the term 'essential oil' or 'ethereal oil' was defined as the volatile oil obtained by the steam distillation of plants. With such a definition, it is clearly intended to make a distinction between the fatty oils and the oils which are easily volatile. Their volatility and plant origin are the characteristic properties of these oils and it is for this reason more satisfactory to include in our definition volatile plant oils obtained by other means than by direct steam distillation. Bitter almond and mustard oil, obtained by enzymatic action, followed by steam distillation; lemon and orange oil isolated by simple pressing and certain volatile oils obtained by extraction are, therefore, included among the essential oils. In the early stages of development of organic chemistry, the chemical investigation of oils was limited to the distillation of a great number of plants and the oils which were obtained in this way were used to compose perfumes according to recipes, some of which are still used at the present time; e.g. the eau de Cologne prepared in 1725 by Johann Maria Farina in Cologne.

CHEMISTRY OF ESSENTIAL OILS

Gradually with the advance of science came improvements in the methods of preparing the oils and parallel with this development a better knowledge of the constituents of the oils was gained. It was found that the oils contain chiefly liquid and more or less volatile compounds of many classes of organic substances. Thus, we find acyclic and isocyclic hydrocarbons and their oxygenated derivatives. Some of the compounds contain nitrogen and sulphur. Although a list of all the known oil components would include a variety of chemically unrelated compounds, it is possible to classify a large number of these into four main groups, which are characteristic of the majority of the essential oils.

1. Terpenes, related to isoprene or isopentene.
2. Straight-chain compounds, not containing any side branches.
3. Benzene derivatives.
4. Miscellaneous.

Representatives of this last group are incidental and often rather specific for a few species (or genera) and they contain compounds other than those belonging to the three first groups (Fig. 2.1).

$$CH_2{=}CH{-}CH_2{-}N{=}C{=}S \qquad \text{allyl isothiocyanate}$$
$$CH_2{=}CH{-}CH_2{-}S{-}CH_2{-}CH{-}CH_2 \qquad \text{diallyl sulphide}$$
$$CH_3{-}CH_2{-}CH{-}S{-}S{-}CH{=}CH{-}CH_3 \qquad \text{sec.-butyl propenyl disulphide}$$
$$| \qquad\qquad CH_3$$
$$CH_3{-}CH_2{-}CH_2{-}CH_2{-}SH \qquad n\text{-butyl mercaptan}$$
$$CH_3{-}CH{=}CH{-}CH_2{-}S{-}CH_2{-}CH{=}CH{-}CH_3 \qquad \text{dicrotyl sulphide}$$

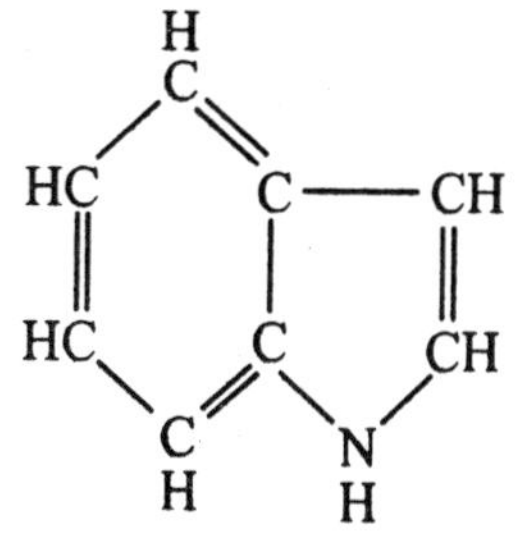

Indole 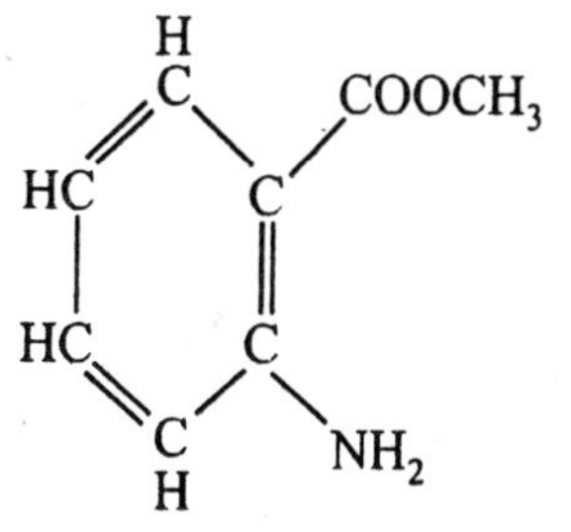   Methyl anthranilate

Fig. 2.1. Natural occurring volatile sulphur and nitrogen containing compounds.

For example, the mustard oils, containing allyl isothiocyanate, are found in the family of the cruciferae; allyl sulphides in the oil of garlic. The oil from *Ferula asafoetida* L., belonging to the family of the *Umbelliferae*, gained reputation from its active component, secondary butyl propenyl disulphide, a competitor of the odouriferous principles of the skunk, primary *n*-butyl mercaptan and dicrotyl sulphide. The more pleasant smelling orange blossom and jasmine perfume betrays the presence of small amounts of anthranilates and indole, both compounds related to the amino acid, tryptophane.

Although it is possible to list a considerable number of such singular cases, the most characteristic group present in many essential oils contains hydrocarbons, as a rule of the formula $C_{10}H_{16}$ and a group of oxygen-containing compounds with the empirical formula $C_{10}H_{16}O$ and $C_{10}H_{18}O$. The English word 'terpene' and the German 'Terpen' are derived from the German word 'Terpentin', English 'turpentine' and French 'térebenthine'. The name 'Terpen' is commonly attributed to Kékulé, who is said to have introduced it as a generic term for hydrocarbons $C_{10}H_{16}$ to take the place of such words as Terebene, Camphene, etc. The name 'camphor' formerly was used to indicate the crystalline oxygen compounds, such as thyme camphor and peppermint camphor; these are now known respectively as thymol and menthol. The name 'camphor' is at present limited to a specific compound and its more general meaning, covering the oxygenated derivatives, has been taken over by the term 'terpene'. With an increase in our knowledge, this broadened definition in its turn became too narrow and had to be modified to cover new and more distantly related compounds. Not all terpenes are represented by the formula C_5H_8; there exist compounds which contain less hydrogen, still others which are more saturated. We also find terpenes, like santene (C_9H_{14}), which have only 9 carbon atoms. The close resemblance to and probable connection with the C_{10} compounds through the terpene acid, santalic acid, make it impractical to omit such a compound from the terpene literature.

At the present time, therefore, we use the term terpene both in its broadest sense to designate all compounds which have a distinct architectural and chemical relation to the simple C_5H_8 molecule and in a more restricted sense to designate compounds with 10 carbon atoms derived from $C_{10}H_{16}$. When confusion with the general designation is possible, members of the C_{10} group are often referred to as monoterpenes. Compounds having a more distant connection with the terpenes, but still containing features which link them with terpene structures, are sometimes called terpenoids or isoprenoids in analogy with the term steroids, which includes not only sterols, but many more remotely connected relatives.

Characteristic for many of these oil constituents is their instability and the ease with which intramolecular rearrangements occur. These properties have been a great hindrance to the study of these compounds. Another drawback in the analysis of these oils is that most of the compounds are liquids so that thorough fractionation is necessary to separate the constituents which boil within a restricted temperature range. Since in the early stages of research it was difficult to define sharply the isolated fraction, a great number of terpenes were named after the plant from which they were obtained.

Order was brought into this chaos by Wallach, who saw clearly that the first task in the study of the oils was the identification of the terpenes with the help of crystalline derivatives, this being the only practical way we possess at present to identify chemical substances with certainty. Based on Wallach's investigation, about 500 compounds have since been isolated and characterised in the essential oils. After a general idea was obtained of the great number of distinct chemical compounds in oils, Wallach and others started the second part of his working programme, i.e. studies of the relationship between the terpenes and the camphors. By reason of their fundamental nature and the clear presentation of the problems they involved, these studies provided great stimulus not only to his contemporaries—Semmler, Harries, Tilden and others—but had a pronounced influence on the development of chemistry as a whole. The establishment of the constitution and the relationship of the terpenes revealed a certain regularity in their structures. Berthelot had discovered how the hydrocarbons $C_{10}H_{16}$, $C_{15}H_{24}$ and $C_{20}H_{32}$ are related to the hydrocarbon isoprene (C_5H_8) isolated by Williams a few years before. However, it was through the combined work of the aforementioned investigators that this hypothesis was established on a firm basis.

The compounds which we find in the monoterpene series can be figuratively divided into 2 isopentene chains; such a hypothetical combination gives substances of the empirical formula $C_{10}H_{16}$. If three of these isopentene units can be recognised in the molecule, the name sesquiterpene is given. In the course of time there have been added diterpenes derived from $C_{20}H_{32}$, triterpenes, $C_{30}H_{48}$ and tetraterpenes, $C_{40}H_{64}$ and finally polyterpenes with an indefinitely large number of these units (Fig. 2.2).

A saturated acyclic hydrocarbon with 10 carbon atoms would have the formula $C_{10}H_{22}$, possessing six hydrogen atoms more than a compound $C_{10}H_{16}$. This lower hydrogen content may be caused by the occurrence of double bonds, by ring structure or by both, giving rise to acyclic, monocyclic and bicyclic representatives, with 3, 2 and 1 double bond, respectively. Therefore, the following possibilities for a molecule with the formula $C_{10}H_{16}$ (monoterpene):

Acyclic	No ring	3 double bonds
Monocyclic	One ring	2 double bonds
Bicyclic	Two rings	1 double bond
Tricyclic	Three rings	No double bonds

All these structural variations of the same empirical formula are found in the constituents of volatile plant oils. A chemical shorthand, developed by terpene chemists, has been introduced to show more clearly the principal structural details.

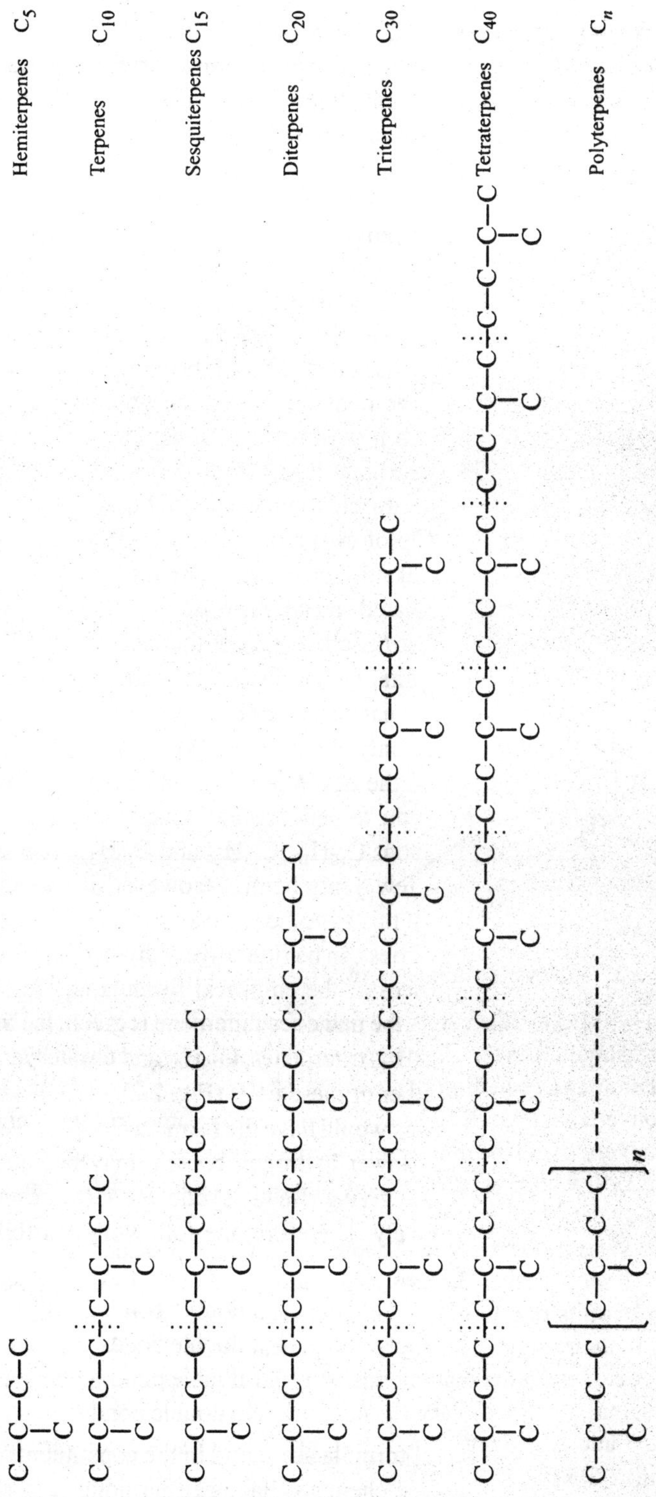

Fig. 2.2. Carbon skeletons of terpenes.

This greatly simplified way of writing formulas consists in assuming a carbon atom at a place where valency lines end, or form an angle. As many C's and H's as feasible are omitted and only double bonds and substituents, such as hydroxyl and amino groups, are written in full (Fig. 2.3). Others prefer to indicate all end groups such as methyl and methylene groups in full.

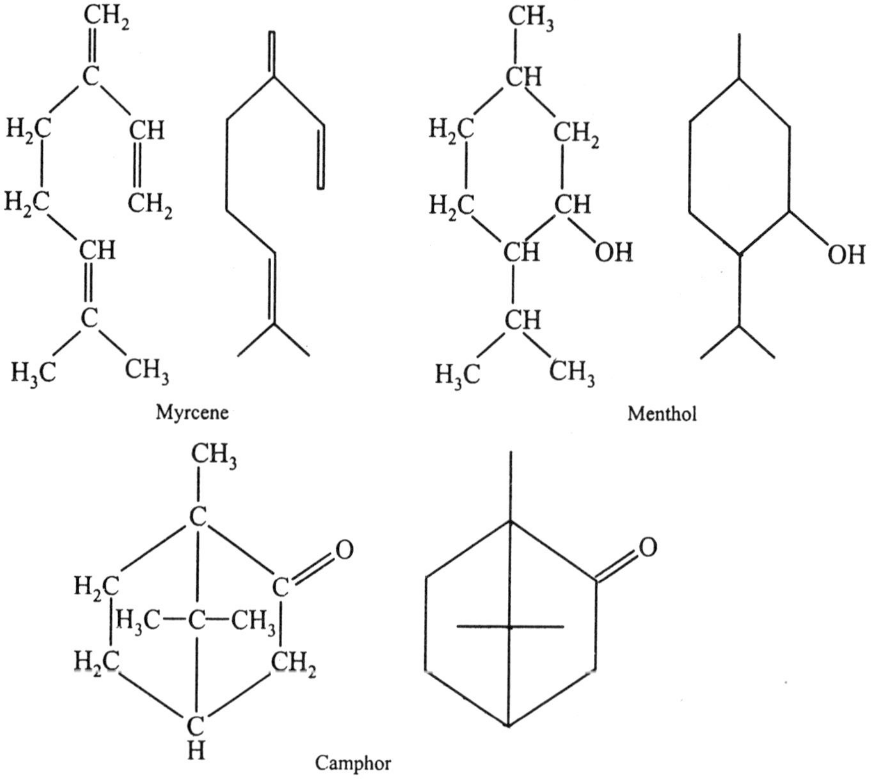

Myrcene   Menthol

Camphor

Fig. 2.3. Abbreviated formulas of terpenes.

As examples of the acyclic terpenes with 3 double bonds, we find ocimene and myrcene. In the frequently occurring acyclic alcohols geraniol and linalool, in the aldehydes citronellal and citral and in dehydrogeranic acid we see several stages of oxidation and reduction of this type of terpene hydrocarbons (Fig. 2.4). Many of these compounds can be converted into each other with great ease. Geraniol, the chief constituent of rose and geranium oil, is easily converted into the monocyclic alcohol α-terpineol, the chief constituent of the oil of hyacinth and into linalool, which as acetate constitutes the characteristic component of lavender oil.

Geraniols of variant origin have variant constants and odours, due to the presence of isomers. The double bond between carbon atoms 2 and 3 makes the existence of cis- and trans-isomers possible and the relative ease of ring formation permits one to distinguish between these forms, which have been called nerol and geraniol according to their origin. The double bond near the terminal carbons is another source of isomerism. Thus geraniol, nerol and other compounds with similar structure, such as citronellol and rhodinol and citronellal and rhodinal, consist of varying quantities of isomers containing the double bond, between either carbon atoms 7 and 8 or 6 and 7, resulting in a further source of variation in the constants of the oil constituents (Fig. 2.5).

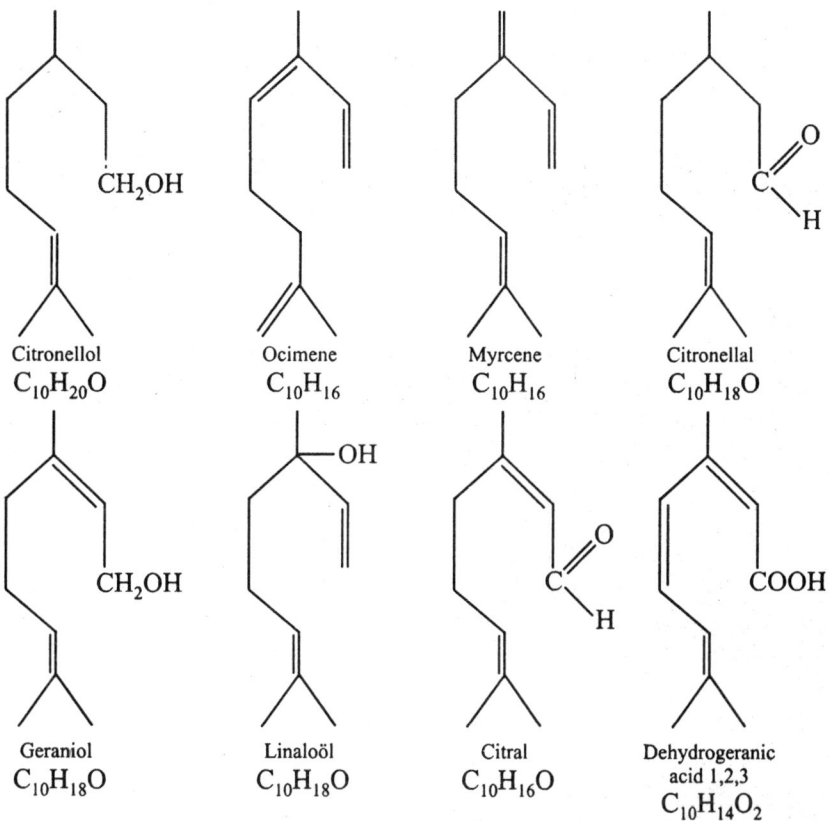

Fig. 2.4. Oxidation stages of acyclic terpenes.

Most of these compounds easily form cyclic derivatives under the influence of acids and the formulas are usually written intentionally in such a way as to indicate where the ring closure takes place. A saturated monocyclic terpene has the formula $C_{10}H_{20}$ and is called menthane. If the compound has the empirical formula $C_{10}H_{16}$, there must be 2 double bonds, since the ring occurs in the place of one of the 3 double bonds present in aliphatic terpenes. Such hydrocarbons are called menthadienes and the method of indicating the position of the double bond given by Baeyer makes use of the Greek capital letter Δ (delta) and an index number indicating the carbon atom from which the double bond starts. If the double bond is in the side chain, then it will be necessary to indicate toward which carbon atom the double bond goes. This number is placed in brackets behind the number of the first carbon atom, as is indicated in Fig. 2.6. (It is customary to indicate a double bond from C_8 to one of the atoms 9 or 10 as $\Delta^{8(9)}$, although with unsubstituted end groups no confusion could arise using the index Δ^8. In the modern American literature the Δ sign is generally no longer used with monocyclic terpenes, but it is still employed in the nomenclature of the bicyclic terpenes and derivatives.)

We find many representatives of this class of menthadienes among the terpene fractions in essential oils. For example, dipentene, formed by the polymerisation of isoprene under the influence of acids, is such a compound. The official name of this compound would be $\Delta^{1,8(9)}$-menthadiene. Carbon atoms, indicated by an asterisk in Fig. 2.6 have four substituents, each of different nature and these substituents can be arranged in two different ways around the carbon atom, thereby forming mirror images.

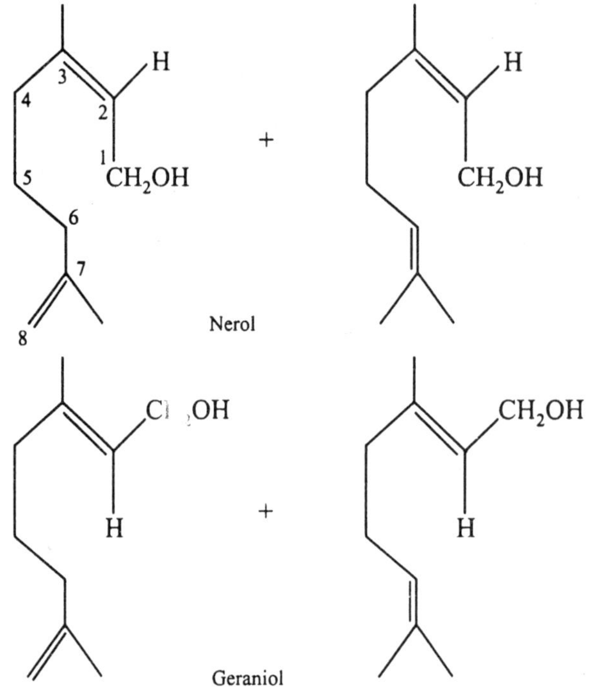

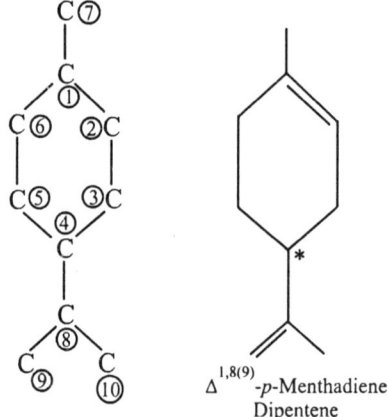

Fig. 2.5. Isomerism of geraniol.

$\Delta^{1,8(9)}$-*p*-Menthadiene
Dipentene

Fig. 2.6. Greek letter Δ (delta) and index number indicating the carbon atom from which double bond starts.

These two forms show similar chemical properties and have the same melting and boiling points, but differ in their behaviour toward light. When plane polarised light is passed through this type of compound, the plane in which the light vibrates is rotated and the amount of this rotation is determined in a polarimeter. The two forms give a rotation of equal magnitude, but in opposite directions. Often equal amounts of the two forms crystallise together and this combination acts in many ways as a third isomer. These so-called 'racemates' or their derivatives have melting points, solubilities, etc. different from the two components, but do not show any optical rotation.

In the $\Delta^{1,8(9)}$-menthadienes all forms and mixtures of these optical isomers and racemates occur in nature. In pine needle and lemon oil we find a laevorotatory isomer called *l*-limonene; the *d*-form we find in oil of lemon and caraway, whereas the racemate, viz. dipentene, occurs in the oil of turpentine.

When we arrange the double bonds in a different way we can make a total of 32 isomers, which include possible optical antipodes and their racemic mixtures and *cis- trans-* forms. Therefore, for this one type of terpene alone, a great number of possibilities exists. Some of these structures occur in nature, as is indicated in Fig. 2.7.

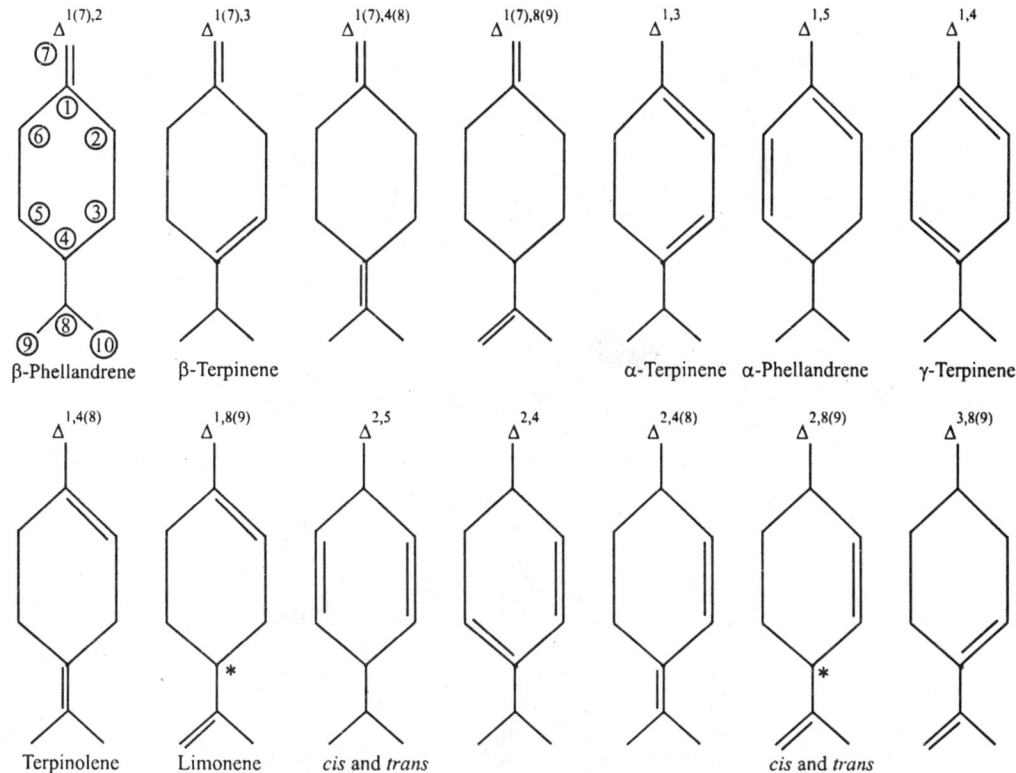

Fig. 2.7. Isomeric *p*-Menthadienes.

The number of possibilities is further increased if the methyl and the isopropyl group occupy positions other than 1,4 on the cyclohexane ring. We find representatives of this structure in sylvestrene a terpene derived from the commercial oil of *Pinus sylvestris*.

The monocyclic terpenes also occur in many stages of oxidation and after we have seen the diversity in the aliphatic series, it is not surprising to find compounds with less and with more hydrogen than the general formula $C_{10}H_{16}$ requires, i.e. 1-methyl-4-isopropenylbenzene $C_{10}H_{12}$, in hashish oil; *p*-cymene $C_{10}H_{14}$, in eucalyptus oil; and Δ^3-menthene $C_{10}H_{18}$, with only one double bond, in thyme oil (Fig. 2.8). Oxygen-containing derivatives (alcohols and carbonyl compounds) of these hydrocarbons also belong to the monocyclic terpene group and many of these structures can be converted into each other by relatively simple chemical reactions (Fig. 2.9).

In all these derivatives we see a so-called head-to-tail union of the branched C_5 chains. The first discovered deviation from this structural scheme was looked upon with a great deal of suspicion.

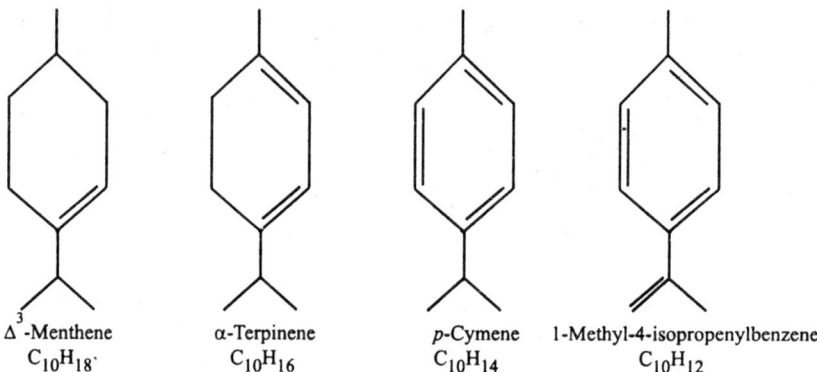

Fig. 2.8. Oxidation stages of monocyclic terpenes.

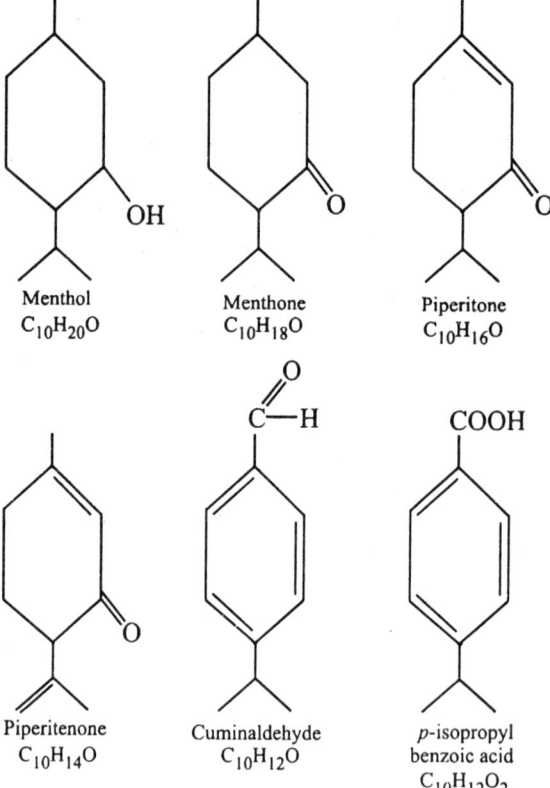

Fig. 2.9. Oxidation stages of monocyclic terpenes.

However, after the synthesis of a derivative of one of these compounds (i.e. tetrahydroartemesia ketone) was achieved, there could no longer be any doubt about the possibility of irregular build-up in the terpene series. The formula of artemesia ketone can still be divided into branched C_5 chains, but no head-to-tail union is found. Recently two similar cases have become known, senecic acid, which occurs bound in senecio alkaloids in some *Compositae*, and lavandulol in oil of lavender, which is accompanied by the ester of the regularly built linaloöl (Fig. 2.10).

Linaloöl
$$H_3C-C=CH-CH_2-CH_2-C-CH=CH_2$$
with CH_3 groups above and OH below

Artemesia ketone
$$H_2C=CH-C-C-CH_2-CH=CH_2$$
with CH_3 groups and CH_3 O below

Senecic acid
$$H_3C-CH=C-CH_2-CH-CH-C=O$$
with CH_3, $COOH$, CH_2——O

Lavandulol
$$H_3C-C=CH-CH_2-CH-C=CH_2$$
with CH_3, CH_2OH, CH_3

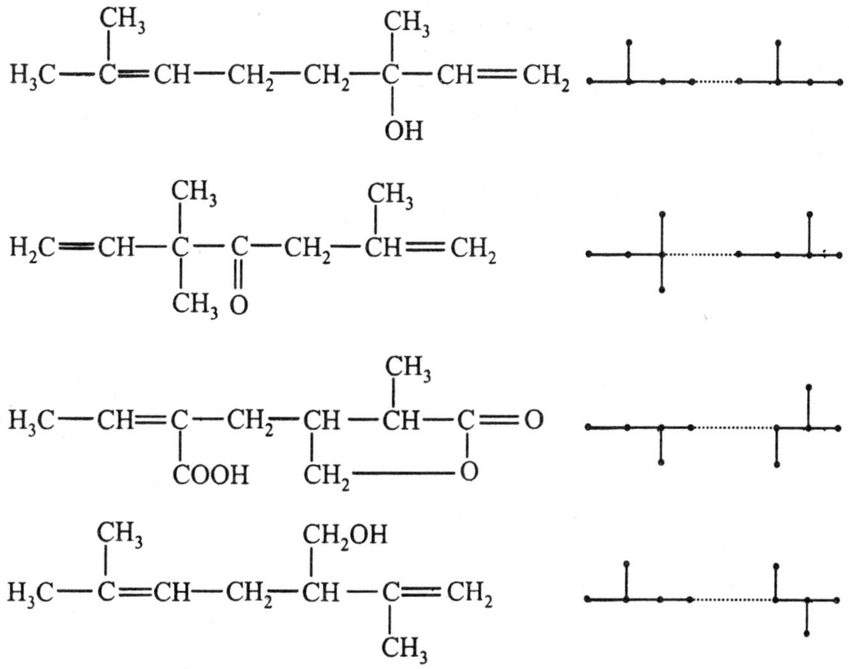

Fig. 2.10. Lavandulol in oil of lavender accompanied by the ester of regularly built linaloöl.

Still another way of connecting the two branched C_5 chains is observed in chrysanthemum acid which, esterified with pyrethrolone, is a part of the ester pyrethrin, the active component of insect powder made from *Chrysanthemum cinerarefolium*. The origin from a regular built carane-like bicyclic terpene through oxidation is indicated (Fig. 2.11).

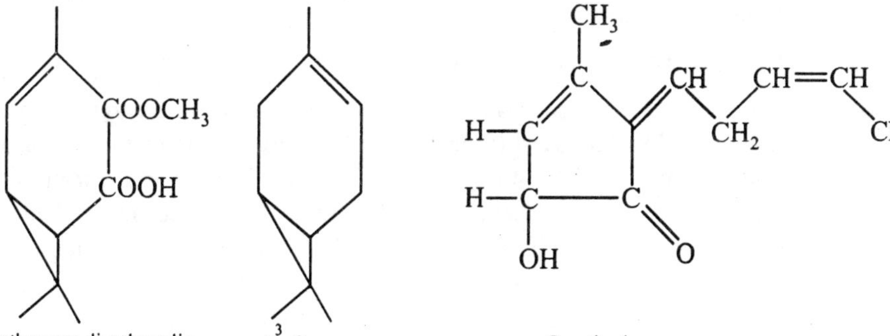

Chrysanthemum dicarboxylic ester — COOCH$_3$ / COOH

Δ^3-Carene

Pyrethrolone

Fig. 2.11. Pyrethrin in its relation to terpenes.

The third group of (bicyclic) monoterpenes has two rings, leaving room for only one double bond for a formula $C_{10}H_{16}$. This type of structure we find in compounds such as carane, pinane, camphane, bornylane, isobornylane and fenchane. Through rearrangements of these different structures (Fig. 2.12), other ring systems can be derived. Molecular rearrangements, shifting of double bonds to other places in the molecule, oxidation or dehydrogenation and hydrogenation occur more or less readily, whereas treatment with acids may open these rings.

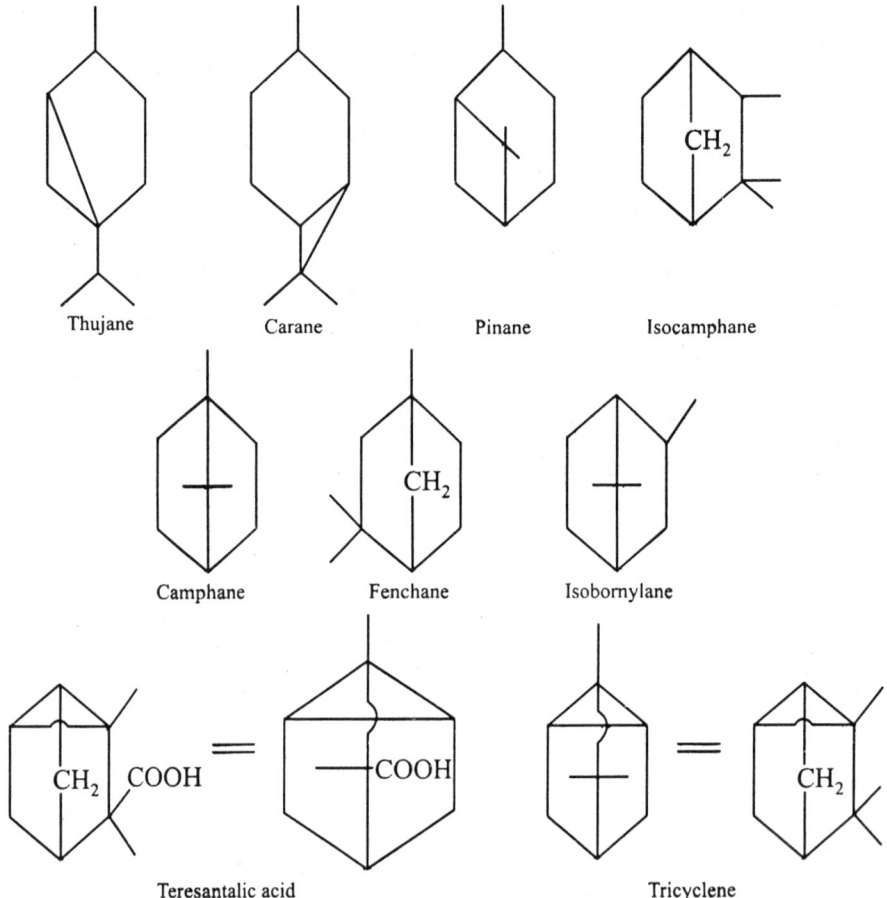

Fig. 2.12. Carbon skeletons of bicyclic and tricyclic terpenes.

The fourth group of (tricyclic) monoterpenes has as its only natural occurring representative teresantalic acid. Molecular rearrangements, leading to a shifting of the connections between the carbon atoms, made the investigations of these compounds very complicated. On the other hand, through these many rearrangements, a considerable number of conversions of great importance occur. The oxidation of α-pinene to camphor includes a simultaneous reattachment of the carbon atom carrying the two methyl groups to the carbon atom carrying one methyl group as indicated in Fig. 2.13. Comparable is the conversion of α-pinene into derivatives of the fenchyl series, i.e. fenchyl alcohol and fenchone. A most ingenious application of this versatility is the complete conversion of *l*-camphor into *d*-camphor and *vice versa* by Houben and Pfankuch.

The next class of terpene compounds contains three of our building stones and its members are called sesquiterpenes, since they contain one and a half times as many carbon atoms as the monoterpenes. Here, as in the terpene series, we can predict what type of compound we might expect from their general formula, $C_{15}H_{24}$, i.e.

4 double bonds, no rings, aliphatic
3 double bonds, one ring, monocyclic

2 double bonds, two rings, bicyclic
1 double bond, three rings, tricyclic
0 double bonds, four rings, tetracyclic.

Representatives of the first four groups are known, and here, as in the C_{10} series, we see representatives of different stages of oxidation and reduction. We count among these some valuable perfume constituents like the aliphatic sesquiterpene alcohols, farnesol and nerolidol. These C_{15} alcohols have the same relation to each other as geraniol and linaloöl in the monoterpene series. Ruzicka has, therefore, called them the geraniol and linaloöl of the sesquiterpene group. This similarity is expressed by their interconversions and ring-closures to monocyclic sesquiterpenes of the bisabolene type, analogous to the formation of terpineol and dipentene in the terpene series (Fig. 2.14).

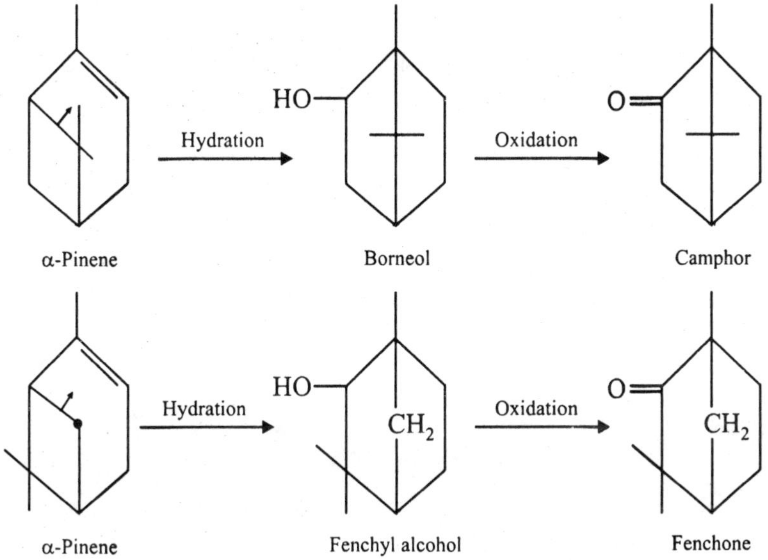

Fig. 2.13. Conversion in the bicyclic terpene series.

By the addition of the unsaturated C_5 chain, the number of possibilities for secondary ring-closure has been increased, and the formation of a bicyclic sesquiterpene takes place easily. These ring-closures can often be effected by treatment with acids or by dehydrogenation with sulphur, selenium and catalysts, such as platinum and palladium. By applying these methods, Ruzicka has done much of the ground work in the sesquiterpene group. It has been found that three chief classes of compounds were formed, one belonging to the ring structure characteristic for a group of blue hydrocarbons sometimes found in essential oils and two to that characteristic of the naphthalene group, i.e. cadalene and eudalene. Although the cadalene formation is easily explained on the basis of a ring-closure, as described for bisabolene, eudalene, a C_{14} compound, could only have been formed from a C_{15} compound by loss of an angular CH_3 group. The structure of the sesquiterpene belonging to this eudalene group shows an architecture which we find quite often in the higher terpenes, resin acids and carotenoids, i.e. a cyclogeraniol or cyclocitral structure. These ring compounds can readily be prepared from aliphatic terpenes under the influence of concentrated acids, such as phosphoric and sulphuric. Derivatives of this type of cyclisation are found among the ionones. The bicyclic sesquiterpenes of the eudalene type may be described as being of this cyclogeraniol ring-closure structure followed by a ring-closure of the linaloöl ⟶ terpinene type (Fig. 2.15). To this group belong the alcohol, **eudesmol** and the lactone, santonine (the active principle of Levant wormseed [*Flores cinae*], well-known for its anthelmintic properties).

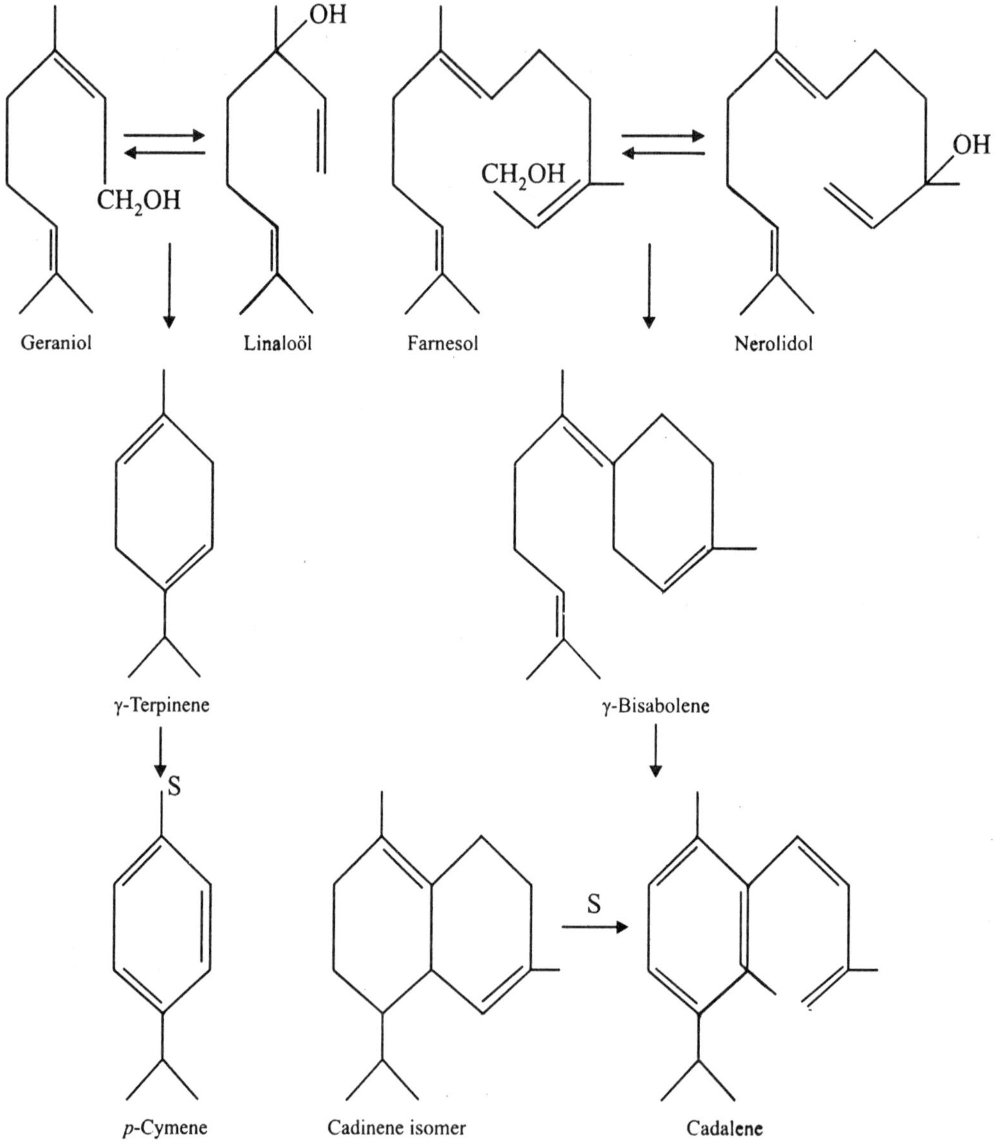

Fig. 2.14. Cyclisation in the sesquiterpene series, cadalene formation.

The third method by which we may derive certain natural sesquiterpenes from an aliphatic chain results in compounds which are present in some oils and which give a blue colour on dehydrogenation. Such bicyclic terpene derivatives, guaiol and vetivone for example, when treated with sulphur or selenium, are oxidised by removal of hydrogen; a stable system of conjugated and cross-conjugated double bonds in the rings is established and intensely blue hydrocarbons are formed. These so-called azulenes, mixed with yellow components, are responsible for the green colour of many oils. This colour is not caused by the presence of copper compounds from the stills as was formerly believed.

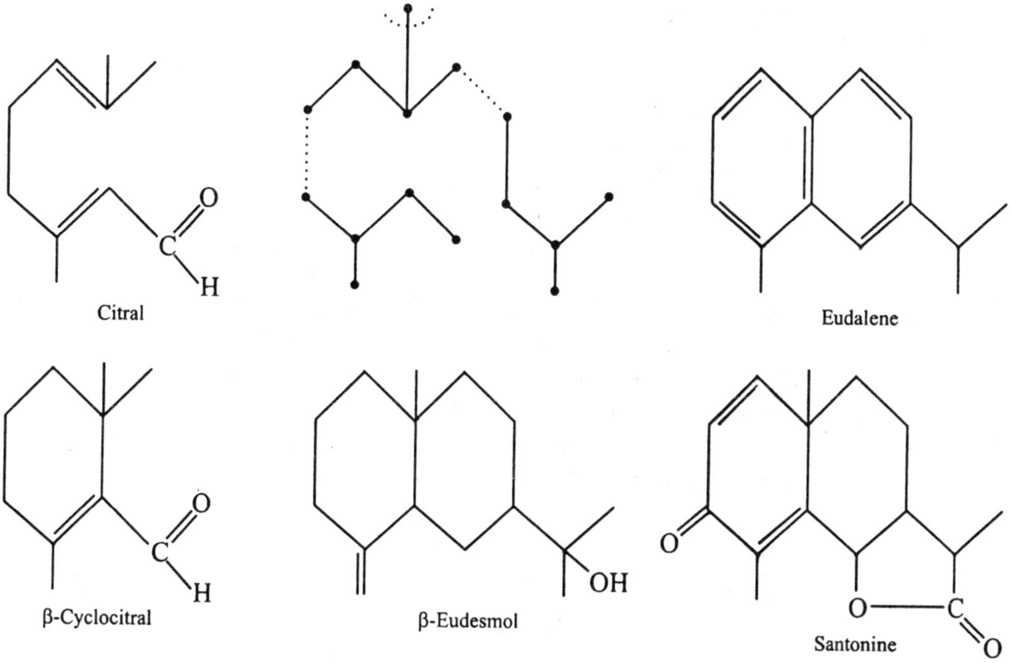

Fig. 2.15. Cyclisation of the sesquiterpene series, eudalene formation.

It is worthy of remark here that the blue colour which appears on the freshly cut surfaces of some mushrooms is due to the formation of the same azulene as that obtained from the guaiol in the oil of guaiac wood and from many sesquiterpenes in other oils, i.e. guaiazulene. The investigations of Ruzicka and of Pfau and Plattner have shown that these azulenes or their hydrogenated precursors consist of a five and a seven-membered ring fused together, wherein the methyl and isopropyl side chains are placed in such a manner that we may describe the compound as being formed from an aliphatic sesquiterpene such as farnesol. This unrolling and connecting of different carbon atoms of a C_{15} chain can be done in several ways. At present, the structures of two of these azulenes (Fig. 2.16) derived from vetivone of vetiver oil and guaiol of guaiac wood are definitely established and syntheses of many azulenes have made this type of compound easily available. Through the formation of well-characterised molecular addition products with picric acid and trinitrobenzene, the azulenes, in addition to cadalene and eudalene, have become a welcome tool for identification of the carbon skeletons of a number of unknown sesquiterpenes.

If the rule of the regular head-to-tail union of the C_5 units fails, and if no known dehydrogenation product betrays the general structure, the difficult road of gradual degradation has to be followed. Such has been the case, for many years, with the investigations of the structure of caryophyllene and cedrene.

After the general structure has been established, important details such as position of double bonds and substituents have to be settled. By the use of certain methods (chiefly oxidation) on original, dehydrated or on partially hydrogenated products, we obtain compounds for the most part complex and unknown. They may, however, indicate combinations of groups such as carbonyl and carboxyl and thus facilitate the choice among a number of proposed formulas.

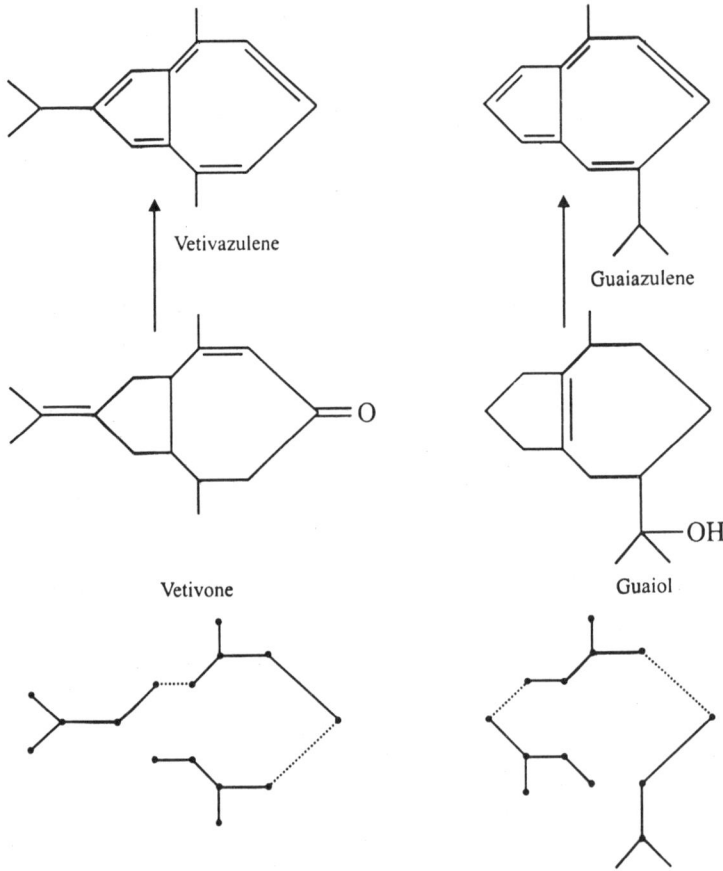

Vetivazulene

Guaiazulene

Vetivone

Guaiol

Fig. 2.16. Cyclisation in the sesquiterpene series, azulene formation.

This elimination procedure has been very fruitful in the sesqui- and higher terpene groups. Its obvious limitation makes us welcome new direct methods of attack, such as that employed in determining the position of the nuclear double bonds in dextro pimaric acid, which consists in marking the position of the double bond by oxide formation followed by substitution with a methyl group and dehydrogenation to a methyl substituted aromatic compound.

Campbell and Soffer used this method to revise the position of the double bonds in the cadinene and isozingiberene formulas of Ruzicka. Ruzicka's degradation acids obtained from cadinene agree with the new formula as well as with the old one, but the new formula does not agree with the oxidation results on the tricyclic sesquiterpene copaene which gives the same dihydrochloride as cadinene. In such cases doubt arises about the homogeneity of the copaene and the cadinene, since it is possible that cadinene hydrochloride obtained from fractionated copaene actually belongs to cadinene, the latter being present as an impurity (Fig. 2.17).

This example emphasises the great need for care in the purification of the substances under investigation. Crystalline derivatives rarely form quantitatively, and hence we cannot be sure that we are dealing with a homogeneous compound. It is to be expected that the application of chromatographic adsorption will contribute a great deal to the clarification of these problems.

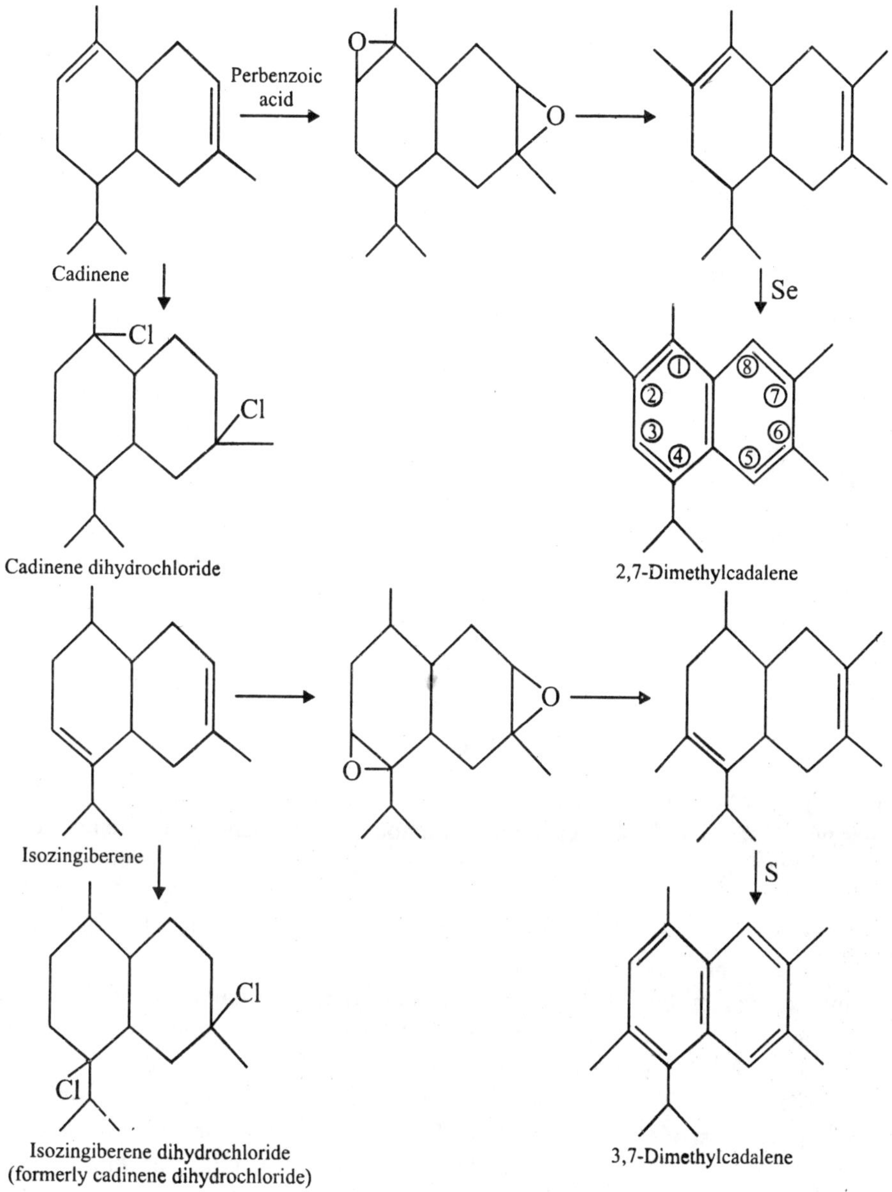

Fig. 2.17. Structure of cadinene.

The members of the next group of compounds contain 4 isopentane units; hence the possibilities of coupling such units are much more numerous than they were in the previous groups. These compounds are difficult to study, since the separation techniques are limited through the high boiling points, the increased chances for isomerisations and the similarity of their physical properties. Fully established structures in the diterpene series are, therefore, few and belong chiefly to some commercially important products—among them the resin acids from rosin, galipot and kaurikopal and compounds like vitamin A and the chlorophyll alcohol phytol (Fig. 2.18).

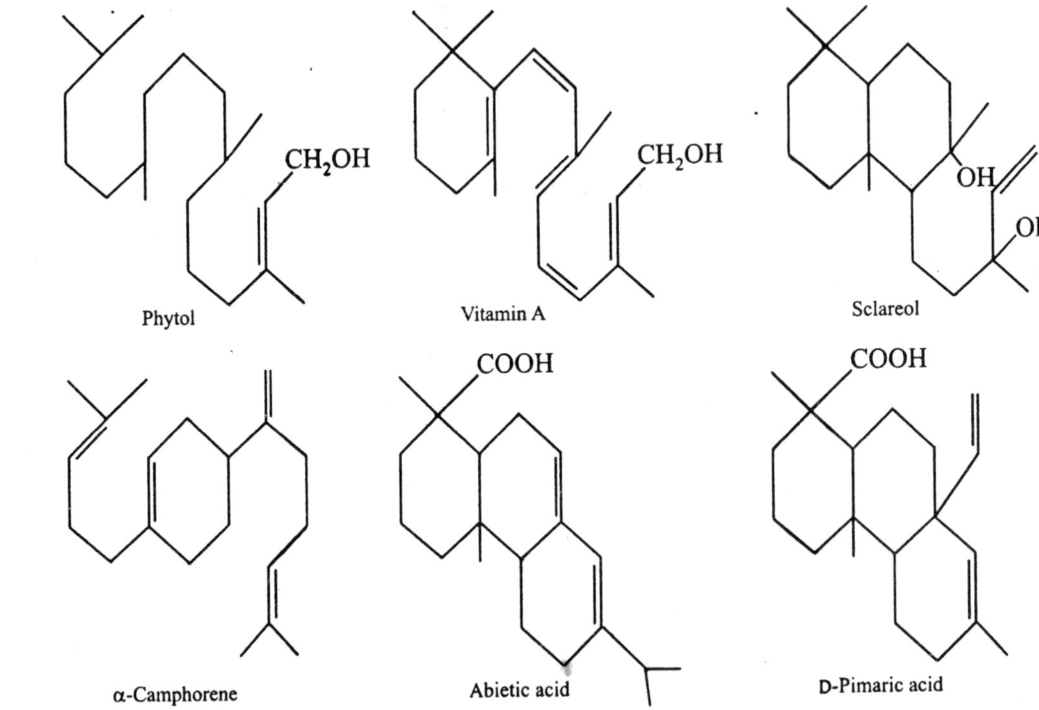

Fig. 2.18. Diterpenes.

With the exception of α-camphorene, sclareol and related manoyl oxide and manoöl, the structures of the diterpenes which occur in the highest boiling fractions of the essential oils are not yet satisfactorily established. This group is at present going through the same early stages of development, i.e. a sharper characterisation, as the monoterpenes fifty years ago. A crystalline diterpene phyllocladene has been found, which appears to be identical with sciadopitene and dacrene isolated from other sources and isomeric with podocarpene and isophyllocladene.

Dihydrophyllocladene is found to be identical with the lignites (fossil resins): hartite, bombiccite and hofmannite. To find still higher isoprene homologues, the separation technique with steam distillation is unsatisfactory and we have to resort to reduced pressure distillation or solvent extraction techniques. Through the use of these methods, products have been isolated which show a continuation of the branched C_5 building plan and consist of six C_5 units. Some of these we find in the non-volatile part of the resins — like β-amyrin; other examples are boswellic acid from incense and betulin, the white pigment of the bark of birch. Interesting members are found in woolfat as lanosterol, in quinine bark as chinovic acid, in cloves and olive leaves as oleanolic acid (Fig. 2.19). This acid is also known to be present as glycoside in several plants. These types of glycosides, as a result of their detergent reaction, have received the name of saponins. Many drug plants, such as sarsaparilla and smilax, owe their pharmacological action to the presence of these C_{30} compounds. The structure determination of these tetracyclic triterpenes relies heavily on the formation of picene derivatives through dehydrogenation. Since all angular methyl groups are removed in this process, special degradation reactions should provide proof of their position. This difficult structural detail has not yet been accomplished for all methyl groups, and their present fluctuating position in the proposed formulas rests largely on the application of the 'isoprene hypothesis'.

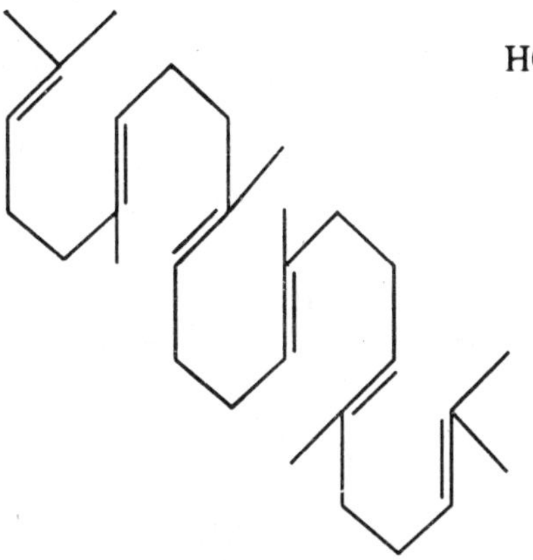

Fig. 2.19. Triterpenes.

The simple symmetrical constitution of the triterpene squalene (Fig. 2.19) present in liver of sharks and many vegetable oils permitted rapid progress in the elucidation of its structure, and even its synthesis has been accomplished by combining 2 mols of the acyclic sesquiterpene alcohol farnesol.

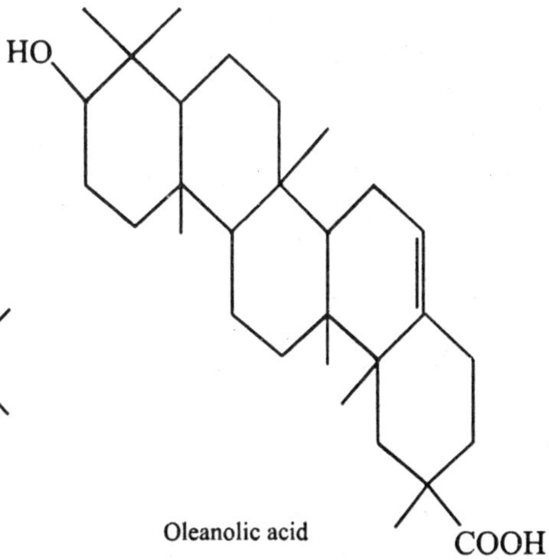

This symmetrical build up, which we see for the first time in squalene, is quite common in the next group, viz. the tetraterpenes. The known members of this group belong to the yellow and red crystalline carotenoid pigments from plants and animals. The carbon skeleton of these compounds can be described as a doubling of a regularly built diterpene. In lycopene (Fig. 2.20), the red pigment of the tomato, we find a chain of 32 carbon atoms with 8 methyl side chains. In most carotenoids the ends of the long chain have formed a cyclogeraniol type of cyclisation, as in β-carotene and xanthophyll (Fig. 2.20).

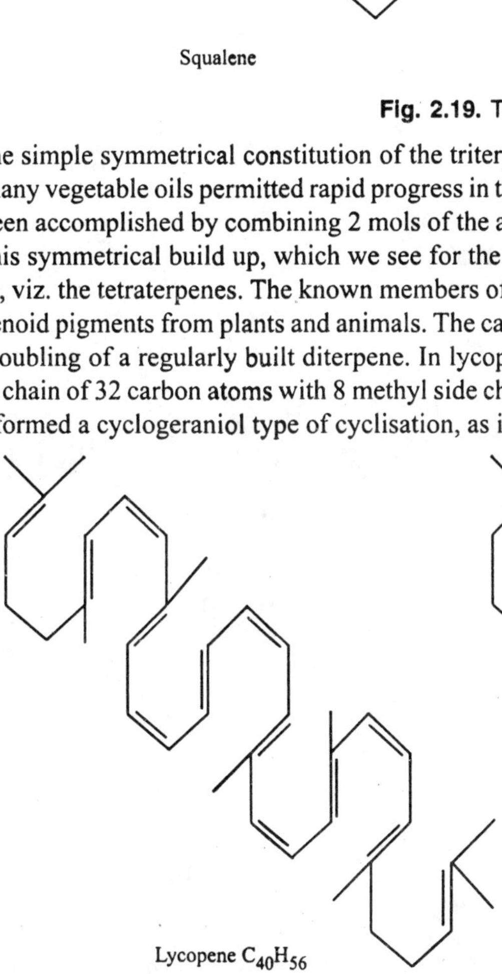

Lycopene $C_{40}H_{56}$

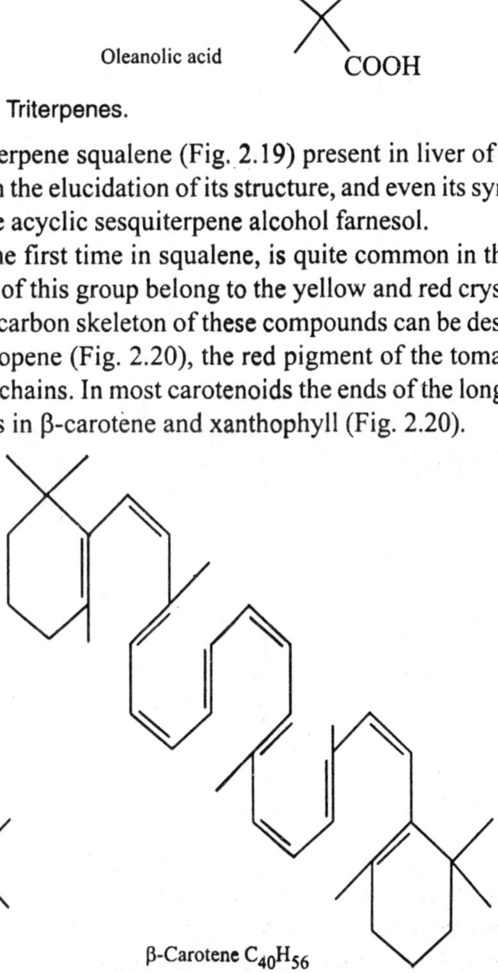

β-Carotene $C_{40}H_{56}$

Fig. 2.20. Tetraterpenes.

The presence of a large number of conjugated double bonds (14 in lycopene) distinguishes this group from other terpenoids and is responsible for the red and yellow colours which are so characteristic of this group of substances. As a result of our lack of knowledge of representatives belonging to the intermediate groups, we must look for the next higher terpenes in a number of compounds which have attracted the attention of investigators on account of their elastic properties. The different rubbers from Hevea, Guayule, etc. belong to this polyterpene group and contain up to several thousand C_5 units.

While all of these compounds can be divided completely into branched C_5 chains, a number of natural products contain structures in which we can recognise one or more of these units, but which we cannot fully describe in this way. In such cases some of the carbon atoms are left over; these form often a straight chain, as in cholic acid and cholesterol. Also in humulone (Fig. 2.21) the connection with the terpene compounds is unmistakable; nevertheless, we cannot fully divide the molecule into branched C_5 chains.

Cholesterol

Humulone

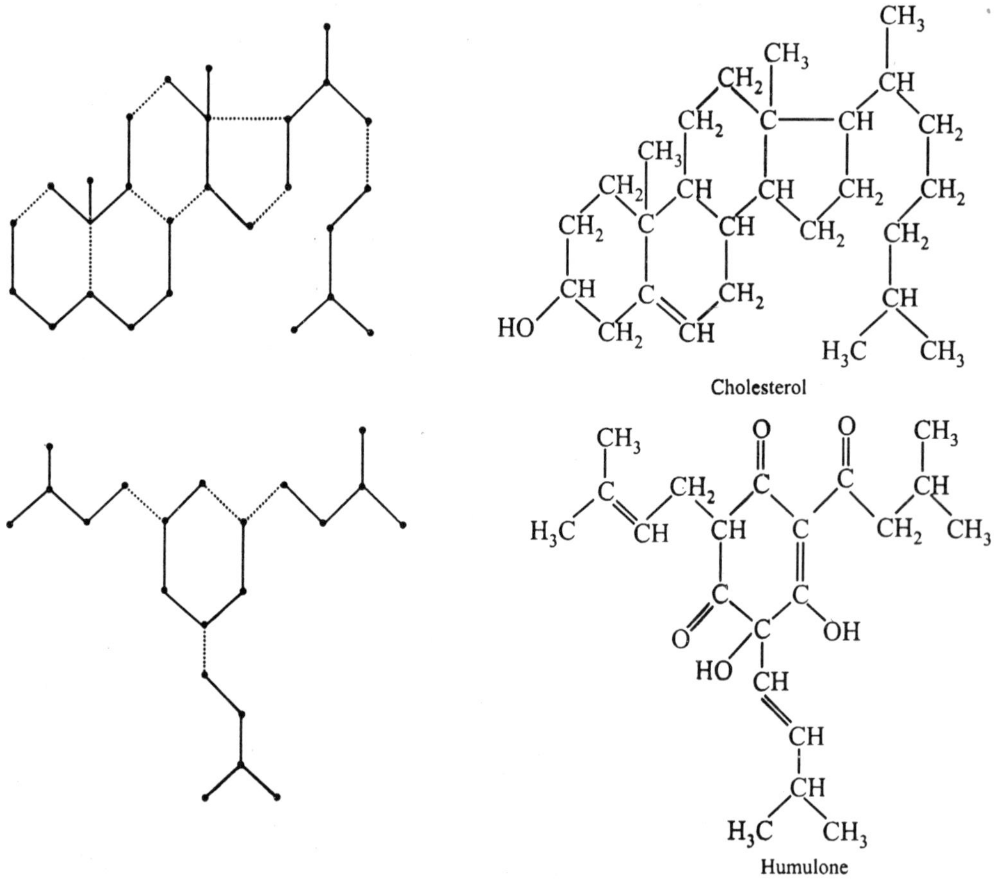

Fig. 2.21. Mixed building schemes.

In some cases the recognition of such building principles serves as a guide in the laboratory synthesis, and also indicates a possible biogenesis. An interesting illustration is furnished by the structure of cannabidiol, one of the constituents of Egyptian hashish. One can easily recognise in this molecule the structures of cymene or 1-methyl-4-isopropenylbenzene, the first of which form the main part of the essential oil of hashish (Fig. 2.22). Similar considerations led to the synthesis of the antisterility vitamin E which is formed by coupling phytylbromide with trimethylhydroquinone, whereas the antihemorrhagic vitamin K_1 is synthesised by condensing the same bromide with the sodium salt of 2-methyl-1,4-naphthoquinone.

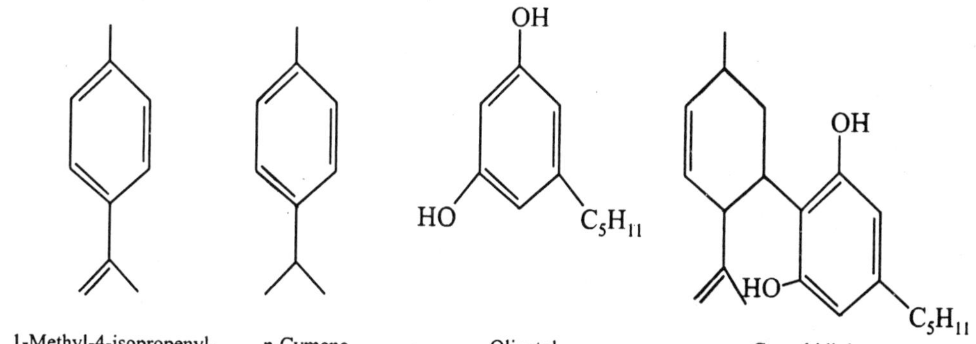

1-Methyl-4-isopropenyl-benzene   *p*-Cymene   Olivetol   Cannabidiol

Fig. 2.22. Constituents of oil of hashish.

The second major group of oil components contains only straight chain hydrocarbons and their oxygen derivatives: alcohols, aldehydes, ketones, acids, ethers and esters. These essential oil hydrocarbons range from *n*-heptane, which forms 90 per cent of the oil of *Pinus sabiniana* and *P. jeffreyi*, to compounds with 15–35 carbon atoms. The higher paraffin-like materials may crystallise out during cooling and storage of the oils and are called 'stearoptenes'. The number of carbon atoms in some of these hydrocarbons suggests a connection with the natural occurring fatty acids through decarboxylation or ketone formation. The formation from the wax alcohols through dehydration and reduction is also held possible.

The alcohols, aldehydes and ketones are quite often contained in the low boiling fraction of the volatile oil. A typical example is found in the so-called leaf alcohol (*cis*- or *trans*-hexen-3-ol-1), carrier of the odour of grasses, green leaves, etc. Oxidation of the alcohol with chromic acid furnishes a hexenal which has been recognised in many green plants, including tea, ivy, clover, oak, beech, wheat, robinia, black radish, violet leaves and cucumbers. However, the volatile oil of cucumber consists largely of nonadiene-2,6-ol-1 with some nonadiene-2,6-al-1 (Fig. 2.23). This aldehyde has also been recognised in the leaf oil of violets.

$$CH_3-CH_2-CH=CH-CH_2-CH_2\cdot OH$$

Leaf alcohol

$$\overset{\textcircled{9}}{CH_3}-\overset{\textcircled{8}}{CH_2}-\overset{\textcircled{7}}{CH}=\overset{\textcircled{6}}{CH}-\overset{\textcircled{5}}{CH_2}-\overset{\textcircled{4}}{CH_2}-\overset{\textcircled{3}}{CH}=\overset{\textcircled{2}}{CH}-\overset{\textcircled{1}}{CH_2}\cdot OH$$

Nonadiene-2,6-ol-1

$$CH_3-CH_2-CH=CH-CH_2-CH_2-CH=CH-C\overset{\displaystyle O}{\underset{\displaystyle H}{\Big\backslash}}$$

Nonadiene-2,6-al-1

Fig. 2.23. Volatile oil of cucumber showing largely of nonadiene-2,6-ol-1 with some nonadiene-2,6-al-1.

In this group are also included the many fatty acids which occur free or esterified with alcohols of different chain length and different degrees of saturation. This group is present in a number of volatile oils from fruit.

The third major group of essential oil components comprises a number of important flavour and perfume constituents derived from benzene and more specifically from *n*-propyl benzene. As in the preceding groups, we find these compounds in many stages of oxidation. The aromatic ring may carry hydroxy, methoxy and methylene dioxy groups; the propyl side chain may contain hydroxyl or carboxyl groups, or form a part of a lactone group, as in coumarin and its many derivatives (Fig. 2.24). Many members of this group are related through simple chemical reactions. For example, on isomerisation followed by oxidation, eugenol is converted to the corresponding vanillin (Fig. 2.25), the flavouring principle of the vanilla bean.

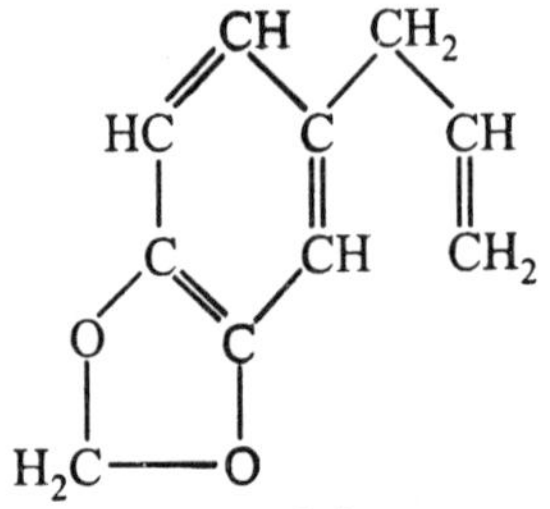

Safrole
(Sassafras oil)

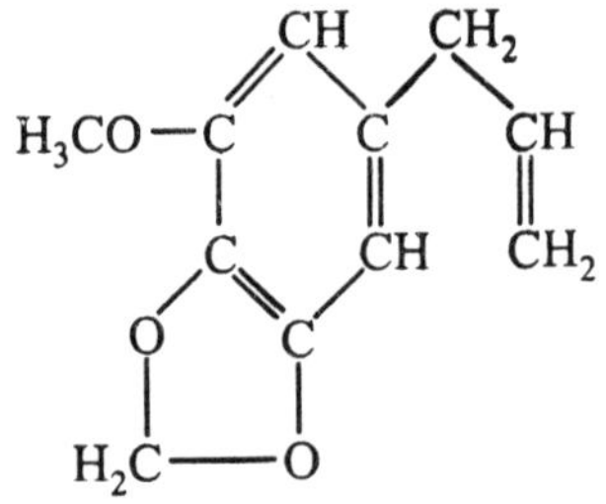

Myristicin
(Nutmeg oil)

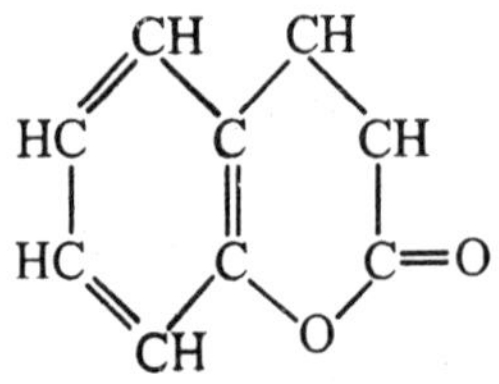

Coumarin

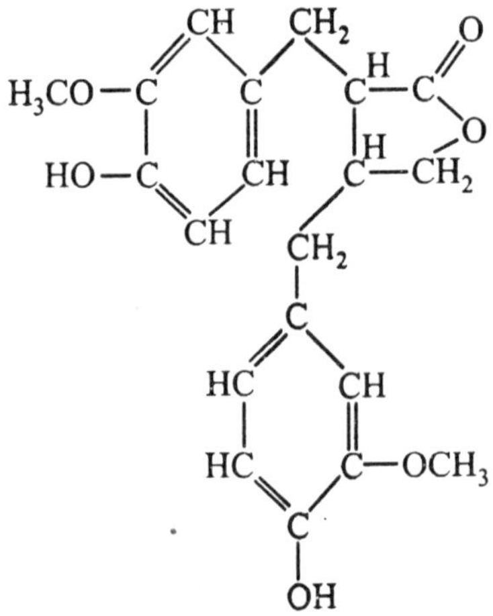

Matairesinol

Fig. 2.24. Aromatic oil constituents.

Eugenol

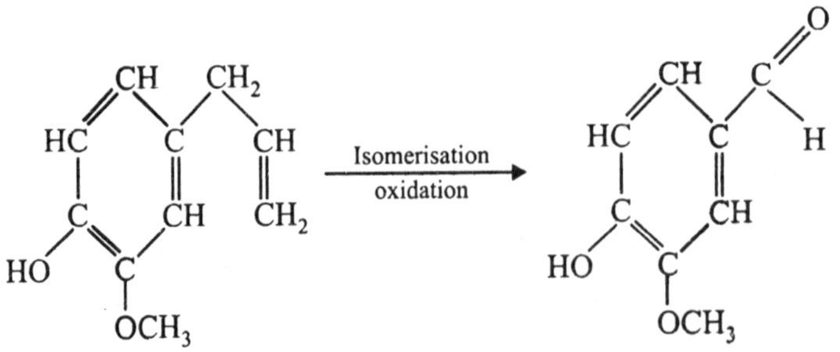

Isomerisation
oxidation

Vanillin

Fig. 2.25. Relations between aromatic oil constituents.

   This group of compounds shows a definite relationship to some of the resins with aromatic structures, like matairesinol, which represent a doubling of the propyl benzene structure. This dimerisation has been demonstrated *in vitro* for isoeugenol methyl ether which is doubled into *bis*-isoeugenol methyl ether (Fig. 2.26). It is probable that a condensation of a large number of analogous units has led to the formation of lignin, the widely distributed component of woody tissues. Such a relation is comparable to the formation of rubber from the smaller terpene building units. A somewhat more distant connection can be seen in the formation of the anthocyans and flavones, since propyl benzene derivatives have been postulated as taking part in the biosynthesis of these plant pigments.

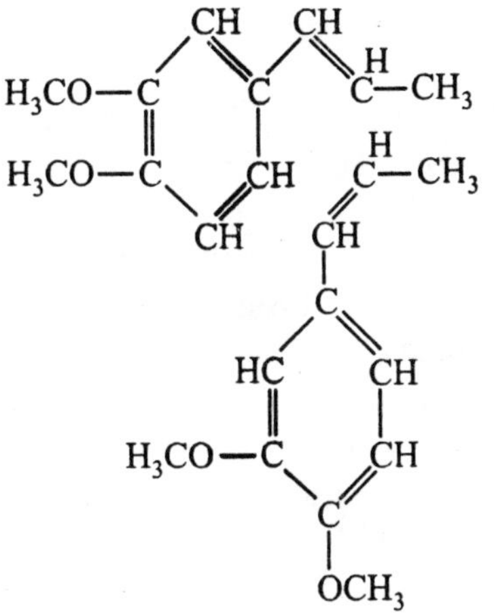

Isoeugenol methyl ether

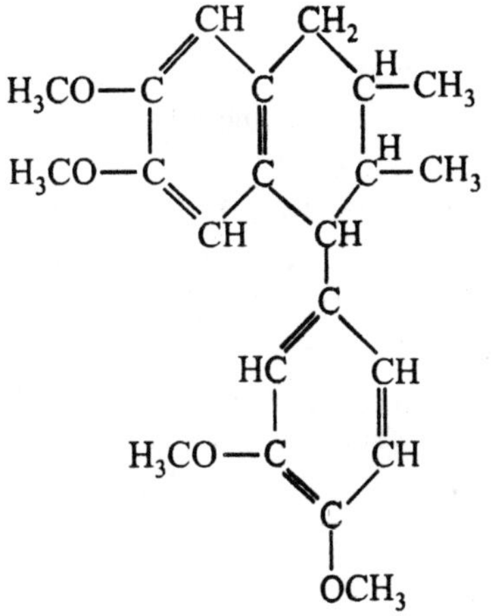

bis-Isoeugenol methyl ether

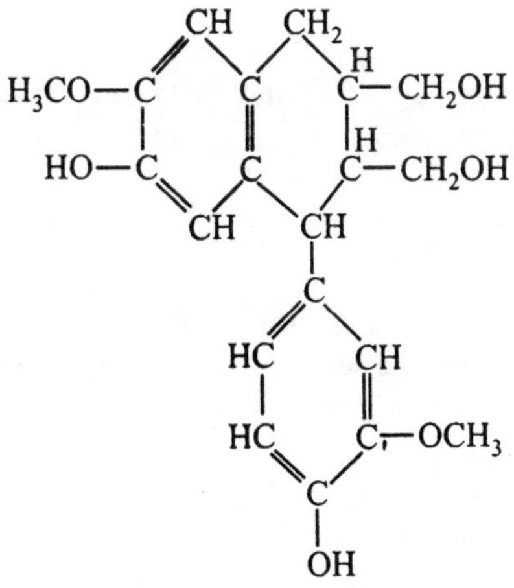

Isolariciresinol

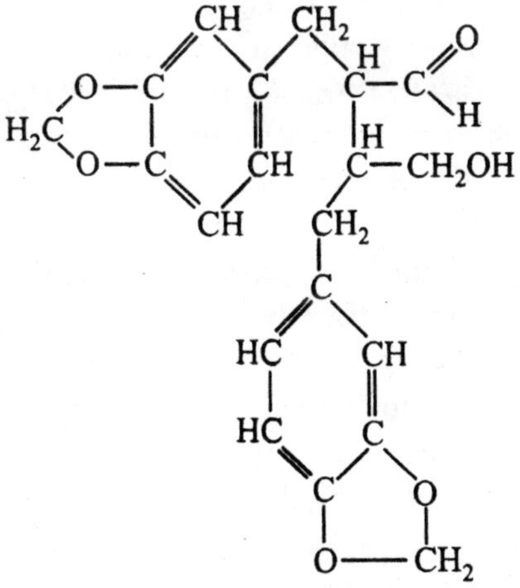

Cubebin

Fig. 2.26. Relation between aromatic oil constituents and resinols.

   From this short account of our chemical knowledge of the essential oil components and their near relatives, it is clear that their study must have occupied the minds of a large number of chemists interested in natural products. In numerous cases the purification, characterisation, structural determination and synthesis of a single terpene has been the lifetime work of many of the terpene chemists.

The difficulties are immediately apparent when the starting material arrives in the laboratory. Separation has to be accomplished on a large diversity of compounds, since the only links between them are their plant origin and their volatility. In addition, many of the constituents are easily converted into other compounds with similar properties. The investigation of the essential oils has, therefore, served as a hard schooling in chemical separation techniques, in which none of the existing methods, physical or chemical, can be neglected. When the oils are obtained from the plant by steam distillation, the steam carries over the volatile component at a temperature of somewhat less than 100°C. This, however, does not represent the actual boiling point of the oil components. At the boiling point of a mixture of oil and water, the sum of the partial pressures of oil and water is equal to the atmospheric pressure. The boiling temperature of the steam and vapour mixture is, therefore, lower than the boiling temperature of water alone.

In a mixture of oil of turpentine and water, which boils at 95.6°C at 760 mm pressure, the vapour pressure of the oil contributes 113 mm, the water 647 mm. Without the help of the water vapour, the bulk of most oils would distil at 150°–300°C at which temperature labile substances would be destroyed and a strong resinification would occur. With the aid of steam distillation, the majority of these compounds are carried over a few degrees below the boiling point of water. Vapour pressure data of single components make it possible to calculate their boiling points by steam distillation and the proportion of oil and water which is distilled at different pressures. While steam distillation is a simple procedure, we cannot *per se* assume that a steam distilled oil is identical with the oils as occurring in the plants. Several cases are known where certain compounds are formed by the action of the steam. These are for the most part degradation products of carbohydrates, like ferfural. Loss of water from alcohols and hydrolysis of esters will result in the formation of new hydrocarbons and acids. Likewise, nitrogen compounds often have a secondary origin. This destruction usually runs parallel with the loss of the delicate nuances in smell and is a certain indication that changes in the original composition of the oil have taken place, a matter of concern for both production and research departments. Since the oils contain chemical compounds of many classes, it is often desirable to remove at least those groups of substances that contain more reactive groupings than the hydrocarbons, among them acids, bases, phenols, ketones and aldehydes. The oils are, therefore, treated with dilute aqueous alkali solutions to remove the acidic substances or with bases to remove the acids, with sulphite, bisulphite or Girard's reagent to isolate ketones and aldehydes, and sometimes with phthalic anhydride to remove the alcohols.

In the oil layer or in the solvent extract of the steam distillate (including that of the distillation water), compounds boiling lower and higher than water are found and the desirability of fractionating the original, or the treated oil, into fractions which preferably contain only one component is indicated. When we assemble the fractionation data in a graph and plot the quantity of oil distilled within a certain temperature interval along the ordinate, although the abscissa shows the boiling points, we notice in the fractionation curve of different oils maxima indicating the presence of distinct components of the oils. In the fractionation of the American oil of peppermint (Fig. 2.27), a typical terpene oil, the first volatile components which distil are small quantities of two compounds which were postulated by some investigators as the building stones of the branched C_5 chains, viz. acetone and acetaldehyde, accompanied by dimethyl sulphide, a compound containing sulphur. These are followed by the hemiterpenes, isovaleraldehyde and isoamyl alcohol; and these in turn are followed, at a temperature of approximately 150°C, by a number of compounds, which by analysis are shown to consist of carbon and hydrogen only. Several small maxima in the boiling point curve indicate the presence of several of these terpenes. At this stage the determination of physical constants, such as specific gravity, refractive index and optical rotation, may aid considerably in indicating the nature of the terpenes.

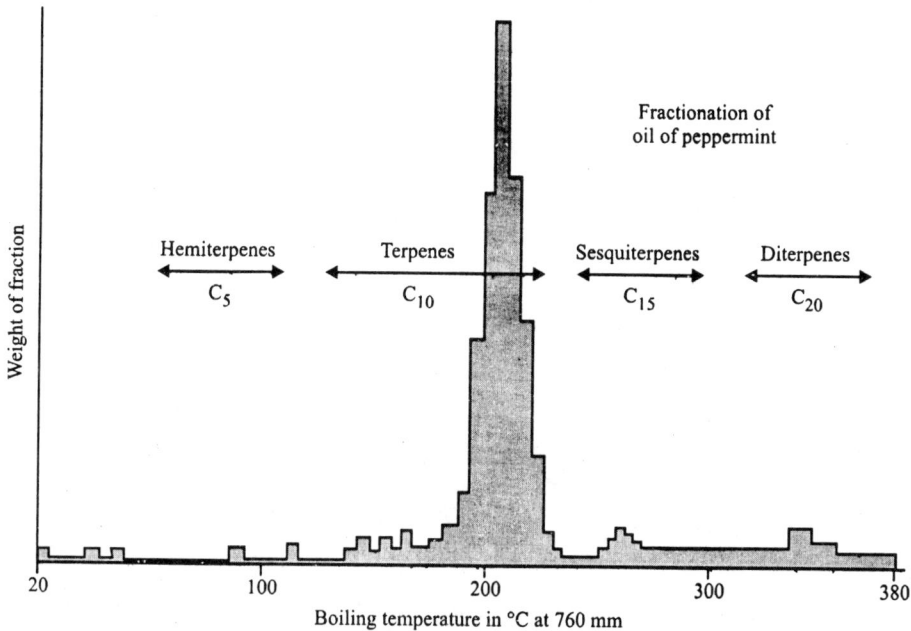

Fig. 2.27. Fractionation of American oil of peppermint, terpene oil and volatile components.

With the exception of camphene and bornylene, all the terpene hydrocarbons are liquid at ordinary temperatures and their tendency to crystallise at lower temperatures is negligible. The tendency to form a distinct crystalline pattern can be greatly increased when polar groups are introduced into the molecule. The first crystalline derivative of a hydrocarbon to be prepared in this way is the so-called 'artificial camphor' obtained by Kindt, when he passed hydrogen chloride into oil of turpentine. The systematic study of these methods is, however, due to Wallach, who about fifty years ago introduced several more of these procedures. Since the double bonds are the only reactive points in the terpenes, these groups are introduced into the molecule by simple addition reactions to the double bond. In this way, halides, dihalides, nitrosohalides, nitrosites and nitrosates are formed. Through these reactions, the hydrocarbon derivatives may crystallise even from impure fractions and their identification is possible through comparisons of the melting points of the same derivatives of known terpenes. Modern chemistry has added only a few more reagents to this list, among them, maleic anhydride for the characterisation of compounds with conjugated double bonds (Fig. 2.28).

When the distillation is continued, the next large group of fractions boils at about 200°–230°C. They consist mainly of the oxygen derivatives of the terpenes, $C_{10}H_{18}O$ and in our fractionation example of peppermint oil, a fraction of menthone is obtained, followed by a larger fraction of menthol. While some oxygen derivatives in peppermint oil are crystalline, in many other oils these have to be characterised by reaction products with certain identifying reagents, such as phenylisocyanate and nitro benzoylchlorides for alcohols and nitrophenylhydrazines for ketones and aldehydes.

The next group of compounds we encounter in the fractionation is again of a hydrocarbon nature. The region of sesquiterpenes C_{15}, and these C_{15} compounds are again followed by their oxygen derivatives which in turn are followed by diterpenes. If the oils contain a number of benzene and aliphatic compounds their fractions will be superimposed on this general scheme.

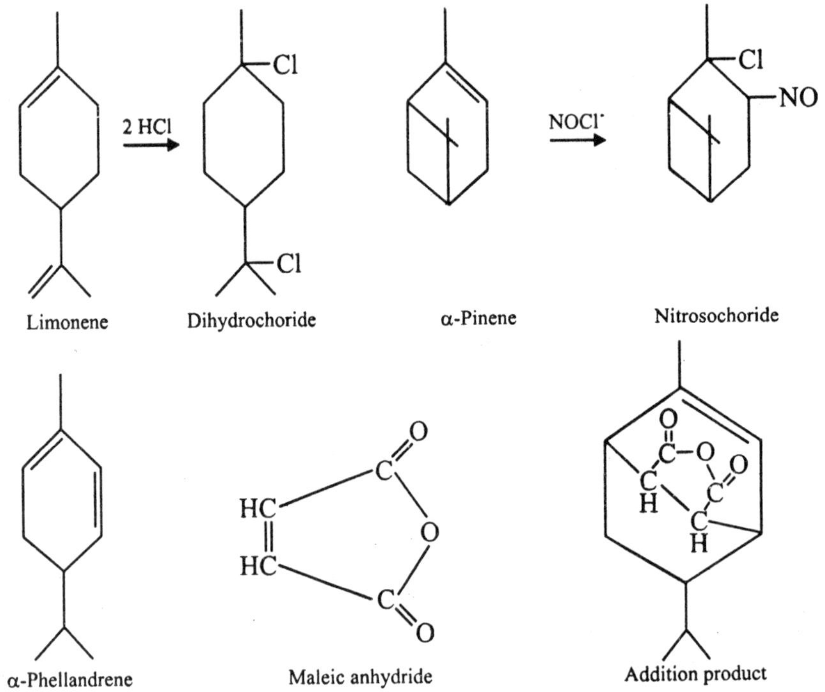

Fig. 2.28. Crystalline reaction products of monoterpenes.

The boiling point regularities observed in the fractionation of the oils are clearly expressed in a graph showing the boiling points of the normal hydrocarbons of different chain length (Fig. 2.29). If the ordinate is plotted on a logarithmic scale nearly straight lines are obtained. The boiling temperatures of the essential oil hydrocarbons are usually lower than those of the straight chain compounds, since branching of the chain tends to lower the boiling point. This counterbalances the possible rise in boiling point through the introduction of unsaturation. The net result is a boiling interval, for the majority of monoterpenes, from 155° to 185°C (representing the range of boiling points from pinene to terpinolene), whereas the straight chain normal decane boils at 175°C.

A further look at the graph shows some irregularities at 300°C, which indicate that even the normal saturated hydrocarbons are destroyed. To avoid this disagreeable behaviour, a reduction in pressure, resulting in a lowering of the boiling point, is resorted to when we intend to continue the fractionation beyond this point. In the case of the much more sensitive terpenes, this phenomenon will appear much earlier and it is usually not safe to raise the outside bath temperature to higher than about 180°C. Thus a fraction containing sesquiterpenes (C_{15}) boiling at 250°C at ordinary pressure can be investigated by distilling at aspirator vacuum of 15 mm at about 120°C, or at a still lower pressure of 0.1 mm at about 60°C.

In this way and by applying ultra high-vacuum, it is possible to study still higher terpene homologues. But gradually these compounds become too complicated and too fragile to give satisfactory fractionation data. For this reason, it is desirable to obtain these compounds, not by steam distillation, but by extraction with solvents, such as alcohol, acetone or petroleum ether or by chromatographic adsorption analysis. Following these procedures we will also find the compounds of the isoprene structure which have taken part in reactions which made them nonvolatile, such as the combination of the diterpene alcohol, phytol, with the complex phorbine ring system of chlorophyll.

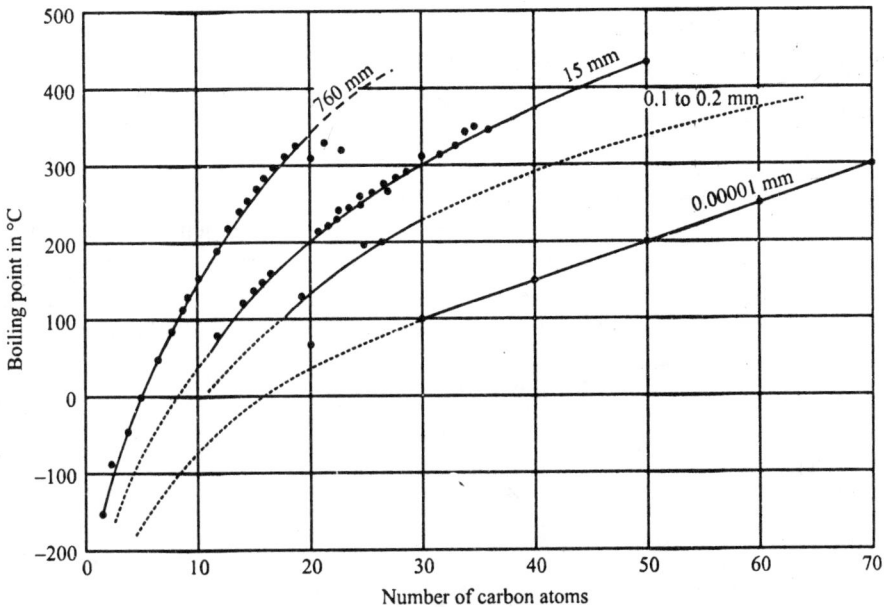

Fig. 2.29. Boiling points of straight-chain hydrocarbons.

When the purified fractions are characterised by preparation of crystalline derivatives and when these are compared by melting point and mixed melting point with the known derivatives, there remain always some fractions which cannot be characterised in this way. In such cases, chemical degradations of the molecules have to be applied. The principle involved in these degradations consists of breaking up the molecule into smaller parts until the pieces have become so simple that they can be recognised. For this purpose, oxidation with ozone, potassium permanganate and chromium trioxide is often used. Sometimes several of these degradations may be necessary before the pieces obtained are small enough to be identified. On the basis of these degradations, a possible structure is postulated and attempts are made to confirm this structure by synthesis. This work has been carried out on about 500 constituents of essential oils. One-fifth of this number is made up of monoterpenes, and only a start has been made on the investigations of sesqui and higher terpenes. In view of the greatly increased possibility of structural isomerism, every time 5 carbons are added to a molecule we may look forward to the addition to our present knowledge of a great number of the higher terpene homologues when a more extensive survey is made.

ORIGIN OF ESSENTIAL OILS

In the foregoing discussion of the components of the volatile oils, we saw that they consist of a variety of compounds which belong to all chemical classes. We cannot expect to find a common history for such varied substances. We do observe, however, certain chemical relations between a number of the components. Indeed, it was this similarity that led us to discuss the results of chemical research in terms of four groups, i.e. straight chain hydrocarbons, benzene derivatives, terpenes and miscellaneous compounds. In view of their structural similarity straight chain hydrocarbons are generally considered as connected with fatty acid metabolism, while benzene and propyl benzene derivatives are connected with carbohydrate metabolism. The group which gives rise to most of the speculation, however, comprises the terpenes.

We have seen that members of this series could conveniently be described as divisible into branched C_5 chains. This statement refers to an established fact, but we enter the field of speculation and hypothesis in assuming that such a structure as a C_5 chain actually represents the basic unit in the formation of the terpenes in the plants.

Many terpene investigators have risked guesses as to the nature of this basic unit, but few have tried to support their hypothesis by experiments. One of the oft-mentioned precursors (as we may call them) is isoprene (C_5H_8), belonging to the group of hemiterpenes. This compound in its turn is postulated to arise from the condensation of acetone or derivatives like dihydroxyacetone and acetaldehyde. Through polymerisation and addition of isoprene to higher terpenes, terpene homologues can be prepared. Among several condensation products dipentene and a bisabolene-like sesquiterpene can be identified (Fig. 2.30).

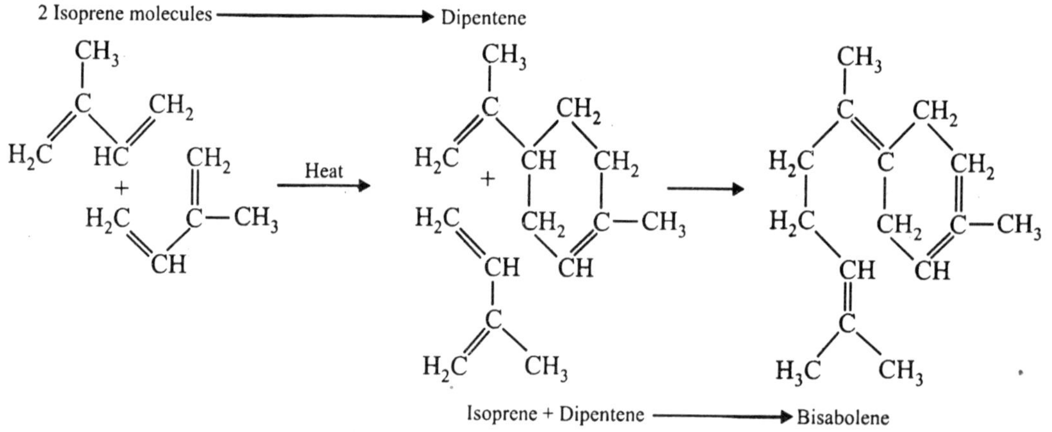

Fig. 2.30. Polymerisation of isoprene.

When such reactions are carried out under simultaneous hydrogenation or hydration, the reactive ends of the molecules are saturated and further condensation and resinification are thereby largely prevented.

Following this principle, Midgley carried out the condensation of isoprene under reducing conditions with sodium amalgam and obtained the terpene hydrocarbon 2,6-dimethyloctane. Wagner-Jauregg condensed two mols of isoprene in the presence of sulphuric and acetic acids. Under these conditions water is added to the double bonds and geraniol can be isolated from the condensation mixture (Fig. 2.31). Ingenious as these experiments are, they do not furnish proof of the isoprene hypothesis.

The same can be said for the hypothetical precursor 3-methylbutenal (Fig. 2.32). This compound would very well satisfy the demands for a reactive precursor. *In vitro* experiments with 3-methylbutenal, with its conjugated carbonyl group and double bond, clearly demonstrate great reactivity and readiness to react with many other molecules.

Fischer succeeded in this way in building up dehydrocitral which might easily serve as the basic substance for aliphatic, as well as cyclic, terpenes.

An added proof would be the synthesis of 3-methylbutenal from acetaldehyde and acetone. Unfortunately, this follows a different addition scheme *in vitro*; and others have, therefore, suggested the formation of 3-methylbutenal by condensation of acetone with pyruvic acid, followed by decarboxylation. This would also furnish an explanation of the presence of isovaleric acid and pyroterebic acid in the oil of *Calotropis procera*, where the latter acid occurs esterified with a diterpene alcohol (Fig. 2.33).

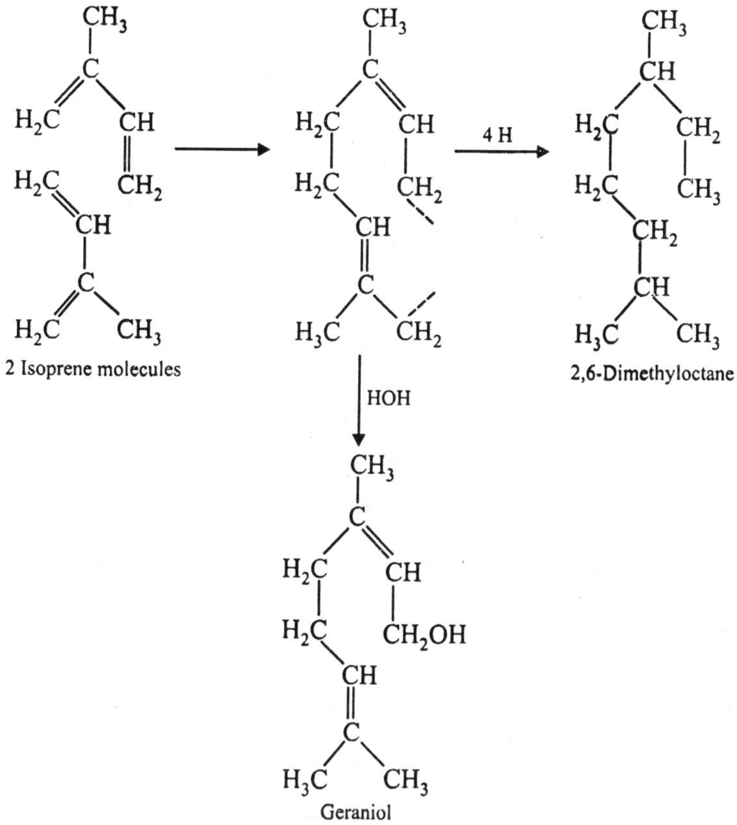

Fig. 2.31. Dimerisation of isoprene.

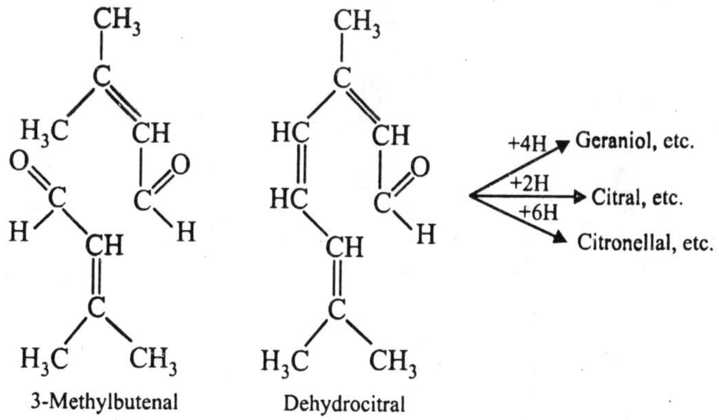

Fig. 2.32. Terpene synthesis from 3-methylbutenal.

However, Francesconi can claim these compounds for his scheme in which isoamyl alcohol has a prominent place. This alcohol is obtained through degradation of carbohydrates, proteins or amino acids like leucine. From leucine, pyroterebic acid and isovaleric acid can be derived with great ease.

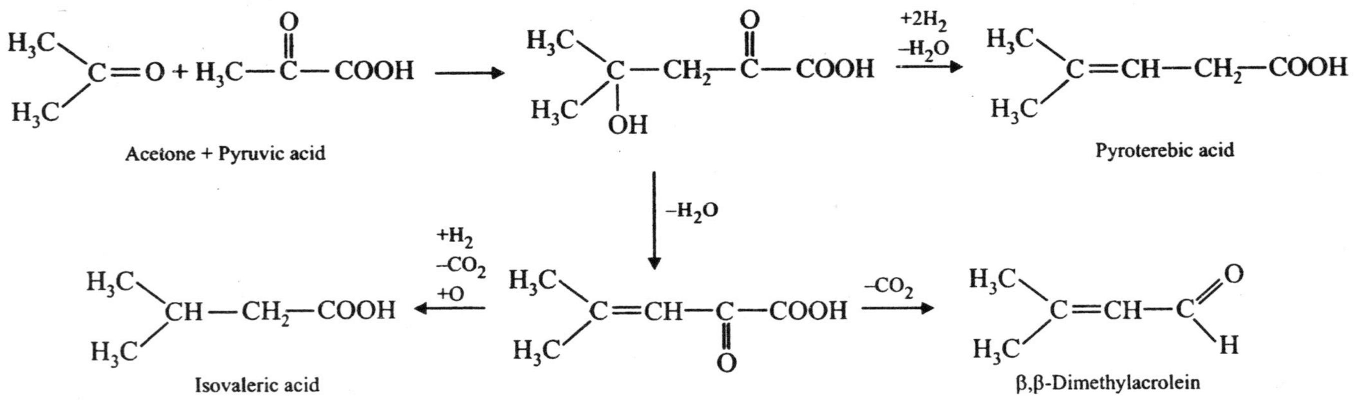

Fig. 2.33. Hypothetical terpene formation from acetone and pyruvic acid.

Huzita follows Ostengo in considering isovaleraldehyde to take a prominent place among the number of proposed precursors. Still another possibility is mentioned by Simpson, who couples acetoacetic acid with 2 mols of acetone to obtain the monocyclic terpenes. The aliphatic terpenes are constructed on paper by linking 3 mols of acetone with one of formaldehyde (Fig. 2.34). Available experimental data on these reactions speak against these types of condensation and special factors and conditions have to be postulated in order to account for the directive nature of the plant processes (Fig. 2.34).

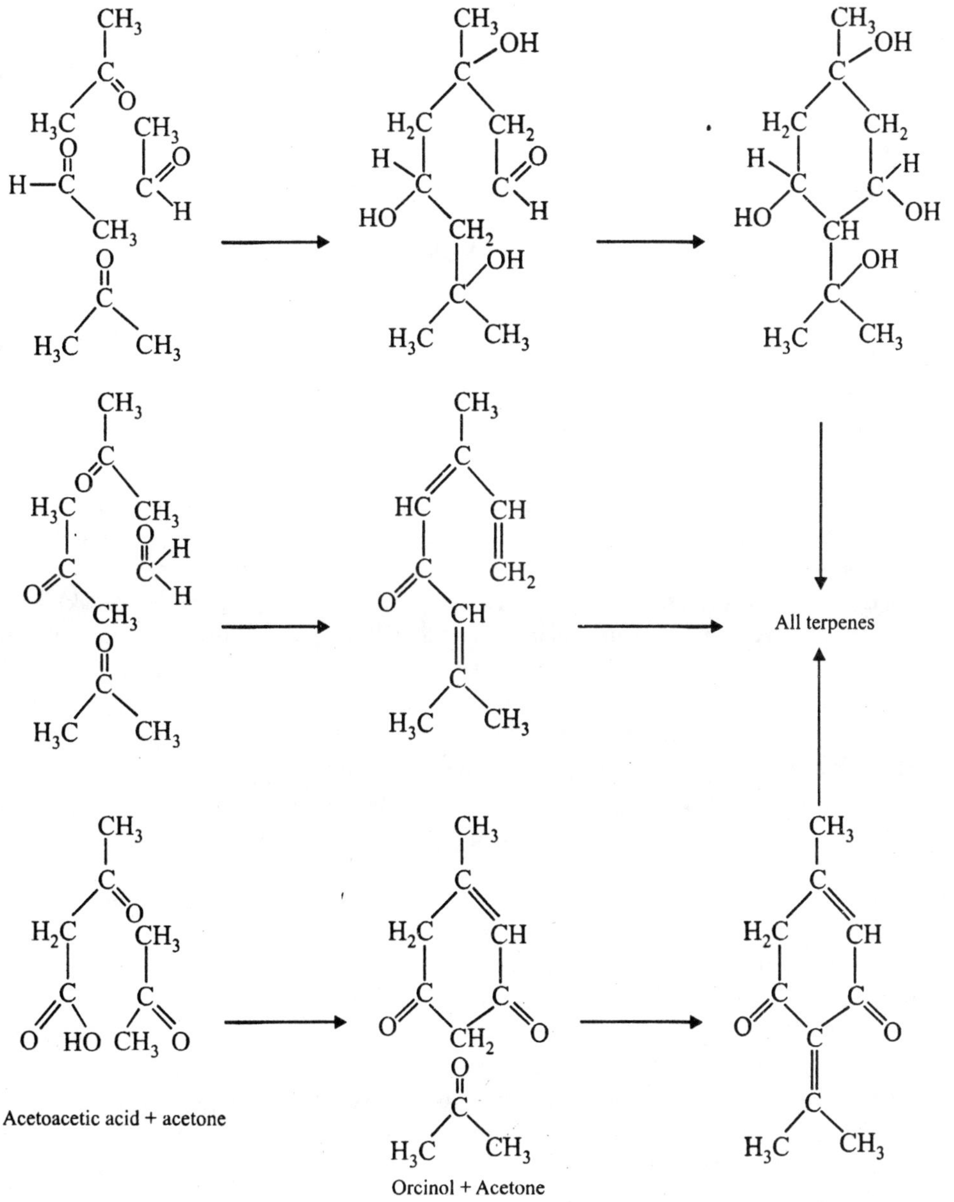

Fig. 2.34. Hypothetical terpene synthesis from acetone, acetaldehyde and acetoacetic acid.

Since none of these theories can be definitely rejected or accepted, it is clear that the presence of the branched chain represents a weak foundation on which to build hypotheses on the formation of the terpenes. We also have to admit the possibility that the 5 carbon units into which we can divide the molecules of the terpenes may have their origin in larger units. This suggestion was made by Emde, who postulated a physiological synthesis from sugars, through a coupling of levulinic acid-like molecules, followed by loss of CO_2 and the addition of smaller fragments of sugar metabolism when necessary (Fig. 2.35). The chief value of this clever hypothesis is probably that it points to other ways of constructing branched molecules. This applies especially to the theory of Hall, who attributes the formation of terpenes and benzene derivatives to the condensation and degradation of sugar derivatives. In this way different hypothetical 'half molecules' were postulated which are finally combined to give the desired structures.

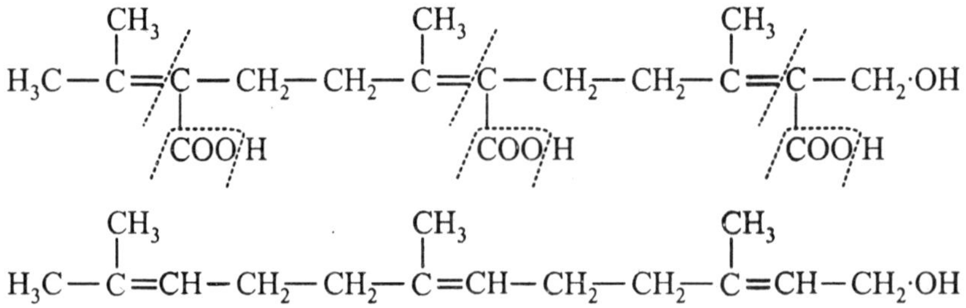

Farnesol formation

Fig. 2.35. Terpene synthesis according to Emde.

Extensive schemes for the derivation of other terpenes and the further synthesis of higher terpenes can hardly contribute to the acceptance of any one of these theories, because once a terpene-like compound is synthesised on paper it is not difficult to explain the many combinations of terpenes we encounter in nature. Oxydases, reductases, esterases and even special ring-closing enzymes ('Kyklokleiasen' of Tschirch) are therefore welcome instruments in the hands of theorists. *In vitro* many of the terpenes have been converted one into the other by simple chemical reactions, which take place under physiologically possible conditions. Under the influence of light, air and water, we can expect reactions to take place which we observe *in vitro* in improperly stored essential oils, i.e. oxidation and polymerisation. Free acids, if present, may cause loss of water, cyclisation and esterification.

Considering the long storage of these oils in the plant, it is not astonishing that analyses of the oils indicate a gradual change in the expected direction with the maturing of the plant. Experiments on peppermint show an increase in the menthone content with an accompanying decrease in menthol content due to oxidative processes. At the same time, the percentage of compounds other than menthol and menthone increases, indicating a splitting off of water and polymerisation.

It is very probable that, in a number of cases, especially in oxidation and reduction reactions, enzymes play an important role. Neuberg succeeded in the reduction of citronellal to *d*-citronellol and of citral to geraniol with yeast. These experiments, extended by Fischer, disclosed certain laws which govern the enzymatic hydrogenation of double bonds between carbon and carbon, and carbon and oxygen. The double bond conjugated with the aldehyde group in citral is slower in its hydrogen uptake than the carbonyl group; and we see, therefore, that the formation of geraniol takes precedence over the formation of citronellal. When geraniol is subjected to further hydrogenation, citronellol is formed, leaving the double bond at C_6 untouched. Citronellol produced in this way from optically inactive geraniol is optically active-dextrorotatory (specific rotation $[\alpha_D] = +6$) as in citronella oil. No further hydrogenation of the isolated double bond can be effected in this way, and it is interesting to note that in plants also, the hydrogenation has come to a halt at the citronellol stage (Fig. 2.36).

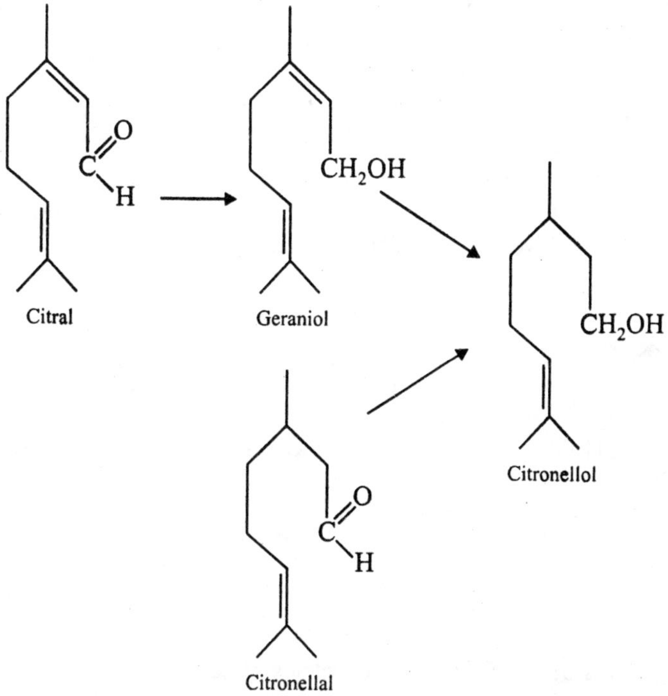

Fig. 2.36. Enzymatic reductions.

Substituents greatly influence the speed of the enzymatic hydrogenations, as seen in the slower hydrogen addition to keto groups, and to double bonds on tertiary carbon atoms. Carvone, main constituent of caraway oil, when subjected to enzymatic treatment, is reduced with difficulty to dihydrocarvone, another constituent of this oil (Fig. 2.37).

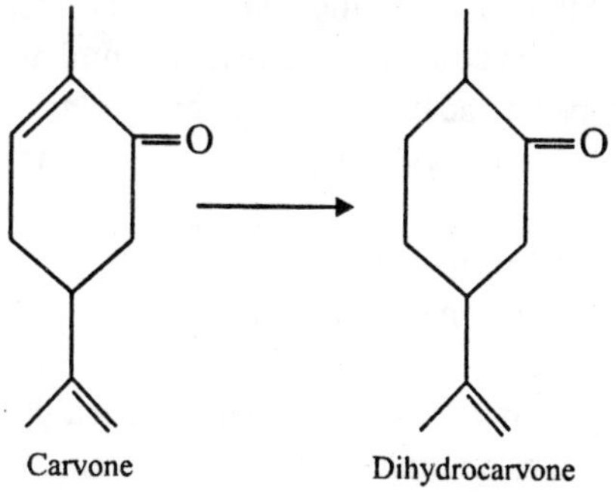

Fig. 2.37. Enzymatic reductions.

The absence of the totally hydrogenated carvomenthol suggests that similar laws are followed in the production of these terpenes in the plant.

These biological reductions can also be followed by studying the excretion products in urine during feeding or injection experiments. While in general, advanced oxidative degradations outweigh hydrogenation processes, a careful analysis of the excretion product shows similar reactions, as in the more simple experiments with yeast or enzyme-systems. Perhaps due to the branching of the chains, the reaction products of terpenes, such as citral, geraniol and geranic acid, can be recognised in the urine of rabbits after feeding or injection experiments. Figure 2.38 shows that, notwithstanding the simultaneous oxidation in other parts of the molecule, the double bond in α,β-position to alcohol, aldehyde or acid groups is hydrogenated. Similar experiments on citronellol confirm these observations; no reduction of the double bond in the isopropylidene group can be observed, but further oxidation produces dihydro Hildebrandt acid and hydroxydihydrogeranic acid (Fig. 2.38).

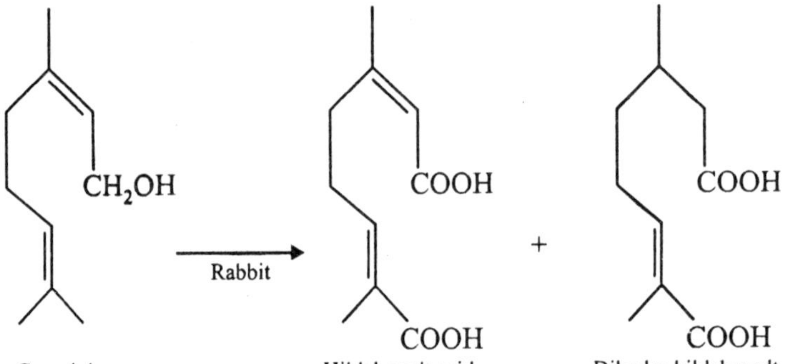

Fig. 2.38. Oxidation and reductions of geraniol in animals.

In β-ionone, however, where the double bonds are conjugated, reduction of the carbonyl group and its neighbouring double bond takes place, leaving the double bond between the two tertiary carbon atoms unchanged. Further oxidation introduces a hydroxyl group at one of the methyl groups (Fig. 2.39). The agents responsible for similar oxidations in the plant are suspected to be of enzymatic nature, but this has not been established experimentally.

Based on the not too improbable assumption that the terpenes present in a specific oil are interrelated, several building schemes were developed involving a stepwise conversion of the components, starting with a common precursor. In this way, Francesconi explained the simultaneous presence of citral, citronellal, linaloöl, dipentene, methyl heptenone and acetaldehyde in lemongrass oil. Likewise, Kremers correlated the components of American peppermint oil, acetone, acetaldehyde, citral, citronellal, isopulegol, menthol and menthone.

The following biogenesis of the two groups of substances found in the oils of American black mint and spearmint was suggested by Kremers. The names of substances actually found in the oils are italicised, while the two reducible groups in the citral molecule are underlined (Fig. 2.40).

Structural relationship and frequent occurrence in mint and eucalyptus oils has been noticed by Read for the terpenes, piperitone, piperitol, α-phellandrene and Δ⁴-carene. Piperitone is always accompanied by geranyl acetate, from which many cyclic terpenes can be formed. Smith, therefore, has expressed the opinion that the geraniol is a possible intermediate precursor of a number of terpenes. In *Eucalyptus macarthuri* the chain of reaction apparently stopped at the formation of geraniol, since the oil contains 77 per cent geranylacetate, while in most other species (under different conditions in the plant), more advanced transformations take place.

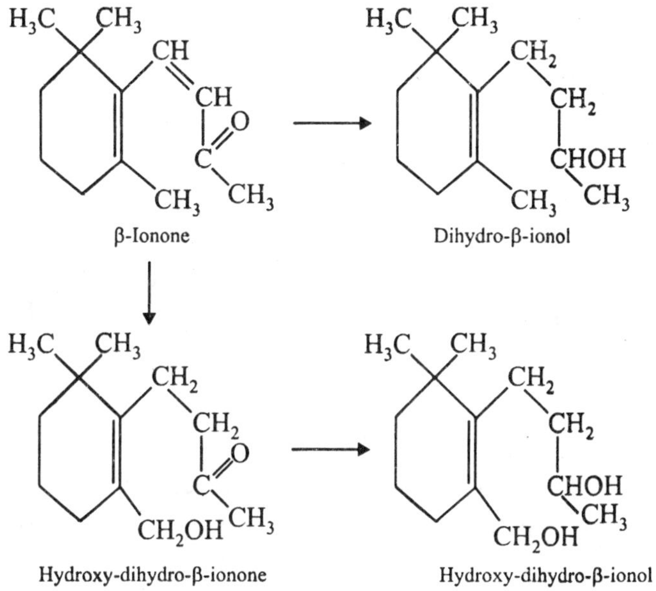

Fig. 2.39. Biological oxidations and reductions of β-ionone.

Similar relations are discussed in the genus *Orthodon* (family Labiatae). These oils mostly contain major quantities of thymol, carvacrol, cymene, cineole, thujene and thujyl alcohol. However, one species, *Orthodon linalooliferum* Fujita, contains 82 per cent linalool. This compound can be converted into many oil components of other species of the same genus. Huzita, therefore, considers this linalooliferum plant as the parent species of the genus *Orthodon*. It is, however, equally well possible that the reactions become blocked at the linalool stage through a mutation process.

Although the tendency has been to explain the formation of the terpene compounds from a C_{10} precursor like geraniol or citral, it is quite feasible that the condensation of the units takes a different and individual path for a number of terpenes.

We are naturally forced to accept this for irregularly built compounds such as artemesia ketone and lavandulol, but it might also be equally true for a number of the regularly built terpenes, e.g. pinene. α-Pinene is one of the most frequently occurring oil constituents and although the preparation of this ring structure from an aliphatic terpene is unknown, easy roads lead from pinene to a number of mono- and bicyclic compounds, such as terpineol, borneol, camphene, camphor, fenchone, fenchyl alcohol, dipentene, 1,4-cineole, terpin, pinol, myrtenol, dihydromyrtenol and verbenone (Fig. 2.41).

Laboratory experiments may indicate groups of compounds which can easily be converted into each other, but we have always to refer to the composition of the natural oils to give these groups a physiological meaning. It appears likely that in different oils the synthesis of specific compounds (such as limonene) might have taken place in several ways—such as by ring opening from pinenes or ring closure of citral, geraniol or other cyclic terpenes or by even direct synthesis.

This individuality of many couplings is further supported by our experience in the higher terpenes, where often, as in abietic acid, one unit is in an irregular position. For an explanation of the different groups of higher terpenes, we have to accept formations from single units, single and double units, doubling of double units, and doubling of triple and quadruple units.

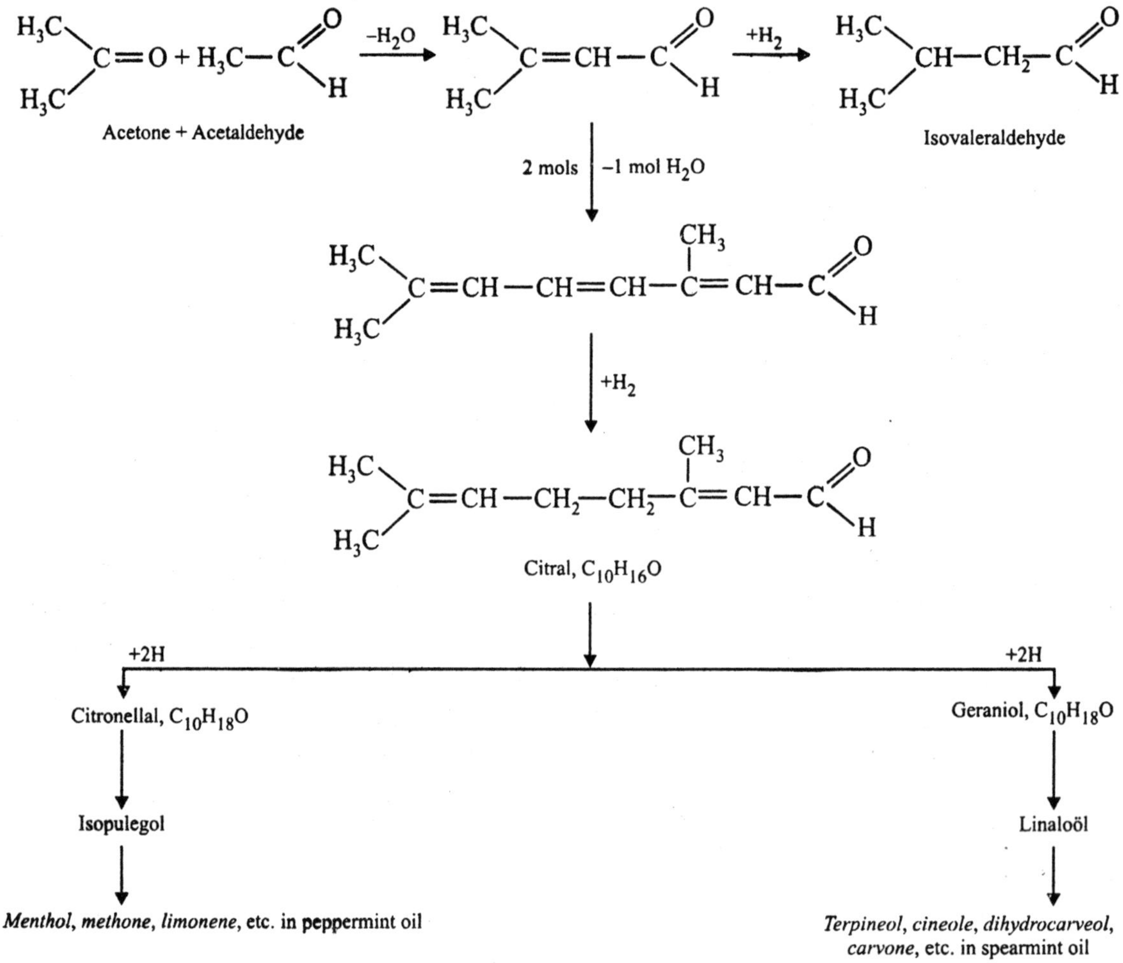

$$H_3C \atop H_3C \!\!\!\diagdown\!\!\! C = O + H_3C - C\!\!\diagup^{O}_{H} \xrightarrow{-H_2O} H_3C \atop H_3C \!\!\!\diagdown\!\!\! C = CH - C\!\!\diagup^{O}_{H} \xrightarrow{+H_2} H_3C \atop H_3C \!\!\!\diagdown\!\!\! CH - CH_2 - C\!\!\diagup^{O}_{H}$$

Acetone + Acetaldehyde   Isovaleraldehyde

2 mols | −1 mol H_2O

$$H_3C \atop H_3C \!\!\!\diagdown\!\!\! C = CH - CH = CH - \overset{\overset{\textstyle CH_3}{|}}{C} = CH - C\!\!\diagup^{O}_{H}$$

+H_2

$$H_3C \atop H_3C \!\!\!\diagdown\!\!\! C = CH - CH_2 - CH_2 - \overset{\overset{\textstyle CH_3}{|}}{C} = CH - C\!\!\diagup^{O}_{H}$$

Citral, $C_{10}H_{16}O$

+2H   +2H

Citronellal, $C_{10}H_{18}O$ Geraniol, $C_{10}H_{18}O$

Isopulegol   Linaloöl

Menthol, methone, limonene, etc. in peppermint oil   *Terpineol, cineole, dihydrocarveol,*
carvone, etc. in spearmint oil

Fig. 2.40. Biogenesis of terpenes in oil of peppermint and of spearmint.

Having reviewed all of these theories, let us summarise the established facts, in order to draw a conservative conclusion regarding the possible synthesis in the plant. We know that:

1. The structural formula of a large number of the compounds in plants can be divided up into branched C_5 chains.
2. The arrangement of the branched C_5 units is in most cases a head-to-tail union, but exceptions occur in the monoterpene group and are common in sesqui-, di- and triterpenes.
3. Ring compounds are easily formed from aliphatic terpenes, whereas the reverse can only be accomplished with difficulty.
4. Oxidation, reduction, shifting of double bonds and polymerisation take place readily.
5. The branched C_5 unit is distinguishable in the formulas of a number of non-terpenes coupled with non-branched structures.
6. The terpenes are often accompanied with propyl benzene derivatives and straight chain hydrocarbons.

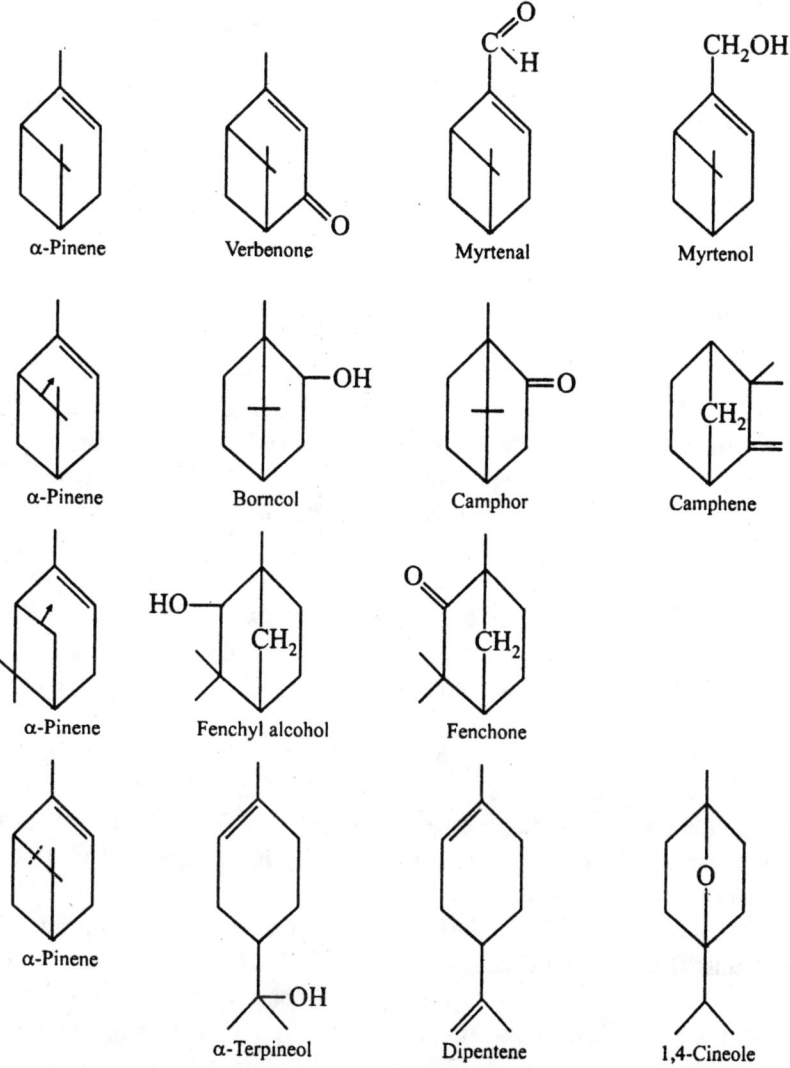

Fig. 2.41. Terpene family.

On the basis of these facts, we may safely conclude that a number of terpenes are formed from a unit which can give rise to one or more branched C_5 chains before or after the condensations. It is possible that the C_5 unit is not the actual structure undergoing condensation and that more complex compounds are involved, which split off certain groups after condensation has taken place. This would include the precursors as described by Hall and Emde, viz. phosphoric acid esters as the sugar precursor, and their degradation products, and protein complexes carrying the condensing structures which release the terpene compounds when formed. The regular head-to-tail union may be predetermined in the compound from which the terpene is formed, or the mechanism of the condensation may be such that this type of union occurs. The terpenes already formed readily undergo secondary changes, such as reduction, oxidation, esterification and cyclisation and this fact may explain the large variety of derivatives of the same pattern.

These families of terpenes may have their origin in independently formed key terpenes, such as geraniol, citral, pinene, etc. Higher terpenes may have been formed through a condensation of lower terpenes of the same or different chain length, whereby quite often derivatives from the regular and symmetrical architecture can be observed. No indications are available that would justify connecting the terpenes directly with other essential oil components, such as straight chain hydrocarbons or propyl benzene derivatives. Although the majority opinion favours a connection through the carbohydrate metabolism in the plant, there is no reason to assume that these products are formed in the same phase of these processes. Other essential oil components show structural features strongly suggesting connections with fat and nitrogen metabolism. From chemical evidence we can draw the conclusion that the complexity of the oil composition is caused by excretion or secretion of products formed in many metabolic processes taking place in the plant.

Since the volatile oils are intimately connected with vital processes in the plant, the presence of these specific components has been used also in the determination of the evolutionary status of plant families.

A continued, thorough chemical study of the volatile and especially of the nonvolatile components will undoubtedly give us a more complete picture of the processes which take place and of the structures which are formed in the metabolic activities of the plant. Although this knowledge must be the basis for any speculation on the mechanism involved, we have to turn our attention again to the living plant itself in order to collect experimental support for our theory of what actually happens. One of the ways in which the plant physiologist tries to solve these problems is to study the cells in which the oils are deposited, and the circumstances under which oil formation takes place.

The observation has been made that some of the cells or spaces in plant tissue are filled with oily droplets, difficult to distinguish from fatty oils.

These oils can be detected by staining with Sudan and osmic acid, and a distinction from fatty oils is best made by taking advantage of the presence of substances with a chemically more active character than the unsaturated hydrocarbons and alcohols, i.e. aldehydes and phenols. For example, droplets containing phenols can sometimes be stained with phloroglucinol hydrochloride. The presence of aldehydes is shown with fuchsin and sodium bisulphite reagents.

The oil secretion appears in different cell groups and distinctions have been made between external and internal gland cells. The external glands are epidermal cells or modifications of these, such as the excretion hairs. The secretion product is usually accumulated outside the cell between the cuticle and the rest of the cell wall. The cuticle is a thin skin covering the secretions and a slight touch suffices to break this thin piece of skin. Thus, on touching the plant, we observe immediately its well-known scent.

The internal glands are located throughout the plant; they are formed by the deposition of the oils between the walls of the cells. This schism of cells has been called a schizogenous formation. If this is followed by dissolution of the surrounding cells, morphologists speak of a schizolysogenous gland formation. Often these intracellular glands have grown to form long canals, coated on the inside with a layer of thin-walled cells.

This coating is said to have a double function, viz. the separation of other tissues from the oils and the formation of oils and resins. The secretion forms in the epithelial cells or in the membranes and passes through the cell wall into the interior of the gland. The secretion crosses a mucilagenous material produced by the outer membranes of the secretion cells which has been called the resinogenous layer by Tschirch. This layer does not possess any of the secretory functions ascribed to it, and the designation 'resinogenous layer' is inapplicable, at least in the cases of the *Umbelliferae* and *Rutaceae* studied by Gilg and collaborators.

Studies on the number and distribution of the glands show unequal distribution. The count of the glandular scales in *Mentha* species shows that the lower surface contains 10–25 scales per sq. mm the upper surface 1–6 per sq. mm. Dimensions and number of the scales increased near the large vein.

If we search the literature regarding the exact place of formation of substances like terpenes, we find that a few disputed observations are available, wherein it has been noted that secretion vacuoles suddenly appear in the cell, then increase in number and size, while cytoplasm and nucleus degenerate. These oil globules appear to be surrounded by a membrane. Some observers have seen small droplets of oil, formed in or near the chloroplast, which unite later and form the large oil drops. Others have not observed any oil drops at all in the cells, but found the oil in the membrane layers adjoining the secretion pockets.

Certain observations along these lines seem to point toward the region of photosynthetic activity, where carbon dioxide is reduced and synthesised to carbohydrates. Some support is lent to this thesis by experiments which attempt to establish correlations between oil secretion and known metabolic processes in the plant. Examples of this angle of research are to be found in studies on the effect of climatic and growth conditions on oil content.

A typical example of such investigations is contained in a report on the oil content and composition of Japanese mint (*Mentha arvensis*) grown in the United States, in which it was established that conditions in southeastern states do not favour the formation of menthol to the same extent as those in the northern and western states. The average differences in large sections of America are of the order of 74.5–81.0 per cent for combined menthol. Data on the individual oils obtained in the different regions show a spread for total menthol of 65.2–88.7 per cent and for combined menthol of 1.7–11.1 per cent. Sievers and Lowman rightly stress, therefore, the importance of a critical attitude toward the evaluation of results obtained in such surveys. More reliable evidence is obtained when the handling and oil determinations are carried out under strictly controlled conditions.

Although such statistical experiments are important from a commercial and agricultural point of view, it is difficult to draw any theoretical conclusions as to the physiological effect of climate, soil and other variables. These data, moreover, give an overall picture of the oil content and composition of young and old leaves, branches and flowers alike. We know, however, that different parts of the plant contain oils which are often of very different chemical composition. As an extreme and almost classical example, the composition of the oil of Sri Lanka cinnamon might be given. The bark yields oil with a high cinnamic aldehyde content, the leaf oil consists chiefly of eugenol, and the root oil contains a high percentage of camphor. Orange and lemon in flowers and fruit contain oils of different composition, and numerous are the examples where only certain parts of the plant contain oil: oil of iris, valerian and calamus occur only in the roots; sweet birch and cinnamon oils are found in the bark; whereas in the case of *santalum album* and cedar, the core wood contains the valuable oils.

Better controlled experiments on the influence of climatological conditions, such as sunlight on the oil formation, are found in a series of articles by Charabot and others. Experiments on shaded and unshaded plants indicate that light favours formation of oil. These observations cover a period of several weeks. We possess at least one observation on the daily fluctuations recorded on the oil content of nutmeg sage, the oil yield being 1.5 per cent during the night and in the afternoon only 0.6 per cent. The content of esters is highest toward the evening and least at night. The yield is lower during windy, dry weather.

To study oil formation as affected by plant development, it is necessary to select one type of organ and carry out the experiments under rigidly controlled and non-variable external circumstances. Since this is usually not feasible, the next best results may be obtained in experiments during a stable weather period on fast growing plants or through the other extreme of very long periods on slow growing plants, thereby averaging the effect of climatic changes.

Although no experimental data exist which will satisfy the most rigid requirements, the second type of experiment is represented by the analysis of oil from the peppermint plant during different stages of growth. Bauer analysed the oils of *Mentha piperita* at four stages—before and during, bud formation; and during and after, flowering. His findings are recalculated and summarised in Fig. 2.42, in such a way that the curves represent the percentage of the components relative to the fresh weight of the plant. The different corresponding growth stages are indicated, I, II, III and IV representing the period before budding, during bud formation, flowering stage, and after flowering stage.

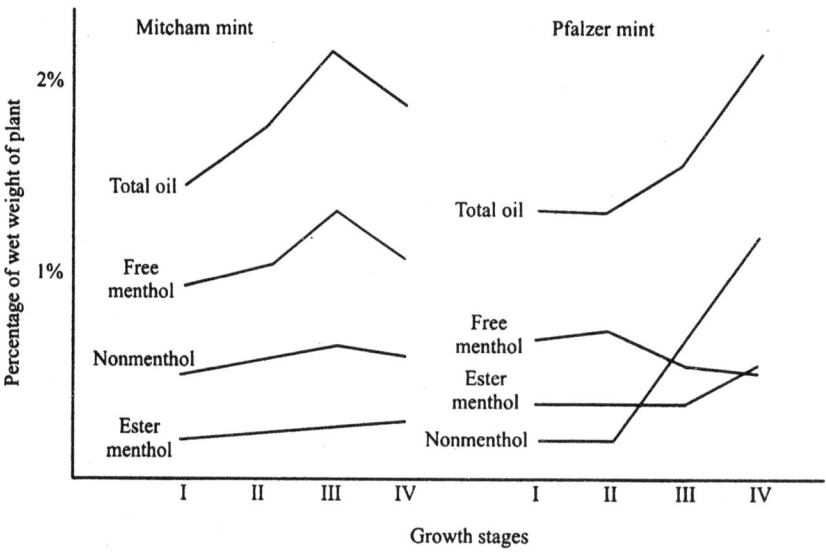

Fig. 2.42. Percentages of mint oils and their components at various stages of development.

The percentage of oil increases until flowering, when it either drops or remains constant. This is due chiefly to a decrease in free menthol formation, although the ester menthol continues to increase slowly, but steadily, probably at the cost of the free menthol. The constitution of the oil of a related mint, 'Pfälzer mint', shows the same behaviour during development in regard to the increase of ester content. Typical for this mint, however, is the increase in compounds other than the alcohol, probably menthone or dehydration products. Similar conclusions can be drawn from the investigations of Charabot on leaves of *Lavandula*, *Mentha piperita*, *Ocimum basilicum*, *Verbena tryphylla*, *Artemisia absinthium* and *Pelargonium*. In the later stages of growth the alcohols decrease probably at least partly through ester formation and dehydration to hydrocarbons. This process in turn is followed by oxidative reactions wherein aldehydes and ketones are formed. A decrease in oil content of the leaves during flowering has been observed by Charabot on *Verbena tryphylla*. In Table 2.1 is listed the mg oil present in different parts of the plant, during the flowering and after the flowering period. In this period the leaves lost a considerable amount of oil, as compared with other parts of the plant. Analysis of the flower oil showed that the material lost from the flower consisted chiefly of citral. Charabot attributed this decrease in oil content of the leaves in *Verbena* and *Artemisia absinthium* to a consumption of the oil constituents by the flowers, and postulated, therefore, a flow of oil from the leaves to the flowering parts.

Table 2.1. Mg of oil in parts of *Verbena tryphylla* per whole plant.

Description	Flowering	After flowering		
Root	10	16	Increase	6
Stem	8	16	Increase	8
Leaves	242	192	loss	50
Flowers	77	56	loss	21
Weight of plant in gm	366	259		

When we take into account the way the oils are stored in the plant, and their toxic action when released, this transfer seems unlikely. It is, however, possible that material which otherwise would have contributed to the formation of the oils is used up in the flowering stage and that the reduced formation of oil is unable to compensate for the constant loss through evaporation. The same explanations can be made for Charabot's experiment in which it was shown that *Mentha piperita* and *Ocimum basilicum* plants, after debudding, contain more oil in the leaves than under ordinary circumstances.

Long-term experiments stretching over two years, and averaging the climatic influences, have been carried out by Charabot and Laloue on *Citrus aurantium*. From their extensive data, the total oil present in a twig with an attached leaf can be followed through its development. Figure 2.43 shows clearly the large increase in absolute weight of the oil during the early period of growth. During the later period the formation in the branches is not even intense enough to compensate for the losses, due to consumption, transportation to other parts and evaporation. An increased production of limonene is observed. This is probably formed by the dehydration of the initially present, free and esterified linaloöl and geraniol. Similar experiments on the oil content at different stages of development were carried out on the oil of bergamot. A tendency in the expected direction was actually observed, i.e. an increase of esters and an increase of terpenes, through the loss of water and through cyclisation.

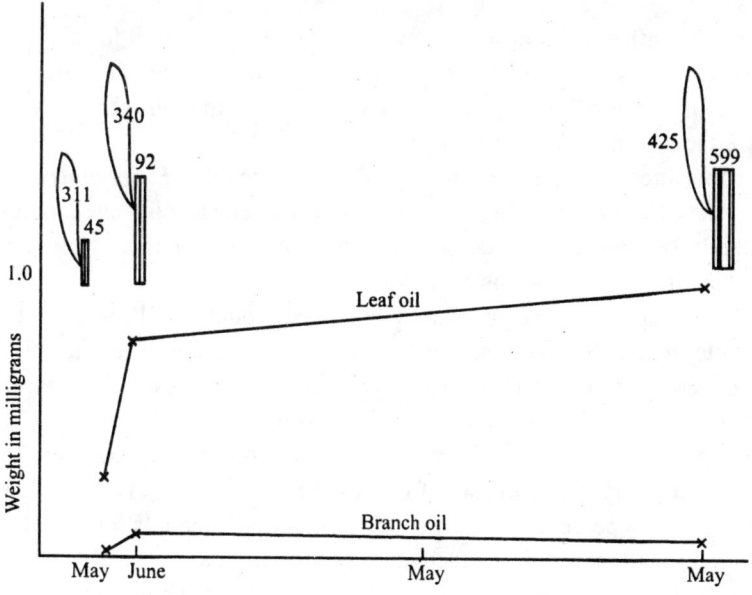

Fig. 2.43. Total oil content in growing leaf and branch of *Citrus aurantium*.

The essential oils extracted from the trunk of the young *Chamaecyparis formosana* tree contain a large amount of *d*-myrtenol and smaller amounts of *d*-α- and β-pinene. *d*-Dihydromyrtenol, which is only present in very small amounts in the young tree, is a major constituent of the older tree. The simultaneous disappearance of the pinenes and myrtenol strongly suggests that the tree converts these substances into the characteristic and rare alcohol, dihydromyrtenol, by oxidation and reduction processes (Fig. 2.44).

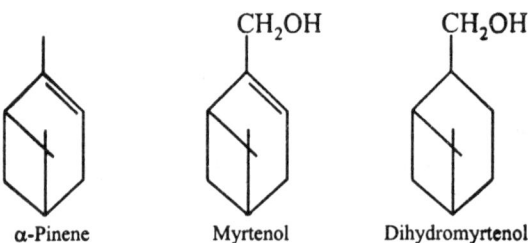

Fig. 2.44. Related bicyclic terpenes in *Chamaecyparis formosana*.

A fourth method for the determination of the effect of growth on the oil content consists of the comparison of the analysis of the oils of leaves harvested at the same time, but representing different developmental states. The influence of preceding variations in weather conditions on the older leaves has to be reduced in a way similar to that mentioned previously in describing experimental methods. It has been shown of peppermint oil that the percentage of yield decreases from the upper to the lower leaves. In agreement with the findings of Charabot and others, Nilov and Ponta found the ester and oxygen content higher in the older leaves. The ester content is also increased through the effect of hydrogen sulphide or ethylene.

The same gradient in oil content is seen in *Pogostemon patchouli*, where the oil is chiefly located in the upper three pairs of leaves, confirming the general rule that the production of the oil coincides with the most active growth.

If we want to study the influence of different environmental factors on oil formation, it appears from the preceding discussion that we have to choose plant material of the same physiological age. It is also advisable to study the oil composition of young tissues which, due to their intense synthesis, are better suited to reflect any effects of the environment.

Careful studies in this direction have been made by Berry on the oil of *Eucalyptus cneorifolia*. The oil of this eucalyptus consists chiefly of cineole, the hydrocarbons pinene and *l*-β-phellandrene, the carbonyl compounds *l*-phellandral, cuminal, cryptal, *l*-4-isopropyl-Δ^2-cyclohexene-1-one; also present are *l*-α-phellandrene and some alcohols such as australol.

Although no marked change in the composition or in the amount of oil can be noted in the mature leaves, the case is quite different in the younger stages of development. The total oil content and the amount of the different components from the growing tips of the branches at different times of the year are shown in Fig. 2.45, expressed in percentage of the wet weight of the plant.

It is thus possible to show the absolute formation of each group of terpenes per unit weight of the plant, uninfluenced by an increased synthesis of one of the components, as would be the case if we expressed the composition as a percentage of the oil. The amount of alcohols formed at different periods does not seem to be greatly affected. More aldehydes are formed in autumn than in spring. During the period of maximum growth in spring and summer the formation of oil is highest.

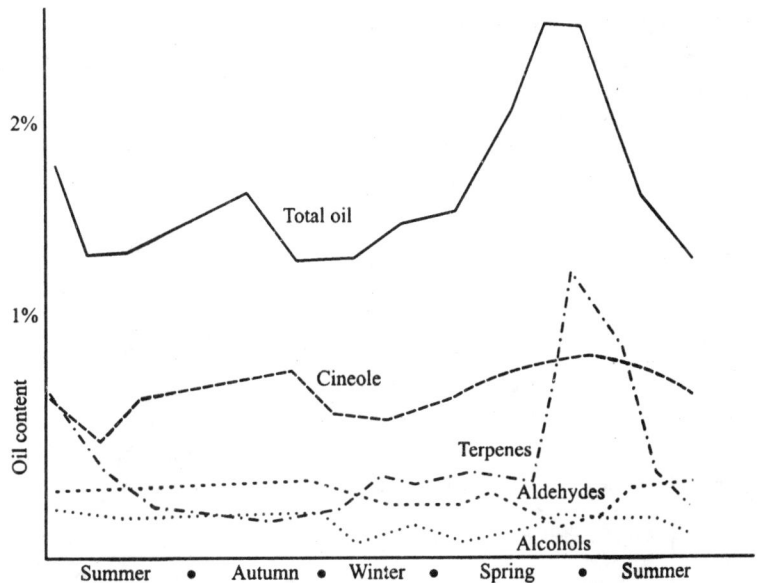

Fig. 2.45. Composition of oil from growing tips of *Eucalyptus cneorifolia*.

This increase cannot be attributed to a greater production of alcohols and aldehydes, because the alcohol content at different periods is not greatly affected; and in the case of the aldehydes we notice even the opposite effect: a decrease during spring. The real contributors toward the increased oil production are the terpene hydrocarbons, viz. β-phellandrene and cymene and in a lesser degree the terpene-oxide cineole. From analytical data on mature leaves, it is known that the phellandrene content of the oil is greatly reduced, and that the cymene content was only 3–4 per cent, as compared to 19 per cent in the young leaves. From these analyses Berry concludes that α- and β-phellandrene might be the precursor of certain terpenes, such as *p*-cymene, phellandral, cuminal and 4-isopropylcyclohexene-2-one-1. In the laboratory these conversions can be carried out with great ease (Fig. 2.46). The optically active compounds present in this oil are stereochemically related and belong to the laevorotatory series, constituting additional evidence of their common genesis. A similar relationship for *d*-phellandrene has been noted by Berry in *Phellandria aquatica*, viz. d-α- and d-β-phellandrene and the corresponding *d*-ketone.

Many more observations made on the yield and composition of plants grown under different conditions of soil, climate and treatment, and in different stages of development could be added, but most of these are of such a specific and often experimentally vague nature that they can justify only the general conclusion that the more actively the plant grows, the larger the quantity of oil formed.

To gain a deeper insight into the physiological processes involved in formation of essential oils, we have to limit our experimental subjects to well-defined organs of well-defined species of plants. The experimental work on the composition of the eucalyptus group is a warning that the oils from closely related species may be widely-different. Even species indistinguishable by ordinary morphological techniques can be distinguished on the basis of the production of oils of different chemical composition.

In many cases, the abnormal behaviour is due to hybridisation of different species. Extensive genetic work has been carried out by Russian workers, and has led to the conclusion that considerable changes in the synthetic activity of the plants can be observed under the influence of hybridisation, so that compounds may appear in the oil which were not present in the parent plants. On the other hand, Mirov in his investigations on the turpentine from the genus *Pinus* describes a Ponderosa-Jeffrey hybrid which contains terpenes inherited from the Ponderosa parent, and heptane from the Jeffrey parent.

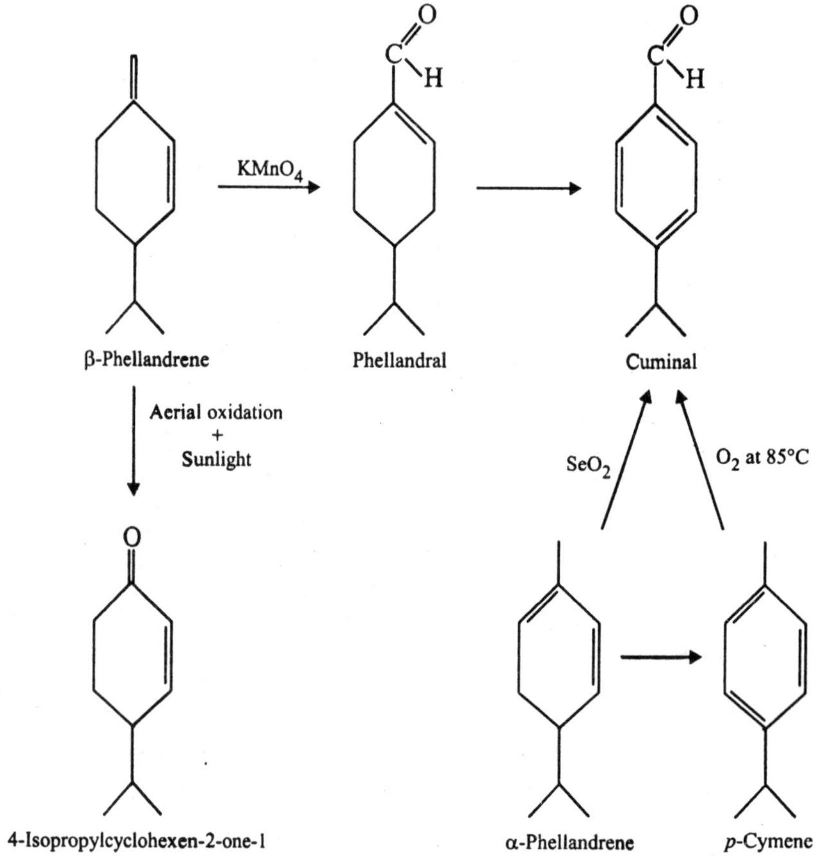

Fig. 2.46. Relations between terpenes in *Eucalyptus cneorifolia*.

Polyploidy and other types of mutations, such as heteroploidy and chromosome aberration, may cause changes in the quantity and composition of the oils, as has been demonstrated in *Pelargonium roseum*.

Many factors are, therefore, involved which change the composition of the oils; and for a successful study of these effects and the solutions of problems of oil formation it is imperative not to add further complications, such as are caused by drying, distilling and harvesting procedures. Storage for a few hours even in the shade may in special cases cause a considerable decrease in the oil content. Russian workers found for nutmeg sage that its volatile oil content decreases 33 per cent after storage for 3 hours, and 55 per cent after 6 hours in the shade, while in the sun it decreases 62 per cent after 6 hours. Their conclusion in this case is that the material should be collected at night and immediately distilled. The losses in volatile components from intact plants are well-known and have been measured quantitatively through micro combustion. The number of excreted products is considerable. These results serve as a warning that external circumstances may easily modify quantity and quality of oils, with the result that changes due to other variables cannot be distinguished. On exposure to air, and especially to sunlight drying of the plant material in the fields; a considerable amount of volatile oil may be lost by oxidation, polymerisation and resinification.

For practical purposes, certain compromises have to be made; nevertheless it should be our goal to choose conditions and experimental material so carefully that reproducibility is assured and the many factors involved can be changed individually. Only in such a way can we expect to unravel the fate of the plant metabolites secreted as essential oils. Such experiments might well throw light on another intriguing problem, i.e. the function of the essential oil in the plant.

A discussion of this subject invites a look at plant metabolism from a more general viewpoint.

FUNCTION OF ESSENTIAL OILS IN PLANTS

When the plant organism is alive and in process of development, external substances are constantly absorbed and transformed into 'building stones'. This reshaping of the foreign substances and their incorporation into the plant system, known as assimilation, requires energy, which is obtained by a series of reactions, whereby a part of the assimilated products is oxidised. The balance of these two series of reactions appears in the growth of the plant. Therefore, while some of the plant material is in a continuous flux, undergoing degradation and rebuilding, another important part of the reaction products can be expected not to take part in an uninterrupted chain of reactions.

Some of these products—such as cellulose—will be deposited in cell walls, the plant thereby acquiring a more rigid structure. Other substances—such as starch—are stored as energy and organic material sources, to be drawn upon when circumstances arise which cause the re-entrance of these substances into the reaction chain. We can thus assign a certain function in the plant to these particular compounds; but we find it much more difficult to do this with a number of other substances, such as alkaloids, anthocyanins and flavones, essential oils, resins and rubber latex.

It is a well-known fact that some plants emanate, besides carbon dioxide, a considerable amount of organic material, chiefly the carriers of the smell of the plant. In some rare cases so much oil is excreted that the oil can be set afire, as in *Ruta graveolens* and *Dictamnus*. At the same time, relatively large amounts of these essential oils are deposited in the plant, and our only evidence for the assumption that such compounds are unimportant sources of energy to the plant is the fact that, prior to leaf abscission, the oils are not transferred to the stem, as is the case with a large part of the carbohydrates.

The question has, therefore, repeatedly been asked: Does the plant derive any specific benefit from these oils? Opinions in this field are based on the observations that some oil-bearing plants are attractive to certain animals, whereas others are repellent. In individual cases, therefore, a contribution is made toward more effective pollination through insect visits. In a number of other cases a degree of protection against the depredations of animal and plant parasites may be afforded by the irritating effect of many oils. Some observers maintain that the oils function as reserve food, as a means of sealing wounds, or as a varnish to prevent excessive evaporation of water (cell fluid). These opinions are not beyond question, and do not appear to be supported by experimental evidence often having their origin merely in a teleological approach to the subject. Most investigators, including Tschirch, the famous resin chemist, hold the view that the functions attributed to those substances are more often of accidental, than of essential, importance to the plant. Those who consider these products a result of phenomena accompanying the growth process have used the term 'waste product'. This, however, rather underrates the value of these secretion products, which, through their formation, may contribute to syntheses important in the continued existence of the plant. Some carbohydrate precursors may serve as hydrogen acceptors, and in doing so may become unusable for further synthesis: Their function, therefore, may arise in their formation, and not in a later stage. Thus we might compare the oils to 'Hobelspäne', the shavings of a plane. As reason for their disposal, the opinion has been expressed that substances such as terpenes, mostly hydrocarbons, are so far remote in their chemical and physico-chemical conduct from the properties of the living substances that they are excreted as 'körperfremde' or alien materials.

There are others who refuse to believe in the waste product origin of the essential oils, and Lutz suspects that these oils have constituents which can be hydrogen donors in oxido-reduction reactions. Although they are thereby transformed into neutral compounds as far as catalysis is concerned, they might re-enter the reaction scheme through a reduction in the presence of light. To prove this theory, experiments were carried out on a fungus belonging to the *Hymenomycetes* on which Lutz determined the antioxidant or hydrogen-donor action of oil constituents. Phenols were found to be excellent donors, as is well-known from the investigations of Moureu, but secondary and tertiary alcohols and aldehydes also showed strong activity. Hydrocarbons are inactive in the dark, but become active in the light. On the other hand, primary alcohols, terpene oxides like cineole, and ketones are inactive; and perhaps are from this viewpoint the real waste products. Lutz considers the oil components as moderators in intracellular oxidation to protect against the action of atmospheric agents. He also includes the possibility that some of the components may be used as an energy source during a deficiency state caused by an interruption of the normal assimilation of carbon dioxide.

It has also been suggested that plants which emanate a considerable amount of oils are prevented from becoming too warm since heat is absorbed in the vapourisation of the oils. In this way the oils would function as a water-sparing mechanism. However, measurements of the relatively large amounts of water and small amounts of oil involved, show clearly that such a contribution would be negligible. In the search for some useful function for the terpenes, Teodoresco was one of the few who carried out experiments on the effects of oils on plants. He showed that the absorption of sun radiation by the essential oil atmosphere around the plant was negligible and certainly did not have any influence on the water evaporation. This oft-debated point, based on a misinterpretation of Tyndall's work, was solved by admitting oil vapour around the plant without, however, making direct contact, and determining the loss of weight through transpiration. Neither direct weighing of the loss of water, as shown in Fig. 2.47, nor transpiration measurements with a potometer demonstrated any heat-screening effect. If, however, the oil was allowed to come in contact with the plant, a considerable reduction in transpiration was evident. Although the damaging effect of prolonged exposure to the oils had been observed before, Teodoresco showed that when the vapour is removed soon enough, recovery follows in a few hours. This action is not confined to the oils obtained from the same plant, but is a more or less non-specific effect for the volatile oils in general.

It would, therefore, appear that a number of essential oils exercise directly or indirectly a definite action on the transpiration in plants. However, experiments carried out on partial saturation of the atmosphere surrounding the plant, simulating more closely the outside conditions, showed that the concentration of essential oil vapour would rarely be high enough to cause any significant decrease in transpiration.

The oils inside the plant, although enclosed by special tissues, might have an influence on the transpiration and other important functions of the plant rather than the vapour of the excreted oil, since there is reason to believe that cell walls would not be an insurmountable obstacle for the oil. This effect would result in a general retardation of a number of the plant activities. Teodoresco mentions specifically a decrease in the nyctinastic, seismonastic, phototropic and geotropic movements. The oils inhibit also the formation of chlorophyll in etiolated plants when exposed to light and cause a decrease in permeability.

Continued exposure to the oil vapours causes damage to the living substance, producing a greater permeability, which is in turn followed by death. General toxic action on plants has been observed by Bokorny with oil of turpentine in concentration of 1:50,000.

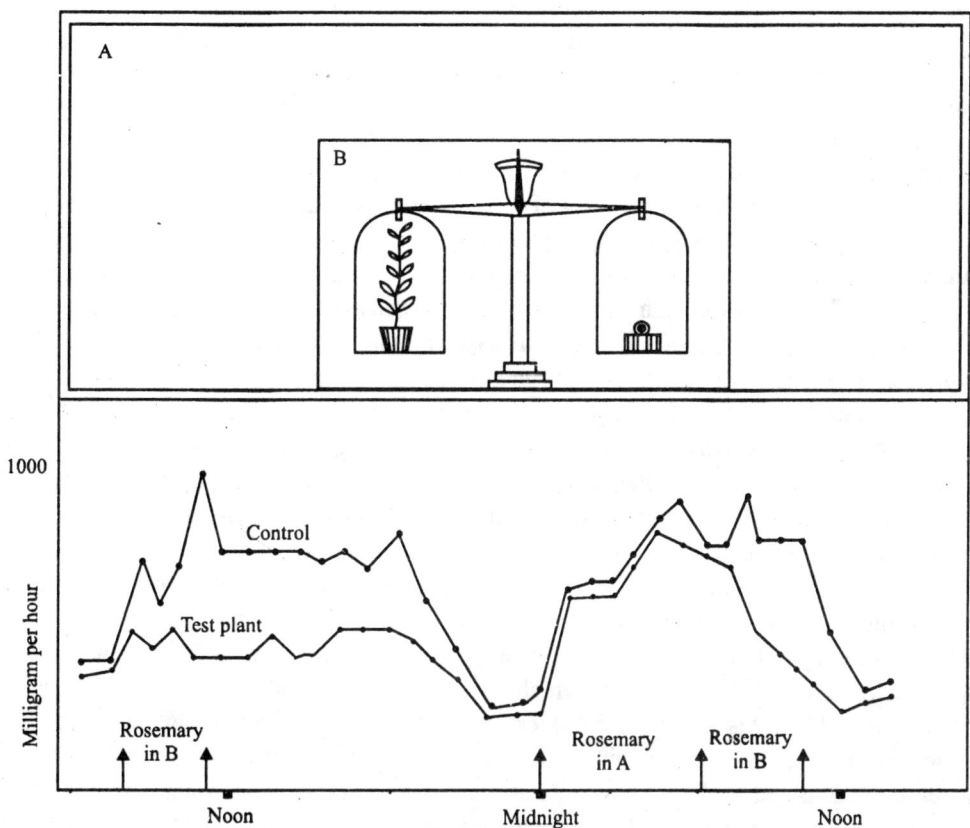

Fig. 2.47. Vapour of *Rosmarinus officinalis* on *Dracocephalum moldavica*.

The action of some essential oils is similar in certain respects to that of anaesthetics on animal cells. This problem of anaesthesia is one of the fundamental problems in general physiology and the results obtained in these studies might well contribute to the understanding of similar effects in plants. The first effect of fat solvents, narcotics and stimulating agents is identical and it may be assumed that they cause a reversible lowering of the permeability for water and water-soluble substances, in harmony with the findings of Teodoresco and others on the pronounced inhibition of transpiration in plants.

The inhibiting and damaging effect of the oils on many life processes has been turned to our advantage in the use of these compounds as bactericidal and fungicidal agents. However, from the diversity of the compounds in essential oils, it is clear that we have to regard with suspicion any general statement on the bactericidal action of the essential oils. From specific cases which have been studied, it can be concluded that the terpene derivatives, while possessing action bactericidal to certain organisms, are not able to inhibit growth in all of the numerous types of micro-organisms. It is, therefore, not astonishing to see aqueous infusions of, for example, lavender, peppermint and juniper drugs fall victim to putrefaction after several days of standing. On account of their bactericidal action, a number of volatile oils have been employed in the past for the treatment of urogenital infections. The simultaneous irritating effect on animal tissue applied, in measured degree may stimulate repairs of tissue and assist in the removal of mucous from trachea and bronchia and relieve tension of the stomach and colic.

Other toxic effects are reported on cultures of fibroblasts and further examples of their inhibitory effect on life processes can be seen in the anthelmintic effect of different oils, especially chenopodium oil. The effect of this American wormseed oil on roundworms, hookworms and intestinal amoebas is very similar to that of santonine, a sesquiterpene lactone present in *Semen cinae*. The toxicity of these oils for certain organisms cannot be measured simply by their bactericidal action. Thymol, for example, is much stronger antiseptically but is much less active as an anthelmintic than santonine or ascaridole, the active components of wormseed oil. The toxic effect of some essential oils and oil components is not limited to the organisms which have to be destroyed, and excessive use in higher animals and man causes depression of the higher centres followed by convulsions. A few cases are known where an apparent stimulating effect is observed. This is the case with terpene compounds such as camphor and menthol, which are used as circulatory stimulants in cases of collapse. It is assumed that when the action of the heart muscle is depressed, camphor may improve the cardiac condition and remove arrhythmia. On the basis of recent investigations, these effects seem also to be due to an inhibitory action on nerve fibres which counteract other fibres belonging to the sympathetic nervous system. Through this effect on the inhibitors, certain muscles are stimulated. A similar explanation might well hold for the acceleration and strengthening of the peristaltic movements of the small intestines of rabbits, according to Haffner and Sone and Shiro.

In general, we observe a definite toxic effect on the important life processes and excessive doses, because of depression and paralysis of the central nervous system, are followed by death. The essential oils probably interfere with delicate mechanisms, through their chemical and physical effects, either by entering and disturbing colloidal systems or by taking part in certain reactions. The oils themselves are at the same time exposed to many influences, which may change them in such a way that removal through the kidneys is possible. This so-called detoxication process takes many forms, and may consist of esterification, oxidation, reduction, or conjugation with compounds such as glycuronic acid and amino acids. When borneol is fed to dogs, it appears as glycuronide in the urine; when vanillin is ingested, oxidative processes are responsible for the excretion of vanillic acid. A combination of both processes is evident when camphor is removed in oxidised form. When such a removal is not possible, as, for example, by accumulation of the oils through injection, the organisms react by walling off the foreign material and tumours and sterile abscesses are reported.

This reaction is in principle similar to what happens in a plant lacking the elaborate detoxication and excretion mechanisms present in the higher animals. A considerable part of the metabolites which are not immediately taken up in further reactions or are not removed by evaporation will have to remain in or near the secretion cells. The interfering action of the oils may then cause lysis of the surrounding cells and changes in the normal metabolism, resulting in the formation of cork and mucilagenous layers, with low permeability for the oil. We may safely conclude that once removed from the continuous chain of reactions, these compounds are a potential danger to all living tissues, and both plant and animal react by walling off the oil from the other tissues. If this is not possible, reactions will take place until the compounds are so transformed that they can be excreted or until they have become harmless from the point of view of the surrounding tissue. From a general viewpoint, essential oils, alkaloids, resins, rubber, anthocyanins and many other secreted substances may have in principle a similar history. Their precursors, linked with essential processes in the organism, undergo secondary and further changes when exposed to the medium in which they are left behind.

Chapter 3

Spice Essential Oils and Oleoresins

INTRODUCTION

Spices (and condiments) are plant products which contribute distinctive flavour and aroma to foods. A variety of spices are used as flavouring agents and for seasoning of food. Spices are parts of plants such as buds, flowers, fruits, barks, roots or seeds obtained from a variety of plants. Spices may be classified into several groups taking into consideration their origin and the characteristic flavour or aroma. Accordingly, the same spice may be classified into more than one group: (i) aromatic fruits like black pepper, paprika or red pepper, vanilla, chillies, dill, juniper berries, coriander, anise, fenugreek, celery, cumin, fennel and caraway, (ii) aromatic seeds such as cardamom, nutmeg and mustard, (iii) Aromatic barks including cinnamon and cassia, (iv) aromatic flower such as clove, (v) rhizomes such as ginger and turmeric, (vi) leaves such as parsley, marjoram, rosemary and sage, (vii) pungent spices such as pepper, ginger, chillies and mustard, (viii) phenolic spices such as clove, eugenol and allspice, and (ix) coloured spices such as saffron, turmeric and paprika.

The characteristic flavour and aroma of spices are due to steam volatile essential or volatile oils and organic solvent soluble oleoresins. The main constituents of essential oils include mono and sesquiterpenes, phenols and phenolethers, aromatic hydrocarbons, alkaloids and pyrazines.

Eugenol, carvacrol, thymol, estragole, anethole, safrole and myristicin are some of the important phenols and phenolethers. Aromatic hydrocarbons such as p-cymene, 1,3,8-menthatriene and 1-methyl-4-isopropenylbenzene also occur in spices. A variety of mechanisms are responsible for the generation of the characteristic flavour and aroma compounds in spices.

Thus biosynthesis of cinnamaldehyde, the main constituent of cinnamon bark and of eugenol and safrole originates from phenylalanine. Terpene oxidation produces some aromatic hydrocarbons in spices. For example, 1-methyl-4-isopropenylbenzene is derived from 1,3,8-menthatriene and (+)ar-curcumene is derived from zingiberene or β-sesquiphellandrene. Character impact compounds include cinnamaldehyde in cinnamon, anethole in anise, d-carvone in caraway, eugenol in cloves, 1-methyl-4-isopropenylbenzene and 1,3,8-menthatriene in parsley leaves, turmerone and ar-turinerone in turmeric.

Spices such as mustard (and horseradish) contain glucosinolates in the cells. After the rupture of the cells, thioglucosidase enzymes act on glucosinolates yielding isothiocyantes such as allyl isothiocyanate from sinigrin and p-hydroxybenzyl isothiocyanate from sinalbin, which are responsible for the pungent burning taste of the mustard and horseradish. The aroma of capsicum pepper is mainly due to pyrazines, particularly 2-isobutyl-3-methoxypyrazine.

The hot, burning pungent flavour of paprika, pepper and ginger are due to alkaloids such as piperine, piperanine, piperylin, ginerol, shogaol, zingerone, capsaicin and its derivatives.

Spices such as paprika, saffron and curcuma also contain pigments which find use as food colourants. Paprika contains carotenoid pigments with capsanthin as the main compound. Curcuma contains curcurmin as the pigment. Antioxidants, mainly the cyclic diterpene diphenals such as carnosolic acid and carnosol, are also found in the extracts of spices such as sage and rosemary.

AROMA OF SPICES

Spices have mainly 2 flavour attributes. The one that catches the immediate attention of a consumer is the spicy aroma. This is contributed by the essential oil (known in the case spice as spice oil) and detected by the olfactory apparatus of the nose. The other is the hot pungent taste felt in the mouth while masticating.

The spice oils and oleoresins industry in India has undergone phenomenal growth in recent years. Due to increasing awareness about the health hazards associated with synthetic chemicals which are mostly petroleum-based, use of natural/essential oils is increasing. Due to biotic contaminants and pesticide residues in whole spices, oleoresins are gaining significance. Encapsulated spice extractives extended on a salt or dextrose carrier, encapsulated spice oils and oleoresins, homogeneous free flowing oleoresins, etc. are currently available. India is the world's largest producer, exporter and consumer of spice oils and oleoresins.

It has near monopoly in pepper, small cardamom and ginger oils and oleoresins. Total quality management (TQM) will be very critical in the coming century. India is preparing itself to face the challenges in quality standards of the major importing countries and also other biotechnological advancement which may lead to development of alternative products. With the emergence of 'nature food', 'ethnic food', 'yogic food' and emphasis on 'back to nature', uses of spices-based oils, oleoresins, pigments and flavourants would be in a bullish market during the coming years.

Spices are so important in our lives that even without really acknowledging its role, we simply say, 'variety is the spice of life'. Spices have played a vital role in world trade due to their varied properties and applications. They are used for adding flavour, fragrance and colour. They possess preservatives and inherent medicinal qualities. India with its favourable climatic and soil conditions for growing spices and other semi-tropical herbs, is in the forefront among the spice-producing countries. Spices that India can offer in abundant quantities are pepper, ginger, turmeric, chilli, cardamom, celery, fenugreek, fennel, cumin, dill, coriander, cinnamon, ajowan, cassia, cloves, nutmeg and mace.

SPICE EXTRACTS

Spice extracts have been developed to meet the new demands of the food processing industry. They have the following advantages: (i) consistency in flavour, (ii) not affected by bacterial contamination, (iii) much longer shelf-life, (iv) easier storage and handling, (v) full release of flavour during cooking, (vi) can be easily blended to achieve the desired characteristics, (vii) new flavour systems can be developed, and (viii) new products development facilities to confer competitive advantages.

SPICES IN VARIOUS FIELDS

A spice is used as dried whole spice or ground spice. Ground spice on distillation yields oils or oleoresins. Other products prepared from ground spices are emulsions and dispersed and microencapsulated products. The common spice oils and oleoresins are listed in Table 3.1.

Table 3.1. Spices oleoresins and essential oil.

Spice oleoresins	Spice essential oil
White pepper	Pepper
Black pepper	Cardamom
Cardamom	Cassia
Capsicum	Cinnamon
Turmeric	Celery
Ginger	Clove
Fenugreek	Coriander
Celery seed	Cumin
Nutmeg	Dill
Clove	Fennel
Fennel	Ginger
Coriander	Turmeric
Dill	Mace
Garcinia	Mustard
Vanilla	Nutmeg
Garlic	Garlic

Spice extracts are used in various preparations. Some of the common applications are listed in Table 3.2.

Table 3.2. Uses of spices extracts.

Processed meats
Soups and vegetable soups, sauces, chutneys and dairy products
Baked goods
Confectionary
Snacks
Beverages
Cosmetics
Perfumes
Hygiene products
Aerosols
Pharmaceuticals

Among the oils, pepper oil is exported in bulk. Paprika oil and mace oil are also exported from India. Among the oleoresins, those of pepper, paprika chilli, turmeric, nutmeg and cassia are major items of export.

DIFFERENT FORMS OF SPICES

Comparative evaluation has been done of various forms of spices, viz. whole spice, ground spice, spice oil, oleoresin, dispersed oleoresin and microencapsulated oleoresin (Table 3.3).

Table 3.3. Advantages and disadvantages of spice forms.

Spices or spice forms		Spices	Ground spice	Spice oil	Oleoresin	Dispersed oleoresin	Micro-encapsulated
a.	Form	S	S	L	L/P/S	Pd.	Pd.
b.	Flavour quality/aroma						
	Complete/balanced	1	2	4	1	1	1
	Consistent/standard	3	3	1	1	1	1
	Storage stability	3	4	4	3	3	1
	Free from contamination	4	4	1	1	1	1
	Bacterial quality	3	3	1	1	1	1
c.	Application						
	Strength	2	2	1	1	2	1–2
	Fast release	4	3	1	2	1	1
	Slow release	1	2	4	4	4	1–3
	Dusty/irritant	3	4	2	1	2	2
	Visual-specks	3	3	1	1	1	1
	Dispersibility	4	4	1	2	1	1
	Ease of metering	2	1	2–3	2–3	1	1
d.	Cost (very approx.)*	9	10		5–20		

Key: a : S = solid; L = liquid; P = paste; Pd. = powder; b : 1. very good; 2. good; 3. poor; 4. very poor; c : ground spice = 10 and * in final product.

This again illustrates that spice oil, oleoresin, dispersed oleoresin and microencapsulated oleoresin are complete, consistent, free from contamination, capable of giving fast release of flavours and have high dispersibility. The ranges of pungent principles and volatile oils in the oleoresins are many and wide (Table 3.4).

Table 3.4. Ranges of pungent principles and volatile oils in oleoresins.

Spice	Essential oil content (%)[1]	Other key constituents	Suggested dispersion rate (%)
Pepper	5–26 (20–26)	Piperine 30–55% (40–42%)[2]	6
Ginger	12–35 (28)	Pungency factor	5
Capsicum (chilli)	Not applicable	Capsaicin 2–20% (3–5%)[3]	2–10
Turmeric	Not applicable	Curcumin 35–98%[4]	–
Cardamom	1 to 60	–	6
Celery seed	7 to 14	–	5
Nutmeg	–(50)	–	8
Coriander	–(40)	–	6
Fenugreek	Not applicable	–	3
Cumin	–(65)	–	3

Notes: 1. Percentages in brackets represent normal range; 2. also available decolourised; 3. colour range 1200–10,000 colour units; and 4. colour range 5000–15,000 colour units.

GENERAL ASPECTS OF PRODUCTION

The best way to produce spice oil is by steam distillation as carried out for any essential oil. However, some special care is required in the case of volatile oil of spices. Being a food flavour, it is necessary to use food grade stainless steel for construction of the equipment especially for contact parts. Spice oils being generally expensive, the process can afford the extra capital cost required for SS equipment. There is also another reason why SS equipment has to be used.

Many spices have phenolic constituents, some of which are volatile like euginol. These on contact with iron will give dark colour to the spice oil.

Spices are generally dried by sun-drying. The next step is size reduction. Very fine powder may result is channeling during steam distillation. It is common to ground to a coarse powder. In some cases after a coarse grinding and other cases directly, spice is passed through a roller mill to flatten the particles into flakes. The exact process of size reduction is decided by the nature of spice and convenience of handling.

The actual process of steam distillation is similar to the case of any essential oil. Therefore only significant aspects especially those important to spice oil will be given in detail. For more details it would be worthwhile looking to classical books, since there is very little change in design or process during the last half a century.

Spices are manufactured in a typical still consists of a distillation chamber, a condenser and a florentine flask arrangement to serve as the receiver. In view of the high cost of oil, recovery of every drop is important. For this reason it is better to use a boiler as an external source of dry steam. The capacity of the chamber can vary between 100 kg to 1000 kg of ground spice. Lower capacity still is useful for oils of high value and where extraction of non-volatile pungent fraction is not important like cardamom oil. For pepper, ginger, celery seed, etc. which are required to be solvent extracted later, a higher capacity still will be appropriate. Larger than above stills are not common. Very high stills are not to be encouraged since unlike fragrance oils, flavour oil are valued highly for heavier sesquiterpenes.

Water cooled condensers are used. It is common to use a cluster of 10 to 20 SS tubes for the passing of vapours to be cooled. These tubes are covered with a shell inside which cool and circulate water. In order to recover every bit of oil, the number, length and diameter of the tubes used are to be based on the cooling area required. This is calculated from the average specific heat of the vapours, latent heat of vapourisation of steam and the temperature of water available in the region concerned.

The receiver is a stainless steel (SS) florentine flask arrangement of 2 to 3 compartments. 3 stage receiver is preferred for full recovery. The condensed water is allowed to overflow. When distilling heavier-than-water oils, it is necessary to provide enough volume for oils to collect in the bottom below the overflow arrangement. The overflow siphons are taken from around middle portion of each compartment. The end of the tube from condenser carrying oil and water should dip well into the water. In heavier oils there is possibility of some lighter constituents to collect at the top. Both these fractions have to be collected.

RECOVERY OF OIL

When the steam distillation is over, water is drawn out and oil collected. At the interphase, it may be difficult to separate oil and water. This is taken in a separating funnel where separation can be obtained. Where there is emulsion formation, use of salt to increase the density of water can be resorted to in the case of lighter-than-water oil. Anhydrous sodium sulphate gives a clear oil. The dry clear oil is packed in high density polyethylene drums or barrels. Epoxy coated steel drums are also usable.

EMERGING TRENDS

New trends like clean spice oil and oleoresin are emerging. To achieve this, the raw material has to be pure. Packing materials should be biodegradable. Information technology in spices trade is growing by leaps and bounds. Use of various quality standards, modern techniques to preserve aroma, extraction, packing, transport, storage and retailing are receiving attention.

SUPERCRITICAL FLUID EXTRACTION

One of the advanced technologies in extraction is supercritical fluid extraction (SCFE). The use of supercritical fluid extraction and chromatography for extracting and measuring spice components has vast potential. Supercritical refers to the specific temperature and pressure above which a fluid has the solvating properties of organic solvents, but the diffusivity of a gas.

The combined solvating and diffusing properties make it possible to extract compounds from solid matrices with little or no pretreatment of the solid.

The most common supercritical fluid used in the food industry is carbon dioxide, due to its non-toxic nature, low supercritical temperature, low cost, and non-flammability. In addition, carbon dioxide volatilises once the extraction is complete, leaving only the extract.

Currently, supercritical extraction and chromatography are not used extensively. Companies that sell this type of equipment need to do more method development work to make it less expensive and practical. It has a lot of advantages over the conventional distillation technique. The product obtained has longer shelf-life, no residual solvent, no residual pesticide, excellent blending characteristics, high potency of active components and freedom from biological contaminants.

NEW SPICE VARIETIES RICH IN QUALITY

Indian Institute of Spices Research, Calicut, Kerala has also contributed to varietal improvement and quality upgradation. Many varieties/hybrids are now available in black pepper, cardamom, ginger, turmeric, and cinnamon. Many of these varieties are rich in essential oil, oleoresin, colour and pungent principles (Table 3.5).

Table 3.5. New varieties of spices and their major constituents.

Name of variety	Major active constituents (%)		
I. Black pepper	Piperine	Oleoresins	Essential oil
Sreekara	5.1	13.0	6.0
Subhakara	3.4	12.4	6.0
Panchami	4.7	12.5	3.4
Pournami	4.1	13.8	3.4
Panniyur–2	6.6	10.9	3.5
Panniyur–3	5.0	12.7	3.7
Panniyur–4	3.8	9.2	4.0
Panniyur–5	3.8	12.3	3.8
Palode–1	3.0	15.4	4.8

(Contd ...)

Name of variety	Major active constituents (%)			
2. Cardamom	Essential oil	1,8 cineole		α-terpene acetate
CCS–1	8.7	42		37.0
Mudigere–1	8.0	36		42.0
PV–1	6.8	33		46.0
ICRI–1	8.3	29		38.0
ICRI–2	9.0	29		36.0
ICRI–3	6.6	54		24.0
3. Ginger	Oleoresin	Ess. oil	Crude fibre	Dry recovery
Varada	6.7	1.8	3.3	20.7
Suprabha	8.9	1.9	4.4	20.5
Suruchi	10.0	2.0	3.8	23.5
Suravi	10.2	2.1	4.0	23.0
Himgiri	4.3	1.6	6.0	20.6
4. Turmeric	Essential oil	Oleoresin	Curcumin	
Suvarna	7.0	13.5	4.0	
Suguna	6.0	13.5	4.9	
Sudarshana	7.0	15.0	7.0	
Prabha	6.5	15.0	6.5	
Pratibha	6.2	16.0	6.2	
5. Cinnamon	Bark oil	Bark oleoresin	Leaf oil	
Navashree	2.7	8.0	2.8	
Nityasree	2.7	10.0	3.0	

Thus, spices occupy an important position in the history of world and they have been finding wide applications in various fields. Spices extracts like oils and oleoresins have captured a wide market over the years. India has great advantage in this field, as it is the centre of diversity of these crops. However, a lot of new innovations are emerging in production, quality standards and packaging. The total perception towards food preparation in the world is undergoing rapid change. With the available potential in R & D and raw material availability, India would regain its past glory and emerge as a global leader in quality spices.

QUALITY ASPECTS

The quality of the oil is checked by refractive index, specific gravity and optical rotation. Unlike in fragrance oil solubility in alcohol is not important. For detailed quality check, organoleptic examination and gas chromatographic pattern are commonly employed.

Essentially, flavour industry wants more oxygenated derivatives as against hydrocarbons, as is available in terpeneless citrus oils. This is achieved in spice oils by fractional steam distillation at the time of manufacture of spice oil itself. Also in oils used in food flavouring, sesquiterpenes are valued more than in fragrance oil. Savoury food using spice flavours are generally eaten when warm. Higher temperature make sesquiterpenes more volatile and consequently more receptive organoleptically. Besides, food is held for as much as a minute in the mouth while chewing. This nearness to olfactory apparatus also make nose to sense heavier fractions very well. This quality of oil is ensured by continuing the distillation for longer time and wherever feasible, by cutting off the more volatile early fractions. It is pertinent to point out that high quality of some spice oils are measured in terms of amount of characteristic sesquiterpenes, e.g. selinene, the dicyclic sesquiterpene in celery seed oil and myristicine, the oxygenated sesquiterpene in nutmeg oil. In pepper oil â caryophyllene and in ginger oil zingiberene and ar-curcumene are important.

OLEORESIN

An oleoresin is a material made by solvent extraction of herbs and spices followed by solvent removal. Solvents extract essential oils, fixed oils, flavour compounds, pigments, and vegetable oils from plant material. An oleoresin can be considered a concentrated mixture of natural colours, aromas, and flavours in vegetable oil. Most herbs and spices are commercially available as oleoresins. Although herbs are defined as leaves and spices are defined as all other parts of a plant, common usage often includes herbs in the general term spice.

The greatest advantages to the use of an oleoresin in food applications are the standardisation of flavour strength, the complete utilisation of flavour, the ability to blend, modify, and customise the product for specific applications, and the elimination of mould, bacteria, filth, insect fragments, and foreign matter of raw spices. In food products where the visibility of particulate matter is undesirable, oleoresins are preferred. The disadvantages of oleoresins result from the physical differences of these products from the raw spice. A liquid concentrate may require different handling and methods of addition than a ground spice. Absence of visible particles of ground or chopped spice with a liquid extract may not be acceptable in some foods. The flavour imparted by an oleoresin, due to the greater availability of the flavour compounds, is more dramatic than the spice so that sophisticated application knowledge is required. The increased solubility of the flavour compounds may also lead to losses or chemical changes in food processing and cooking. It may require a significant number of trial formulations of oleoresins to duplicate an existing flavour.

Soluble spices first originated in the 1930s, when the oleoresins of black pepper and ginger were developed. These original oleoresins were produced by extracting ground spices with a solvent, removing the solvent under vacuum and disposing off the inert material. The first oleoresins were heavy masses of material, but as improvements in extraction technique and knowledge of solvents grew, product quality and demand increased.

Oleoresins consist of both the volatile and non-volatile portion of spices and, therefore, have a flavour balance characteristic of the ground spices or herbs. Advantages include instant flavour release, standardised flavour and aroma to meet precise specifications, good economy and sterilisation through the manufacturing process.

Process of Manufacture

The details of the manufacturing process of oleoresins depends on the plant material to be processed and the solvents used, four stages are involved: (i) grinding, (ii) extraction, (iii) desolventisation, and (iv) standardisation.

Grinding

Grinding or a similar process (such as chopping, maceration, etc.) is used to make extraction of the plant material more rapid or more efficient. The optimal type of grinding depends on the plant material, or, more specifically, its physical structure. Some herb leaves are dried and gently crumbled before extraction. Other spices, in which the oils are contained in hard-to-extract glands or in a woody matrix, are ground to very fine particles. Grinders may include a cooling mechanism to prevent degradation of heat-sensitive compounds and loss of volatile components. The grinding operation must be designed to have minimal deleterious effect on the flavour and aroma components as well as on the vegetable oils extracted.

Extraction

In extraction, the ground spice is washed with a solvent to dissolve the pigments, flavour, and aroma components and separate them from the nonsoluble residue (marc or spent). Extraction equipment can be of various designs but are of two basic types: batch extractors and continuous extractors.

A batch extractor, in its simplest form, is a container that can be filled with ground spice and solvent. A stainless steel tank with a steam jacket to heat the solvent is typically used. After sufficient time has passed to dissolve the soluble materials, the mixture is separated by filtration. The oleoresin in the soluble fraction is recovered by removal of the solvent. The marc is also desolventised to recover the solvent for re-use. Extraction and filtration can be combined by use of baskets to hold the spice within the extractor. In this design the solvent flows by gravity through the bed of ground material, dissolving the flavours and oils and carrying them out of the extractor for recovery.

Variations of batch extractors include centrifugal extractors, where the solvent is forced through the ground material in a spinning container, and high-pressure extractors, where the solvent is pumped at high pressures. Efficiency of extraction is greatly influenced by adjustable parameters such as solvent temperature, contact time, ground particle size and so forth.

The design of a continuous extractor differs in that ground material continuously enters the extractor through an air lock, passes through the solvent stream and then exits as marc through an opposing air lock. Extraction is usually a multistage process. These extractors are most efficient when flow is 'counter current', with fresh solvent in contact with the ground material in the last stage of extraction.

A two-step extraction is sometimes used to obtain two fractions from a spice. This uses a non-polar solvent to remove essential oil, followed by using a polar solvent to extract other, more polar compounds. By this procedure, black pepper, for instance, can be extracted with hexane to obtain the essential oil followed by extraction with methylene chloride to obtain a more pungent fraction.

Solvents approved for the manufacture of oleoresins in the United States are hexane, acetone, methanol, ethanol, isopropanol, and methylene chloride. Although oleoresins produced with chlorinated solvents are allowed in the United States, many other countries, such as the European Community and Japan, do not allow food products made with chlorinated solvents—a serious consideration for exportation.

Carbon dioxide, when liquified under high pressure, is also used as an extraction solvent. Such extraction is usually done by batch extraction due to the technical difficulty of admitting ground material into a pressurised extractor. Extraction is often done at temperatures and pressures high enough to produce superfluid conditions. The extraction solvent then has properties of both a gas and a liquid. This greatly increases the solvent power and the efficiency of extraction. Because liquid and supercritical carbon dioxide are not satisfactory solvents for polar compounds or compounds of high molecular weight, traditional solvents may be added to the carbon dioxide to increase the solvent power and increase the efficiency of extraction. The disadvantages of the technical complexity of the high-pressure extraction equipment, the small extractor size, and the low efficiency of extraction must be balanced against the potentially milder extraction conditions, the ease of solvent removal, and the perceived 'naturalness' of the solvent. The organoleptic properties of products obtained by this method are somewhat different from the equivalent products obtained from traditional solvent extract and distillation.

Desolventisation

Desolventisation is the distillation process in which the extraction solvent is removed from the oleoresin. Although this can be done at atmospheric pressure with relatively high heat, preservation of sensitive, more volatile flavour compounds usually requires the use of vacuum conditions and lower temperatures. When carbon dioxide is used as the extraction solvent, reducing the pressure to atmospheric evaporates the solvent.

If the oleoresin does not contain any desirable volatile compounds, desolventisation may be vigorous, removing all volatiles. A wiped-film evaporator, in which the solvent-laden oleoresin passes as a thin film on a heated surface, can be used to strip off all the solvent as well as any other components that will evaporate. Turmeric oleoresin, in which the nonvolatile extractives are natural colourants, is often desolventised in this manner. The volatile oil contained in this oleoresin is often considered an undesirable aroma component and its loss during desolventisation may improve the quality of the oleoresin.

In many oleoresins, volatile components such as terpenes contribute an important part of the flavour profile. Their loss during desolventisation would lessen perceived product quality. In this case a still with reflux or fractionation capabilities is used. The less volatile essential oil is separated from the solvent and returned to the oleoresin. Alternately, a significant fraction of the essential oil can be removed with the solvent and the distillate then fractionated to recover the oil.

In the United States, the maximum residue for solvents used in extraction of oleoresins is listed in 21 CFR, part 173. For the most commonly used solvents, these levels are as follows:

Solvent	Level (ppm)
Acetone	30
Methanol	50
Hexane	25
Isopropanol	50

Residual solvent level is measured by a codistillation technique followed by gas chromatography (GC) analysis of the distillate. One of the difficulties of this technique is that it does not distinguish between the chemicals of the solvent and the same chemicals derived from plant material. The common solvents are readily detected in plant tissue. Hexane, for instance, is one of the many degradation products of vegetable oil. It would not be feasible to produce an oleoresin with zero hexane content, even if hexane was not used in extraction. Another difficulty arises from the fact that the standard assay requires the steam distillation of a sample of oleoresin. Heating oleoresin in boiling water produces many small organic compounds that may interfere with chemical identification by GC.

Standardisation

Standardisation produces consistent flavour, colour, and aroma in oleoresins—this is one of the major advantages of such products over raw spices. By blending different batches and adding recovered or additional essential oil, an oleoresin of defined characteristics can be produced.

The addition of edible oils, such as soyabean or cottonseed oil, can be used to adjust flavour intensity to within specifications. Other ingredients may be emulsifiers to improve homogeneity and ease of application and diluents to decrease viscosity. Such additives, if used, should be clearly stated on the manufacturer's label. These additives should follow Food and Drug Administration (FDA) guidelines for natural products if the oleoresin is to retain its status as a natural product.

Physical Characteristics

Oleoresins may be liquids or solids depending on the specific nature of the flavour compounds they contain and the amount of essential oils, fixed oils, and triglycerides in them. Oleoresin cinnamon, if extracted with hexane, for example, is a thin liquid consisting of over 90 per cent cinnamaldehyde. Only a trace of vegetable oil is extracted from the bark from which it is made. Paprika oleoresin, made from the fruit of *Capsicum annuum L.*, is usually greater than 85 per cent vegetable oil and has the viscosity of vegetable oil. The carotenoid pigments are predominantly esters of fatty acids. In contrast, nutmeg oleoresin is a pasty solid because of the high content of trimyristin, the triglyceride of myristic acid.

The flavour intensity of oleoresins is 6–40 times as strong by weight as the corresponding herb or spice. Extraction concentrates the flavour chemicals. The degree of concentration depends on the percentage of extractables in the raw spice. In food applications, oleoresins often provide a stronger flavour impact than would be predicted on the basis of a chemical comparison to the raw spice. The flavour components have been extracted from the plant matrix and are more readily incorporated into food and available to the palate. The majority of oleoresins are stable when stored at room temperature. Low water activity and high content of components that are naturally bacteriostatic minimise microbiological growth. Many oleoresins are sterile. Some oleoresins may undergo oxidation due to the highly unsaturated components in them; these require refrigeration or storage under an inert atmosphere. Manufacturers' directions, such as mix before use, should obviously be followed.

Chemical Composition

It is not possible to describe the chemical composition of oleoresins in general terms. Some contain various terpenes and sesquiterpenes dissolved in vegetable oil while others are terpene free. The fixed oils, the non-volatile oils, are an important part of the chemical and flavour profile. The important components may be carotenoids, curcuminoids, phenolics, aldehydes, or many other classes of compounds. The chemical composition of oleoresins is determined by the plant material used and the solvent used for extraction. Oleoresins do not contain carbohydrates, protein, cellulose, and other materials not extracted by solvents.

Quality Control

Physical properties of oleoresins, such as specific gravity, refractive index, optical rotation, and viscosity, are not important for determination of the quality of these materials. However, they may be very important for proper dosage and ease of addition with some process equipment. Some oleoresins require heating and stirring before use to ensure a homogenous product.

Analytical methods for quality control purposes must be chosen for the specific oleoresin or components of interest. For many oleoresins used to provide aroma, the percentage of essential oil can be determined by steam distillation with chemical composition determined by a hyphenated gas chromatographic technique: gas chromatography-mass spectroscopy (GC-MS), gas chromatography-Fourier transform infrared (GC-FTIR), etc. various methods of compound detection and identification.

For other oleoresins, specific assays have been developed to measure the components of interest. Examples are capsaicinoids in capsicum oleoresins, curcuminoids in turmeric oleoresin, piperine in black pepper, and others that can be found in a literature search based on the specific oleoresin.

It remains true, however, that the most important assay for a flavour material is taste. There is no substitute for sensory evaluation. Despite the high cost of maintaining flavour standards, training and testing sensory panelists, and testing all products upon receipt or before shipment, this is a necessary part of quality control.

Application Examples

Oleoresins are usually very much soluble in vegetable oil. This makes their use in oil systems simple; they are often added to the oil before it is added to the food. Oil solubility aids in the distribution of flavour throughout a food product. Oleoresins, which are very concentrated flavours and colours, should be dissolved completely and mixed thoroughly into the food to avoid areas of excessive flavour or colour. With the use of capsicum oleoresin, concentrated extractives of chili peppers, such areas would be 'hot spots' in the literal sense. Capsicum oleoresins are available that are more than 1000 times hotter than hot sauces sold in grocery stores.

The oleoresins with the largest use as colourants are paprika, turmeric, and annatto. Colours of these oleoresins are limited to yellow and red-orange hues. These are listed as colours exempt from certification by the US FDA as distinct from the certified colours, which are synthetics. In other countries, such as the European Community, turmeric and paprika oleoresins are generally regarded as spices or flavours.

The chromophores in paprika oleoresin are carotenoid pigments, particularly capsanthin esters. This oleoresin is used in bread crumb coatings, processed cheese, processed meats, salad dressings, sauces, and snack food coatings where it provides a yellow-orange to red-orange hue. Method of use ranges from as simple as spraying the surface of a cracker to as complex as formulating a dry powder containing flavours, gums, cheese powders and other ingredients to coat a cracker chip Paprika oleoresin is stable to aseptic retort, and extrusion processing and not affected by variation in pH. It may be stored in closed containers at ambient temperature. Oxidative degradation can be a concern. Degradation can be catalysed by light, by heat, and by trace metals. Paprika oleoresin stabilised with other plant extracts is commercially available.

Turmeric oleoresin is an extract of the root of *Curcuma longa* L. It contains three related pigments known as curcuminoids. It is used to provide a bright yellow hue comparable to that of FD&C Yellow No. 5. Turmeric is very heat stable but not stable at high pH. Curcuminoid pigments are also sensitive to ultraviolet (UV) light exposure; foods made with turmeric oleoresin usually require protective packaging. This oleoresin is widely used in bakery mixes, breading, cereal, process cheese, margarine and soup. Most mustards and pickles contain turmeric.

The extract of annatto, *Bixa orellana* L., is sometimes termed annatto extract and not annatto oleoresins because some forms of the product do not contain a significant amount of vegetable oil. The extract may even be obtained as powder although liquids are more common. The primary pigment, bixin, is a carotenoid containing dicarboxylic acid functional groups. It is oil soluble but can be saponified to make the water-soluble pigment, norbixin. When dissolved in oil or water, annatto provides yellow-orange to red-orange hues, depending on concentration. The precipitation or agglomeration of norbixin in cheese and cheese products gives the well-known 'pinking' of the colour. Low pH is usually a factor in this colour change. Dairy products and snack foods are the major applications of annatto extracts, although other foods may also be coloured with this natural product. Annatto is also blended with paprika and turmeric oleoresins to make other hues. Annatto has sufficient heat stability for aseptic and extrusion processing, but short heating cycles are recommended. The extracts can be sensitive to oxidation and UV degradation.

An interesting use of oleoresins is in cooking oils. Paprika and turmeric oleoresins can be used to colour an oil such as popcorn oil. The coloured oil is then used both for popping the popcorn and for colouring it as it pops. With the addition of spice oleoresin blends to the oil, flavour can also be added to produce a flavoured, coloured product. This is easily adapted to home cooking for products such as microwaved popcorn.

Oleoresins have further applications in systems in which high oil solubility is not an advantage. They can be blended with emulsifiers to make them water dispersible or, with the use of polysorbate esters, even water soluble. As an example of this, a vinaigrette, in its simplest form, would consist of vegetable oil, vinegar in water, natural colour and herb flavour. Paprika oleoresin can be used to provide an orange colour and mixed oleoresins of basil and other herbs can be formulated to provide flavour. If oleoresins are used in this two-phase system, both colour and flavour will dissolve in the oil layer. After mixing, the layers will quickly separate into two layers of significantly different colour and flavour. If the oleoresins are first blended with emulsifiers to make water dispersible products, the emulsified products will disperse into both layers. After the layers separate, both will contain colour and herb flavour giving a more satisfactory salad dressing. Emulsified oleoresins are effectively used in reduced-fat sauces, spreads, and dressings where oleoresins would not be soluble. The flavour evenly disperses with direct addition of the emulsified oleoresin to the food product.

Antioxidant Properties

Although oleoresins have been widely used to flavour and colour oils and foods, there are other applications of oleoresins in foods. The well-known preservative effects of spices and herbs also apply to oleoresins made from them. Components that have the ability to inhibit oxidation are extracted with colour and flavour components, producing a spice extract that inhibits oxidation in foods.

Rancidity in fats and oils is caused by a complex set of oxidation reactions; free radical reactions are particularly important. An antioxidant is a substance that is capable of retarding or preventing oxidation.

Various factors accelerate or inhibit oxidation. A classification system has been established to group these factors by mechanism. The primary inhibitors are phenolics. These compounds intercept and neutralise free radicals preventing the propagation step in oxidation. The basic structure of a phenol is illustrated in Fig. 3.1; it is a hydroxy group on an aromatic ring. Other substituents on the aromatic ring determine the efficiency of the compound as an antioxidant. The phenolic hydrogen atom of a substituted phenol readily reacts with highly reactive free radicals that develop early in the oxidation process.

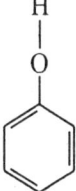

Fig. 3.1. Phenol structure.

This quenching reaction transfers energy producing a phenolic radical, which can either lose this energy thermally or undergo further, less damaging reactions. In some cases, the antioxidant phenol is regenerated in subsequent reaction.

Many spices contain phenolic compounds with potential uses as antioxidants. Those most commonly cited in the literature are rosemary, sage, thyme, turmeric, oregano, mace, nutmeg, ginger, and members of the mint (Labiatae) family. Of these, rosemary has had the most widespread commercial application. There are many phenolics in oleoresins of rosemary. Although carnosol and carnosic acid are present in highest concentration, many others have also been identified. These phenolic compounds act synergistically as antioxidants. Standardisation of rosemary oleoresin by concentration of individual compounds such as carnosol is not accurate. Protection from oxidation is due to all the phenolic compounds present. Various commercial products based on these oleoresins have been used to protect foods against lipid oxidation, pigment fading, and flavour degradation. In a liquid oleoresin, phenolics have a much larger effect than they would have when bound within the cell structure of the ground leaf.

The type and amount of oleoresin needed in an application depends strongly on the type of fats in the system, the synergistic effects of other ingredients, and processing conditions. Effectiveness in a given fat can be measured by various techniques such as the active oxidation method and the peroxide value. A more rapid method, which has become common in the last few years, is the use of a Rancimat to measure the induction time for the onset of rancidity. Studies using a Rancimat have good correlation to shelf-life studies with results produced in a fraction of the time. A synergist increases the effectiveness of an antioxidant. Such a synergist may even be an antioxidant itself in some applications. Compounds such as ascorbic acid and citric acid may increase the effectiveness of rosemary oleoresin by an amount greater than simple additivity would predict. These acids are chelating agents capable of binding to trace metal ions, removing their pro-oxidant influence. Iron and copper are particularly strong pro-oxidants. Polyphosphates and even lecithin, which contain phosphates, can chelate metals. These materials can be incorporated into the oleoresin or added separately to help protect lipids in a food product.

Topopherols are phenolics present in most crude vegetable oils. Although they are not present in a significant amount in rosemary oleoresin, they are oil soluble and easily incorporated.

The phenolics in spice oleoresins have characteristics that make them significantly different from the synthetic phenols like BHA and BHT. With their higher molecular weights, they are much less volatile; they are not lost at frying temperatures. Rosemary and related oleoresins are flavouring extracts and may be labelled as such or, as is more common, the phrase 'natural flavouring' may be used.

Spice oleoresins are extracts of botanical origin. They are considered GRAS (generally recognised as safe). Although they may have secondary benefits because of their antioxidant properties, they remain plant extracts. The commercially available rosemary oleoresins are not flavourless. This flavour may limit their use in some systems where high concentrations are necessary to give the desired degree of stabilisation. In other food systems, the flavour may be desirable and may improve sensory appeal.

NUTRITION

The contribution of oleoresin and essential oils to nutrition can usually be ignored; the level of usage, as a fraction of the diet, is extremely small. Obviously the vegetable oils in them are fats. Essential oils would also analyse as 'fat'. There may be a contribution to nutrition from oleoresins containing carotenoid pigments that have measurable vitamin A activity.

Ongoing research has indicated that diet plays a significant role in the risk of cancer and other diseases. Many herbs and spices contain antimutagens and anticarcinogens. Compounds with anti-inflamatory and antioxidant properties may inhibit tumor initiation, promotion, and progression when consumed as part of the diet. The potential of phytochemicals has led to the concept of 'designer foods' in which products are selected or formulated to provide for increased intake of beneficial, non-nutrient constituents.

SPICE OIL IN OLEORESIN

During the last two to three decades, one of the positive developments in the country has been the emergence of spice extraction industry, which is patronised by the world flavour fraternity very well. When extraction industry was developed in India some special features were added on. Primarily process became a 2-stage operation. The essential oil is first removed by steam distillation. The residue is then extracted with a suitable solvent to get the non-volatile fraction principally hot, pungent constituents and in some cases, colour giving compounds. Extraction is carried out by batch counter-current technique in SS percolators, where the active principles are collected as miscella by cold percolation. By removing the solvent by distillation, resin containing all the valuable non-volatile constituents is obtained. Required quantities of resin and spice oil are blended as per customer specification.

As mentioned earlier, flavour industry wants spice oil rich in oxygenated and sesquiterpene compounds. This can be achieved by resorting to fractional steam distillation. Tailor-made aroma extractives can be obtained by regulating time and conditions of steam distillation. Harsher mono terpene-rich early fraction find a ready use for blending in oleoresin. The resin portion will have all the higher boiling sesquiterpenes and diterpenes which are difficult to steam distil. Blending with harsher early fractions of oil helps to maintain the total bouquet of oleoresin at acceptable level.

Thus oleoresin also contains spice oil. The usual level of oil in different oleoresins are pepper 18 to 25 per cent, ginger 25 to 30 per cent and celery seed around 10 per cent. Nutmeg and cardamom oleoresins are demanded at wide range of oil content from 20 to 90 per cent.

Although pepper, chilli, ginger, turmeric and cardamom are India's major spices especially in export trade, as far as spice essential oils are concerned, only pepper, ginger and cardamom out of above are the major items. Chilli has no essential oil and turmeric oil has only limited value. To these nutmeg oil and celery seed oil can be added as the major spice oils.

Pepper oil used to be top earner, but in the last couple of years the unit value has decreased considerably. Besides this 20 per cent of the pepper oleoresin is oil. Pepper oil is mainly used for flavouring of meats, vegetable curries, savoury snacks, soups and dressings. However in food, the hot taste of pepper is more valued than its aroma. A small quantity is used in men's cosmetics, as the oil is believed to bring strong male fragrance note. Aroma of ginger is slightly more valued than its hot pungency. Cochin ginger is valued for its excellent aroma. In world trade next in importance is Nigerian ginger. Ginger from other sources including from other regions in India are considered inferior. Ginger oleoresin on an average contains about 30 per cent essential oils. Aroma of ginger is particularly liked in baked foods like ginger biscuit and soft drinks like ginger, etc. Cardamom has a high unit value and hence quantities of export are less. In recent times oleoresin is also moving. The oil content of oleoresins can vary from 10 to 90 per cent. Cardamom oil is used in cream biscuits, sweets, masala tea and coffee and even in savoury items. But the oil which has picked up a lot is nutmeg oil. The flavour of this is liked both in sweet and savoury foods. In Europe nutmeg flavour is used widely in meat preparations. Similarly celery seed oil also has found favour for use in food. A large number of other spice oils are produced and exported. The more important ones are cumin oil aniseed oil and cinnamon oil. Indian coriander has low oil content. It would be worthwhile exploring the possibility of introducing coriander with high oil content like the varieties grown is Russia and Morocco. Ajowan and dill oils have better potential, if superior varieties are introduced. Juniper berry is mainly grown in the Himalayan region.

A number of spice oils have become prominent in recent years. Mustard essential has high value and its production has come up well. Mustard has both fixed and essential oils. Because of the high pungency of the essential oil, its recovery is beset with health and environmental problems. But the oil has good price and has demand in Japan and Western countries where it is used to give the special pungent taste of mustard. Traditional mustard paste is now-a-days made using essential oil. Indian garlic is low in oil content compared to Chinese, but has high and welcome flavour. Clove used to be imported to India through a protected channel. With liberalisation of import, clove oil is being produced in India. Indonesia, Zanzibar and Madagascar produce large amount of clove oil at a cheaper price. With more clove plantations, India can compete in a big way. Apart for flavouring, clove oil with high eugenol content, has demand in dental preparations as an anti microbial agent. There is some growing interest in minor oils like galangal oil and caraway oil in India.

There are a large number of spices and herbs which are generally native to Europe. India has made token entry in manufacture and export of oils like rosemary, thyme, basil, parsley, etc. A wide range of herbs are of Mediterranean origin. They include laurel, sage, oregano, marjoram, etc. These herbs should be imported and oils and oleoresins manufactured in India for reexport to Europe where there is good demand. With a well recognised spice extraction industry, Indian production and export of spice oils and oleoresins are expected to grow to near monopoly level.

Flavour

Taste buds offer a limited means of detection, however, compared with the human olfactory system, which can perceive thousands of different chemical aromas. Indeed, 'flavour' is primarily the smell of gases being released by the chemicals you have just put in your mouth. The aroma of a food can be responsible for as much as 90 per cent of its taste.

Processed Spices

The earliest form of processed spices was ground spice. Ground spices find their biggest use in foods when a visual effect is desired (i.e. a red fish curry with capsicum and an yellow dal curry with turmeric), while liquid forms of spices offer consistency, sterility and uniformity. Often, both forms are combined in a food product. For example, corn chips may have specks of ground spices, while the salt and powdered cheese are coloured with oleoresin dispersions.

Other Forms of Spices

The other forms of spices include:
1. Standardised oleoresins: Oleoresins to which essential oils and/or solubilising agents are added to meet product requirements.
2. Liquid soluble spices: Extracts to which solubilising agents have been added so they are dispersible in oil or water systems.
3. Dry soluble spices: Dispersions of extracts on a free-flowing carrier such as salt, dextrose, sugar or maltodextrins. Some suppliers have dispersed up to 45 per cent extractive onto the carrier.
4. Encapsulated spices: Emulsification of extracts with starches or gums for spray drying.

The major advantage of spice extractives is cost. The savings are realised since the extraction process results in virtually all of the spices flavour and aroma being released, unlike with ground spices.

Liquid soluble spices, dry soluble spices and encapsulated spices are standardised, resulting in a consistent replacement ratio for ground spices. With oleoresins, the amount needed to replace ground spices differs with each spice. Essential oils offer an advantage when a clear end product is desired, and are used in products such as pickles or alcoholic beverages.

Taste

In order to give a processed food a taste that consumers will find appealing, a flavourist must always consider the food's 'mouth feel'—the unique combination of textures and chemical interactions that affect how the flavour is perceived. Mouth feel can be adjusted through the use of various fats, gums, starches, emulsifiers and stabilisers. The aroma chemicals in a food can be precisely analysed, but the elements that make up mouth feel are much harder to measure.

Colour

Every food designer knows that consumers judge a product not only on its flavour, but on its appearance, as well. One important class of ingredients exists solely to enhance the appearance of what we eat along with food colours. In recent years, product designers have been asked to formulate using so-called natural colours with increasing frequency. This presents a set of challenges that is totally different to those presented when using certified colours. As any artist would say, it's primarily a matter of understanding the palette and correctly applying the colours.

Turmeric

Turmeric is a bright yellow colourant made from the roots of the herb *Curcuma longa L.* The pigments responsible for the colour are known as curcuminoids: curcumin and related compounds. Turmeric's solubility depends on the medium in which the pigments are dispersed and the process. For instance, turmeric oleoresin is water-soluble; but a suspension of turmeric extract in oil can be added to fat-based systems. At high pH this colourant turns orange. There are no usage restrictions, as long as the level conforms to good manufacturing practices (GMP).

Annatto

Annatto is another yellow food colourant. It comes from the seeds of the *Bixa orella* tree. The pigments that produce the yellow to orange colour range are the carotenoids—bixin and norbixin; the concentration is expressed as a percentage of one or both of these compounds and the content varies with the extraction method. The pH, emulsifiers and the overall solubility affect the hue; the greater the solubility in oil, the brighter the colour. Water and oil-soluble, and oil/water dispersible forms of annatto are available. Because it may precipitate or turn pink at a pH less than 5, suppliers have developed specially emulsified acid-proof versions.

Beta-carotene

Beta-carotene is a precursor for vitamin A, in addition to its use for imparting an orange-yellow colour to food. Most beta-carotene is derived from algae or synthesised. Beta carotene is oil-soluble, but can be made into a water-dispersible emulsion. No restrictions have been placed on the level of use and it is listed as GRAS (generally regarded as safe).

Paprika oleoresin

Paprika oleoresin is extracted from the pod of *Capsicum annum*, or *paprika*. It contains three main naturally occurring pigments: capsanthin, capsorubin and beta-carotene. This combination produces a bright orange to red orange in food products. The oleoresin is oil-soluble, but when emulsified becomes water dispersible.

Red cabbage juice

Red cabbage juice produces a bright pink to red colour in products with a pH of less than 4. A higher pH causes the anthocyan-based pigments to turn an unstable purplish blue colour. The product dissolves in water, but not in oil.

Beet juice

Beet juice in either liquid or dehydrated form contributes a bluish-red colour produced by a compound known as betanin which is stable at a higher pH range than red cabbage juice. There are no limits on its usage level. When used at high levels, though, it contributes a characteristic beet flavour.

Grape skin extract

Grap skin extract imparts a reddish purple colour to beverages. However, the FDA restricts its use to alcoholic beverages, beverage bases, still and carbonated drinks, and 'ades'.

Other non-certified colours

Other additives can be used in food products as colourants, but their use is limited because of cost (saffron), limited application (ferrous gluconate—only in black olives), or non-human consumption (Tagetes meal from marigolds is for chicken feed only).

Functional Advantages

Spices can have functional properties in food and beverage systems in addition to being used as seasoning. For example, deheated mustard is being used for its water binding and emulsification properties. Some spices have a long history as colourants, and using the antioxidant properties of other spices is increasing as natural continues to be more important.

Paprika, annatto and turmeric oleoresins can be used alone or in blended form to provide hues of pale yellow to deep red-orange. Derived from natural vegetable sources, they provide a cleaner labelling option. Natural antioxidants found in spices can play a role in providing natural protection against oxidation in foods. Rosemary and sage have been reported to have some of the highest antioxidant activity of spices, while oregano and cloves also have high antioxidant values.

Antioxidants—including vitamin C, vitamin E, lycopene and various carotenoids and polyphenols—appear to positively affect overall health. These compounds are believed to promote immune system function as well, particularly in elderly individuals, and to reduce the susceptibility of LDL ('bad') cholesterol to oxidation, which leads to plaque formation.

These favourable effects have driven industry as well as consumer interest in finding ways to increase dietary levels of various antioxidants.

'In today's society, we take pleasure in defining heroes—we also take great pleasure in shooting these heroes down.' This is true not only for antioxidants as a group, but also for specific compounds. Beta-carotene had its moment of fame; now the focus seems to have shifted towards tocotrienols, the polyphenols found in green tea, and to mixtures containing lutein, zeaxanthin and other carotenoids. Because so much has yet to be learned, it is certain that the function of antioxidants in nutrition will continue evolving, in turn affecting food product design.

Extracts of spices are being used more commonly in medical applications as more and more people are becoming aware of the science we have called 'ayurveda' for the last 3000 years or more. The traditional use of turmeric as an antitoxin is now being used in medicine. Extract of ginger is used in formulations to help overcome nausea, pepper extracts are used as bio availability of medicines.

Oils are used in fine fragrances for perfumes to render that specific aroma of being woody or musky or floral or tender and so on. They are also used in home toiletries as effective insect repellants, fungal inhibitors and so on.

New Technology

Spinning cone column (SCC) distillation

Producing fresh-tasting or 'true-to-nature' flavours has its challenges. Commonly used batch distillations can be inefficient and time-consuming. State-of-the-art distillation technology, such as a spinning cone column (SCC), make it possible to capture fresh flavour substances today. In this process a highly efficient liquid-gas contacting column, also known as a distillation or stripping column, uses gentle mechanical forces to enhance the distillation process. By this means, volatile flavour compounds are rapidly separated from a thin-film liquid system. Viscous slurries with high levels of suspended solids as well as clear liquids can be processed without damage to the flavour or extracted product.

SCC technology originated in Australia, achieving early success as a method of capturing and removing the grassy notes from milk in this region, and has been commercially viable for about 12 years now. Since then, the industry has begun to use it for flavour management to transfer positive flavours from one product to another such as transferring full cream flavour to non-fat products.

Fruits, vegetables, tea, coffee, peppermint, beer, wine and citrus are key flavour categories that are benefited by SCC technology.

Encapsulation

In the flavour industry, encapsulation of a liquid material into a solid matrix is common practice for various reasons as it facilitates mixing of incompatible ingredients:
1. Overcomes binding with the food matrix.
2. Prevents unwanted changes during processing.
3. Improves hydrolytic and oxidative stability.
4. Masks unpleasant odour or taste.

Much as an eggshell protects the inner contents of the egg from the outside environment, a 'microcapsule' protects its inner contents. The use of microcapsules is a way to achieve controlled release of the inner material in the core.

Flavour encapsulation traps a flavour into a matrix to give controlled or targeted release in a food or beverage. Encapsulants also help protect flavours from degradation during processing. While there are many ways to encapsulate flavours for food systems, one method does not work in every system.

Various encapsulation methods include: (i) spray-drying with fat, protein or carbohydrate matrices, (ii) extrusion, (iii) coacervation, (iv) molecular inclusion, and (v) liposome entrapment.

Controlled release of flavours has been the 'Holy Grail' in food science. You can take the flavour and mix it with an oil-soluble flavour in the bilayer or a water-soluble flavour in the core. Research has shown that this protects the flavour from degradation in some systems and gives longer flavour and better flavour, depending on the application.

While in the pharmaceutical industry, controlled release may refer to release in the bloodstream and controlled release of flavour only happens in the mouth when combined with air and saliva.

Chapter 4

Flavour and Fragrances

INTRODUCTION

Mother nature's greatest gift to humans has been her plants. Plants have always fascinated humans down the ages and fulfilled their basic need of food, clothing and shelter. In addition nature continues to also provide humans with plants for medicine and pleasure. Aromatics and intoxicants, both of them derived from plants, affect the human central nervous system in their own unique ways, one giving munificent pleasure and the other an addicting one. Aromatics keep a person in a congenial frame of mind, while the latter acts on the higher centre of the human brain to imbalance one from normalcy, making plants and plant-based products a forerunner for scientific research.

In this chapter we will discuss only on the benevolence of aromatics that keeps the human brain in the right state of equilibrium, and helps in conferring delight and magnificence in fulfilling the three 'Purushartas', viz. 'Dharma', religious merit, 'Artha', material benefits, and 'Kama', personal desires, in addition to achieving 'Arogya', good health.

We are aware that the use and enjoyment of fragrances have endured a tradition as old as humans down the ages and continue to play a purposeful role to enhance our lifestyles.

Fragrances, as we know today, are complex mixtures of natural and synthetic ingredients. Natural ingredients originate from materials found in nature, like roots, bark, leaves, flowers, etc. Natural ingredients are obtained by use of physical processes such as pressing/cold expression, tapping, by *enfleurage*, distillation, hydro diffusion, extraction, etc. whereas synthetic ingredients are manufactured through chemical processes. Fragrances are by themselves multifaceted; eliciting feelings of joy, confidence and a sense of well-being to those who wear them, providing an opportunity to create a virtually unforgettable, personal signature.

A subtle spray of fragrance can spark cherished memories and emotions to lift spirits, augment relationships, improve a person's mood, light up romance, to overwhelming enjoyment and happiness. In personal care, fabric care and household care consumer products, fragrances enhance its sense of cleanliness/freshness and serve to mask the unpleasant odour of base ingredients. In short, 'fragrances help make life complete'.

ORIGIN AND HISTORY OF FRAGRANCES

Fragrances originated in India in early times and regular barter trade by the Arabs carried it to the western shores like Egypt, Persia, Greece, and Rome. Aromatics and their uses have been profusely mentioned in 'Ayurveda', India's medicinal tradition of almost 3000 years. Ayurveda explains the various ways that aromatics can be engaged to create useful products for humans to savour. Individual fragrant substances, like flowers, aromatic leaves or roots can be used directly or can be used to produce fragrances or 'Gandha dravyas'. The art of blending various fragrant substances in right proportions to concoct a likeable fragrance was considered to be one of the 64 learning arts that a person needed to be proficient in ancient Indian society.

Several literary works in Sanskrit, our epics the Ramayana and Mahabharata, technical treatises like Gangaadhara's 'Gandhasara—The essence of scent making', and 'Gandhavaada—Hypothesis on Odours', Varahamihira's 'Vrhatsamhita', Somesvara's 'Manasoallasa', Chavundaraya's 'Lokoparakaram', in Kannada, have detailed information on perfumery and fragrance creation.

'Gandhashastra—The science of odours', deals with cosmetics and fragrances. It being a branch of Ayurveda, the fragrance ingredients mentioned therein are also said to possess medicinal properties. It also mentions the usefulness of the ingredients in improving skin complexion, lustre and its appearance, to overall enhance beauty.

'Gandhayukti—The science and strategies to make odoriferous substances' discusses all technicalities of perfumery and fragrance creation. Sanskrit texts written during the Mauryan rule also describes the method of fragrance preparation and its development. For example, it says that sandalwood is grated on a wet stone and mixed with grounded spices to get a paste. The paste obtained is further crushed along with fragrant flowers and leaves and mixed well with oil. The oil so obtained is applied all over the body to keep it pleasant smelling.

Somesvara in his encyclopaedic treatise 'Manasoallasa' mentions an interesting detail on the fragrances and cosmetics used by kings, in their royal bath.

Fragrances Used by Royals for Bathing

According to Somesvara, perfumed body massage oil should be prepared as given below:

Sesame seeds, perfumed with the strong aroma of Ketaki flowers (*Pandanus* sp.), Yati (*Jasminum grandiflorum*), Punnaga (*Calophyllum inophyllum*) and Champaka (*Michelia champaka*) is taken and crushed to extract oil from them. The oil extracted is used first to massage the body.

After massaging is complete, a fragranced ointment is applied. The fragrance ointment is prepared as detailed below:

Part A

1. Palaka (*Spinach*) roots.
2. Tagara (*Catunaragum spinosa*).
3. Mamsi (Fleshy root of *Nardistachys jatamansi*).
4. Ashvagandha (*Withania somnifera*).
5. Puskara (*Inula racemosa*).
6. Kushta.
7. Patolaka/Snakegourd (*Trichosanthes dioica*).
8. Musta.
9. Nishadvayam (a combination of *haridra—turmeric* and *daru haridra—berbaris aristata*).
10. Granthi parana (glandular leaves of *Artemisiavulgaris*).

Part B

1. Neem.
2. Rajavraksa/Aragvadha (*Cassia fistula*).
3. Tulsi (*Ocimum sanctum*).
4. Arjaka (*Ocimum basilicum*).

Part C

1. Cardamom.
2. Jati (*Myristica fragrans*).
3. Sarshapa.
4. Sesame.
5. Coriander.
6. Bakuchi (*Veronia anthelmintica*).
7. Cakramardu (Cassia tora).

Part D

1. Clove/Lavanga.
2. Padmaka (*Prunus puddum*)
3. Lodra.
4. Sandal.
5. Suradru (*Devadaru*).
6. Agurusorala (*Pinus roxberghi*).

Part E

1. Nagakesara (*Mammea longifilia*).
2. Punnaga (*Calophyllum inophyllum*).
3. Kanta (*Aglaia roxburghina*).
4. Kumkuma (Saffron).
5. Champaka (*Michelia Champaka*).

Part F

1. Guggulu (*Balsamodendron*).
2. Saindhava salt (Rock salt).
3. Bola (*Myran*).
4. Sarjarasa (Yellow resin).

Procedure

1. Part A materials are dried in shade. It is powdered and mixed thoroughly.
2. Part B materials are grounded to make a paste. The paste is then added to 1.
3. Part C items are mixed and powdered. The powder obtained is mixed to 2 above.
4. Part D plant weeds are shade dried and powdered. The mixture obtained is mixed with 3.
5. To the mixture 4 obtained above add Part E flowers and mix further.
6. Pound Part F in rice water and vinegar (Kanjika).
7. Mix 6 to 5 above and finish the ointment.

Turmeric (*Haridra*) pulp scented suitably is applied on the body. Ointments made out of the aromatic pulp of *Amalaka/Amla* is applied to hair for growth of luxuriant black long mane. Soap (*Khali*) for bathing is made by the mixture of wheat flour, fermented rice gruer (*arnala*), Madana (*Randia dumetorium*) root powder and pisuna (*Saffron powder*).

Ketaki and Champaka Fragrances

The Chinese traveller, Fa-Hien describes India as a land or exotic aromatic flowers, fruits, resins and grass. He describes the role of *Ghandikas* or perfumers who created the fragrances and marketed it.

Natural essential oils traditionally have been used to make attars or natural fragrances.

Ketaki oil and champaka oil were other scented oils that were a connoisseur's delight in ancient India. Ketaki (*Pandanus odoratissimus*) and Champaka (*Michelia champaca*) are popular flowers in India right from olden times. Ancient Sanskrit literatures mention them very extensively. Ketaki and Champaka are used in cosmetics and perfumery as perfumed oils, body powders, incenses, etc. Champaka oil is extolled and even referred to as liquid gold by Varahamihira. The early European botanist, Buchanan reports that majority of Indians in 1811 AD used Sesame oil infused with Punnaga and Champaka flowers as bathing oil. Champaka Oil in combination with mallika, uptala, surabhi or patala was also very popular during that time.

Fragrances during the Mogul Rule

Yashodhara in his treatise *Yashah prakasha sudhokara* has described the use of *Adhahpathana yantra* to produce fragrances. The method is comparable to the method mentioned in *Ain-e-Akbari*, a chronicle by Abul Fazal 1590 AD to make *Chuwah* a very popular fragrance used by Emperor Akbar and his courtiers.

Small pieces of lignum aloes are taken in a narrow vessel, luted with clay cotton and rice bran. A small space is left at the neck of the vessel, which is placed in a dish of water so that the mouth of the first vessel touches the surface.

A gentle fire using cow dung cakes is made around the vessel. The heat generated melts the aloes till it distils into the water. It is then collected and washed with water or rose water to remove the smoky odour.

In olden times, Attars were very popular with the well-to-do sections of society. Some attar is pure oil, while some are mixtures of different essential oils, resins and concentrates in a natural base or carrier oils. The unique aroma of attar is due to the condensed vapours of individual flowers directly into the base oil, generally sandalwood oil. The aroma of sandalwood oil has the unique property to complement with the aroma of other plant oils, combined with it and act as a preservative to other essential oils without getting rancid.

Varahamihira's 'Ghandayukti'—Practical Perfumery

Varahamihira describes two important aspects seen in fragrance preparations. Firstly, a practical method for preparation and secondly exploring the possibility of using the information in another field of research with setting botanical identity of the plants as mentioned in *Brhatsamhita*.

Ghandayukti can be easily understood by reading along with a commentary based on it called *Bhattopapala's vivrtti*. 'Ghandayukti' is a practical art of blending fragrance ingredients to prepare valuable fragrances that are stable for long. *Ghandayukti* describes a method of manufacturing a large number of fragrances, but utilising only a few standardised, basic aromatic ingredients by changing the relative proportion in the final fragrance formulation.

Ghandharnava is the term coined by Varahamihira for this method of manufacturing fragrances. Varahamihira claims that innumerable fragrances of diverse odour profiles can be created. An ingenious method of tables or *Koshtaka* is used in deciding the proportions concisely and precisely to create popular fragrances.

For understanding, let us consider a simple fragrance made by using only 16 standardised aroma ingredients. In this case the 'Koshtaka' consists of a permutation table of 16 cells of 4 cells each in a single line. One aroma ingredient is represented in one cell. By permutation and combination of these aroma ingredients innumerable fragrances are made as shown below:

Ghanam	Balakam	Shaileyakam	Chamaka
Ushira	Nagapushpa	Sprkka	Aguru
Tulsi	Damanaka	Nokha	Tagara
Dhanya	Karpura	Chola/Choroka	Malaya

Each formulation takes an ingredient from each of the four quarters at different proportions and a large number of formulations can be obtained, as required. Supposing we need to make a fragrance containing only four ingredients we can formulate as Ghanam 1, Balakam 3, Shaileyakam 2, and Malaya 3. Many such combinations are possible with larger number ingredients of varying ingredient proportions. A lot more details in fragrance formulations are mentioned in *Ghandhayukti*.

Why India lost its leadership position in the world perfume market?

The science of perfumery and fragrance creation were so developed that India was placed in a pivotal place in the ancient cosmetic and perfumery world economy.

The botanist Buchanan, in his detailed informative paper 'account of the manufacture of rose water and other perfumes at Patna in 1811 AD and its bearing on the history of the Indian perfumery industry', gives very interesting insights on the state of the perfumery industry in Kannauj of Mythili (Kanyakubja as mentioned in Sanskrit literature) and the importance given to it by the Europeans.

He further states that the industrial revolution that took place in Europe was largely due to the awakened interest of the European nations to the excellence of the Indian perfumery industry and their zest to compete with India.

Buchanan's paper infers that their keenness to compete with India and dislodge its premier position resulted in the successful penetration of the world fragrance market that was once a domain of the Indian perfumery industry, where India enjoyed complete monopoly.

Interestingly, India, which was once a world leader of the fragrance industry, is today one of the world's largest consumers of foreign fragrances and fragranced products. The rapid advancements made by the European industry in the 20th century due to modern scientific thought and knowledge made sure that India lost out on all that it had treasured over centuries.

Fragrances today

Fragrances earlier were made up of wholly natural ingredients. Perfumers used essential oils, resins, absolutes, extracts from plants and ingredients obtained from animal origin. All materials used were obtained by physical processing, with no change occurring in the ingredients during the extraction process. The dwindling agricultural forest-lands because of encroaching civilisation, ever-increasing world population, have all reduced the natural flora and fauna. The declining natural vegetation has invariably lowered the supply of natural fragrance ingredients for fragrance manufacture. Limited availability, of natural fragrance ingredients has now led to their lower relative concentrations in fragrance formulas.

Sadly, nowadays almost 90 to 95 per cent of the raw materials used in fragrance creation are synthetically manufactured and only 5 to 10 per cent are of natural origin.

The consumers' fascination of fragrances has only increased with time as the manufacture of fragranced personal care, laundry care and household care products is ever growing. In addition, fragrances are now added to a number of other commercial products such as tissues, candles, baby diapers, etc. Fragrances have also made their way into scented stationeries and even trash bags.

Nowadays, products are being sold with fragrances as its main selling point, with the entire advertising campaigns centered on the odour of a product. The consumer trend too has been towards more powerful and long lasting fragrances.

Fragrance dilemma

'The fragrance foundation', a nonprofit educational arm of the global fragrance industry, says that there are more than thousand body fragrances alone in the world market today. While many people enjoy wearing fragrances and using fragranced products, the gamut of related advertisements carries some away.

There is a growing outcry by some people who claim that exposure to some synthetic fragrances and fragranced products adversely impacts health. Symptoms like headache (especially migraine), sneezing, watery eyes, sinus problems, anxiety, nausea, wheezing (especially in asthmatics), shortness of breath, inability to concentrate, brain fog, dizziness, convulsions, sore throat, cough, chest tightness, hyperactivity (especially in children), tremor, fatigue, lethargy and drowsiness are experienced by some users. People, suffering from MCS (Multiple chemical sensitivity), a health condition in which exposure to one chemical is thought to lead to adverse reactions with others, claim that exposure to fragrances triggers various symptoms, leading to the point that sufferers become incapacitated or have to forego many of their routine activities to avoid fragrance exposure.

Fragrances influence the human body positively, as well as, sometimes, negatively. The human body is amazing as it tolerates exposures to many substances all in a day's time. The factors that determine what will be tolerated without adverse effects and what will be not are very many. Variations can exist even in the same individual, depending on a number of factors. In general, a healthier person is more tolerant towards conditions that are less than optimal.

Females are usually more prone to problems from synthetic fragrances, than males. Individual genetic factors, body chemistry and age also have a bearing on human tolerance towards chemicals. It is often difficult to pin down the cause of several symptoms when the triggering substance is one that is common in the environment.

We are aware that fragrances are a complex mix of art and chemistry. The chemicals used in the fragrance formulation must not only be compatible, but also be aesthetically pleasing to the nose.

More than 5000 chemicals are used in the manufacture of fragrances. Synthetic organic chemicals constitute 80–90 per cent (by weight and value) of the raw materials used in fragrance formulations today and very little is known about the impact synthetic fragrances have on human health.

Synthetic fragrance ingredients and its sensitivity to humans

The International Fragrance Research Association (IFRA), a consortium of associations from most countries of the developed world, leads the industry initiative in regulating the use of fragrance materials.

Individual fragrance companies belong to IFRA through their membership in national associations, as there is no direct company membership in the association. At present IFRA includes national associations from the Asia-Pacific (Australia, Singapore, and Japan), North America (United States, Canada), Latin America (Brazil, Mexico) and Europe (France, Germany, Italy, Netherlands, Spain, Switzerland, and United Kingdom). India is not a member of IFRA.

Another body that plays a role in regulating the industry is the Research Institute of Fragrance Materials (RIFM), set up in 1968 by the fragrance industry. The Institute has an independent research and testing programme handled by an expert panel of academicians. It is recognised internationally for its expertise in toxicology, pharmacology, dermatology, environmental sciences and biochemistry. RIFM maintains a database of safety information of ingredients and liaises with regulatory scientific authorities. IFRA relies on RIFM's scientific judgement in establishing guidelines and restrictions on use of fragrance ingredients by fragrance suppliers. The two organisations play a supporting role to each other.

IFRA is responsible for risk management, while RIFM is concerned with the assessment of risks in fragranced products. To date, RIFM has tested more than 1300 fragrance materials, and published results in scientific journals such as food and chemical toxicology. The results of the aroma chemical screening are then submitted by RIFM to the international fragrance association (IFRA). If a fragrance material is found to have adverse health effects, IFRA categorises the material as: Prohibited (P), restricted (R), sensitising (S), etc. and recommends amounts of the material to be used in fragrances and fragranced products. Categorisation of aroma chemicals by IFRA based on their safety profile is shown in Table 4.1.

Table 4.1. Categorisation of aroma chemicals by IFRA based on their safety profile.

Name	Category
1,3-Dibromo-2-methoxy-4-methyl-5-nitrobenzene (Musk KS)	P
1,3-Dibromo-4-methoxy-2-methyl-5-nitrobenzene (Musk alpha)	P
2,2-Dichloro-1-methylcyclopropylbenzene	P
2,4-Dihydroxy-3-methyl-benzaldehyde	P
2-Methoxy-4-methylphenol	R
2-Pentylidene cyclohexanone	P
3,7-Dimethyl-2-octen-1-ol	P
3-Bromo-1,7,7-trimethylbicyclo[2.2.1]heptane-2-one	P
4,6-Dimethyl-8-t-butyl coumarin (Butolia)	P
4-Methyl-7-ethoxycoumarin (Maraniol)	P
5-Acetyl-1,1,2,3,3,6-hexamethyl Indan (AHMI, Phantolid)	R
6-Isopropyl-2-decalol	P
6-Methylcoumarin (Toncarine)	P
7-Methylcoumarin	P
Acetyl ethyl tetramethyl tetralin (AETT, Versalide)	P
Acetyl isovaleryl (5-Methyl-2,3-hexanedione)	P
Acetylated Vetiver oil	S
Allantroot oil	P
Allyl esters	S
Allyl heptine carbonate	R
Allylisothiocyanate	P

(Contd ...)

Name	Category
alpha-Methyl anisylidene acetone	P
Amylcyclopentenone	R
Angelica root oil	R
Anisylidene acetone [4-(4-methoxphenyl)-3-buten-2-one]	P
Asarone [(E)-and(Z)-2,4,5-trimethoxypropen-l-yl benzene]	R
Benzene	P
Benzyl cyanide	P
Benzylidene acetone (4-phenyl-3-buten-2-one)	P
Bergamot oil expressed	R
Birch wood pyrolysate	S
Bitter orange peel oil expressed	R
BMHCA (p-t-butyl-alpha-methylhydrocinnamic aldehyde)	R
Bromostyrene	P
Butyl-dihydrocinnamaldehyde (bourgeonal)	R
Cade oil	S
Carvone oxide	P
Cedar moss	R
Chenopodium oil	P
Cinnamic alcohol	R
Cinnamic aldehyde	R
Cinnamyl nitrile	R
Cinnamylidene acetone	P
Citral	R
Citrus oils and other furocoumarins containing essential oils	R
Colophony	P
Costus root oil, absolute and concrete	P
Cumin oil	R
Cyclamen alcohol (3-(4-isopropylphenyl)-2-methylpropanol)	R
Diethyl maleate	P
Dihydrocoumarin (Melilotine)	P
Dimethyl citraconate	P
Diphenylamine	P
Esters of 2-nonynoic acid, exceptmethyl octine carbonate	P
Esters of 2-octynoic acid except methyl and allyl heptine carbonate	P
Ethyl acrylate	P
Ethylene glycol monoethyl ether and its acetate	P
Ethylene glycol monomethyl ether and its acetate	P
Eugenol	R
Farnesol	R

(Contd...)

Name	Category
Fig leaf absolute	P
Furfurylideneacetone	P
Grapefruit oil expressed	R
Hexahydrocoumarin	P
Hexylidene cylcopentanone	R
HMPCC (3 and 4-(4-hydroxy-4-methylpentyl)-3-cyclohexene-1-carboxaldehyde)	R
Hydroabietyl alcohol	P
Dihydroabietyl alcohol	P
Hydroquinone monoethylether (4-ethoxy phenol)	P
Hydroquinone monomethylether (4-methoxy phenol)	P
Hydroxycitronellal	R
Isocyclogeraniol	R
Isoeugenol	R
Isophorone	P
Lemon oil cold pressed	R
Lime oil expressed	R
Limonene	S
Linaloöl	S
Massoia bark oil	P
Massoia lactone	P
Melissa oil (genuine *Melissa officinalis*)	P
Menthadienyl formate	R
Methoxy dicylopentadiene carboxaldehyde (scentenal)	R
Methoxycoumarin	P
Methyl beta-naphthyl ketone	R
Methyl crotonate	P
Methyl heptadienone (6-Methyl-3,5-heptadienone)	R
Methyl heptine carbonate	R
Methyl methacrylate	P
Methyl N-methylanthranilate	R
Methyl octine carbonate (MOC)	R
Methyl-2(3)-nonenenitrile (citgrenile)	R
Methyleugenol	R
Moskene	P
Musk ambrette	P
Musk tibetene	P
Nitrobenzene	P
Nootkatone	S
Oak moss extracts	R

(Contd ...)

Name	Category
Octen-3-yl acetate (amyl vinyl carbinyl acetate)	R
Opoponax	R
Other materials	P
p-Methylhydrocinnamic aldehyde	R
p-tert-Butylphenol	P
Perilla aldehyde	R
Peru balsam	R
Petitgrain mandarin oil	R
Phenyl benzoate	P
Phenylacetaldehyde	R
Phenylacetone (Methyl benzyl ketone)	P
Pinacea derivatives	S
Propylidene phthalide	R
Pseudoionone (2,6-dimethylundeca-2,6,8-trien-10-one)	P
Pseudomethylionone	P
Rue oil	R
Safrole, isosafrole, dihydrosafrole	R
Santolina oil	P
Savin oil	S
Sclareol	S
Styrax	R
Tagetes oil and absolute	R
Tea leaf absolute	R
Toluene	P
trans-2-Heptenal	P
trans-2-Hexenal	R
trans-2-Hexenal diethyl acetal	P
trans-2-Hexenal dimethyl acetal	P
Tree moss extracts	R
Trimethylcyclohexa-1,3-dienyl methanal (safranal)	R
Trimethylcyciohexenyl/cyclohexadienyl)-2-buten-1-ones (rose ketones)	R
Verbena absolute	R
Verbena oil	P

Note: P (Prohibited), R (restricted), and S (sensitising).

Nitromusks are important and relatively inexpensive fixatives for soap perfumes. IFRA guidelines state that they are potentially toxic and so prohibited for use in fragrances. In line with the guidelines issued, the use of nitromusks has been declining in recent years. Other classes of musk chemicals like macrocyclic musk or polycyclic musks are replacing it.

While many companies voluntarily adhere to the IFRA safety guidelines, it is not required by law to follow any of the group's recommendations, or to limit the use of any fragrance materials. It may also be noted that RIFM tests only raw materials and not finished fragrance products.

The environmental health effects of synthetic fragrances are complex. However a study by the United States environment pollution authority (EPA) in 1991 has shown that some common synthetic fragrance chemicals are hazardous to humans in many ways.

1. Benzaldehyde is a narcotic sensitiser, a local anaesthetic and a CNS depressant. It causes irritation to the mouth, throat, eyes, skin, lungs, and GI tract, resulting in nausea and abdominal pain and may cause kidney damage.
2. Benzyl acetate is carcinogenic (linked to pancreatic cancer). Vapours are irritating to eyes and respiratory passages, exciting cough. In mice hyper-anaemia of the lungs has been noticed. It can be absorbed through the skin, causing systemic effects.
3. Benzyl alcohol is irritating to the upper respiratory tract. It causes headache, air-nausea, vomiting, dizziness and drop in blood pressure, CNS depression, and death due to respiratory failure in severe cases.
4. Camphor is local irritant and a CNS stimulant. It gets readily absorbed through body tissues. Its vapours cause irritation of eyes, nose and throat, dizziness, confusion, nausea, twitching muscles and convulsions.
5. Ethyl acetate is on the EPA hazardous Wwste list. It is irritating to the eyes and respiratory tract. It may cause headache and narcosis. It can cause a defatting effect on skin, drying and liquid cracking of skin, anaemia with leukocytosis and damage to liver and kidneys.
6. Linaloöl is a narcotic and causes respiratory disturbance. In animal tests, reduced spontaneous motor activity and depression, development of respiratory disturbances leading to death, depressed frog-heart activities have been observed. It can also cause CNS disorder.
7. α-pinene is a sensitiser and damaging to the immune system.
8. γ-terpinene causes asthma and CNS disorders.
9. α-terpineol is highly irritating to mucous membranes. Aspiration into the lungs can produce neumonitis or even fatal edema. It can also cause 'excitement' ataxia (loss of muscular coordination), hypothermia, CNS and after respiratory depression and headache.

Similarly, the European Union Cosmetics Directive identifies 26 fragrance ingredients as allergens (Table 4.2).

Table 4.2. Fragrance ingredients as allergens.

Amylcinnamic aldehydes
Farnesol
Amylcinnamic alcohol
Geraniol
Anisyl alcohol
Hexylcinnamic aldehyde
Benzyl alcohol
Hydroxycitronellal
Benzyl benzoate
Isoeugenol
Benzyl cinnamate
Lilial
Benzyl salicylate

(Contd ...)

d-Limonene

Cinnamic alcohol

Linaloöl

Cinnamic aldehyde

Lyral

Citral

Methyl heptine carbonate

Citronellol

γ-Methylionone

Coumarin

Tree moss

Eugenol

Oak moss

Studies have shown that some synthetic fragrance chemicals can cause ill health effects, primarily to skin, lungs and the brain. Synthetic chemicals absorbed by the skin, break down into products that are stronger sensitisers than the original chemicals. The olfactory/limbic tract is the most direct connection between the human brain and the air that we inhale. As there is no blood-brain barrier, the fragrance chemicals have the potential to effect, and possibly damage, brain tissue, resulting in neurotoxicity syndrome.

Fragrance chemicals can enter the human body through inhalation, ingestion or absorption. On entering the body, they get absorbed into the bloodstream and spread throughout the body.

Individual sensitivity to fragrance chemicals varies widely right from zero or no effect, to severe symptoms. It may be noted that many people who report sensitivities to synthetic fragrances also report sensitivities to other chemicals. This makes the claims of adverse reactions to synthetic fragrances difficult or impossible to link to a particular fragrance chemical.

Fragrances without synthetic aroma chemicals

Interestingly, most synthetic fragrances generally contain similar basic ingredients, with the exception of certain speciality chemicals. The speciality materials, some of them captive for organisational perfumers, impart certain uniqueness to the fragrance odour profile.

It is quite likely that odour effects and chemical stability possible by use of synthetic aroma chemicals are near-impossible to get with only natural stuff.

Natural plants have always played significant role as medicines. At one time, it was felt that the chemical synthesis would completely replace drugs of natural origin. However, in spite of various synthetic drug discoveries the use of plant drugs continues unabated. Even today, the medicinal needs of about 80 per cent of people in developing nations are met by herbal drug preparations. Furthermore, in spite of the emergence of many wonderful synthetic drugs, the problems of senescence and 'civilisation' diseases, e.g. immuno deficiency syndromes, arthritis, mental disorders, cancer, etc. are still not tackled completely.

Naturally, there is a greater demand for natural medicines and 'health-foods' today than ever before. In analogy to the above, the fear of synthetics having unwanted side effects or being potential carcinogens, without any therapeutic benefits, regular scientific updates on the understanding of adverse effects of synthetics, is having its toll on consumers preferring naturals.

In view of these developments, aromatic plants producing essential oils become significantly important from the functional point of view. At this juncture, natural fragrances made by use of only organic ingredients and essential oils, an amazing phenomenon of plant metabolism, may rank as the next best alternative.

Today, India has 16 per cent volume share of the world essential oil market and 21.5 per cent share in value terms. India's share of natural isolates/chemicals is only about 14 per cent in the global market.

These being the industry scenario, just imagine the requirements of natural aroma ingredients necessary to completely replace or eliminate synthetics and the scope it holds for India (Tables 4.3 and 4.4).

Table 4.3. Some essential oils producing Indian plants with potential in the flavour and fragrance industry

Ambrette	Curcuma leaf	Mentha citrata
Angelica	Dhavana	Mint
Artemisia	Dill	Mogra
Asafoetida	Eucalyptus	Nagarmotha
Basil Indian	Fennel	Nishigandha
Bergamot	Fenugreek	Nutmeg
Birch sweet	Garlic	Oak moss absolute
Cajeput	Geranium	Ocimum canum
Capsicum	Ginger grass	Orange bitter
Caraway	Ginger	Orange sweet
Cardamom	Grapefruit	Palm rosa
Cedar wood	Gurjam balsam	Parijat
Celery	Jasmine absolute	Patchouli
Camomile	Jamrosa	Pepper
Champaka	Juniper	Peppermint
Cinnamon	Kewda	Rose
Citronella	Lavender	Rosemary Indian
Clary sage	Lemon	Sandalwood
Clocimum	Lemongrass	Screwpine
Clove bud	Linaloe	Spearmint
Clove leaf	Lily	Tuberose
Cocoa	Lime	Tulsi
Coriander	Liquorice	Turmeric
Cumin seed	Marigold	Valerian
Curcuma aromatica	Marjoram	Vetiver

Table 4.4. Essential oils producing plants in different States of India.

State	Essential oil bearing plant
Andhra Pradesh	Sandalwood
Bihar	Mentha, basil, lemongrass, palmarosa
Gujarat	Palmarosa, kewda

(Contd ...)

State	Essential oil bearing plant
Himachal Pradesh	Mentha, patchouli
Karnataka	Sandalwood, citronella
Kerala	Citronella, lemongrass
Madhya Pradesh	Lemongrass, citronella, basil, sandalwood
Northeast	Lemongrass, citronella, patchouli, eucalyptus
Orissa	Kewda, palmarosa, lemongrass, citronella
Punjab	Mentha, basil
Rajasthan	Vetiver, basil, lemongrass, palmarosa
Tamil Nadu	Jasmine, sandalwood, lemongrass, geranium
Uttar Pradesh	Mentha, rose, basil
Uttarakhand	Lavender, geranium, mentha
West Bengal	Lemongrass, palmarosa

TYPES OF FLAVOURS

Natural Flavours

Natural flavours are products made using some of the different single compounds of natural origin. There are about 2000 different products in this category. These natural chemical compounds are separated by physical process from mixtures by distillation, extraction, or solidification. Sometimes, a combination of microbiological or enzymatic process are also employed. Some examples of natural flavours include menthol derived from peppermint oil, citral from lemon grass oil, methylsalicylate from winter green oil, amyl acetate distilled from banana, etc.

Natural Identical Flavours

Natural identical flavours are the most important category that comprises about 3000 substances that are synthetically created. The substances that are artificially created are identical with the chemical composition of compounds found in the natural product and found suitable for human consumption. A typical example is the vitamin C tablet that we consume. Chemically it is ascorbic acid. It is found in lemons, but can also be prepared artificially from D-glucose, which is, in turn, produced from sugar. The chemical molecule of vitamin C obtained from lemon and sugar are structurally identical and same. Similarly amyl acetate distilled from banana and the one synthetically produced by mixing vinegar with amyl alcohol in presence of sulphuric acid are structurally identical and smell and taste the same. Menthol, citral, and vanillin, etc. are other examples.

Artificial Flavours

Artificial flavours are nonidentical flavour ingredients that have been discovered by scientists and researchers. These substances are not naturally present in foodstuffs. If, at any future date, the chemical is identified in any natural food product, then it is re-classified as natural-identical. Artificial flavours discovered are about 200 and are prohibited in use till it is proved to be completely harmless for human consumption through a series of evaluation and clinical testing. It is believed that the first artificial flavour was accidentally discovered in Germany. A scientist at work while mixing a group of chemicals in his laboratory suddenly found that his lab was filled with a sweet smell of grapes. It was only later discovered that the chemical obtained by the accidental mixing was methyl anthranilate, now a very important flavour ingredient in grape flavours.

The inventions of equipment like gas chromatographs and mass spectrometers that are capable of detecting volatile gases at low levels, helped in the synthesis of a number of synthetic flavours during early 1960s. Today, spectrometers, gas chromatographs, headspace vapour analysers and other sophisticated instruments are available to help provide details of flavour components by detecting the chemical present in amounts as low as ppb. Although human nose is more sensitive, with an ability to smell at ppt levels, instruments help scientists to work continuously with the same efficiency. This is not possible with the human nose that gets tired in continuous usage and has to be rested and be refreshed intermittently.

Complex smells and tastes like roasted Indian coffee are composed of volatile gases from nearly a thousand different chemicals. A simple smell of strawberry is obtained by the interaction of about 350 chemicals that are present in strawberry flavour in very small or infinitesimal amounts. Although flavour normally is obtained from a mixture of different volatile chemicals, often a single compound provides the dominant smell. A typical example is that of ethyl-2-methyl butyrate that smell just like apples, amyl acetate smells like bananas.

One question that always rankles in the mind of the consumer is whether natural flavouring agents is preferable to natural-identical or artificial flavours and so safer to use than synthetic substitutes. Consumers prefer to see natural flavour on any labels of processed food, believing it to be safer for health. There is nothing further from the truth than this. A natural flavour is not necessarily healthier or purer than an artificial one. Differences between artificial and natural flavour can be arbitrary, and absurd if one only looks whether it is natural or artificial, and not what it contains or how the flavour has been made.

In principle, there is no difference between the safety of natural and nature identical flavour. In some case, the naturally derived flavour may be harmful than the synthetic one. Almond flavour predominantly contains benzaldehyde. When benzaldehyde is derived from natural fruits like peach and apricot, trace amounts of hydrogen cyanide, a deadly poison, is also extracted along with the natural flavour. However, benzaldehyde derived synthetically by mixing clove oil and amyl acetate does not contain any cyanide and is completely safe for use. Nevertheless it is considered an artificial flavour and sells cheaper to the dangerous natural one, that is expensive, and contains cyanide that can kill.

Thousands of flavouring agents are used in food preparation. According to experts who have evaluated the products, flavouring substances are generally recognised as safe when used in recommended dosages and as advised by the manufacturer. Ironically, however, some naturally occurring substances are restricted. Naturally containing substances when consumed beyond a specified level are harmful. Typical examples include solanine in potatoes, myristicin in nutmeg (Jaiphal) and coumarin in strawberries, raspberries, tea, and cinnamon. All the above materials are permitted if the quantity used is low, but not allowed at higher concentrations. However, use of coumarin, both natural and synthetic, in flavour is not permitted.

All flavouring substances are regulated by legislation, issued by FDA. Government departments that control the safety of foods are also responsible to control the safety of flavours used in the food products. The flavour industry too, over the years, have accumulated a lot of information and data regarding use, occurrence, biological properties and all the information have been used to carry out independent safety evaluation by various experts.

The manufacturers of flavour ingredients around the world have set up the International organisation of the flavour industry (IOFI) based in Geneva, Switzerland. IOFI issues guidelines to the members, makes recommendations, draw up rules and make available their expertise, to harmonise the diverse rules in various countries for the betterment of the industry and for the benefit of the consumer.

Intergovernmental organisations like European flavour and fragrance association (EFFA), european council (EC), the scientific committee for food of european commission (SCF), the food and agriculture organisation (FAO), and the world health organisation (WHO) of the United Nations also conduct independent study group to evaluate the safety of the flavouring substances. Fragrances and flavour association of India (FAFAI), essential oil association of India (EOAI) are similar bodies set up by the Indian industry.

Tens and thousands of flavouring ingredients occur naturally in food and it is practically impossible to establish safety on an individual basis of all substances in the near future. If such a prohibition does come through, we all will have to stop eating completely and life will truly become unbearable. Imagine if one has to forgo all the tasty items that have been consumed from the beginning of human civilisation, but not sufficiently tested as safe. People believe that natural flavours are safe and good to be used. Synthetics are synonymous to second rate poor quality stuff. The high degree of confidence an individual exhibits towards natural stuff tends to mistrust and lack of faith towards synthetic. A good example is the flavouring of ice cream with vanilla flavour. Natural vanilla flavour is rare and prohibitively expensive.

If a rule is implemented that only completely natural vanilla is to be used to flavour ice-cream, then it can be consumed only by the very rich as this luxury can only be affordable to them. Organic chemistry and modern technology has now made it possible to produce synthetic vanilla flavour and ice-cream made out of this can be enjoyed by all at a very reasonable and affordable price.

Although absolute safety can never be guaranteed for any food item or flavour, the flavour industry does promise with assurance that approved and properly manufactured flavours do not present any risk in use. However, the industry and manufacturers recommended dosage levels have to be strictly adhered. Individual intake of solid food products annually amounts to about 900 to 1000 kg. Of this total amount about 500 grams of flavouring is found to occur naturally in our foodstuff. These amounts to less than 0.05 per cent dosage of flavouring consumed. To make the menu more interesting, attractive and palatable concentrated aromas are added to foods that either do not have their own natural aroma and taste or have very little of them. This extra addition too does not add up to more than 25 grams per person per year, as the quantity used is very low usually less than 0.05 per cent.

We consume food and drink to get the much-needed energy to survive and live life at the fullest. Taste is a very important component during the consumption of food and drink.

The taste of the selected food and the aroma released by it is responsible for recognition and acceptance. A tasty food that appeals to our brain contributes to our general sense of well-being by assisting the digestive process. Supposing flavours are eliminated from our food, life will become dull and boring, not good enough to live. That is the importance of flavours in our day-to-day life.

FLAVOUR ENHANCERS

Traditional flavours activate two of the senses, taste and odour. A compound with no intrinsic flavour of its own, but with the ability to enhance the perception of flavour is termed a flavour enhancer or flavour potentiator. In a broad sense, the definition encompasses ingredients such as salt for savoury products and acids for fruit flavours. In reality, the term is reserved to describe certain compounds in the food industry, whose sole purpose is flavour enhancement in meats, fish, poultry, vegetables, fruits, cakes, breads and beverages.

The largest volume flavour enhancer is monosodium glutamate (MSG), the sodium salt of the naturally occurring amino acid, L-glutamic acid. Hydrolysed vegetable protein (HVP) and autolysed yeast extracts contain relatively high levels of MSG, glutamic acid and other amino acids, and so are used as flavour enhancers. Two derivatives of ribonucleic acid (RNA) that serve as flavour enhancers are the disodium salts of inosine-5'-monophosphate (IMP) and guanosine-5'-monophosphate (GMP). When used in combination, MSG and the 5'-ribonucleotides provide a synergistic effect on flavour enhancement.

Maltols and mono-ammonium glycyrrhizinate (MAG) intensify the perception of sweet flavours. Maltol, which occurs naturally in bread, coffee and other products subjected to browning reactions, produces a caramel like flavour. Ethyl maltol has a similar, but much stronger effect. Other related compounds, furanones and pyranones, possess similar properties and produce distinctive notes described as burnt pineapple or maple.

MAG the other compound of interest as a sweet flavour potentiator, is derived from the liquorice root. It has a synergistic effect with sucrose and contributes a mild liquorice character to the flavour. The liquorice intensity is concentration dependent. At high levels MAG masks certain undesirable flavours, such as background bitterness, acidity and off flavours. In recent years there has been considerable research and development activity on flavour enhancers free from glutamic acid or the ribonucleotides. These are based on natural products like soya flour, yeast extracts, jambu oleoresin and others.

Monosodium Glutamate

Monosodium glutamate (MSG) is a widely used food additive and flavour enhancer. It is the sodium salt of glutamic acid, an amino acid that exists naturally in plants. Mushrooms, carrots and some seaweeds are full of it. MSG (now sold as *Aji-no moto, Ac-cent*) has been in use for more than two thousand years since the Japanese isolated it from sea tangle, a type of seaweed, realising that these odourless, almost tasteless white crystals intensify the flavour of sweets, sours and savouries.

The Chinese use MSG very widely and this explains as to why the headaches, burning and twitching it sometimes causes is called 'Chinese restaurant syndrome'. For a number of years the FDA has been testing MSG and continues to rate it in the GRAS category (in 1995, the scientific advisers to FDA agreed that MSG was safe for almost everyone). However, as a concession to those few who are sensitive to it, the FDA requires that all food containing MSG be so labelled, even if the MSG is only a component of hydrolysed vegetable protein or soya protein (some of these contain 20 per cent MSG).

Fermentation processes are the most economical and widely used routes for manufacturing MSG. Virtually all production of MSG worldwide is via fermentation of the glucose present in various vegetable substrates.

Specific micro-organisms can biosynthesise L-glutamic acid from a carbon source, such as acetic acid or glucose preparation, and a nitrogen source such as gaseous ammonia or a solution of urea. A suitable culture medium requires inorganic salts, biotin, and additives such as antibiotics and antifoaming agents. The glutamic acid is recovered by crystallisation and is then converted to MSG.

Only the L-form of MSG is important in food technology as the D-form lacks any flavour enhancement properties. MSG is used as a flavour enhancer by itself or with various other compounds. Typical food types using MSG are gravies, meats, oriental foods, soups, stocks and bases, and prepared vegetables. Many convenience foods contain MSG to counterbalance the loss of flavour caused during processing.

Ribonucleotides

The derivatives of ribonucleic acid that are important as flavour enhancers are the disodium salts of inosine-5'-monophosphate (IMP) and guanosine-5'-monophosphate (GMP). Japanese researchers have isolated IMP from bonito and later found GMP in shiitake mushrooms. When added to food, especially in the presence of MSG, the ribonucleotides increase flavour 20–200 times, depending on the type of food and the concentrations at which they are used.

A 50:50 co-crystallised mixture of 5' inosinate (IMP) and 5' guanylate (GMP), two of nature's most potent flavour enhancers, Ribotide is produced mainly by fermentation, with glucose as the raw ingredient.

Ribotide is free-flowing and is readily soluble in water. Because of the small amounts used, it may be advantageous to add Ribotide in a pre-mix with salt, MSG, or other dry ingredients, or in a water solution. Because it is co-crystallised, Ribotide will not separate during handling, impart uneven flavours in complex formulations, or manifest overtones of its own. It is always uniform in strength. Under ordinary storage and processing conditions, Ribotide remains stable. Most foods have a neutral or slightly acid pH; only a very few have a pH <3 or >9. Also, food-processing temperatures usually fall within a range of 100°C to 110°C, and few processed foods are heated for longer than 60 minutes.

Using Ribotide with foods having strong phosphatase activity such as wheat flour, full fat soya flour, mushrooms requires proper procedures. Phosphatase is readily inactivated by heating for 10 minutes at 80°C or several minutes at 100°C. One can safely add Ribotide after this heating process. As an alternative, Takeda recommends the use of Ribocoat, which is Ribotide coated with edible hydrogenated oil and fat, which melts at the temperature that inactivates phosphatase. Once this protective coating melts, Ribotide's flavour-potentiating power is released. Moisture also affects Ribotide's stability; and it is most stable under dry conditions. Ribotide's flavour enhancing effect, powerful on its own, is intensified in combination with MSG. One can obtain equivalent flavour while significantly reducing cost by replacing a portion of the MSG in the formulation with Ribotide. Replacement will also significantly reduce sodium content in the final product. The replacement ratio will depend on many factors, but from an economic viewpoint, 5 per cent Ribotide use is recommended.

Uses of Ribotide

Ribotide, can be used as true flavour enhancer:
1. To replace beef extract.
2. Suppress metallic and other 'off flavours'.
3. Overcome bitterness.
4. Enhance sweet, salty, and meaty flavours.
5. Give improved mouthfeel or smoothness.

As more and more international cuisines gain in popularity, processors are finding new applications for Ribotide. As a stand-alone flavour enhancer, it intensifies the characteristic flavours of these ethnic cuisines. Many of the popular prepared foods taste even better by the use of Ribotide and among these are: pizza, frozen entrees, ranch-style dressings, flavoured rice and noodle dishes, tortilla chips, nacho-flavoured chips, barbecue sauces, frankfurters, instant and canned soups and broths, cheese sauces, cajun seasonings, stuffing mixes, seasoned bread crumbs and breading mixes.

Maltol/Ethyl Maltol

Maltol and ethyl maltol can improve overall flavour, potentiate sweetness, increase the sensation of creaminess, mask bitterness and suppress an acid bite or burn. Maltol is a flavour enhancer that is especially effective in enhancing fruit-like flavours in soft drinks, jams, gelatines, cakes and other foods containing high levels of carbohydrates. It has functions of preventing acidity and bitterness, removes smell of fish, and reduces irritation. It is produced with furfural from farm by-products and has biological activity more than 88 per cent. In addition to food it is used in cigarettes and cosmetics.

One part of maltol can replace four parts of coumarin. It is much more expensive than MSG or the ribonucleotides and hence its market is limited. Ethyl maltol has chemical properties similar to those of maltol. It is also produced the same way as maltol. It has gained attention worldwide as its flavour increasing power is 4–6 times that of maltol. One part of ethyl maltol can replace 24 parts of coumarin. Ethyl maltol is an effective flavour extender and multifunctional modifier, which can be used in food, beverages, cigarettes, wines, perfumes, cosmetics, and medicines.

People's Republic of China, is a large manufacturer of ethyl maltol. Ethyl maltol is the only product given the international food chemical codes (FCC) clearance in China. The use levels of ethyl maltol in various products are given in Table 4.5.

Table 4.5. Use levels of ethyl maltol in various products.

Products	Levels (ppm)
Biscuits	25–150
Bread	25–150
Cakes	30–50
Candy	40–50
Pastry	15–30
Meat	30–60
Cocoa, tea	5–10
Cooked and instant puddings	10–75
Fruit style soda water	2–10
Fruit wine	15–25
Gelatine desserts	10–75
Ice-creams	5–10
Bottled and canned soft drinks	1–10
Dry beverage mixes	5–30
Malted milk	10–40
Wines and liquors	10–50
Tomato soft drinks	15–25
Tomato soup	5–15
Tomato sauce	15–30
Soya sauce	15–20
Others	10–200

Ammoniated Glycyrrhizin

Ammoniated glycyrrhizin, enhances the flavour of chocolate and increases the perceived sweetness of sucrose in a number of products. Licorice extracts, derived from the roots of the liquorice plant *Glycyrrhiza glabra*, also possess flavour potentiating properties. Marketed under the name, *Magnasweet* by MAFCO Products, Camden, NJ, is the ammonium salt of glycyrrhizic acid.

Two forms are available: ammonium glycyrrhizinate (AG) and mono-ammonium glycyrrhizinate (MAG). MAG is a white, crystalline powder, stable, in low pH systems, and retains less of the liquorice flavour making it applicable for a range of products. A brown powder, AG has more of the characteristic liquorice flavour, which can impart an appealing, difficult-to-detect flavour nuance when used at low levels. At higher levels, it can strengthen and improve flavours such as chocolate or maple. AG and MAG are 50 times sweeter than sucrose, and due to *Magnasweet's* synergistic action with sweeteners, it becomes 100 times sweeter than sucrose when combined with cane sugar. It also will react synergistically with other nutritive and non-nutritive sweeteners. Other attributes of *Magnasweet* are its ability to enhance natural and artificial flavours; mask bitter and astringent aftertastes; and soften harsh notes. It can also be used for flavour modification at very low levels. *Magnasweet* is approved as FEMA GRAS.

Intensate Flavours

Intensate flavours are based on new chemical research and work with both traditional and novel botanicals. Blended for balance, the flavours are all on the GRAS list. Unlike traditional flavours they do not have distinctive aromas and as such have the flexibility to combine successfully with all types of sweet and savoury flavours.

The products are derived from sources like menthol, capsicum, jambo oleoresin, green tea catechins, black tea tannins, and proanthocyanins and without the characteristic flavour of the parent sources. Some of the flavour effects of intensate flavours and their applications are given in Table 4.6.

Table 4.6. Some effects of intensate flavours and their applications.

Flavour effect	Applications
Heat or pungency	Snack seasoning
Tingling or cooling	Salad dressings, beverages (alcoholic and nonalcoholic)
Cooling or heating	Confectionary products
Lingering heat	Sauces and salsas
Astringent or drying	Used with a variety of substrates

Miscellaneous Flavour Enhancers

Although MSG, the 5'-ribonucleotides, and maltol are considered as primary flavour enhancers in the food market, there are several other developments of considerable interest in the flavour enhancers arena. Some of these developments are the following:

Dioctyl sodium sulphosuccinate

It imparts a fresh milk flavour to canned milk. It has also been used in soups, seasonings, imitation crab meat, sauces, snacks, and cheese powder.

N,N'-dioctylethylenediamine

It is a flavour enhancer for margarine and reconstituted nonfat milk solids.

Cyclamic acid

It is a flavour enhancer for margarine.

Soyarome

It is a product of basic research conducted at Gist-Brocades headquarters in Delft, the Netherlands. It is based on fermented soya flour and is labelled as such. In addition to flavour enhancement it extends the length of time that flavours are perceived on the tongue, nearly three times. Soyarome enhances the flavour of·soups, especially when they have a substantial vegetable component. It has no glutamic acid or

5′-ribonucleotides, which are often found in savoury flavour enhancers. Soyarome makes ice-cream and creamy puddings taste richer, and lifts all spice notes.

GB select cheese booster

It is a combination of soyarome and yeast extract. This combination intensifies the flavour of cheese solids, and imparts a buttery, creamy character and aged cheese notes. Due to the increased cheese impact in cheese crackers, it is possible to use less cheese powder in these preparations. The cheese booster has also been used as a topical seasoning for snacks.

Amiflex AL-G

It is a product derived from wheat gluten and marketed by Takeda vitamin and food USA Inc. This product has a clean, mild, savoury flavour, free from unpleasant tastes. It has high content of glutamic acid and nitrogen, is low in sodium chloride, mixes easily and evenly ensuring better *umami* (mouth feel) effect. It can be used to replace MSG completely or can be used with the 5′-ribonucleotides such as Takeda's Ribotide.

Amiflex AL-G2

It is a product derived from corn gluten, and marketed by Takeda. It has similar characteristics and flavour potential as Amiflex AL-G.

Prymeast

These are autolysate yeast extracts marketed under different brand names by Takeda. They are 100 per cent primary yeast extracts with a distinctive taste. They are recommended for vegetable soups, dehydrated soups, and sausages. They are also used to optimise the taste of meat, poultry, sauces, and seasonings. The different products in this category are given in Table 4.7.

Table 4.7. Prymeast type flavour enhancers manufactured by Takeda.

Product	Particulars
Prymeast Type SD	It has a distinctive taste and concentrated flavour profile, which is recommended for improving soups, dehydrated soups, and sausages. It is also used to optimise the taste of poultry, sauces and seasonings
Prymeast Type LS	It has low sodium (as 1% sodium chloride), while maintaining a strong profile with yeasty characteristics. It is suitable for low sodium soups, seasonings, sauces, and prepared foods. It improves taste in healthy, reduced-sodium formulations
Prymeast type IG	It is a special primary yeast extract with a high natural 5′-ribonucleotide content. It has strong flavour enhancing properties, and is very effective in soups, seasonings, sauces and prepared foods. It can be formulated at very low usage levels. Its relatively low sodium content allows reduced sodium levels in most applications
Prymeast Type MTS	It is a product with an intense meat flavour, and an economical replacement for expensive natural meat extracts. Its boullon-like characteristics are recommended for most meat, soup and sauce applications
Prymeast Type IGS	It is a speciality yeast extract with a high 5′-ribonucleotide content. It has strong flavour enhancing properties and at the same time imparts a savoury taste of its own. It optimises flavour in soups, seasonings and various prepared foods

(Contd ...)

Product	Particulars
Type Cheddar	It has smooth cheddar-cheese-flavour characteristics and provides desirable cheese flavour for snack foods, sauces, soups and other prepared foods. It is recommended for all applications requiring flavour profiles with a cheese note
Prymeast type Tom	It has excellent tomato flavour characteristics and is especially effective in enhancing the flavour of tomato-based processed foods, sauces, soups, and seasonings. It exhibits a mild, brothy taste, which is recommended for low sodium soups and sauces
Prymeast type MTSM	It is a light brown, granular yeast autolysate product with an intense meat flavour. It is an economical replacement for expensive natural meat extracts
Prymeast type Stock	It has mild brothy character. Its stock-like flavour characteristics allow extensive applications in soups, sauces, seasonings, and gravies
Prymeast type Veggie	It has distinct vegetable flavour characteristics and effectively enhances the taste of vegetable soups, stews, sauces, seasonings, and meat products. It adds outstanding vegetable flavour notes to all recommended applications
Prymeast type Smoke	It has an intense smoke flavour and improves the taste of meat and poultry products, while providing a smoked flavour profile. It is recommended for soups, especially pea and bean soups, sauces, seasonings and other processed foods

ENZYMES AND ACIDULANTS

Enzymes

Food in its natural state is full of countless varieties of delectable flavours and textures. Plants have a complex array of enzymes necessary for their life process and raw food is filled with enzymes, which are the biochemical foundation for thousands of digestive and metabolic functions within the body. Lipase breaks down fat, protease breaks down protein, cellulase breaks down cellulose, and amylase breaks down starch, to mention only a few.

Enzymes not only produce characteristic flavour, but also cause flavour deterioration. The latter enzymes must be inactivated in order to stabilise and preserve a food. Freezing depresses enzyme activity and pasteurisation eliminates the activity completely.

The characteristic flavours of food, such as vegetables and fruits, are considered to result from enzymatic action. Flavours generated by enzymes in vegetables and fruits consist mainly of aldehydes, ketones, esters, alcohols, terpenes, terpenoids, and S-containing aliphatic and aromatic volatile compounds. They can be produced from non-volatile precursors by the action of different enzymes in the intact tissue before harvest or due to the disruption of the cell tissue so that the compartmentalised endogenous enzymes and the substrates interact.

Alternatively, flavours can be produced by the action of exogenous enzymes or micro-organisms during fermentation. Enzymatically produced flavour is evident in vegetables, fruits, and dairy products. Food enzymes, generally classified as carbohydrases, proteases, liposes, pectic enzymes and cellulases have specific functions, namely:
1. Speed up reactions.
2. Reduce viscosity.
3. Improve extractions.
4. Carry out bioconversions.
5. Enhance separations.

6. Develop functionality.
7. Create and intensify flavour.
8. Synthesise chemicals.

Traditionally, the creation of flavours by enzymes is used in the fermentation process to prepare products such as alcoholic beverages, cheese, pickles, vinegar, bread, and sauerkraut. Several essential oils are also created by enzyme action. In the case of sweet birch oil, the oil is released from the bark by the action of the enzymes. In bitter almond, the enzyme emulsion attacks the glucoside (amygdalin), and releases the oil of bitter almond. More varied applications of enzymes are in the hydrolysis of lactose, preparation of modified fats and oils, processing of fruit juices, conversion of corn starch into high-fructose corn syrup (HFCS), and other processes.

Enzymes are produced from animal tissues, plant tissues, and most frequently from micro-organisms. The majority of enzymes are produced by submerged fermentation using bacteria, yeast, and fungi. Some application of enzymes in the food industry are indicated in Table 4.8.

Table 4.8. Some applications of enzymes in the food industry.

Area	Enzyme type	Application
Alcohol production	Amylases	Starch liquefaction
Baking	Fungal proteases	Dough conditioning, flour bleaching, anti-staling
Brewing	Microbial proteases, papain, pectinase	Low-calorie beer, barley-alternative
Confections	Invertase	Cream candy centres
Coffee	Pectinase, cellulase	Separation of beans, viscosity control of extracts
Dairy	Rennins, lactase, lipase	Cheese-making, accelerated cheese ripening, natural cheese flavour concentrates, whey utilisation, removal of burnt flavour in ultra heat-treated milk
Fats and oils	Lipase, phospholipase	Cocoa butter substitution, flavour ester synthesis, hydrolysis of oils and fats
Flavours	Protease, lipase	Synthesis of savoury flavours, natural flavour esters
Fruits and vegetables	Cellulase	Breakdown of cellulose structure
Fruit juices and wines	Pectinase	Mash treatment, citrus pulp wash, viscosity reduction
Protein	Bromelin, papain, pepsin, pancreatin	Soya milk production, egg white replacement, functional hydrolysates
Sugar processing	Amylase, cellulase	Removal of undesirable starches and polysaccharides in the processing of cane sugar
Starch processing	α-amylase, glucose	High-fructose corn syrup, maltase syrups, dextrin syrups
Others	Proteases	Meat tenderising, coffee soluble-extract viscosity reduction

Acidulants

Chemicals used as food acidulants are citric acid, phosphoric acid, malic acid, lactic acid, fumaric acid, adipic acid, and tartaric acid. These chemicals have several functions in food, namely,

1. Adjusting the pH of foods.
2. Enhancing and modifying flavour.
3. Serving as preservatives.

4. Adding sourness and a desired tartness to many food products.
5. Reducing the growth of micro-organisms, that might spoil food.
6. Preventing rancidity and discolouration of foods by functioning as synergists to antioxidants.
7. Acting as buffers during various stages of food processing in finished products.

The role of various acidulants in foods is given below.

Citric acid

It is the most versatile and widely used food acidulant with excellent solubility, extremely low toxicity, chelating ability, and pleasantly sour taste characteristics. It is used as a flavour enhancers, as a preservative in beverages and syrups, as a synergist antioxidant for fresh and frozen fruits and vegetables, and as a pH regulator in gelatine desserts and jellies.

Citric acid and its sodium salt are extensively used in carbonated beverages as a flavour enhancer, preservative, as a buffer to regulate tartness if the acid level is high. In candy it is used primarily to enhance the flavour of fruits and berries. In jams, jellies, preserves and gelatine desserts it adjusts the pH for maximum gel formation and enhances the flavour. In conjunction with erythorbic acid it helps in preventing the rancidity in fish and discolouration in shellfish.

In canned vegetables (tomatoes, onions, pimientos) and fruits (prunes and grapefruit) it optimises the flavour and enhances the activity of antioxidants in preventing colour and flavour degradation. Citric acid treatment protects the colour and flavour of bacon, sausage and cured ham against changes due to oxidation. It prevents crystallisation of honey, stabilises spices and prevents discolouration of onions. In sherbets and water ices it is used as a flavour adjunct.

Phosphoric acid

It has a characteristic flavour and tartness and is used almost exclusively in cola-flavoured carbonated beverages.

Malic acid

It is used mostly in fruit-flavoured sodas such as those with apple and berry flavour. It enhances flavour and stabilises the colour of carbonated and non-carbonated fruit-flavoured drinks and cream sodas. In sugar-free drinks, it masks the off-taste produced by sugar substitutes. It is chiefly suited in dietetic fruit-flavoured sodas containings aspartame because of its synergism and ideal blending properties. Blends of malic acid and citric acid exhibit better taste characteristics than either separate acidulant.

Fumaric acid

It has strong acid taste and low solubility restricting its applications. It is principally used in fruit juices, gelatine desserts, refrigerated biscuit dough, cured meat, and poultry products.

Adipic acid

Principally used in jams, jellies, gelatine desserts, bottled beverages, and powdered concentrates for fruit-flavoured beverages.

Lactic acid

Used to adjust the pH of beer, wine, and dairy products. Because of its mild taste, it is also used to enhance flavour in fruit drinks and confectionary. Ethyl lactate is used in flavourings.

Tartaric acid

It has a strong, tart taste and augments natural and synthetic fruit flavour. Used mainly in grape-flavoured foods, and in candies in conjunction with citric acid to produce the sour apple, wild cherry, and other especially tart flavours.

Flavour Compositions

Flavour compositions are mixtures of aromatic chemicals that are added to foods and beverages to improve palatability. Excluded from this group are compounds like vanilla and peppermint, which can be used directly as flavours and other products such as acidulants, sweeteners, and flavour enhancers, which are used to enhance taste. Originally flavours were compounded to duplicate natural aromas by the blending of essential oils, aroma chemicals, and concentrated fruit juices.

Now-a-days flavour compositions include those products produced by heat processes such as baking and roasting. These flavours arise from the Browning or Maillard reactions giving the products the characteristic caramelised colour. Such flavours can be concentrated or used as ingredients in other flavour formulations for meat, savoury, etc.

Flavour compositions are also prepared by the extraction of basic foods such as fish and meat to produce concentrated natural extracts with standardised flavour strength and containing the most subtle of flavour notes. Commercial flavours like cheese flavours are produced by enzymatic modification of food substrates. Flavour compositions are often diluted for practical reasons to an approximate use of strength of 1:1000 (1 gram of flavour added to 1 kg of food or beverage). In chewing gums the use level of flavours is ten times higher than this level of dilution. The use strength of flavour compositions can be higher or lower as desired for various applications and as such they are available as concentrated flavours and diluted flavours. Commercial flavour composition is shown in Table 4.9.

Table 4.9. Commercial flavour compositions.

Flavour composition	Classification	Manufacturing process	Raw materials	Product form
Compound flavours	Natural/ synthetic	Blending, mixing	Essential oils, natural extracts, natural aroma chemicals, concentrated fruit juices	Liquid, spray-dried, encapsulated
Thermally processed flavours	Natural	Heating/cooking under pressure	Amino acids and sugars, hydrolysed proteins	Paste, powder
Enzymatically modified flavours	Natural	Enzymatic/microbial treatment	Food substrates such as cheese	Paste, powder
Natural extracts	Natural	Aqueous extraction, heating, enzymatic treatment	Food substrates such as seafood, fish, meat	Liquid, paste

Solvents are used in flavour compositions to dissolve the ingredients and to adjust the strength of liquid flavours. These are food grade ethanol, isopropanol, propylene glycol, and glyceryl triacetate. Edible oils are also used for diluting flavour compositions. In powdered flavours, vegetable gums, starch or other polysaccharides are used to act as carrier as well as for dilution.

Flavour compositions can be premixes (such as concentrated juices, sugar syrups, dry beverage mixes), semi-manufactured flavours containing mixed fruits, sugar and flavours (used in yogurt and ice-cream), and snack flavours comprising spices, salt, flavour enhancers, and hydrolysed vegetable proteins.

Taste is the single most important factor, followed by texture and mouth-feel in the manufacture of processed foods. Health and nutritional concerns come into prominence only after the taste criterion is satisfied. The growing affluence of consumers, the acquired international taste for exotic foods, the ease of preparation, variety, and convenience provided by new food processing and packaging technologies have created an environment for the creative development of flavour compositions.

The back-to-nature trend is increasing in compounding flavours, although natural raw materials are costlier than the alternative synthetic aroma chemicals. Flavour compositions are also dependent on the way the food is cooked, namely, use of microwave ovens, and food modifications such as low fat food. The development of new flavour compositions is a combination of scientific inputs, creative compounding abilities by flavourists and appropriate tasting/application trials by food technologists.

The significance of tasting and prototype development is increasing importance in the new food and beverage concepts. Some commercial units practice captive manufacturing of flavour concentrates. These include beverage manufacturers like Coca-Cola, Pepsi Co. and Tobacco companies. In the 1990s, vanilla, citrus and savoury flavours have accounted for 18 per cent, 8 per cent, and 18 per cent respectively totaling slightly below two–thirds of the total value of flavour compositions worldwide.

Flavour compositions have been experiencing an average annual growth rate of 6–8 per cent in recent years. Commercial flavour compositions are given in Table 4.9 and the amount of flavour used in already some food products and beverages is indicated in Table 4.10.

Table 4.10. Amount of flavour used in some food products and beverages.

Food items	Amount of flavour used (%)
Hard candies, biscuits and other roasted foods	Oil soluble flavours: 0.2
Carbonated beverages and other drinks	Flavours in propylene glycol solvent: 0.2
Carbonated beverages, other drinks, wines and ice-creams	Water soluble flavours: 0.07–0.12
Carbonated beverages and other drinks	Emulsion flavours: 0.1
	Clouding agent: 0.08–0.12
Carbonated beverages and other drinks	Paste flavours: 0.2–0.25
Candies, biscuits	Fruit flavours: 0.2
Dry beverage mixes	Fruit flavours: 0.5–1.0
Convenience foods and soups	Meat, vegetable, poultry powder flavours: 0.3–1.0
Dry beverage mixes, puffing foods, troche	Encapsulated flavours: 0.05–0.3
Wherever applicable	Wine flavours: 0.04–1.0
Wherever applicable	Tea flavours: 1.0

Fragrance Compositions

Fragrance compositions are complex blends of essential oils, aroma chemicals, and natural derivatives (absolutes and concretes). The relative value of a fragrance composition is a function of the product being scented. High value fragrances are used in the high end of the market (fine perfumes, colognes). Quality, functionality and reasonable cost are criteria for the fragrance compositions used in cosmetics, detergents, and household products. In general, the less expensive compositions contain more of the synthetic materials. Prices of fragrance compositions depend on the end uses and the buying power of the end user. Development of fragrance compositions involves perfume formulators, quality control experts and product application specialists. Fine fragrances are still created based on experience, skill, and intuition of the perfume formulator.

Laboratories of flavour and fragrance companies as well as large soap and consumer product companies with in-house perfume formulators are involved in the development of fragrance compositions. The top note, middle note, and bottom note in fragrance compositions influence the perceptiveness of the olfactory bulbs in the nose, make the odour more perceptible and long-lasting.

Globally, the use of fragrance compositions is growing in line with the economic development of the region. There are several variations in the use pattern of fragrances such as culture, consumer preferences for lightly or heavily scented products, odour types, and climatic conditions. However, the increase in population in middle income group world-over and their greater consciousness towards personal hygiene are contributing towards sustaining established markets and accelerated growth in niche areas. The average fragrance content of perfumed products is indicated in Table 4.11.

Table 4.11. Average fragrance content of perfumed products.

Perfumed products	Fragrance content (%)	Diluting media used
After shaves	1.0–2.5	40–50% aqueous ethanol
Air fresheners	2.0–10.0	Solvents, bases, propellants
Bath oils	4.0	Aqueous ethanol
Candles	1.5–5.0	Wax
Creams	0.3–0.5	Fatty cream bases
Decorative cosmetics	0.02–0.50	Bases
Deodourants	1.0–2–0	Bases, propellants
	0.20–0.40	Sprays
Detergents	0.10–0.30	Benzenoid alkylsulphonates
Eau de cologne, Eau de perfume	2.0–8.0	70–80% aqueous ethanol
Hair care products	0.30–0.50	Aqueous ethanol
Industrial soaps	0.30	Soap bases
Mouthwashes	5.0	Water
Perfumes	8.0–25.0	80% aqueous ethanol
Powders	0.50–1.0	Powder bases
Shampoos	0.40–0.50	Water
Soaps	1.0–2.0	Soap bases
Sun lotions	0.20–0.80	Cream bases
Technical products (industrial and household)	0.20–0.40	Solvents, bases, propellants
Toothpastes	1.0	Inorganic salts (wet)

SWEETENERS AND FAT SUBSTITUTES

Sweeteners

Sweetness is a subjective perception influenced by a multitude of variables including temperature of the food being tasted, pH, other flavours and ingredients in the food, physical characteristics of the food sweetener, concentration, rate of sweetness development, and permanence of sweetness and flavour.

Sweeteners of one kind or another have been found in human diets since pre-historic times. They are used in formulated foods for many functional reasons as well as to impart sweetness. Their major functions are the following:

1. Render certain foods palatable and mask bitterness.
2. Add flavour, body, bulk and texture.
3. Change the freezing point and control crystallisation.
4. Control viscosity, which contributes to body and texture.
5. Prevent spoilage.
6. Bind the moisture (in certain cases) in food that is required by detrimental micro-organisms or alternatively serve as food for fermenting organisms that produce acids, which preserve the food, thereby extending the shelf life.

Sweet flavours are obviously used most often in sweetened products, and the sweetening system is typically a large percentage of a formulation. Sweeteners affect the flavour by enhancing the profile; providing differing degrees of sweetness; offering their own contributing flavour; and by changing flavour character and delivery in the mouth. This was a problem for the beverage industry when it went from sucrose-sweetened products to dietetic beverages and drinks sweetened with high fructose corn syrup. The same flavour systems no longer delivered as they had previously, resulting in different-tasting beverages that required flavour reformation.

The way sweeteners interact with flavours and deliver to the human olfactory system is quite complex and almost totally unpredictable. When flavouring is based on sweetness concentration, mildly sweetened products require the use of less flavour compounds as the flavour comes through more clearly. At very high levels, sweetness becomes intense and begins masking the overall flavour. As a result, higher flavour compound levels are required.

Sweeteners have been classified in a number of ways, namely, nutritive or non-nutritive, natural or synthetic, regular or low-calorie/dietectic/high intensity, and as foods (fruit juice concentrates). Commercially there are several sweeteners with varying degrees of sweetness and having different regulatory status. A list of sweeteners, their sweetness and regulatory status in the industrial triad, is given in Table 4.12.

Table 4.12. Sweeteners, their sweetness and regulatory status.

Sweetener	Sweetness	Regulatory status		
		US	EU	Japan
Sugar (sucrose)	1	A	A	A
Acesulphame-K	200	A	A	NA
Alitame	2000	P	P	P
Aspartame	200	A	A	A
Crystalline fructose	1.2–1.7	A	A	A
Cyclamate (sodium salt)	30	P	A	NA
Dextrose	0.75–0.85	A	A	A
Glycyrrhizin	50	NA	NA	A
High fructose corn syrup (HFCS)	1–1.5	A	A	A
Lactitol	0.3–0.4	P	A	A

(Contd ...)

Sweetener	Sweetness	Regulatory status		
		US	EU	Japan
Mannitol	0.7	A	A	A
Neohesperidin DC	2000	NA	A	NA
Saccharin	300	A	A	A
Sorbitol	0.5–0.7	A	A	A
Stevioside	300	NA	NA	A
Sucralose	600	P	P	P
Thaumatin (Talin)	3000	NA	NA	A
Xylitol	1	A	A	A

NA: Not approved; A: approved; P: pending.

Notes: Alitame is approved in Australia, New Zealand and Mexico; Cyclamate is approved in Canada; Glycyrrhizin is approved as a flavouring agent, but not as a sweetener in the US; Saccharin is permitted in Canada only in personal care products and pharmaceuticals, but not in foods and beverages; and sucralose is approved in Australia, Canada, Russia and Mexico.

Flavours associated with sweeteners are of several categories. Obviously, molasses, honey, malt syrup and brown sugar all contribute a desirable or undesirable characteristic flavour, in addition to sweetness. But some not-so-obvious sweeteners also contribute their own flavour. Sucrose possesses a flavour that can be overpowering when used at high levels in delicately flavoured systems, and glucose can begin contributing a burning or bitter taste in higher concentrations. Some of the polyols (sugar alcohols) impart bitterness and a cooling sensation to varying degrees. Amongst the non-nutritive sweeteners, aspartame has a relatively clean flavour but tends to flatten flavour slightly; saccharine and sucralose can contribute bitterness or metallic notes, and acesulphame K can have bitter notes at higher concentrations.

The sweet brown flavours have the annotations of roasted, burnt or caramelised flavour systems. They are created from botanicals and supplemented with natural or artificial flavours, or created by reaction processes. Flavours in this category include brown sugar, malt, honey, maple, molasses, caramel, butterscotch, coffee, and chocolate. Flavour profiles for the base notes in many sweet brown flavours are similar. The sweeteners used in food systems in the categories sweet syrups, sugar alcohols, and high-intensity sweeteners with their salient features are given below.

Sweet syrups

High fructose corn syrup (HFCS)

HFCS is an excellent sweetener for carbonated and non-carbonated beverages, replacing all or part of the sugar. Its clear intense sweetness allows true fruit flavours to develop naturally in all soft drinks. Fermented breads made with HFCS have better qualities of crust colour, flavour, texture, and sweetness than those made with sugar.

Honey

It is considered as a sweetener, but has a characteristic flavour. The complex flavour results from the sugars, acids, volatile and non-volatile components present in it. The characterising flavour is from the source of the plant pollen such as clover, alfalfa, raspberry, blueberry, orange blossom, buckwheat, sage, thyme, and rosemary.

Typically, darken-coloured honey has a stronger flavour than that from the lighter-coloured one. Honey, being sweeter than sucrose, can lead to oversweetness, and its humectant qualities can cause problems with product texture. The blend of honey with other sweeteners boosted with artificial honey flavour provides the desired flavour characteristics at a lower cost and without texture problems.

Maple syrup

The sap of black maple and sugar maple trees is another sweetener containing a characteristic sweet brown flavour. The syrup right out of the trees is mostly sucrose. Evaporation produces some glucose and fructose upon inversion at low pH. One group of flavouring components comes from the ligneous materials in the sap. A second group is formed by the caramelisation of sugar. Maple syrup also is a humectant and can give rise to texture problems in food products.

Molasses

This concentrated extract of sugarcane is strongly flavoured, slightly sweet syrup. Molasses flavour has a niche for itself in some speciality baked goods and those foods flavoured with sweet spices, such as cinnamon and ginger. Lower, uncharacterisable levels of molasses make an excellent tool for building base notes in many sweet brown flavours. Molasses colour, flavour, and composition greatly depend on the region and climatic conditions of sugarcane growth. Blending helps to ensure consistent and uniform colour, flavour, and ash control.

Polyols (Sugar alcohols or polyalcohols)

Sorbitol

It occurs naturally in many edible fruits and berries. It is only 70 per cent as sweet as sucrose. It has many functional properties desirable in a sweetener. In general it is used in foods to aid retention of product quality during ageing, or to provide texture or other product characteristics. New sugarless foods and confections, sweetened solely with aspartame are substantially boosting sorbitol sales.

Lactitol

Lactitol monohydrate, a sugar alcohol, has physico-chemical properties different from those of sugars. It is derived from milk sugar and is used as a sweetener in Japan, Israel and Switzerland. Lactitol's sweetness value approximates one-third that of sucrose and hence it is suitable where bulking with low sweetness is required. It can be blended with high-intensity sweeteners to increase the sweetness.

Mannitol

Mannitol is only about 70 per cent as sweet as sucrose and is also non-carcinogenic. It is non-hygroscopic and so is used as a dusting agent for chewing gum and as a bulking agent in powdered foods. 95 per cent of the mannitol used is in powder form and the rest is granular. Its market is growing for sugar-free confections. The seaweed *Laminaria digitara* containing upto 10 per cent mannitol is the raw material for its manufacture.

Xylitol

Its sweetness is similar to that of sucrose. It is found in small amounts in a variety of fruits and vegetables. The good solubility, uniform blending with foods, lower melting point than that of sucrose, and the non-carcinogenic (does not promote tooth decay) properties of xylitol, are taken advantage of in the manufacture of confectionary products. Xylitol is expensive and as such is used in small amounts in combination with other sweeteners. Blending with xylitol minimises the hygroscopicity or the laxative effect of sorbitol, and improves the solubility of mannitol. Xylitol also has an excellent synergistic effect with aspartame.

High-intensity sweeteners

Aspartame

First appeared in the soft drink market in combination with saccharin (30 per cent aspartame and 70 per cent saccharin). It is approved world-wide in several applications such as non-alcoholic beverages, frozen desserts, refrigerated flavoured milk beverages, fruit wine beverages containing less than seven per cent alcohol, yoghurt-type products, gelatine desserts, confectionaries, baked goods, and low-alcohol beer. Aspartame is 200 times as sweet as sucrose. It has a sugar-like taste and enhances some flavours.

Saccharin

It is approximately 300 times as sweet as sucrose and has been used as a food additive since the early 1990s. It combines well with other sweeteners and has an excellent shelf-life. Its main disadvantages are a bitter, metallic after taste and concern over its safety. However, it is the most widely used non-nutritive sweetener, and is the least expensive on a sweetness basis. Saccharin has been used non-primarily in soft drinks and also as a tabletop sweetener in a wide range of other beverages and foods. It is currently in use in more than eighty countries in the dietectic soft drink market.

Acesulphame-K

It has a rapidly perceptible sweet taste 200 times as much as that of sucrose. Since its approval in 1988 it is used in chewing gums, dry beverage-mixes, instant coffee and tea, gelatines, puddings and non-dairy creamers. It has a good shelf-life, good pH and temperature stability and is approved for use in foods and beverages.

Cyclamate

It is thirty times sweeter than sucrose, a sugar-like taste, a good shelf-life and a synergistic effect with saccharin or aspartame. Although its usage has been involved in controversies, it is currently permitted in Canada and the European Community (excluding UK). Its use with saccharin gives a better taste to beverages than saccharin alone.

Alitame

It is reportedly 2000 times as sweet as sugar with the same taste as sugar. It is a dipeptide made up of L-aspartic and D-alanine amino acids. It is patented in thirty-two countries and is approved in Australia, New Zealand, China, Indonesia and Mexico. For use in food, beverage and tabletop applications, it has market potential in bakery products, snack foods, candies, confectionary, ice-creams and frozen dairy products.

Sucralose

It is a chloro-derivative of sucrose reportedly 600 times sweeter than sucrose. In Canada it is marketed under the brand name *Splenda* and is approved for use in soft drinks, dairy products, biscuits, cakes, puddings, breakfast cereals, jams and jellies, canned fruit and chewing gum. It is also approved in Brazil, Mexico, Australia, New Zealand, Qatar, Russia, and Romania.

Thaumatin

It is a mixture of sweet-tasting proteins from the seeds of *Thaumato coccusceus daniellii*, a west African fruit. It is 2000–2500 times sweeter than sucrose. It has synergistic effect with other sweeteners like saccharin, acesulphame-K, and stevioside. Its taste develops slowly and it leaves a liquorice after-taste. It is a GRAS chemical in the US for chewing gum use. In Japan it has been permitted as a natural food additive since 1979. In the UK and Australia it is primarily used as a flavour enhancer, although approved for use as a sweetener.

Stevia

It is 400 times sweeter than sugar with a longer-lasting sugar taste. It is approved for use in Japan but is still under consideration in the US. It has high temperature stability and is suited in baked or cooked foods. The stevia extract arises from *Stevia rebaudiana*, a plant native to South America.

Miscellaneous

Other high-intensity sweeteners considered for use in foods are glycyrrhizin extracted from liquorice root and used as a flavour enhancer, morellin from the African serendipity berry, hermandulcin (a oil from a Mexican plant), and bioflavonoids from citrus fruits.

Fat Substitutes

Fat is an important ingredient in many foods and most consumers enjoy the taste, texture and aroma fat gives to foods. Chemically it is a triglyceride containing both saturated and unsaturated fatty acids. Fat is the most concentrated energy source in the diet providing nine calories per gram compared with four calories from carbohydrate or protein.

In recent years fat from vegetable sources has increased accounting for 43 per cent of the fat available in the diet. Vegetable fat is consumed mostly in the form of plant oils such as soyabean, corn, sunflower, safflower, canola, cottonseed, palm, coconut, etc. Fat in foods originates from meat products, fried foods, butter, margarine, dairy products, cheese, nuts, baked goods, salad oils, shortenings, mayonnainse, salad dressings, frostings, gravies, and sauces. Most oils used in foods, shortening, and in institutional cooking are partially hydrogenated. High proportion of these partially hydrogenated oils, semi-solid fats, are used in some food preparations to give them flaky texture, taste, and mouth-feel. The amounts of total fat contributed from various food groups in the diet are indicated in Table 4.13.

Table 4.13. Amount of total fat contributed from various food groups in the diet.

Food group	Total fat from food group (%)
Meat, poultry, and fish	30
Grain products	25
Milk and milk products	18
Fats and oils (mainly table spreads and salad dressings)	11
Vegetables	9
Others	7

Fat contributes to 34 per cent of the total energy in the diet, and approximately 12 per cent of this total energy are as saturated fat. Most health authorities advise that the fat consumption in our diets should be reduced to 30 per cent or less total calories, with saturated fat providing 8–10 per cent or less of the total calories. The main concern about excess saturated fat in the diet centres on its potential role in raising blood cholesterol and thereby the risk factor in incidence of coronary heart disease (CHD).

Fat substitutes (replacements or mimetics as they are called) provide an opportunity for individuals to reduce intake of high-fat foods and enjoy reduced-fat formulations of familiar foods while preserving basic food selection patterns. Many of the fat replacements in use today can be incorporated into foods that reflect the changing tastes of consumers. Traditional and new ingredients and technologies provide flavourful, satisfying foods, such as salad and cooking oils, cheeses, ice-creams, bakery products, and salty snacks and crackers, that are reduced in fat or contain no fat. When limiting dietary fat, consumers still need to satisfy their basic nutritional needs. No product is a panacea. Additional reduced-fat products will not replace a person's need for moderation and good nutrition. However, they do provide palatable alternatives, which can make the difficult task of compliance with a reduced-fat and/or reduced-calorie diet easier. Thus, when incorporated into an overall balanced, nutritious diet, reduced-fat foods and beverages can play an important role in helping consumers reach and maintain their goal of reducing consumption of dietary fat, cholesterol and calories.

The fat replacements developed to date generally fall into one of three categories: (i) carbohydrate-based, (ii) protein-based, and (iii) fat-based.

Carbohydrate-based fat substitutes

Many of the low-fat products introduced in recent years contain carbohydrate-based fat replacements (e.g. cellulose, malto-dextrins, gums, starches, fibre and polydextrose). Carbohydrates have been used safely for many years as thickeners and stabilisers. These ingredients are also effective fat substitutes in many formulated foods, including heat applications. They are not suitable for frying foods. Nearly forty starch-based products have been recommended as fat replacements. Most of these are used to form a gel containing modified starch and water.

The gel is then substituted for fat on an equal-weight basis. These starch-based fat substitutes have many different properties depending on the degree of cross-linking, substitution and acid modification. In many cases two or more starch products have to be used together to give the desired effect. Starches can also be combined with other polymers and emulsifiers. Maltodextrins, the products of acid hydrolysis of starch act as bulking agents, giving the mouth-feel qualities of fat. Other most widely used fat substitutes are cellulose derivatives, gums, and hydrocolloids.

Protein-based fat substitutes

Protein-based fat replacements have tremendous potential for use in a variety of products, especially frozen and refrigerated products. Although protein-based fat replacements are not suitable for frying foods, they can be used in many heat applications (e.g. cream soups, pasteurised products, baked goods). A mixture of egg white and milk proteins, water, sugar, pectin and citric acid is subjected to high shear to form a gel of protein spheroids. Termed *Simplesse*, it was developed by Nutra Sweet Kelco. The small spheres produced by micro-particulation simulate the mouth-feel of fat. This product is used in frozen desserts. A similar version, *simplesse* 100, is made from whey protein and is approved for use in baked products. One gram of micro-particulated protein supplies only 1–2 calories and can replace one gram of fat, which provides 9 calories per gram. Several other protein-based fat substitutes are on the market and are used in both cooked and uncooked products.

Fat-based fat substitutes

Scientists have been able to chemically alter fatty acids to provide fewer or no calories, making fat-based fat replacements possible. Some fat-based fat replacements actually pass through the body virtually unabsorbed (e.g. olestra). These ingredients have the advantage of heat stability and offer excellent versatility. Some may be used in frying; others as cocoa butter substitutes. The four important products in this category are olestra, capranin, salatrim and medium-chain triglyceride (MCT).

Olestra

Olestra, with a brand name olean, was developed by Procter and Gamble (P & G) and approved in 1996 by the FDA in the US for use in preparing potato chips, tortilla chips, and other savoury snacks. It is a sucrose polyester made from a sucrose backbone and 6–8 fatty acids. The number and type of fatty acids vary depending on the desired performance characteristics. The fatty acids are derived from soya, cottonseed, or corn oils. Olestra's molecules are much larger than those of ordinary fats and as such the body's digestive enzymes cannot break them down. Olestra is thus neither digested nor absorbed and passes straight through the body. It does not provide any calories and does not impart any sweetness. There are some concerns about olestra regarding its blocking of the absorption of fat-soluble vitamins such as A, D, E, and K. FDA, therefore, has specified that these vitamins should be added to foods prepared with olestra. In spite of this opinion on the use of olestra is divided amongst dietectic associations and consumer advocates.

Caprenin

Caprenin, or caprocaprylobehenin, is a fat substitute introduced by Procter and Gamble (P & G) in 1991. It is a triglyceride composed of naturally occurring fatty acids, namely, caprylic (C_8), capric (C_{10}), and behenic (C_{22}). Caprylic and capric acids are derived from coconut and palm-kernel oils. Behenic acid is derived from hydrogenated rapeseed oil. Caprenin provides five calories per gram and according to P and G's patent can replace 70 per cent of the fat in confectionary products, which usually contain 25–45 per cent fat. Caprenin is recommended as an alternative to cocoa-butter and other confectionary fats. Instead of the traditional FDA clearance, caprenin's approval is based on an expert panel convened by the Life Sciences Research Office of the Federation of American Societies for Experimental Biology based on P and G's published research data.

Salatrim (Benefat)

It is an esterified monostearin consisting of short-chain (acetic, propionic, butyric) and long-chain (stearic) fatty acids. Salatrim is derived from ingredients found in nature and provides five calories per gram instead of the nine calories per gram provided by the traditional fats. It was developed by Nabisco and is now marketed by Cultor Food Science, USA. Since salatrim is a fat product, it delivers the taste and performance of conventional fats. The first product using Salatrim was Hershey's reduced fat baking chips introduced in 1995. A more recent product is Snackwell's granola bar.

MCT (medium-chain triglycerides)

These are esters of fractionated coconut oil fatty acids, marketed by Stepan Co., USA and ABITEC Ingredients (formerly Karishamns food ingredients), USA. MCT provides 8.3 calories per gram, only marginally less energy than the traditional fats. However, recent physiological studies suggest that they are burnt readily for energy and have little tendency to be incorporated into tissue lipids that are deposited as fat. MCT is in the GRAS list but its use since several years has been mainly in medical and infant feeding products due to its high cost. Of late, its usage has been expanded into sports/nutrition foods.

APPLICATIONS OF FLAVOURS AND FRAGRANCES

Applications of Flavours in Toothpaste

The need for flavours is obvious, and mint has always been the preferred choice for toothpaste. Mint flavours impart a feeling of freshness for two reasons, namely:

1. The general public associate a mint taste with freshness, cleanliness and relief.

2. Mint flavours, especially when combined with menthol, contain oils that are volatile in the warm environment of the mouth.

The evaporation needs energy, which is extracted from the tissues of the mouth as heat, thereby imparting a cooling sensation. Toothpaste, which is usually sweetened and flavoured to provide palatability and consumer acceptance, contains either sorbitol or glycerine as humectants. Sorbitol, which has a high negative heat of solution, extracts the heat for its dissolution from the tissues of the mouth and imparts the cooling sensation.

Sugar-based mints do not impart this coolness. This cool sensation is also experienced when one chews sorbitol based tablets. Conventional toothpaste and natural toothpaste use the same type of flavours, mostly mints like peppermint, spearmint and wintergreen. However, conventional pastes use artificial flavours while natural pastes use herbal extracts as well as essential oils. Natural pastes also use mints, but they have more unique flavours such as anise, ginger, fennel, cherry, and cinnamon.

Applications of Flavours in Tobacco

Today tobacco is grown in more than 120 countries. The largest growers are China, United States, India, Brazil, Turkey, and several European countries. As plants mature, the chlorophyll pigment rapidly decreases and virtually disappears. This is true of tobacco also after harvest. Many important carotenoid aroma constituents are formed during the post-harvesting and curing of tobacco. While there are more than 2700 components identified in various tobacco varieties, amongst those contributing to the aroma of cured tobacco, the two important ones are β-damascenone and megastigmatrienones (four isomers).

The most common uses of tobacco are for cigarettes, cigars, pipe tobacco, chewing tobacco and snuff. In spite of the health hazards attributed to tobacco in recent years and the associated litigation, the global tobacco industry is yet a sizable one.

The secret to great tasting tobacco is in the flavouring. Tobacco companies use flavourings to smooth out tobacco, remove harshness and stinging and deliver a mellow flavoured smoke. Flavour enhancers and top notes are also used by the tobacco industry.

Various substances are added to tobacco components to affect the flavour and palatability of smoke, alter smoke composition and yield, modify burn rate, and alter pH to optimise nicotine delivery. The major contribution of the tobacco flavour specialist is help to provide a rich, clean, full-bodied tobacco flavour, to keep to a minimum hotness and irritation in the mouth, and to ensure high satisfaction from an adequate level of nicotine per puff, requirements that guarantee the consumer a pleasurable smoke. The so-called casings are solutions of usually water-soluble ingredients that provide a means of incorporating flavourings and other additives into the tobacco blend. Casings are often used in tobacco processing to reduce the harshness of nicotine in high-nicotine tobaccos, thus permitting greater use of these tobaccos in cigarette manufacture. This use of casings is based on the assumption that nicotine is one of the primary satisfaction factors for which tobacco products are used. However, in air-cured tobaccos (cigars, for example), the pH of the smoke is generally alkaline and the flavour effect of nicotine is harshness, which can be choking and unpleasant. In the case of tobaccos containing sugars (flue-cured, oriental), the tobacco is weakly acidic, the effect of the nicotine is greatly modified, and the harshness is dramatically reduced. This same effect is often achieved by addition of sugars to air-cured tobaccos to mellow the smoke and/ or by the blending of air-cured tobaccos with flue-cured and oriental.

The tobacco flavours include four types, namely, Virginia, burley, cigar and reaction. The Virginia type can blend the tobacco odour with green, wine-like and sweet odour but not too strong. The odour of burley type is very strong and can decrease the irritation of tobacco. The cigar type can modify and blend the cigar odour to maintain original characteristic odour and decrease the irritation of cigar. The reaction type is odourless. When cigarettes are smoked, the reaction flavours get decomposed and go out with the odour of tobacco. Reaction flavours can modify the smell, mask other odours, enhance tobacco odour, as well as soften the tobacco leaf. The normal dosage of tobacco flavours is 0.15–0.35 per cent for all the four types.

TYPES OF FRAGRANCES

Fragrances are usually considered in two broad categories, as either fine fragrances or functional fragrances. Fine fragrances include perfumes, colognes, after-shaves and fragrances for cosmetic products. They are classified in different ways, namely, men's, women's, unisex, signature, designer, etc. Functional fragrances include all personal and household cleaning products. Apart from these fragrances have some outlet in a few miscellaneous applications.

Fine Fragrances

Exotic, sophisticated blends of fragrant oils from every corner of the world create an ambience and an aura that is refreshing, inspiring, and exhilarating. Fine fragrances must work on the skin and blend with body odour. They must be pleasant, diffusive and substantive (long-lasting). They must also have the quality of genuine beauty and signatures that distinguish them from each other. For most fine fragrances, the perfumes themselves are the products. They are sold to the consumers at various concentrations in alcoholic or aqueous-alcoholic solutions, depending on the type of application intended. Women's perfumes are typically 20–35 per cent fragrance oil in 95 per cent ethanol. Women's colognes are offered in the range 15–25 per cent fragrance oil. Men's colognes and after-shave products usually contain 2–12 per cent of fragrances. The creation of fine fragrances allows for the highest degree of freedom in terms of ingredient choice and economics. Consequently, fine fragrances are often trendsetters and eventually find their way into other products. Perfumes are grouped into broad odour categories showing their relationships to each other and are available as men's, women's, and unisex fragrances.

Signature Fragrances

Speciality fragrances (signature fragrances) are carefully balanced blends of functional and perfumery ingredients. They have strong aesthetic as well as functional properties and can be adapted for a wide variety of products, ranging from space deodourants to cosmetics and toiletries.

Designer fragrances

Fine fragrances are also classified as designer fragrances based on the fragrance house or perfumer, who has created the fragrance.

Functional Fragrances

Functional fragrances are used in detergents, soaps, fabric softeners, household and industrial/institutional cleaners, cosmetics and toiletries, plastics, candles, waxes and polishes, and sanitation goods.

Detergents

In the household sector, a major value based market is that for detergents. The major product types in household detergents are the following:
1. Heavy duty laundry powders.
2. Heavy duty laundry liquids.

3. Light duty hand dishwashing liquids.
4. Automatic dishwashing liquids.

Consumers have come to enjoy pleasant-smelling, personal and household cleaners. Amongst these, there are a great variety of laundry detergent and dishwashing formulations on the market, and new ones are introduced every year. Significant factors to be considered for the choice of the fragrance in detergents are the following:

1. The presence of malodours in the product bases.
2. Possibility of reaction between the detergent constituents and fragrance constituents.
3. Presence of bleaching agents in the detergents.
4. Stability of the fragrance material in the detergent.
5. Rate of evaporation of the fragrance from the sales package.
6. Performance of the detergent in the wash water and on the laundered-cloth.
7. Ability to impart a pleasant scent to the clean and dried fabrics.

Detergent fragrances must be particularly powerful and effective because they are incorporated in detergents at a rather low level of 0.3 per cent. In products like dishwashing liquids, where grease removal is a major criterion, they have to withstand the effect of other ingredients in the formulations. The level of fragrance used may be higher than 0.3 per cent in concentrated products. Substantive ingredients such as galaxolide, lilial, lyral, and ambroxan are used to obtain residual fragrance on the fabrics. Typically floral fragrances are used in laundry as well as dishwashing detergent formulations. The odours in these fragrances are cosmetic floral, jasmine aldehyde, green herbaceous, green citrus, fresh floral mouguet, rose mouguet bouquet, intense floral citrus, and others. Some common fragrances used in laundry detergents are given in Table 4.14.

Table 4.14. Some common fragrances used in laundry detergents.

Lemon grass	Linalool	Linalyl acetate	Methyl cedrylone	Methyl salicylate
Moskene	Musk xylol	Myrcenyl acetate	Nerol	Nonalactone
Oakmoss 25%	Octanal	Olibanum resinoid 80%	Opoponax oleoresin 70%	Orange oil cold pressed
Para hydroxy phenyl butanone	Para tertiary bucinal	Patchouli	Peppermint	Peru balsam
Petitgrain	Phenylethyl alcohol	Pine oil steam distilled	Rose otto synthetic	Rosemary
Spearmint natural	Spruce	Terpineol	Terpinolene	Terpinyl acetate
4-tertiary butyl cyclohexyl acetate	Tetrahydrolinalool	Tonalid	Thyme white oil	Trichloromethyl phenyl carbinyl acetate
Vanillin	Vertivert	Vertivert acetate	Ylang ylang	–

Soaps

The function of the soap is to clean. However, the fragrance at a concentration of 1–2 per cent plays a large role in the perceived quality of the soap bar. Aesthetically a beauty-soap requires a different type of fragrance from that used in a deodourant soap or a freshness bar. Besides the aesthetic aspect, technical limitations in the choice of fragrances for soaps are the characteristics of the soap base, presence of additives, higher pH (generally 9.5–11.0) of the soap which can lead to hydrolysis followed by discolouration, odour quality, stability of the fragrance, and cost involved. The proper fragrance in a bar of soap can make the difference between just getting clean and having an enjoyable experience. The correct fragrance at the recommended use level of 1–2 per cent will not discolour and most importantly will give forth an appealing scent from the bar prior to its use and vital, yet not too strong, odour during use. The odour types used in soaps can be single florals or complex compositions in which fine fragrances' have been the models for the soap creation. Typical fragrances used in soaps are given in Table 4.15.

Table 4.15. Typical fragrances used in soaps.

Apple (green, red, spice)	Arabian dreams	Banana	Black tea
Carnation	Cedar	Chloe type	Gardenia
Jasmine neroli	Lavender	Lemon floral	Linden
Mayan gold	Moroccan memories	Musk (Egyptian)	Oriental
Patchouli	Tangerine	Tropical wood	Various fruit essences

Fabric softeners

The principal functions of fabric softeners are to minimise the problem of static electricity and to keep fabrics soft. Fragrances are very important ingredients for fabric softeners. They have to be intense, persistent, withstand high temperature, and reinforce the sense of softness. Most liquid fabric softeners have a pH of 3.5, which limits the choice of fragrances. Products based on acetals, schiff bases, oakmoss extracts, and other speciality chemicals can create malodour problems or cause discolouration.

A special requirement of fragrances for fabric softeners is the ability to leave a residual of odour on the fabric after line- or machine drying. Substantive materials in the fragrance satisfying the criteria must not only blend into the fragrant type as well as the odour from the product base but also must survive rinsing. In tumble-dry softeners, wherein a nonwoven fabric, foamed plastic, or a cotton string contains the active softener ingredient and the fragrance, the fragrance partly disappears with the drying hot air and is partly absorbed into the fabrics. For this application stability of the fragrance over many drying cycles is important. Several variations of floral type fragrances are generally used in fabric softeners.

Household and industrial/institutional (I and I) cleaners

The household cleaners segment includes scouring cleaners, wall, woodwork, floor, and glass cleaners, spot and soil removers, bathroom and toilet bowl cleaners, and hand cleaners. Some of the cleaners may contain ingredients like ammonia, bleaches, and disinfectants. The fragrance should withstand the effect of such chemicals and present a pleasant odour during the storage, handling, and after-use of the cleaner.

Industrial and institutional (I and I) cleaners market segment has been growing considerably due to demographic factors. The cleaners used in this category are hard surface cleaners, laundry and dry cleaning materials, commercial dishwashing products, food industry cleaners, metal cleaners, and miscellaneous cleaners. Fragrances find a place in these areas predominantly in sanitorial products, hand cleaners, laundry (in hotels and motels, hospitals, nursing homes, retirement complexes, cafeteria, bars, and restaurants), and transportation cleaning materials.

Since the cleaner formulations in general are alkaline, contain surfactants, sanitisers, disinfectants and other additives, the choice and use level of the fragrance to impart the desired effect is important.

Cosmetics and toiletries

Cosmetic products comprise of perfumes, colognes, toilet water, decolognes, pre/after-shave, skin-care, face powders and make-up products. Fragrances used in cosmetics are of two general types, essential oils, and fragrance compositions, which are by far the larger of the two types in monetary value and importance. Fragrance compositions are compounded mixtures of essential oils and other raw materials and synthetic aroma chemicals. Such compositions contain a few to literally hundreds of these components, blended with great effort and skill to produce the aesthetic and technical performance characteristics desired. The selection of fragrances by cosmetics customer companies is almost entirely subjective after meeting certain minimum technical requirements. In products like talcum powders, problems can arise due to the presence of alkaline impurities. In such cases aldehydes and terpenes fail to contribute to the desired odour and the fragrance choice is to be carefully made.

Toiletries consist of mouthwash, toothpaste, bath oil, body oil, body spray, deodourants, soap, shampoo, and hair-care products. Fragrances are used in all these products. Some essential oils such as peppermint and menthol are used directly without compounding in toothpaste and mouthwash.

The stability of a fragrance in shampoo normally does not pose any problems, as the shampoo pH is nearly neutral. However, in some cases, viscosity problems can arise. Generally 0.5–1.05 is the dosage of fragrance for normal shampoos. In products where a strong odour and residual effect are desired, the dosage can be as high as 1.5 per cent. Fragrances used in deodourant and antiperspirant sticks and lotions must have stability similar to those used in soaps due to higher temperatures (~60°C) encountered during manufacture. In antiperspirants, the presence of aluminium salts can reduce the pH to about 2.3 and as such acid-sensitive fragrances will be unsuitable for such applications. In modern approach to deodourants the fragrance should smell good both in its original form and with the addition of body odour as it develops. Body oils are truly multi-purpose. Not only are they a functional cosmetic but they deliver a beautiful fragrance that contributes to their mood setting qualities. Some fragrances used in body oils are listed in Table 4.16.

Table 4.16. Some fragrances used in body oils.

Fragrances for body oils	Characteristics
Blackberry musk	A sensuous combination of dry fruity notes accenting a blend of soft musks
Cedarwood sage	Just like a sauna spiced with invigorating yet calming spice notes
Cherry	Youthful and fresh
Coco mango	A blend of fruit and coconut that is reminiscent of afternoons in the sun
Coconut	An old favourite for summer. Full bodied but not too aromatic
Dewberry	Fruity with some spice notes but without the green bitter notes sometimes found in this fruit
Geranium	Beautiful rose notes, tinged with a hint of minty green
Jasmine neroli	Reported to be the favourite fragrance of the harems in the Ottoman empire. The soft bouquet of the night blooming jasmine enhanced by the sweet floral of neroli
Musk	A classic reported to have aphrodisiac properties. Its subtle lingering fragrance appeals to one and all
Musk Egyptian	Cleopatra's secret? The musk base is enhanced with exotic florals, woods and touches of spice
Orchid	It is reported that orchids do not have an odour but this fantasy fragrance smells as good as orchids. A creation based upon a merging of the perfumer's perception of the odours of several orchid varieties

(Contd ...)

Fragrances for body oils	Characteristics
Patchouli	Imagine a bath in a tropical pool ringed by patchouli. Sweet, floral slightly fruity with a hint of spice
Peach	Just like freshly picked peaches. Slightly green fruity top notes. Leaves a long lasting characteristic peach fragrance
Pine lavender	Great for long, hot soaks. The refreshing odour of pine merged with the feminine softness and longevity of lavender
Tea rose	Very clear, fresh and light. None of the heavy notes of the common rose
Vanilla	Restful and calming. A universal favourite that is good for all ages. Its sweet, subtle slightly woody notes can stand-alone or blend with other fragrance favourites
Ylang	A tropical delight. Light and heavy floral notes, very slightly spicy and long lasting

Plastics

Most fragrances can be adapted to plastic compounding operations. The end-use application, FDA requirements and temperature exposure are important factors in fragrance selection. Typically, fragrances are liquid at room temperature although powdered, granular and pellet physical forms are available.

Aromatherapy

Aromatherapy is one of the most exciting and burgeoning modes of herbalism today. It has become a truly global discipline, different parts of the world contributing varied uses and methods of application for essential oils.

Aromatherapy is not about fragrance, but about healing. In aromatherapy, aromas are therapeutic. The healing properties come from essential oils, highly concentrated extracts taken from herbs, flowers and other plants. Certain properties in essential oils trigger therapeutic effects in one's body. When inhaled deeply, or applied to the skin surface in carrier oils, these properties produce very specific beneficial results. According to Chinese herbal energetics, some herbs have ascending actions, while some descend; some invigorate while others sedate. Some herbs move to the body's surface, or the extremities, while others penetrate deeply to affect organ functioning.

Essential oils in aromatherapy

Essential oils are used in aromatherapy by three methods of application, namely, ingestion, inhalation, and massage. The method of ingestion, the traditional one, requires larger dose or quantity of the aromatic substance. It normally takes a longer time to influence the body, as it has to reach the nervous system along with the circulation of the blood. The dosage or the percentage of aromatic substance is much less, about 1.0–5.0 per cent of the massage oil. The skin may absorb about 0.1 ml of the massage oil, which is a very small quantity as compared to the dose of ingestion. Here the odour of aromatic substance in the massage oil influences the body.

Inhalation, according to the findings of aromatherapists, influences the body immediately. In this method the fragrant material is sprayed or a wad of cotton is kept near the patient's nostrils. The sense of smell by reflex action has immediate and enormous influence on the nervous system. To achieve the maximum benefits, full strength, undiluted essential oils are required.

The term '100 per cent essential oil' is used to describe oils that contain only the extract of a particular plant. The essential oil industry itself actually grades the quality of 100 per cent essential oils on a scale of 1–5, with 1 being the purest, top grade.

The ultimate therapeutic value of the essential oils used is totally dependent on the quality of the live plants, the way the oils are extracted, and the way they are handled after extraction. High standards that focus on product purity are critically important. The best oils come from wild or organically grown plants because the plants themselves are chemical free.

Also, the best oils are extracted using methods that use no heat and take more time, thus preserving the vitality and life essence of the plant. In some cases, such as with citrus oils, it is relatively easy to use these methods to extract a quantity of oil. In other cases, as with rose oil, the process is difficult and the raw material is rare, making the resulting oil quite precious. Common oils that are easy to extract consequently cost less than the more precious oils. It is established that mixtures of essential oils are more effective than individual oils.

When essential oils are distilled, the process actually yields another, totally distinct product known as a hydrosol, or floral water. Floral waters are a natural complement to essential oils because they contain all of the water-soluble properties that were in the original plants. Floral waters offer a more gentle, less concentrated form of the natural elements and are often easier to use. Essential oils are concentrated, highly potent substances and various essential oils are used for aromatherapy. A working knowledge of how to use them safely is essential and the guidelines for this are the following:

1. Undiluted oils should not be used on the skin. Some of the essential oils which are skin irritants are cinnamon, clove, dwarf pine, oregano, pimento, savoury, thyme and wintergreen. The most effective way to dilute essential oils is in a carrier oil of vegetable origin such as almond, apricot, hazelnut, olive, grape-seed, or sesame oil. A safe and effective dilution for most aromatherapy applications is 2 per cent which translates to 2 drops of essential oil for 100 drops of carrier oil (10–12 drops of essential oil per ounce of carrier oil).
2. Only pure essential oils from plants must be used.
3. Before using the oil tests for sensitivity are essential.
4. Essential oils such as angelica, bergamot, bitter orange, cumin, lemon, lime, opoponax, rue and verbena which are photosensitive should be used with caution.
5. Essential oils such as all-spice, cinnamon, clove, oregano, savoury, spearmint, and thyme which are irritating to mucous membrane should also be used with caution.
6. All essential oils must be kept out of reach from children.
7. The essential oil blends used should be varied. The same blend should not be used over the entire body for daily application for more than two weeks.
8. Essential oils should be used cautiously by the elderly, convalescing, or persons having serious health problems such as asthma, epilepsy, heart disease and during pregnancy.
9. Essential oils should not be taken orally for therapeutic purposes.
10 Over-exposure to an essential oil either through the skin or by inhalation may result in nausea, headache, skin irritation, emotional unease, or a 'spaced-out' feeling. Irritation to the skin or accidental splash to the eyes of the essential oil should be treated by diluting with straight vegetable oil and not water.

Miscellaneous applications

Apart from the major markets already highlighted, fragrances find application in some miscellaneous markets such as air fresheners, olfactory marketing, candles and incenses, sanitary goods, waxes and polishes.

Air Fresheners

Traditionally fragrances have been used to get rid of malodour and create a pleasant environment. However, sensitivity issues related to perfumes have led to alternate methods of odour removal. In spite of this, fragrances continue their presence for use in air fresheners, which are deployed in various places.

Fragrances for air fresheners are used in aerosol perfumes, battery operated and metered air fresheners and dispensers, gels, sachets, etc. In these cases scientifically formulated essential oils are slowly evaporated into the atmosphere neutralising unpleasant odours and leaving just a trace of fragrance of one's choice.

Olfactory Marketing

Fragrances become a powerful marketing tool when impregnated in a high quality print of a company or associated logos. Euromat, Dour, Belgium with its know-how uses the direct printing technology and professional perfumes selection to produce olfactory marketing and communication tools. Besides the usual popular perfumes range Euromat offers the capability to create a more subtle and lighter perfume and produce a personalised and proprietary on-demand fragrance. Euromat's standard fragrance palette consists of 65 perfumes.

Candles and Incenses

Candles and incense have always been part of magical and ritual activities and nobody will deny that the burning of incense is also a quite common practice in normal daily life. This is not surprising, because already the scent on its own creates a nice and peaceful atmosphere and a pleasant feeling.

Some concentrated fragrances are soluble in wax while many others are not or are only soluble in small amounts. Different candle manufacturers use different wax formulations, which further complicate the solubility of perfume oils. In order to be sure that fragrances are soluble in all wax formulation, stabilisers which will 'carry in' the perfume oil into the wax are added.

In the past, most scented candles used between 1.5–2 per cent perfume. Today, many scented candles contain from 5–10 per cent perfume oil. One will only get as much perfume out of a candle as one puts into it. Many of the users want to make their fragrances as strong as possible. Almost any fragrance type can be supplied in a specifically formulated version for use in scented candles. Prices vary strictly according to the cost of the raw materials used in each. The most popular scent for scented candles is vanilla. This accounts for 40–50 per cent of the total candle fragrance used. The next most popular scent is cinnamon or spice. Following these, are strawberry, peach, apple or spiced apple.

Incense has been burnt for thousands of years, worldwide. It was burned to mask the odours of sacrificial animals. Incense was also used to carry prayers to the Gods. Incense is still burnt today, by holy men worldwide to promote ritual consciousness, the state of mind necessary to rouse and direct personal energy. Fragrant smoke also is believed to purify the place of worship and the surrounding areas of negative, disturbing vibrations. Fragrances used in incense have been related to so many factors such as Ayurveda, the zodiac, etc. and they are reported to have different significance depending on the incense used. In India, agarbatties are very common. Some of them are scented sticks or perfumed by dipping the unperfumed sticks in the desired perfume solution. The common raw agarbattes come in three types, namely, for any perfume, for rose, and for sandalwood. Typically, in a recipe consists of 2.0 kg of raw-sticks, 0.1 kg of perfume and 0.5 kg of diethyl phthalate.

FLAVOUR ANALYSIS

Chemical analysis or sensory evaluation should be utilised to determine flavour products and the flavour quality of foods; both must be used. Sensory evaluation looks at the whole sample, is very reproducible and the analysis is usually done by averaging individual responses of trained judges. Objective chemical analysis is dependent upon sampling techniques and sample handling and/or separation techniques before measurement. But, as noted previously, some chemicals that cause large gas chromatography (GC) peaks have little or no odour. Thus, instrumental methods can only be utilised to measure flavours when they are calibrated by analytical sensory methods.

Psychophysics and Sensory Evaluation

Psychophysics is the study of the relationship between the psychological perception of a stimulus and the physical stimulus that causes that perception. Sensory evaluation is the utilisation of psychophysical techniques in the food industry to answer three types of questions:

1. *Description*: What does the product taste like? How is one product different from another in quality? How do changes in the process, formulation, packaging, or storage conditions affect its perceived sensory characteristics?
2. *Discrimination*: Would people notice the difference? How many people would detect it? If there is a difference, how great is it?
3. *Affective or hedonics*: How much do people like this product? Is it an improvement over another product? Which attributes are liked or disliked? Which product would the consumer select?

The first consideration in any sensory study is to define the objective of the test. Do we need to know whether two samples are different in character (an analytical question) or which of the two is preferred (a subjective, consumer-oriented question)? The objective will determine the selection of panellists, the methodology employed, the appropriate level of statistical error to permit and the interpretation of results to provide a recommendation.

Panellists can vary from untrained consumers to specially trained flavourists. Target consumers must determine the preference for and acceptance of a finished product, whereas trained panellists are employed to differentiate among samples or to profile samples. All panellists, trained or not, must be screened for specific odour or taste deficits.

The instructions given to the panellists play an important role in any sensory test. The perceived sensory information, upon which memories of the event are based, is believed to be available for only a few tenths of a second. If not dealt with in that time, it is lost. Anticipated information is perceived more readily than that which is unexpected and the panellist's motivation may influence what perceptions are retained. Information that passes through the selective filter of attention can be stored for seconds in short-term (working) memory, but if not rehearsed, it is lost. The limited duration of short-term memory dictates the number of questions that can be answered after one taste or smell of a sample.

Experiences during the panellist's life are an uncontrolled factor in testing. Familiarity with a stimulus will increase the likelihood of its recognition and may bias the panellist towards a greater liking for it.

The sensitivity of the taste and olfactory systems varies enormously across individuals—sometimes by a factor of 100. Moreover, any individual's sensitivity also varies over time. Changes arise from ageing, illness, level of arousal, motivation and expectancy. Body temperature alters taste and smell sensitivity because of blood flow changes across the tongue and olfactory epithelium and this rises and falls with one's circadian rhythm. Sensitivity rises with the oestrogen surge of the menstrual cycle and it rises when atmospheric pressure is low. In short, the psychophysical tests described below are subject to a host of variables, only some of which can be controlled by the sensory analyst and so results must be interpreted statistically and with caution.

Discrimination tests

Discrimination or difference testing is used to determine whether there is a perceptible difference between two or more products and, in some cases, the magnitude of the difference. As these tests involve comparative judgements, they can be very sensitive in determining small differences between products. There are many types of difference tests: the paired comparison test, the triangle test and the duo-trio test are among the most commonly used in the food industry to measure the flavour differences in foods and food products.

Paired comparison

This test is used to determine whether two samples differ in a specific character; it is a directional test with a named attribute. For example, the panellist is presented with two samples and asked which one is more bitter. Positional bias is an important factor; thus, the sample order of presentation must be balanced so that there are equal numbers of AB and BA presentations. The statistical chance of obtaining the correct answer by guessing is 1 in 2 or 50 per cent. Therefore, the detection threshold is normally placed at 75 per cent correct responses, indicating that the difference has been detected on half the trials.

Multiple comparison

Efficiently used to evaluate four or five samples at a time, this test only measures the direction and magnitude of differences in one or perhaps two characteristics. A known standard is labelled as a reference or control and presented to the panellist along with several blind coded samples. The panellists are then asked to compare each coded sample to the known standard on the basis of an identified characteristic.

Triangle test

This test is used to determine an unspecified sensory difference between two products. The panellist is provided with three samples and told that two are the same and one is different. The objective of the test is to identify the different sample. In addition, the panellist is often asked to give the reason for his or her decision.

Taste order is specified because it has been shown to affect the test results: there is a tendency to select the middle sample as being odd. The six presentation possibilities (BAA, ABA, AAB, ABB, BAB, BBA), should be presented equally (the number of panellists being a multiple of six) or at least randomly. Because this is a forced choice test, that is a decision must be made even if no difference is perceived, there is a one-in-three possibility that the odd sample will be identified by chance alone.

The triangle test is popular because: (i) it is rapidly administered, (ii) it is an easily understood task, and (iii) data analysis is simple.

Duo-trio test

This test is used to measure unspecified differences between samples. It is another three-sample difference test, where the panellist is first given a control sample and then asked which, of the next two samples, is the same as the control. The probability of guessing the correct answer in the duo-trio test is one in two or 50 per cent. This test is useful for panellist screening and training. Using immediate feedback, this practice helps teach panellists to discriminate, especially if allowed to retaste the samples and attempt to associate the similarities in the identical combination and then decide what is different in the odd sample.

Ranking test

This test is used to establish a magnitude of difference between samples on a specified attribute. The panellists are presented with 3–5 coded samples and asked to rank them in order according to a single specific attribute, e.g. sweetness. The taste order should be prescribed and a balanced design used.

Magnitude estimation

In this test, two or more coded samples are presented in a specified order, which is balanced across panellists. An arbitrary value for the attribute in question is assigned to the first sample. When panellists analyse (via tasting or smelling) the next sample, they assign a higher or lower value to it according to their estimate of the magnitude of the difference. Scales used could be category scales, line scales or ratio scales. The simplest means of evaluating perceived intensity is to have panellists assign each stimulus to one of several categories, ranging from 'no flavour' to 'very strong flavour'.

The categories can be replaced with a line scale, along which the panellist places a mark corresponding to the intensity of the odourant. This takes more training, as standard concentrations of the attribute to be determined are used as anchors to define the ends of the line. When a highly trained panellist assigns a series of numbers that represent the ratio of the perceived intensities of the presented flavourants to the first presented sample, a taste or odour's psychological magnitude can be related directly to its physical concentration by a logarithmic function. The logarithm of the magnitude estimation (P) is plotted as a function of the logarithm of stimulus concentration (C) as in equation (4.1).

$$\log P = n \log C + \log k \qquad \qquad \ldots (4.1)$$

where, k is the y-axis intercept and n is the slope. Taking the antilogarithm of each side yields a power function, equation (4.2):

$$P = kC^n \qquad \qquad \ldots (4.2)$$

where n is the slope that relates psychological perception to physical concentration. The value of n is nearly always less than one for olfactory stimuli; hence a linear plot of perception versus concentration shows that our olfactory receptors become saturated (Fig. 4.1).

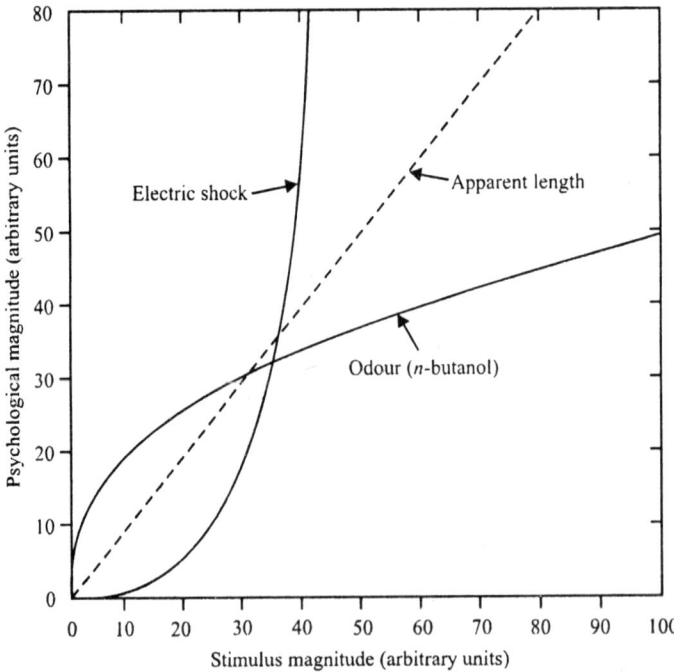

Fig. 4.1. Relationship between perceived magnitude of three types of stimuli, as measured by magnitude estimation and stimulus magnitude.

Magnitude estimation using the ratio scale offers a level of rigour not found in the other approaches, so its use is desirable as a psychophysical method. However, because of the following complications, it is rarely used in sensory testing in the food industry:

1. To generate reliable numbers, the panellist must retain an accurate memory of the entire stimulus series.
2. If odours are presented too slowly, memory fades; if too quickly, adaptation reduces perceived intensity.
3. The concept of ratios is unfamiliar to many people and they use numbers as if they were categories, 10, 20, 30, etc.
4. Finally, a number of non-sensory factors can affect the slope of the power function, including the range of numbers over which the ratings are made, the complexity and intensity range of the stimulant and the order of stimulus presentation.

Threshold tests

A subset of difference testing is the measurement of the lowest concentration of a stimulus that a person can detect or recognise. The detection threshold is the lowest concentration at which a stimulus is capable of producing a sensation, while the concentration at which the stimulus can be identified is called the recognition threshold. As described above, the recognition threshold is higher than the detection threshold. The difference threshold is the extent of change in the stimulus necessary to produce a noticeable difference. This has been labelled the JND for just noticeable difference.

These are not straightforward tests in olfaction, for the concentration of a molecule that actually reaches the olfactory receptors is a function not only of stimulus concentration, but also of solubility, volume, pressure and the respiratory cycle of the subject. In taste, saliva contains some sodium chloride, so the detection thresholds for salt will be elevated to just above the salivary concentration to which the panellist is adapted. Also, taste sensations are commonly confused at threshold levels.

Method of constant stimuli

The method of constant stimuli is the original measuring technique for thresholds. The panellist is presented with a series of randomised concentrations of flavour compounds ranging from imperceptible to clearly recognisable and the point at which the correct response is given on 75 per cent of the trials (i.e. halfway between the 50 per cent chance level and 100 per cent correct) is defined as the threshold. This approach suffers from the need for long times (at least several minutes) between sample presentations to ensure that adaptation effects have dissipated. With the requirement that there be several trials of each concentration, subject fatigue and boredom begin to influence the results. However, the method of constant stimuli retains the advantage of providing not just the threshold value, but also information about detection across a range of concentrations, so it is still used when time is not a factor.

Method of limits

The method of limits is in more common use today. The classic approach was to present alternating ascending and descending concentration series and to take the mean of the transition points as the detection threshold. However, concerns about adaptation during the descending series have led to its deletion from most procedures, leaving only an ascending method of limits. This is efficient, but leads to a slightly higher estimate of threshold, i.e. poorer sensitivity—than does either the fun method of limits or the method of constant stimuli.

Staircase method

The staircase method is a variant of the method of limits whereby an ascending series with large concentration jumps between steps is first given. This grossly determined threshold defines a tight concentration range to be explored intensively by either another ascending series (method of limits) or by a random presentation of concentrations (method of constant stimuli). Many passes may be made across this transition point while avoiding much of the adaptation that accompanies the higher concentrations. This two-stage method of first defining the approximate threshold, then focusing on a tight range around that point to provide greater definition, preserves the best features of both methods.

The approach for calculating the difference threshold (JND) is the same as the method of limits or the method of constant stimuli for determining detection or recognition thresholds, except that the comparison stimulus is an odourant rather than a blank. In sensory systems, the size of the change necessary for a JND is a constant proportion of the intensity from which that change is made. Thus, for example, a 10 decibel (db) tone may become perceptually louder when it is raised to 10.3 db, but a tone of 100 db must be raised to 103 db for a change to be detected. This is a statement of Weber's Law, which can be represented by equation 4.3,

$$\Delta I/I = K \qquad \qquad ... (4.3)$$

where, I is the original physical intensity, ΔI is the change necessary to elicit a JND and K is a constant.

In the example of auditory intensity above, $K = 0.03$ the smaller the value of K, the greater the discriminative capacity of the sensory system. Values of K for olfaction fall between 0.15 and 0.35. The ability of humans to detect changes in stimulus intensity is not as advanced in olfaction as in vision or audition, yet it is not as impoverished as is often supposed. Only a few specialists who evaluate cosmetics, perfumes or wines ever have this capacity challenged and so most people are unaware of their limits.

Flavour units

In a particular food, it is useful to determine the concentration of an odour or taste, even if the chemicals responsible for those perceptions are unknown. The inverse of the determined dilution that produced the threshold level can be used as a flavour unit; for example, a sample having a threshold flavour of 2 ppm would contain 5,00,000 flavour units. The Scoville Heat Unit is a flavour unit used in the food industry to provide a quantitative measure of how much chilli pepper, black pepper or ginger was added to foods.

Descriptive analysis

All descriptive analysis methods involve the identification, description and quantification of sensory aspects of a given product. They require trained personnel who are thoroughly familiar with the sensory attributes of the product being tested and who can accurately and precisely communicate their perceptions. The perceived sensory parameters which define the product are referred to by various terms such as attributes, characteristics, character notes, descriptive terms or descriptors. The choice of terminology for the sensory parameters is arbitrary, but must be agreed upon by all panellists during training sessions and applied in the same way during the testing. However, if the selected sensory attributes and corresponding definitions of these attributes can be related to the real chemical and physical properties of a product, the descriptive data are easier to interpret and more useful for decision-making.

The intensity or quantitative aspect of a descriptive analysis expresses the degree to which each of the characteristics is present by assigning some value along a measurement scale (category, line or ratio). The validity and reliability of intensity measurements are dependent upon the selection of a scaling technique that is broad enough to encompass the full range of parameter intensities, but which has enough discrete points to pick up all the small differences in intensity between samples. Thorough training of the panellists is necessary so that they use the scale in a similar way across all samples and across time.

Descriptive analysis should be used to:

1. Define the sensory properties of a target product for new product development.
2. Define the characteristics and specifications for a control or standard for quality assurance, quality control or research and development applications.
3. Document a product's attributes before a consumer test to help in the selection of attributes to be included in the questionnaire and to help in explanation of the results of the questionnaire.
4. Track a product's sensory changes over time with respect to understanding shelf-life problems.
5. Map a product's perceived attributes for the purpose of relating them to instrumental, chemical or physical properties.

There are three commonly used forms of descriptive analysis and listings of descriptive terms: flavour profile method, quantitative descriptive analysis and the spectrum method.

Flavour profile method

This method involves the analysis of a product's perceived flavour characteristics, their intensities, order of appearance and after-taste. Four to six trained judges are together in the same room, but individually evaluate one sample at a time and record their results. Additional samples can be evaluated in the same session, but samples are not tasted back and forth. The results are reported to the panel leader, who then leads a general discussion of the panel to arrive at a 'consensus' profile for each sample. The data are generally reported in tabular form, although a graphic representation is possible.

Quantitative descriptive analysis (QDA) method

In this method QDA panellists evaluate products one at a time in separate booths to reduce distraction and panellist interaction. The score-sheets are collected individually from the panellists and the data are entered into a computer. Panellists do not discuss data, terminology or samples after each taste session and must depend on the discretion of the panel leader for any information on their performance relative to other members of the panel and to any known differences between samples. The results of a QDA test are analysed statistically and the report generally contains graphic representation of the data in the form of a 'spider web' with a spoke for each attribute (Fig. 4.2).

Spectrum method

This is a custom design approach to panel development, selection, training and maintenance. The aim is to choose the most practical system given the product in question, the overall sensory programme, the specific project objective(s) in developing a panel and the desired level of statistical treatment of the data. The method requires that terminology used as descriptors be developed and derived by a panel which has been exposed to the underlying technical principles of each modality to be described. The panellists must demonstrate a valid response to changes in ingredients and processing by choosing terms (and concrete reference samples for these terms) for flavours that vary with these changes. For quantitative differences in a characteristic, the method requires at least two and preferably 3–5 reference points distributed across the range to anchor the scale (category, line or ratio) used. A set of well-chosen reference points greatly reduces panel variability, allowing for comparison of data across time and products. The basic philosophy of the spectrum method is to train the panel to define each product's sensory attributes fully, to rate the intensity of each and to include other relevant characteristics, such as changes over time, difference in the order of appearance of attributes and integrated total aroma and/or flavour impact.

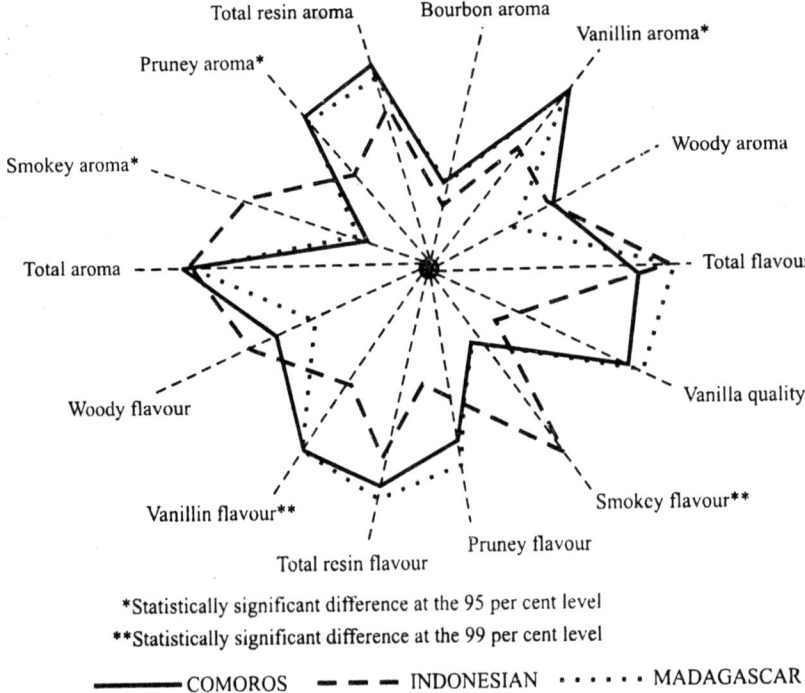

Total resin aroma Bourbon aroma Vanillin aroma*

Pruney aroma*

Woody aroma

Smokey aroma*

Total aroma

Total flavour

Woody flavour

Vanilla quality

Vanillin flavour**

Smokey flavour**

Total resin flavour Pruney flavour

*Statistically significant difference at the 95 per cent level

**Statistically significant difference at the 99 per cent level

———— COMOROS   — — — INDONESIAN   · · · · · · MADAGASCAR

Fig. 4.2. A circular graph illustrating sensory differences in vanilla from different regions.

Time-intensity techniques

As alluded to above, the perception of flavour occurs over real time: aroma, taste, texture and even thermal and pain sensations display dynamic changes in intensity over time. Most sensory analysis techniques have made the panellists estimate their responses before or after expectorating. But with the development of computers able to collect and process large amounts of data, important information such as the rate of onset of sensation, time and duration of maximum intensity and rate of decay of perceived intensity, time of extinction and total duration of the entire process can be made available. This increase in information has been useful in showing the time-intensity (T–I) differences in sweeteners judged to be identical in total intensity.

To the panellist, the test is rather enjoyable. Using a computer with a lever (joystick or mouse) that can go up and down on an intensity scale, the panellist simply pushes up or down as the sensation being measured increases or decreases, while the computer monitors the time axis. A push-button can be provided to indicate the exact occurrence of such things as swallowing and chewing.

Affective tests

Also called consumer testing, affective or hedonic tests are used to assess the personal response (preference and/or acceptance) by current or potential customers. Most people today have participated in some form of consumer tests.

Typically, a test involves 100 to 500 target consumers in three or four cities. Potential panellists are screened by telephone or in a shopping precinct. Those selected and willing are given samples, together with a score-card requesting their preferences and reasons for them, along with past buying habits, age, income, employment and ethnic background. Results are calculated in the form of preference scores overall and for various subgroups.

The most effective tests are based on protocols run among selected subjects of a target population that is anticipated to contain consumers of the specific products. The subjects or panellists are carefully selected to be representative of a larger population about which the investigator hopes to draw some conclusion. In the case of discrimination and descriptive tests, the investigator samples individuals with average or above-average abilities to detect differences. It is assumed that if these individuals cannot find a difference, the larger human population will be unable to detect it. In the case of affective tests, however, it is not sufficient merely to select from the general population. Instead, consumers of the type of product being tested must be recruited for the tests.

Consumer tests come in two forms. If a choice of one item over another is forced, then it is called a preference test. This test does not actually indicate whether any of the products are liked or disliked, only which is preferred; the researcher must have prior knowledge of the current or competitive product which is being tested against to make this judgement. In order to determine the 'affective status' of a product, one must perform an acceptance test, which is similar to attribute quantification in descriptive analysis except that the descriptor here is acceptance or liking. However, care must be exercised in the choice of questions asked and conclusions drawn, e.g. if one asks consumers if they like or dislike the sour taste, one does not know if they are also responding to their perception of bitter or astringent. Samples are usually rated along a hedonic category scale. Neither the numerical (linear) nor multiplicative (ratio) scale should be used, as they are too complicated for untrained consumers.

Instrumental Analysis

Wet chemistry

As instruments have been refined, the analytical field has been retreating from the isolation and purification of flavour compounds. However, wet chemistry is sometimes necessary for the unequivocal identification of the chemical structure of a flavour. Large sample sizes are needed because of the low concentration of a flavour compound in a food. Primary separations are usually done via the traditional partitioning scheme (Fig. 4.3) to separate acidic, basic and neutral flavour compounds from each other.

This is accomplished by varying the hydrogen ion concentration of the water. Acidic compounds are extracted into the aqueous phase at pH 9–10; basic compounds are extracted into the aqueous phase at pH 3–4. Then secondary separations are performed chromatographically, such as with GC, liquid chromatography (LC) or thin-layer chromatography (TLC) on a preparative scale. A tertiary separation would use distillation for liquids and crystallisation for solids. When isolated, the pure flavour compound is identified using at least two of the following techniques: mass spectrometry (MS), nuclear magnetic resonance (NMR), infrared (IR), ultraviolet-visible (UV/VIS) spectroscopies and elemental analysis.

Taking advantage of the chemical reactivity and differences in functional groups of the individual classes of flavour components, separations may also involve liquid/liquid extraction (e.g. acids and bases), derivative formation (e.g. 2,4-dinitrophenylhydrazones of carbonyls) or complex formation (e.g. heavy metal binding to sulphur compounds).

Once the compound has been isolated and identified, quantitative analysis is used to measure intrinsic properties that vary with concentration and also have a minimum of interferences from other compounds in the sample matrix.

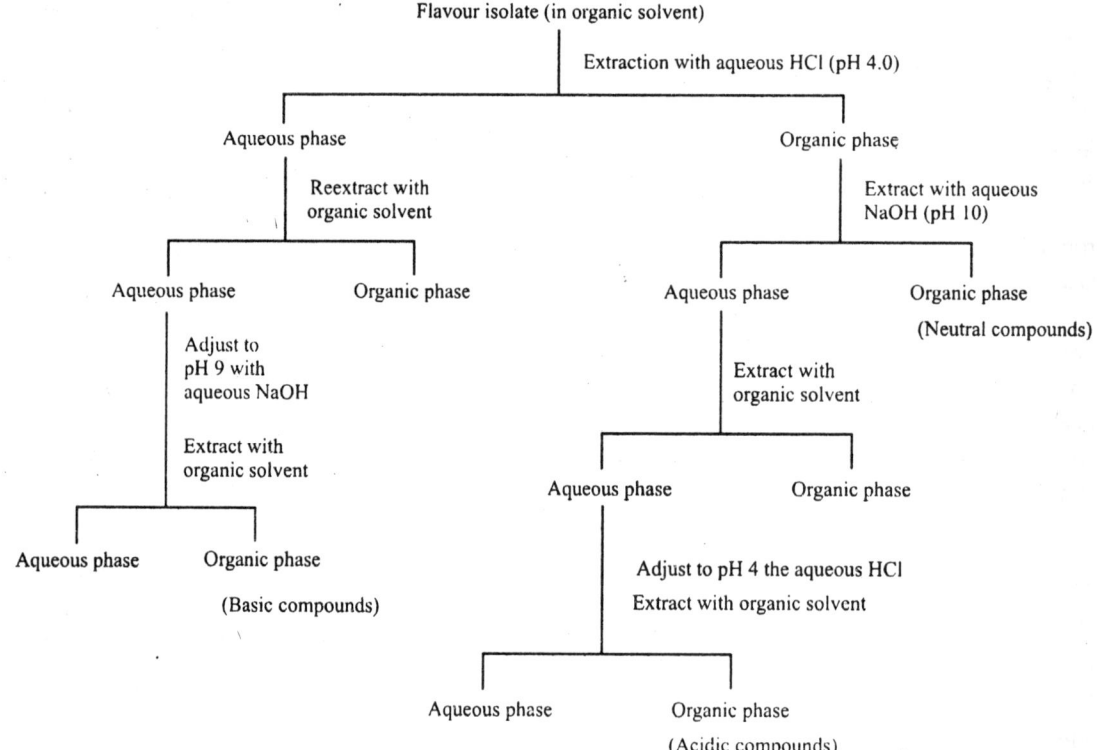

Fig. 4.3. Traditional liquid–liquid partitioning scheme for the separation of acidic, basic and neutral compounds.

Absorption spectroscopy (UV/VIS)

Absorption spectroscopy is based on the absorption of light at a specific wavelength in the ultraviolet (200–350 nm) or visible (350–700 nm) region of the electromagnetic spectrum. In order to determine the concentration of analyte in a given sample solution, the amount of light absorbed from a reference beam of light passing through the sample solution is measured. If the compound naturally absorbs the radiation, it is measured directly. When the analyte does not absorb radiation of the appropriate wavelength, it can be chemically modified during the analysis to convert it into a species that absorbs the appropriate radiation; this is called derivatisation. In either case, the presence of analyte in the solution will affect the amount of radiation transmitted through the solution. Therefore, the relative transmittance, with and without the sample, may be used as an index of analyte concentration.

Absorption spectroscopy is a quick and easy means of analysing many flavours, as long as the sample is a liquid, translucent and not very complex. However, many foods are solid, opaque and chemically complex. When absorption spectroscopy is not appropriate, then a form of chromatography is usually used.

Chromatography

Chromatography is a general term applied to a wide variety of separation techniques based on the partitioning or distribution of a sample (solute) between a moving (mobile) phase and a fixed or stationary phase. It can be viewed as a series of equilibrations between the mobile and stationary phases. In Gas chromatography (GC), the mobile phase is a gas that flows through the stationary phase, which could be a solid or a liquid coated onto a solid matrix. The separation of compounds is determined by the relative rate of the reversible absorption or volatilisation of the solutes into and out of the stationary phase. In high-performance liquid chromatography (HPLC), the mobile phase is a liquid that flows through the stationary phase and the separation of compounds is determined by the relative solubility of the solutes in the two phases. In ion-exchange chromatography (IEC), the mobile phase is usually water that flows through a charged stationary phase and separation is achieved for ionic solutes that bind with the stationary phase. Supercritical-fluid chromatography (SFC) uses CO_2 as the mobile-phase gas which, under pressure, is in its supercritical state, in which the CO_2 has characteristics of both a liquid and a gas. Both stationary phases for GC and HPLC have been employed for SFC.

Volatile flavour compounds are usually analysed by GC and those that are non-volatile by HPLC. Since only ionic species are separated by IEC, it is used to separate organic acids and salts. Volatile flavours found in fats and oils can be measured directly by SFC, as lipids are soluble in supercritical CO_2 and do not foul a column as they do in GC.

Gas chromatography

Since only volatile flavour compounds move in the mobile phase, any non-volatile compounds must be removed before injection, because columns are destroyed by lipids, carbohydrates, proteins and minerals found in most foods. Sample preparation may involve headspace analysis, distillation, preparative chromatography, solvent extraction or a combination of these techniques. Care must be taken during sample preparation to ensure that flavour compounds are not formed or degraded (transformed). In most GC instruments, a liquid sample is injected onto a heating block that volatilises the solutes into the mobile phase. Even if artefacts are not developed during sample preparation, they can be formed in the injection port. For example, it has been shown only recently that onion and garlic flavour compounds cannot withstand the normal temperatures in the injection port.

Originally, GCs utilised packed columns for the stationary phase. However, in the early 1980s, capillary columns were developed that improved resolution and used less sample. Today, packed GC columns are used for preparative-scale separations, whereas capillary columns are used for analyses. There are four main types of columns in use today: non-polar (OV-1, SE-30), intermediate polarity (OV-17, OV-225), polar (carbowax) and chiral (cyclodextrin). Stationary phase selection involves both intuition and knowledge of chemistry and help with both can be obtained from the column manufacturer and the literature. However, selecting the best stationary phase is not as necessary as it once was, since the high efficiency of capillary columns often results in separations even when the phase selectivity is not optimal.

Numerous detectors are available for GC, each one offering advantages in either sensitivity or selectivity. The most common detectors are flame ionisation (FID), thermal conductivity (TCD), electron capture (ECD), flame photometric (FPD) and photoionisation (PID). Detectors with limited applications are nitrogen-phosphorus (NPD) and electron laser capture (ELCD). One can even use the human nose as the detector; a hand-made funnel, called a sniffer port, can be attached to the GC. The commercially available unit has been christened CHARM (combined hedonic and response measurements) analysis.

Hyphenated GC techniques are those that combine GC with another major technique; these include Fourier transform infrared (GC-FTIR), mass spectroscopy (GC-MS) and atomic emission spectroscopy (GC-AES). These hyphenated techniques allow compound identification as well as quantification and are rapidly replacing wet chemical methods for identifying the flavour molecules.

High performance liquid chromatography

HPLC can be used to analyse for any compound that is soluble in the mobile phase. However, because it takes longer and the peaks are broader than GC, volatile compounds are not usually analysed by HPLC. Since more compounds are soluble in a liquid mobile phase, sample preparation is not as rigorous for HPLC. Many times, the food sample can simply be extracted with an organic solvent, diluted with the mobile phase, filtered and shot on the column. As long as a guard column, which can be changed often to remove irreversibly adsorbed material, is attached in front of the analytical column, destruction of the column is minimal. However, the more complex the sample matrix, the harder the chromatography becomes. Thus, it is common to perform a sample clean up using small disposable chromatographic columns prior to the HPLC analysis.

There are two common types of HPLC columns: normal phase and reverse phase. In normal phase chromatography, the stationary phase is polar (silica gel) and the mobile phase is non-polar (organic solvents). In reversed-phase chromatography, the stationary phase is non-polar (C-18, C-8) and the mobile phase is polar [water, CH_3OH, CH_3CN, tetrahydrofuran (THF)]. There are also special columns available with intermediate polarity for rare problems (amine, diol, phenyl) and cyclodextrin for chiral separations.

The workhorse of HPLC detectors is the UV/VIS detector set at a specific wavelength. However, it must be remembered that each individual analyte will have different chromophores and thus absorb different amounts of light at different wavelengths. This means that when developing a new HPLC analysis, it is necessary to isolate and purify enough of a flavour compound to determine the relative response of the detector compared to the standard (either internal or external) before quantitative estimates can be made. A fluorescent detector is more sensitive than UV/VIS, but few flavour compounds possess the ability to emit electromagnetic radiation.

Considered the universal detector, refractive index (RI) measures all compounds that possess a different ability than the solvent to bend light. This type of detection yields both positive and negative peaks and is not as sensitive as most other methods of detection. This frail detector also suffers from temperature and flow-rate variations and cannot be used with gradient elution. But detection by RI is used for sugars, since they are non-volatile and do not contain a chromophore.

Another universal detector uses IR spectroscopy, but this technique is used more for the identification of compound classes than for quantitative analysis.

Electrochemical methods are also utilised for HPLC detection. Measuring the change in current as the analyte is oxidised or reduced, amperometric detectors are very selective and sensitive, especially when the current comes in pulses.

Ion exchange chromatography

This is actually a special case of HPLC, utilising the same physical system of pumps and tubing. In this case, buffered water is used and the pH or ionic strength of the water can be varied for gradient elution. The column is usually charged positive or negative (SO_3^-, NR_3^+) and ions such as salts and acids are separated. A conductivity detector is used to measure the current that can flow through the mobile phase after it leaves the column to establish when ions are coming off the column.

Supercritical fluid chromatography

Supercritical fluid chromatography (SFC) is a relatively new technique that is a hybrid between GC and HPLC. This system can use either GC or HPLC columns and detectors. However, most systems use a GC oven for temperature control and an FID detector with either an HPLC column (packed) or a GC-type capillary column. The FID detector must be modified from those used in GC, as the CO_2 mobile phase acts as a fire extinguisher. Since the chromatography produces peaks that are broader than GC, but not as broad as HPLC, SFC is not used when a sample can be analysed by GC.

Non-volatile polar compounds are not soluble in supercritical CO_2, so they cannot be analysed by SFC and if injected into the system will foul the column. Small amounts of methanol can be added to the mobile phase to increase the solubility of polar substances in supercritical CO_2, but the methanol interferes with FID detection, so a UV/VIS detector is usually used. The best use of SFC using FID detection is for flavour compounds that do not contain a chromophore, but are in a lipid matrix.

Hyphenated techniques

As foods are so complex, with many compounds not separating well using just one technique, pre-purification is often necessary. Simply separating a complex mixture by GC, HPLC or SFC may give overlapping peaks that cannot be resolved well. The column and/or mobile phase can then be changed, which changes the partitioning efficiencies, to remove interfering compounds.

Heart-cutting is when two GCs are hooked up together (GC-GC) and a portion of the eluent from the first GC is placed onto the second GC. This has usually been done with a packed column on the first GC and a capillary column on the second GC because of sample sizes.

HPLC-GC is a technique where a fraction collected from an HPLC containing volatile compounds is injected into the GC.

There are commercial units today that combine supercritical CO_2 extraction with automatic injection into a GC. This is not SFC-GC, because no chromatography is performed prior to injection onto the GC. Because most nonpolar compounds and high molecular weight polymers, like proteins and complex carbohydrates, do not dissolve in supercritical CO_2, this is an efficient method to clean up a sample with minimum effort. However, problems can occur with fatty foods if pressures are too high; lipids are extracted and can foul the GC column.

The hyphenated techniques allow compound identification as well as quantification and are rapidly replacing wet chemical methods for identifying the chemical structures of flavour molecules such as GC-MS, GC-FTIR and HPLC-MS.

Sample Handling and Artefacts

Sample selection

The first step in any analysis is to select the samples to be analysed, which may not be as straightforward as it seems. Sample selection depends first on what the problem is that the analysis is to solve. If one is trying to control the quality of a food product, then a representative sample is absolutely necessary; however, if one is trying to identify a flavour or off-flavour, then the strongest flavoured samples need to be selected. Using the most intense samples will increase the probability that relatively insensitive machines can pick out the compounds of interest. One must also think of the resources available. How accessible are the most ideal samples? Are they available only once or do they occur seasonally or on a routine basis? How much is available? How perishable are they? What is the required turnaround time? Are samples going to be pooled or replicated? Do different portions need different analyses? For example, the surface versus the bulk of a prepared steak contains very different flavour compounds. One of the most important things to consider is how to monitor samples in order to detect and prevent contamination and abuse. Although we can simply put a piece of bread or hot sauce into our mouths and obtain a sensory response, a desirable instrumental response occurs only after the flavour compounds have been extracted from the food, concentrated and placed into the instrument.

Homogenisation

Particle size reduction of a food is usually the first step in extracting flavour. For sensory analyses, the food is cut and chewed well. For instrumental analyses, this is generally accomplished by grinding (dry sample), cutting or slicing (whole foods), shearing or blending (wet samples) or shattering (seeds). Particle size distributions can be observed by sieving (dry samples) or microscopy (wet and dry samples).

Mixing

Only a portion of a sample is actually analysed instrumentally. If the food sample is not well mixed before that portion is removed then the analysis may vary with each portion. Problems to overcome include classification, stratification, phase separation and agglomeration. In heterogeneous samples, such as foods, different particles contain different amounts of flavourants. For example, essential oils in citrus fruits are mainly in cells of the flavedo layer. If the particles differ in shape and size, they can separate during manipulations. This is especially true when the particles are also different in density, electrostatic charge or surface tension. The flavourants can be encapsulated in structures or entrapped by hydrophobic-hydrophilic interactions.

Sample preparation

Sample preparation includes any operation performed on the test portion prior to analysis. Problems to guard against are moisture variations during weighing, incomplete dissolution of the attribute or sample during dilutions and volume changes with temperature fluctuations. Also, since the methodology used for 'clean-up' greatly influences a flavour profile, one needs to determine why the clean-up step is there, how it works and what it does to the sample.

Most fresh plant and animal tissues contain active enzyme systems that, once cell walls are disrupted, quickly alter the flavour profile. Thus, the rapid inactivation of enzymes during sample preparation is essential, but one must be aware of the artefacts or interferences contributed by means of enzyme inactivation. Commonly, thermal processes are used to inactivate enzymes. However, this may result in the loss of unstable or volatile flavour compounds. Homogenising the food in methanol avoids this problem, but it may interfere with isolation by decreasing the polarity of the aqueous food slurry and forming methyl ester artefacts. Enzymes can also be inactivated with the use of heavy metal salts containing Cu^{2+}, though this metallic ion can catalyse lipid oxidation. So far, no obvious disadvantage to the isolation of flavour compounds has been found when foods containing enzymes are treated with high concentrations of neutral salts, such as an equal volume of saturated $CaCl_2$ solution, to inactivate them.

Sometimes enzymes are added or activated to help in the analysis of food samples. Carbohydrases and proteases are often added to digest the foods, so the compounds of interest are more easily freed from the sample. However, during this digestion, many of the flavour compounds can also be transformed. Thus, digestion is not recommended for flavour analysis. Long isolation procedures may permit fermentation to occur. Anti-microbial agents are sometimes added to control this.

Besides enzymatic and microbially induced changes in flavour profile, chemical changes can also occur. It is common practice to add antioxidants or prepare the sample under N_2 or CO_2 to avoid oxidation. High temperatures (> 60°C) for extended periods can promote Maillard browning reactions. Thus, reduced temperatures during sample preparation are recommended.

Since flavours occur at such low concentrations, contamination of the test portion before analysis is a real problem. Most food is now packaged and handled with plastic containers; small amounts of plasticisers can migrate into the foods and be detected by GC-MS.

Isolation and concentration

Direct analysis of the headspace vapours above a food product is the ideal method to isolate flavours, but the primary problem is the low concentration of flavour compounds in the headspace. Headspace analysis has found substantial application in flavour studies where trace analysis is not necessary.

Purge and trap

The equilibrium headspace vapours above a solid food or the food itself may be purged with an inert gas in order to obtain a large volume of headspace gas for analysis. The flavour compounds are then concentrated using cryogenic traps or adsorption columns. The problem with cryogenic traps is that the most abundant volatile in foods is water, so an additional step is generally needed to extract the flavour constituents from the water. Volatile flavours are often trapped on adsorbent materials to avoid this co-condensation of water. If the adsorbent has a minimal affinity for water, this eliminates the need for solvent extraction and the associated problems. Typical adsorbents used are charcoal (activated carbon), Porapak Q (polymer of ethyl vinyl-divinyl benzene), Tenax GC (polymer of diphenyl-phenylene oxide), XAD resins (polymers of divinyl styrene, acrylic ester or sulphoxide).

Distillation

Distillation is a rather broad term that includes any technique that vapourises a liquid mixture through the addition of heat and subsequently collects the vapours by removal of the heat. It takes advantage of the difference between the volatility of flavour components and the non-volatility of the major food constituents. A simple distillation is not usually used in flavour analysis because of the small concentration of flavour components and their delicate nature. Rather, extra water is added to the food sample to lower the boiling points of the flavour compounds and help carry them out into the collection vessel. This technique, called hydrodistillation, utilises co-distillation of water to transfer the flavour volatiles into the distillation head. Steam distillation is when the water is added to the food sample continuously in the form of steam. The distillate is a very dilute solution of volatile flavours and water which must be extracted with an organic solvent and the solvent dried (e.g. anhydrous $MgSO_4$) and concentrated before analysis can be performed. The distillation can be performed directly into a solvent trap to help speed the extraction step.

Likens and Nickerson developed a method that combines both the distillation and extraction steps, called simultaneous distillation/extraction (SDE). As shown in Fig. 4.4, distilling the extracting solvent during the collection of the primary aqueous distillate allows for a very efficient flavour extraction. However, this extended heat treatment may be deleterious to some of the unstable flavour compounds.

Vacuum distillation is another way to lower the boiling points of flavour compounds; the distillation is performed under reduced pressure. When a very high vacuum is used, this is called molecular distillation. Usually utilised in high fat and/or low particulate samples, the vacuum requirements limit this method to food samples containing essentially no water. For molecules to volatilise out of a liquid food matrix efficiently, they must be spread out in a thin film to increase the surface area of the liquid-gas interface, so very short distances must be provided between the condenser surface and the thin film of food. This can be accomplished with two very different designs: (i) falling film, and (ii) spinning disk. In falling film, the lipid rich sample is dripped onto the inside surface of a pipe heated from the outside by rotating wipers that keep the food matrix in a thin film. As the film falls, volatile molecules escape and are collected on a condenser that is found in the centre of the pipe. With spinning disk, the lipid-rich sample is dripped onto the centre of a tilted rotating circle that is in close proximity to a flat circular surface cooled with water (condenser). The speed of the rotation and the viscosity of the sample control how thin the film will be on the surface of the disk. As the sample migrates to the outside of the circle, flavour molecules escape to be collected off the flat condenser. A significant advantage of molecular distillation is the decreased opportunity for artefact formation or contamination.

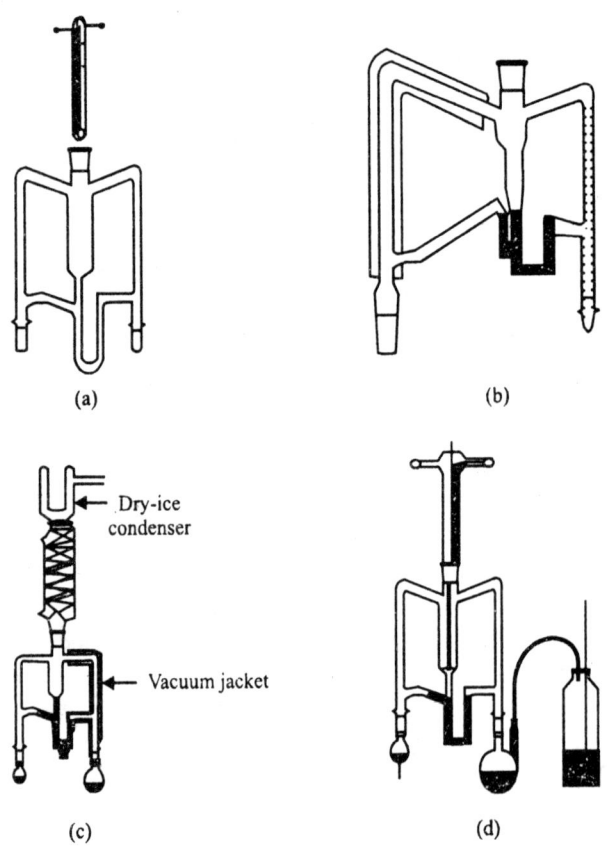

Fig. 4.4. Various Likens and Nickerson devices for the isolation of volatiles by simultaneous steam distillation extraction: (a) original apparatus, (b) modification includes a solvent arm with Vigreux indentations and an insolated solvent arm, suitable for extraction with heavy solvents, (c) modification with vacuum jacket to minimise premature condensation and dry-ice condensor to reduce volatilisation losses, and (d) modification where steam is generated in a separate vessel.

Extraction

Most flavour compounds exhibit substantial solubility in organic solvents, but unfortunately lipids are also soluble in organic solvents. Therefore, in high-fat foods, the solvent extract (fats and flavours) may need to be treated further by steam distillation, molecular distillation, chromatography, dialysis or liquid CO_2 to separate the flavours from the fats. Thus, solvent extraction is best performed on fat-free foods, such as alcoholic beverages, fat-free bakery products, fruit or berry juices and some vegetables. If the food sample is dry, simple percolation through a column works well. To reduce solvent use, it can be recycled via distillation through a Soxhlet apparatus. For liquid food samples, the simplest method is batch extraction using separatory funnels.

The major problem with batch solvent extraction is emulsion formation in the separatory funnel. Emulsions may be broken by the use of centrifugation, addition of a saturated NaCl solution, slow stirring or pH adjustment. Bath solvent extraction is also tedious and labour intensive. Continuous liquid/liquid extraction generally provides more efficient extraction and reduced labour requirements, but at a greater cost in equipment and time.

When CO_2 is liquified under pressure, it is a useful nonpolar solvent. Liquid CO_2 is used to separate volatile flavour compounds from high-fat foods, as it does not extract lipids very well. Liquid CO_2 has also been used to separate the polar and nonpolar constituents of orange oil.

In the presence of water, liquid CO_2 contains a small amount of carbonic acid: $H_2O + CO_2 \rightarrow H_2CO_3$; thus its nonpolar solvent properties are modified to provide some polar character. As pressure is increased, more carbonic acid is formed. Above a pressure of 73 bar and temperature of 31°C, CO_2 becomes supercritical, in which state it becomes a better solvent, holding a much higher concentration of compounds. The solute load of CO_2 can be controlled; the lower the temperature and the higher the pressure, the more soluble polar compounds become. Supercritical extraction (SCE) units fit on GC instruments which perform extraction and analysis of solid food samples automatically.

Dialysis

This technique is good for small molecules in fat samples, such as in the isolation of cheddar cheese flavour. A membrane is used to hold back the large triglycerides and allow the small flavour molecules to pass. However, recovery of flavour molecules decreases rapidly as the molecular size of the sample increases.

Derivatisation

Chemically modifying flavour compounds offers several advantages. Usually the derivative imparts UV-absorbing properties, which thus aids in HPLC analysis using UV detection. Many unstable and highly volatile flavour compounds become stable and non-volatile upon derivatisation. Because derivatives are specific to a functional group, this greatly simplifies the problems of separation and detection.

Concentration

Most of the extraction and isolation methods produce a dilute solution of volatiles that needs to be concentrated for analysis. Evaporation is typically used for flavour isolates in organic solvents and takes advantage of the differences in boiling points between the flavour compounds and solvent. A disadvantage of evaporative techniques is that flavour compounds may be lost by codistillation. Since flavour isolates typically contain water from the food product, care must be taken to remove water prior to concentration to prevent steam distillation and substantial flavour loss.

Flavours can also be adsorbed from dilute aqueous solutions by charcoal, silica gel, alumina, porous polymers and other adsorbents. Typically, an aqueous distillate is passed through a column of adsorbent; the adsorbent is rinsed with water and then eluted with an organic solvent. These same adsorbents are used to concentrate the dilute flavour volatiles in a gas (e.g. headspace).

Data Handling

Design of experiments

When should the various tests be used? This depends upon the objective of the experiments. If quality control is being performed on a product that should not change, then a simple triangle test may suffice. If a new product is being developed and the origin of an off-flavour needs to be known, then both sensory and instrumental tests are needed. Sometimes instrumental analysis of a nonflavoured compound in a food can be used to assess the status of a flavour; for example, both pentane and hexanal have been used as indices of the oxidative flavour deterioration of fats in foods. However, the essentially odourless pentane seems to provide a better index of the actual flavour intensity than does hexanal, which definitely contributes to the flavour. So the best advice is to determine objectives before performing any type of analysis for flavours.

There has been a consistent desire of analytical chemists to equate 'subjective' with sensory and 'objective' with instrumental analysis. However, if the instrumental method is not truly measuring the total flavour, then it may not be helpful to solve the flavour objective of one's experiment. Sensory data have become much more objective as we find ways to permit people to respond in a consistent and predictable manner. A panel of selected and trained people can consistently and quantitatively measure differences that we cannot measure instrumentally. Sensory and instrumental analyses may be correlated in one of two ways. The instrumental information may merely reflect the status of the flavour, such as in the example above of using pentane to determine the extent of lipid oxidation, or it may be analysed to identify the actual compounds that contribute to the flavour.

Chemometrics

Flavour changes frequently result from subtle alterations in many components, rather than drastic changes in a few, so analysis of one variable at a time is not normally sufficient. Chemometrics uses multivariate statistics to determine the correlation between sensory and instrumental analyses. Treating two or more variables simultaneously requires the use of matrix algebra, vectors, eigenvectors and eigenvalues. Techniques such as nearest-neighbour analysis can serve to classify unknown samples if there are samples available from each known category. Techniques such as clique analysis and multidimensional scaling can suggest categories when researchers do not know beforehand what categories exist. Factor analysis can provide clues to unknown underlying variables. Reducing the number of variables is often accomplished by principal-components analysis, which reduces the variability in a limited number of variables and discriminant analysis, which focuses on combinations of variables that distinguish among categories.

Artificial neural networks can be used to train a computer to recognise a pattern, evaluate a new unknown sample and place it within one of previously determined categories. As computers increase in speed and memory, artificial neural networks can be connected to sensor arrays to mimic the human nose.

Electronic nose

A commercial product, AromaScan, emulates the human nose. It is based on an array of sensors that are formed from electrically conducting organic polymers. The sensors function by the adsorption of volatile chemicals onto the polymer surface causing a change in electrical resistance. The extent of this change depends on the chemical compositions of the aroma and the physical and chemical structure of the polymer. The sensor array produces signals which are digitised and processed via computer to produce a distinctive and unique pattern of response for the sampled aroma. When combined with a neural network, this instrument can be taught to recognise the pattern or an aroma of a product. Because both adsorption and desorption of volatiles at the polymer surfaces are quick and all the sensors operate simultaneously, this can be used in quality control or quality assurance programmes as the first line of defence for routine analysis. Thus, only the samples with an identified divergence from acceptable aroma variations need to be analysed further.

Correlations with instrumental and sensory techniques

There is no direct correlation of this new instrumental technique with current instrumental methods. Since a single compound produces a signal in many sensors and a single sensor has a broad sensitivity to different compounds, the identification of specific volatile compounds still needs to be performed via chromatographic methods.

As this instrument is emulating the human nose, it correlates fairly well with sensory panels doing difference testing when the neural network is trained with many samples that contain the variations found acceptable and unacceptable to the sensory panels. As the sensitivity of sensors to specific compounds may be larger or smaller than that of the human nose, there are cases where complete correlations will be impossible using the current commercially available sensor array. In these cases, the conducting polymers on the sensor array may need to be custom developed for such specific applications.

ANALYTICAL METHODS

The analytical methods used for quality assurance of flavours and fragrances can be grouped as physico-chemical, instrumental and sensory analysis.

Physico-chemical Methods

Specific gravity, refractive index, melting or congealing-point, and optical rotation are the physical properties measured to evaluate the specifications for raw materials and intermediates, as applicable.

Many spices are processed to produce essential oils, oleoresins, essences, extracts, resinoids, etc. In addition to subjective physical observation, macroscopic and microscopic examination of the spice is the criterion for the continued analysis of the product to determine adherence to specifications. The American spice trade association (ASTA) has developed a series of official analytical methods which includes sections on general methods and methods for specific spices. General methods include preparation of sample, moisture by distillation and drying, total ash and acid-insoluble ash, steam-volatile oil by modified Clevenger of Lee and Ogg methods, alcohol extract, sieve analysis and nonvolatile methylene chloride extract. ASTA has also made available a manual of microbiological methods for the detection and enumeration of micro-organisms occurring in spices. FDA has published methods for the determination of residual solvents in spice extracts.

Chemical analysis is carried out only if it is necessary, as this requires much more time in comparison with the other methods. Despite impressive data available on the chemical composition of food flavours, there is still a lack of complete understanding of what determines the flavour of many foods. Establishing the chemical composition and structure of flavour compounds found in food is, however, important for correlating structures to sensory properties and for understanding the mechanism by which flavours are formed by their precursors.

Instrumental Methods

The complexity of natural products requires the use of separation techniques having the highest available resolution, such as gas and liquid chromatography. In addition to high resolution, the most sensitive analytical techniques such as mass spectroscopy must be used to detect the highly potent trace components. Major advances in both gas chromatography (GC) and mass spectrometry (MS) have increased the capability of acquisition of useful mass spectral data from the narrowest of GC peaks. Some of these advances are the introduction of inert thermo-stable capillary columns, gentle, non-vapourising on-column injection methods, improved interfaces between GC and MS for spectral acquisition, storage-data manipulation, and library search.

Gas-liquid chromatography is the essential tool for the investigation of fragrant materials because such materials must exhibit some degree of volatility in order to be perceived. The fused-silica capillary columns, are the mainstay of the analytical techniques. Gas chromatography is coupled with mass spectrometry to obtain chemical structural information on the hundreds of materials that may be present in a complex mixture. Advances in computer technology for acquiring, sorting and interpreting molecular fragmentation data from GC/MS runs make it possible to perform thorough analyses with remarkable speed. In cases not readily identifiable from mass spectra alone, gas chromatography coupled with infra-red spectroscopy (GC/IR) is applied. The infra-red spectra are recorded in the vapour phase by Fourier transform methodology. Those components that resist identification by the above techniques are isolated and analysed by nuclear magnetic resonance (NMR).

The analysis of flavours and fragrances involves:

1. Sample preparation (for total volatile analysis, or head-space analysis, which aims at analysis of volatile compounds found at equilibrium in the vapour space above the food).
2. Fractionation of the sample by column chromatography using silica gel.
3. Analysis by the use of GC/MS.

Head-space analysis technique, which was prevalent to investigate the top notes (the most volatile part of essential oils and other naturals) has been applied directly to flowers and other parts of plants. It has been found that this technique can be applied in these cases without removing them from the living plant. This approach has indicated that there are wide differences in the volatile compositions in live and picked flowers. Reconstitution of the analytical data generated this way has provided perfume manufacturers with novel and fresh notes for use in their creations. The head-space technique is applied to many kinds and varieties of flowers, herbs, spices, and fruits.

Since the early 1980s gas chromatography-olfactometry (GCO) has emerged as a quantitative method for the characterisation of odour and aroma. Quantitative-GCO is exemplified by aroma extraction dilution analysis (AEDA) in which chromatograms of a series of dilutions are recorded separately. As each diluted extract eluting from the gas chromatograph is sniffed, the weaker odours drop below the threshold and cannot be detected. The quantitative bioassay data produced by GCO indicate the relative potency of odourants in a complex mixture. While most of the earlier methods involved the scaling of perceived intensity, a most developed method of this type, called Osme, is based on the computerised recording of lever position matched with perception of intensity. The GCO technique is used to focus analytical chemistry on the most odour-potent components of complex foods.

Charm analysis (CA) is a proprietary GCO system developed in the Flavour Chemistry Laboratory at the New York State Agricultural Experiment Station in Geneva, part of the Cornell College of Agriculture. Gas chromatography (GC) is used to separate the flavour component, and a trained flavourist sniffs the effluent of the GC to describe the aroma peak. Charm analysis offers a high-resolution GCO and complementary software, called Charmware. The software takes advantage of a database of flavour compounds, known as Flavournet, compiled from GCO, AEDA and other methods that have detected odourants.

Sensory Analysis

Sensory evaluation as part of the quality-control process has many facets, but if implemented correctly, can be an invaluable part of a company's overall agenda for producing quality food products and perfumes. Many companies have been using human sensory panels to assess the aroma quality of their products. Sensory analysis is concerned with the similarities in human flavour perception using methods that are designed to average out certain differences and to detect others. A panel (group of persons) tastes or smells the same material and reports their perceptions according to set guidelines. Using statistical methods, the similarities in the perceptions of the panel members are isolated. Sensory analysis requires much time to design, execute, and analyse, and is therefore expensive. Consequently, less labour-intensive instrumental procedures are preferred. However, the results from instrumental techniques are indirect and their accuracy must be established using different sensory methods.

Companies need tools that provide the following:

1. Simple and reliable results in seconds.
2. Immediate decisions at the point of production.
3. Reduce turnaround.
4. Overcome analytical bottlenecks.
5. Avoid subjective measurement and provide objective data.

Today, many industries rely on human panels or on analytical techniques (e.g. gas chromatography or liquid chromatography) to evaluate products whose odour or taste characteristics are key to customer acceptance. Both methodologies have shown some major drawbacks:

1. Human sensorial methods are amazingly accurate but people fatigue easily and are somewhat subjective in their evaluation. They are not always as consistent as one would like and transferability from one person to another is extremely difficult.
2. More classical techniques such as chromatography are precise and objective, but relate only to specific parts of the smell or taste and not always to the parts considered most significant by the human senses. Moreover, they need skilled people for the interpretation of the data.

To overcome these main drawbacks, smart sensing technologies are considered to be a viable alternative to routinely distinguish differences, predict acceptability of odours and volatile organic compounds (VOC) from a large range of raw materials, intermediates and finished products. A smart sensing system can be an array of gas or liquid sensors or a fingerprint mass spectrometer that creates an electronic fingerprint from the smell or taste of the product.

Gas sensor arrays (electronic nose and electronic tongue)

These provide either a simple answer like 'recognised', 'good', or 'bad', or a more sophisticated response such as odour intensity or a molecule concentration. The terminology can be simple and qualitative or more specific and quantitative.

The arrays are non-specific electrochemical devices. They are of three categories, namely,

1. Metal oxide sensor.
2. Conducting polymer sensor.
3. Quartz crystal micro-balance.

Metal oxide sensors operate at around 400°C. Oxygen in the air reacts with lattice vacancies and removes electrons from the conducting band. Odour molecules react irreversibly with the oxygen species, liberating electrons and lowering the measured resistance of the sensor. The metal oxide sensors are inorganic in nature. Conducting polymer sensors are made of pyrrole, indole, or derivatives of similar materials, electrochemically deposited on a silicon substrate. They tend to swell in the presence of odours and thus change resistance. Conductive polymers are very responsive to polar molecules, thus making them complementary to the function of metal oxides. They operate at room temperature and display rapidly, reversible reactions leading to rapid discrimination. These sensors of organic nature, however, are susceptible to moisture and humidity as also are three orders of magnitude less sensitive than metal oxide sensors.

Quartz crystal micro-balance is a device wherein the sensor element is a quartz resonator coated with an organic material similar to the stationary phase of a gas chromatographic column. The resonant frequency of the sensor changes as aromas adsorb and desorb from the coating, changing the mass of the resonator, and hence its frequency. The lifetime and drift of these sensors depend on the organic interface. The three basic steps in creating a digital fingerprint of odour/taste are sample preparation, sensory detection, data analysis, and pattern recognition. The sample preparation involves its heating in a vial for a precise interval at a fixed temperature, and injecting the volatile matter in the head-space into a carrier gas (air) of the instrument. All these steps are automatically performed in the commercially available sensory equipment.

Fingerprint mass spectrometry

The quadrupole instruments for electronic olfaction, sometimes called fingerprint mass spectrometry are similar in design to that technology used for GC/MS. The only difference is in the absence of the GC module used to separate the volatile molecules before the detection by the MS. In fingerprint mass spectrometry, the entire aroma enters the quadrupole module without separation. The resulting fingerprint is from the entire, ensemble aroma just as it is presented to a human being.

The sensory technologies are used at different levels in the food, cosmetics and packaging industries, either for research and development, or quality control and process control. In the latter, applications are in the crop-growing stage (to test the maturity, contamination of moulds, parasites), harvesting, the reception of incoming raw materials, process control, finished product inspection, and testing for tainting of the product by packaging. Applications also exist at the distribution level, to check that products received conform to specifications. Typical applications of the electronic nose are the following:

1. Discrimination between single volatile compounds.
2. Tracking of the aroma evolution of ice stored fish or meat.
3. Tracking of the evolution of cheese aroma during the ageing process.
4. Classification of wines produced under the same denomination (in order to find out those productions not fitting with the standard).
5. Classify different varieties of peaches.
6. Classify different ripeness degrees of apples.
7. Classify olive oils according to their country of production.

Fragrance and Sensitivity

Consumers' fascination has increased with the manufacture of a multitude of scented personal products (colognes, perfumes, shampoos, conditioners, hair-spray, shaving cream, make-up, baby-care products, deodourants, soap, feminine products, etc.) and household products (cleaners, air-fresheners, bleach, laundry detergents, fabric softeners, etc.). Furthermore, scents are now added to a number of other commercial products such as tissues, candles, and diapers. Perfumes have made their way into mailboxes, many magazines carry a perfume strip advertisement, and scented stationary are used by some companies for mass mailings. Trash bags and even flowerpots now come in scented versions. The fragrance of a product has become its main selling feature and whole advertising campaigns are built around the odour of a product. Not only many of the products we use are scented, but also there are a number of scents from which to choose. The trend also has been towards more powerful and long lasting fragrances.

According to the 'Fragrance Foundation', a non-profit educational arm of the fragrance industry, there are more than thousand body fragrances alone in the market today. While many people enjoy wearing perfumes and using scented products, some being carried away by the variety of related advertisements, there is a growing outcry from some people who claim that exposure to some perfumes and scented products adversely impacts health. Symptoms experienced by some people include headache (especially migraine), sneezing, watery eyes, sinus problems, anxiety, nausea, wheezing (especially in asthmatics), shortness of breath, inability to concentrate, brainfog, dizziness, convulsions, sore throat, cough, chest tightness, hyperactivity (especially in children), tremor, fatigue, lethargy, and drowsiness. People, who suffer from multiple chemical sensitivity (MCS), a health condition in which exposure to one chemical is thought to lead to adverse reactions to others, claim that exposure to fragrance triggers various symptoms. Often this is to the point that sufferers become incapicitated or must forego many of their usual activities to avoid exposure.

Problems with fragrances

The problems that are considered to be arising from fragrances are associated with several positive as well as negative factors. The human body is quite amazing. It tolerates exposures to many substances in a day's time. There are many factors that determine what will be tolerated without adverse effects and what will not be. There may be variations in the same individual depending on other factors involved. In general, the healthier a person is the more tolerance there is towards conditions less than optimal. Age also affects tolerance. Women are usually more prone to problems from fragrances for various reasons. Individual and generic factors also play an important role. Individual body chemistry varies and so does tolerance to chemicals. It is often difficult to pinpoint the cause of several symptoms when the triggering substance is one that is common in the environment.

The process of developing a fragrance is a complex mixture of chemistry and art. Not only must the chemicals used be compatible, but also the combination must be aesthetically pleasing to the nose. There are more than 5000 chemicals used in the manufacture of fragrances. Synthetic organic chemicals constitute 80–90 per cent (by weight and value) of the raw materials used in flavour and fragrance formulations. Like many other chemicals and chemical mixtures in widespread use today, little is known about the impact fragrances have on human health. A study by the United States environment pollution authority (EPA) in 1991 of 31 fragrance products has shown that they have thirteen common chemicals, which are hazardous in many ways. These chemicals, fragrance products in which they are present and their harmful potential are given in Table 4.17.

Table 4.17. Common chemicals found in fragrance products and their harmful potential.

Chemicals present	Fragrance products	Harmful potential
Acetone	Cologne, dish-washing liquid and detergent, nail enamel remover	On EPA, RCRA, CERCLA hazardous waste lists. Inhalation can cause dryness of the mouth and throat; dizziness, nausea, in-coordination, slurred speech, drowsiness, and, in severe exposures, coma. Acts primarily as a central nervous system (CNS) depressant
Benzaldehyde	Perfume, cologne, hair-spray, laundry bleach, deodourants, detergent, vaseline lotion, shaving cream, shampoo, bar soap, dishwasher detergent	Narcotic sensitiser, local anaesthetic, CNS depressant. Causes irritiation to the mouth, throat, eyes, skin, lungs, and GI tract, resulting in nausea and abdominal pain. May cause kidney damage. Do not use with contact lenses

(Contd...)

Chemicals present	Fragrance products	Harmful potential
Benzyl acetate	Perfume, cologne, shampoo, fabric softener, stick-up air-freshener, dish-exciting	Carcinogenic (linked to pancreatic cancer). Vapours are irritating to eyes and respiratory passages, washing liquid and detergent, soap, cough. In mice: hyper-anaemia of the lungs has been hair-spray, bleach, after-shave, noticed. Can be absorbed through the skin causing deodourants systemic effects. Do not flush to sewer
Benzyl alcohol	Perfume, cologne, soap, shampoo, nail enamel remover, air-freshener, laundry bleach and detergent, vaseline lotion, deodourants, fabric softener	Irritating to the upper respiratory tract. Headache, nausea, vomiting, dizziness, drop in blood pressure, CNS depression, and death in severe cases due to respiratory failure
Camphor	Perfume, shaving cream, nail enamel, fabric softener, dish-washer detergent, nail colour, stick-up air-freshener	Local irritant and CNS stimulant. Readily absorbed through body tissues. Causes irritation of eyes, nose and throat, dizziness, confusion, nausea, twitching muscles and convulsions. Avoid inhalation of vapours
Ethanol	Perfume, hair-spray, shampoo, fabric softener, dish-washing liquid and detergent, laundry detergent, shaving cream, soap, vaseline-lotion, air-fresheners, nail colour and remover, paint and varnish remover	On EPA hazardous waste list. Symptoms are fatigue, irritation to eyes and upper respiratory tract even in low concentrations. Inhalation of ethanol vapours can have effects similar to those effects characteristic of ingestion. These include an initial stimulatory effect followed by drowsiness, impaired vision, ataxia, and stupor. Causes CNS disorder
Ethyl acetate	After-shave, cologne, perfume, shampoo, nail colour, nail enamel remover, fabric softener, dish-washing liquid	On EPA hazardous waste list. Irritating to the eyes and respiratory tract. May cause headache and narcosis (stupor), defatting effect on skin, drying and cracking of skin, anaemia with leukocytosis and damage to liver and kidneys. Wash thoroughly after handling
Linalool	Perfume, cologne, bar soap, shampoo, hand lotion, nail enamel remover, hair-spray, laundry detergent, dish-washing liquid, vaseline lotion, air-fresheners, bleach powder, fabric softener, shaving cream, after-shave, solid deodourant	Narcotic. Causes respiratory disturbance. Attracts bees. In animal tests, ataxic gait, reduced spontaneous motor activity and depression, development of respiratory disturbances leading to death, depressed frog-heart activity have been observed. Causes CNS disorder
Methylene	Shampoo, cologne, paint and varnish chloride	Banned by the FDA in 1988. No enforcement possible remover due to trade secret-laws protecting chemical fragrance industry. On EPA, RCRA, CERCLA hazardous waste lists. Carcinogenic. Absorbed, stored in body fat, it metabolises to carbon monoxide, reducing oxygen-carrying capacity of the blood. Causes headache, giddiness, stupor, irritability, fatigue, tingling in the limbs. Causes CNS disorder
α-Pinene	Bar and liquid soap, cologne, perfume, shaving cream, deodourants, dish-washing liquid, air-freshener	Sensitiser (damaging to the immune system)
γ-Terpinene	Cologne, perfume, soap, shaving cream, deodourant, air-freshener	Causes asthma and CNS disorders

(Contd...)

Chemicals present	Fragrance products	Harmful potential
α-Terpineol	Perfume, cologne, laundry detergent, bleach powder, laundry bleach, fabric softener, stick-up air-freshener, vaseline lotion, cologne, soap, hairspray, after shave, roll-on deodourant	Highly irritating to mucous membranes. Aspiration into the lungs can produce pneumonitis or even fatal edema. Can also cause excitement, ataxia (loss of muscular coordination), hypothermia, CNS and respiratory depression and headache. Prevent repeated or prolonged skin contact

Studies have shown that fragrance chemicals can cause health effects, primarily at the skin, lungs and brain. The fragrance portion of laundry and cosmetic products is the primary cause of allergic and irritant skin reactions to those products.

However, there have been some instances of dermatitis from airborne materials, although actual physical contact with the product never occurred. It has also been found that fragrance chemicals absorbed by the skin break down into materials that are stronger sensitisers than the original chemicals.

Studies conducted to ascertain the effect of fragrances on people with chronic lung disease (particularly asthma) have shown divergent results.

A number of studies have been conducted to show as to how fragrance affects the brain. There is a strong link between the sense of smell and emotion. Many researchers believe that this is due to the proximity of the olfactory bulb to the limbic system, which popular media have dubbed 'emotion central'. The olfactory/limbic tract is the most direct connection between our brains and the air we breathe.

There is no blood-brain barrier and the fragrance chemicals thus have the potential to effect, and possible damage, the brain tissue, resulting in what is termed neurotoxicity. Other studies have shown that fragrances can alter mood and alleviate anxiety and stress, the properties that are modulated by natural chemicals in the brain.

Fragrance chemicals can enter the body through inhalation and ingestion through the nose and mouth, and absorption through the skin. Once in the body they are absorbed into the blood stream and transported through the body. Individual sensitivity to the fragrance chemicals varies widely from no effect at all to severe symptoms. Many people who report sensitivities to fragrances also report sensitivities to other chemicals. Because of the complex and competitive nature of fragrance development, manufacturers were given the right to protect their products through state trade secret laws, which allow them not to disclose the ingredients to anyone. Due to this, claims of adverse reactions to fragrances may be difficult or impossible to link to particular fragrance chemicals. Because of the number of chemicals involved, their differences in volatility, polarities, and other properties, analysis is expensive and technically sophisticated.

Currently, the fragrance industry is essentially self-regulated. Although regulating agencies like the food and drug administration (FDA) in the US have jurisdiction over fragrances under the food, drug, and cosmetics act, they actually administer very little control over the fragrance products, allowing the fragrance industry to police itself. People's claim of sensitivity to fragrances has resulted in efforts to characterise the risk, but the issue has defied a concise identification of a public health risk and a solid scientific definition. Hence, the regulatory authorities are not in a position to propose changes in regulations.

Many manufacturers of fragrance chemicals are reported to be conducting their own safety tests. In addition, the fragrance industry developed the research institute for fragrance materials (RIFM) in 1996 to conduct research on fragrance ingredients in order to ensure the safety of the perfumery chemicals. The ingredients are most commonly tested for allergenicity, phototoxicity, and general toxicity by oral and dermal routes. The issue of environmental health effects of fragrances is complex, controversial, and is slowly garnering more public attention. An indisputable fact is that there is a lack of sufficient research on the issue and the matter needs to be explored by careful study.

PACKING OF FLAVOURS AND FRAGRANCES AND THEIR SENSORY PERCEPTION
Packaging of Flavours

Packaging of relevance to flavours is in the food industry wherein food is packaged to preserve its quality and freshness, appeal to consumers and to facilitate storage and distribution.

Food quality losses may be caused by oxidation, moisture gain or loss, change or loss of flavour, aroma and colour, texture change, exposure to light, enzymatic reactions, heat or cold, spoilage organisms, and pests.

Primary food package materials are those which are in direct contact with food. Some of them are glass, metals (aluminium and steel cans and foils), paper and paperboard, and plastics. Environmental pressure from consumers and government legislation is increasingly demanding the easy disposability and/or recycling of the packaging material.

The food package industry is the largest sector within the package market, which represents one of the top ten industries of the world. Key factors for the growth in the food packaging market are the changing socio-economics and demographics of different global regions.

Among the oldest packaging materials, glass remains popular in spite of its fragility and weight disadvantage. Along with foil and metal, glass is considered inert to flavour compounds.

Consumer desire for conveniently packaged products has promoted a trend in packaging materials away from the inert toward more interactive synthetic polymers. Plastics used for packaging are either simple homopolymers or copolymers. Flavours and packaging interact as a result of three factors:

1. Migration of packaging or food components.
2. Permeation of the package by gas, water and organic vapours.
3. Exposure of the package to light.

The transfer of vinyl chloride monomers from packages made of polyvinyl chloride (PVC), and migration of residual styrene present in polystyrene materials, are both examples of odour-active interactions with plastic that adversely affect food flavour.

Migration of food flavours into packaging also is a concern. The low molecular weights and boiling points of flavour components enhance the rate or extent of this flavour absorption. The loss of flavour to packaging is called 'scalping', and results in significant flavour losses that must be compensated for in the formulation. For example, in toothpaste manufacturing, the advent of flexible tubes made of polyethylene or polyolefins requires 5 to 10 per cent more flavour, due to sorption in the contact layer of the tube.

Orange juice, which contains flavour components such as acetaldehyde, is scalped by polyethylene within a few days. Compensation for natural flavour loss in this type of product is not easily accomplished. Migration of contaminants from outside the package, such as strongly flavoured mints, or perfumes from cosmetics and detergent, is controlled in the retail grocery industry by product segregation.

Permeation of packaging by oxygen and water vapour from the atmosphere can cause flavour degeneration. The transfer mechanisms for flavours are similar to those for gas and moisture, but the gains and losses have more significance because of their lower initial concentrations. If oxygen permeates the package, oxidation may result.

Oxygen also participates in light-induced reactions. Light is responsible for the deterioration of food pigments, vitamins, proteins, amino acids, fats, and oils. Oils are susceptible to more rancid flavour development, due to oxidation, as their degree of unsaturation increases. The resulting compounds directly and indirectly impact flavour by acting as precursors in flavour and off-flavour development.

Oxidation of vitamins and oils, which protect and deliver flavour by serving as antioxidants or flavour carriers, contributes to flavour loss. Limiting the flux of water vapour to keep moist foods moist, and dry foods dry, offers an obvious packaging advantage. Not surprisingly, water activity also represents an important variable that influences the rate of many chemical reactions of flavour compounds.

Packaging of food products in plastic makes use of a number of different plastic materials with different barrier properties. None of these, however, is an absolute barrier, such as glass or metal. This means that gases, flavours, and fragrances can be transported into and through the material and by doing so affect the quality of food and its storage-life.

Apart from the permeation of the gases and vapours, it is also possible that low molecular weight components of the plastics such as plasticisers, catalysts, colourants, and reinforcing agents can migrate to the food and develop off-flavours. For this reason, all plastics used in food contact must have specific approval from regulatory agencies like EC (scientific committee for foods), FDA and national governments.

Studies on the extraction of aromatic substances from plastics by common solvents as well as super-critical carbon dioxide have shown that external conditions such as moisture; and the composition of the food affect the aroma absorption. Normally, the barrier properties of the packaging materials are determined for unused plastic materials without taking into consideration that food will be in contact with the material during transport and storage.

To be able to guarantee the quality of a particular food throughout the desired shelf-life, it is important to test the protective capability of the packaging under real life conditions. As food is complex, simplified model systems are often used to simulate the food. This can still lead to over estimation of aroma absorption. In addition, it is important to use for such tests the very low concentration of aromatic substances found in a food as higher ones affect the plastic and in turn the adsorption characteristics. A further aspect of aroma absorption into the packaging arises with the reuse of packaging.

Polyethylene terephthalate (PET) has become common in the beverage industry and a number of PET bottles are now re-fillable. Organisations like Rapra technology, Ltd. Europe's leading independent plastics and rubber specialist, now offer an alerting service aimed at providing the polymer, packaging and the fast moving food processing industries with the most up-to-date commercial market and technical information on polymers in food packaging.

Packaging of Fragrances

Packaging of perfumes is of special importance related to fragrances. The golden age of perfume packaging was the late nineteen, twenties, thirties, and forties, a time when the French fashion houses reigned supreme. The style and cachet of the designs created during that period may never be surpassed. Today, markets are discovering evocative ways to present consumers with new product forms that will appeal to their ever-changing lifestyles.

Fragrance marketing is all about fantasy, and the bottle is the physical manifestation of this fantasy, the fragrance and its name are meant to create. As long as fragrances reflect upon the aspirations and sexual dreams of men and women, beautiful bottles to contain these fragrances will continue to stimulate those fantasies. With the new millennium giving us a new feeling of buoyancy and excitement about the future, a new definition of luxury may emerge and along with it new consumer profiles.

Unique features of Acousto-Magnetic systems allow fragrances to be protected and openly displayed. This initiative demonstrates a trend which is also gaining momentum in the United States to utilise acousto-magnetic source tagging in order to implement assisted self-serve and open merchandising for fragrances. Sensormatic's acousto-magnetic labels are incorporated directly into the packaging at the point of manufacture. This programme will provide perfumes retailers with greater security since anti-theft labels will be concealed, while also reducing labour costs by eliminating in-store tagging.

Quality Assurance

Flavour characterisation

Human perception creates difficulty in the characterisation of flavour. People often perceive flavours differently due to both physiological and psychological factors. Some of the abnormalities observed are termed as Ageusia, Agnosia, Autosmia, Cacogeusia, Cacosmia, Cryptosmia, Dysosmia, Hyperosmia, Hypogeusia, Hyposmia, Macrosmatic, Merosmia, Microsmatic, Parageusia, and Parosmia.

The sensory properties of food are generally complicated due to many different flavour qualities at different intensities. Flavour characterisation therefore involves an understanding of different interrelated factors such as, flavour perception, psychophysics and flavour intensity.

Flavour perception

As previously indicated human perceptions of flavour are generally defined in terms of odour and taste. Texture also plays a part in this perception, the contributing factors being presence of pain, sense of touch, and the detection of sound. Sensory perceptions are both qualitative and quantitative. Sweet, bitter, salty, fruity, floral, etc. are different flavour qualities produced by different chemical compounds. The intensity of particular sensory quality is determined by the amount of the stimulus present.

Psychophysics

Psychophysics is the study of the relationship between sensory perceptions and the stimuli that produce them. In the early 1800s, Weber observed a mathematical relationship between the perceived intensity of sensation and the physical intensity of the stimulus that produced it. He observed that the minimum detectable difference between the intensity of two stimuli, called the Just noticeable difference (JND), is proportional to the total intensity of the stimulus.

This relationship known as the Weber's law has been found to be applicable to a large number of sensory qualities, such as taste and odour of many different chemical, loudness of sounds, brightness of lights, and pain produced by electric shock. JND was determined by a discriminability test in which people were asked to discriminate between a stimulus at two different intensities. Weber's law took into consideration only physical variables.

The consideration of psychological variables also in flavour perception resulted in the refining of the Weber's law to what is now generally referred to as Stevens law.

As per this law,

$$\Psi = k\phi^{n}$$

wherein Ψ is a measure of the perceived intensity of the sensation, ϕ is a measure of the physical intensity of the stimulus which produced the response, and k, n, being constants dependent only on the units chosen for the variable scales Ψ and ϕ. The exponent n, however, is characteristic of what is being measured and is independent of stimulus intensity.

Different sensory qualities and their corresponding Stevens law exponents are given is Table 4.18. These values have been determined by process called magnitude estimation in which people associate numbers proportional to their perception of the intensity of a situation.

Table 4.18. Different sensory qualities and their Stevens law exponents.

Stimulus	Stevens law exponent, n
Electric shock	3.5
Temperature	1.6
Loudness of sound	0.6
Brightness of light	0.3
Sweetness of sucrose	1.5
Bitterness of quinine	0.6
Saltiness	1.0
Sour	1.0
Odour of n-heptane	0.6

The differences in the Stevens law exponents explain as to why dilution of a product like wine brings about large changes in its acid, sweet, and astringent tastes, while changing the aroma only slightly. Practical implications of Stevens law in the manufacture of food are profound. Aspects of flavour perception not accounted for in the Weber-Stevens laws are threshold, saturation and adaptation.

For every sense there is a minimum detectable stimulus intensity called the threshold. Saturation is the concentration of a stimulus above which no increase in perception can be detected.

Exposure to a flavour over time always results in a decrease in the perceived intensity. This dynamic effect of flavour substances is called adaptation and is the basic process by which people experience flavours in foods as well as in sensory tests.

Measuring the dynamics of flavour perception is an emerging technology. Termed as time-intensity analysis, these methods are finding wide application in taste analysis. Discriminatory sensory analysis is used by manufacturers who want to substitute one component of a product with another safer or cheaper without changing the flavour in any way. Several formulations are attempted until one is found with flavour characteristics that cannot be discriminated from the original or a standard sample.

Flavour intensity

The perception of a substance when sniffed or tasted is represented in four general types of scales, namely, nominal, ordinal, interval and ratio. Each of these scales has different properties and allowable statistics. Table 4.19 lists the characteristics of these flavour intensity scales.

Table 4.19. Characteristics of flavour intensity scales.

Flavour intensity scales	Characteristics
Nominal	Used to determine the qualities of flavour. It has no order, distance, or origin and is just a collection of names such as sweet, sour, bitter, salty, umami, etc. The nominal scaling of odours requires only that the person has frequently encountered the odour, has a long-standing connection between the odour and the name, and has aid in re-calling the name. The nominal scaling of flavour qualities of a real material is complicated due to simultaneous perception of a number of different flavour qualities
Ordinal	An ordinal scale has both name and order but no distance or origin. Weak, moderate, strong, or numbers 1, 2, 3 can form an ordinal scale with three points. There are no intermediate points and the scale only indicates that one point is smaller than the other.

(Contd...)

Flavour intensity scales	Characteristics
	Although ordinal scales are used to measure flavour intensity, they are more often used to determine attitudes towards a sensation. This aspect of flavour is called hedonics and it is an attempt to determine the psychological impact of flavour perceptions. It is distinct from flavour characterisation in which ordinal scales are used to arrange a set of samples in their order of increasing intensity and to estimate the magnitude of these intensities
Interval	The interval scale has meaningful distance as well as name and order but no meaningful origin. The quartermaster nine-point scale used as scale of 1 (like extremely) to 9 (dislike extremely) with a midpoint 5
Ratio	The ratio scale has name, order, distance and a meaningful origin. Magnitude estimation method yields a ratio scale and is frequently used as an appropriate scaling method for sensory data

ISOLATION AND PURIFICATION TECHNIQUES FOR SPECIALITY FLAVOUR AND FRAGRANCE CHEMICALS

The flavours and fragrances chemicals are directly consumed as food flavours and used as personal care, products, detergents, bathing soaps, etc. Hence, the quality of the product plays a very important role. Consistent product quality depends on the correct isolation and purification processes adopted.

Various steps involved in isolation and purification of natural as well as synthetic aroma chemicals are discussed below.

How to Select the Appropriate Isolation and Purification Techniques

A synthetic reaction results in the formation of a mixture of components besides the main component. Appropriate isolation and purification techniques need to be adopted in order to achieve higher yield and purity of the component. Isolation of speciality aroma chemicals depends upon:

1. Volatility (particulary when the solvent has to be removed).
2. Polarity (in case of extraction from an aqueous solvent is to be carried out).
3. Stability in acid, base and water.
4. Stability in heat, light and air.

Isolation of the required aroma chemicals generally involves addition of water, neutralisation with acid or base followed by extraction with a suitable solvent. Acid traces are removed by washing with sodium bicarbonate solution and traces of alkali can be removed by dilute HCl.

Purification

After isolating the main components from the reaction mixture/natural plant products, the next step involves purification which generally involves the following techniques:

1. Crystallisation
2. Freeze drying
3. Distillation
4. Chromatography

The process used for purification will depend upon the physical properties and physical state (i.e. liquid or solid) of the component to be purified. Different techniques used for isolation and purification are briefly discussed below.

Crystallisation

Purification by this technique depends on the solubility of the product in a given solvent or a mixture of solvents. Hence, selection of an appropriate solvent for crystallisation is very crucial for increasing the yield of the crystallised product.

An ideal solvent should have the following properties:

1. The solvent used for crystallisation should dissolve the impurities easily or to a very less extent.
2. It should dissolve the substance completely at higher temperature and form crystals at lower temperature.
3. To a maximum extent the solvent should have a low boiling point and its recovery should be easy.

The boiling point and suitability of a few solvents used for crystallisation are shown in Table 4.20.

Table 4.20. The boiling point and suitability of a few solvents used for crystallisation.

Solvent	Boiling point °C	Suitability
Water	100	Most suitable solvent and should be used whenever possible
Methanol	64.5	Flammable, toxic
Ethyl alcohol	78	Flammable
Acetone	56	Flammable
Ethyl Acetate	78	Flammable
Toluene	110	Flammable
Carbon tetrachloride	77	Non-flammable, vapour toxic
Light petroleum	40–60	Flammable
Cyclohexane	81	Flammable
Ethyl methyl ketone	80	Flammable
Dichloromethane	40	Non-Flammable

Filtration

Purification of the crystallised material through filtration is an important step. Various types of nutsche filters, filter presses and centrifuges are used for this purpose. The choice of the solvent or mixture of solvents depends upon the nature of the component to be separated from the mixture. The recovery of material from the mother liquor as second crop of crystals and recovery of solvent is essential for economic feasibility of the product.

Lyophilisation (Freeze Drying)

This process is used for removal of water by freezing the reaction mixture.

Solvent Extraction

As the crude product from the reaction mixture contains by-products and other impurities like isomers, in addition to the main component, the solvent extraction process can be used for purification. Solvent extraction can be carried out in two ways.

1. Batch extraction: This separation technique is normally used to separate natural aroma compounds that are immiscible in water, from a solution or suspension in an aqueous medium in an organic solvent.

2. Continuous extraction: This technique is used when the substance to be separated is more soluble in water than the organic solvent. This can be carried out by:
   (a) Liquid–liquid extraction by upward displacement.
   (b) Liquid–liquid extraction by downward displacement.

Column Chromatography Separation

Separation and isolation of substances which polymerise on heating is carried out by column chromatographic technique. For example, isolation of various guaicols with vinyl group. The column is made of silica gel or alumina.

After packing the column, the material is poured from the top of the column and upon adorption, eluted by different solvents. This technique is particularly useful for separation of high value flavour and fragrance aroma chemicals.

Distillation

Steam distillation

This consists of volatilising the substance by passing steam through it. The prerequisite for this method is that the substance to be separated should have appreciable vapour pressure. In this technique, distillation takes place below the boiling point of water. Most organic compounds fall in this category. Most of the essential oils are separated by this technique.

Fractional distillation

Aroma chemicals from natural essential oils are isolated by fractional distillation. As these chemicals undergo partial decomposition at elevated temperature, the boiling point is reduced considerably by reducing the external pressure to 0.01–30 mm Hg. This makes it possible to separate the aroma chemicals at lower temperature without decomposition.

Molecular distillation

This technique is used for speciality aroma chemicals having very high boiling point and high molecular weight. In this case, fractional distillation cannot be used. Here, the distillation is carried out in a small distillation column. There is a short direct path between the material to be distilled and the cooled area where the material is collected. This method requires very high vacuum, i.e. 0.01 to 0.001 mm Hg. This is the only method by which substances having high molecular weight can be distilled without decomposition.

Ascertaining the Purity of Purified Speciality Flavour/Fragrance

The purity of the component isolated and purified after the reaction can be calculated by determining its melting point/boiling point, refractive index, etc. and comparing it with the standard material. Small quantities of impurities can be analysed by gas chromatography and high pressure liquid chromatography techniques. Spectroscopic techniques like UV, IR and NMR are used to determine the groups and carbon skeleton. Finally, the elemental analysis and GC/MS could be used to determine the molecular formula and molecular weight. By using these techniques the level of purity could be ascertained and on comparing this with the standard material the decision whether further purification is necessary could be made.

Optimising the Yield of Product during Isolation and Purification

For optimising yield of the product, the reaction has to be conducted in such a way that it involves a minimum number of steps. The lesser the number of steps, the better is the mole economy and hence the overall yield. This could be done by adopting alternative routes for reaction. Modifying the reaction process and use of alternative raw material could also help in optimising the yield of the product. Here again, the isolation and purification step is most critical for the quantitative yield.

The selection of proper solvents/solvent mixtures for crystallisation, type of distillation conducted and extraction affect the yield. There are no set rules for separation and purification of aroma chemicals, but use of literature data along with continuous effort to derive improved process can improve the yield substantially.

New Trends—Green Chemistry Techniques

Adopting green chemistry techniques as described below would have a positive impact on the yield and cost of the product.

Solventless process

Use of solvents could be avoided to the maximum extent, except for crystallisation. Attempts could be made to distil the material after preprocessing, i.e. filteration/removal of aqueous phase/drying in vacuum, etc. and efficacy of direct distillation over the use of solvent could be ascertained. This will improve the yield, as the number of steps are reduced.

Use of liquid and supercritical carbon dioxide

Use of this green solvent could avoid the problems associated with the recovery of the solvent.

Use of phase transfer catalyst

Phase transfer catalysts not only enhance the yield of the reaction but sometimes also make the separation steps easier. Greater mole economy is achieved if PTC is used.

Common Problems Associated with Isolation and Purification of Speciality Aroma Chemicals

Some of the common problems associated with isolation and purification of speciality aroma chemicals are:

1. Slow filtration of the reaction mixture.
2. Repeated washing of organic layer with water and aqueous layer with solvent leading to the loss of solvent and increase in the aqueous waste load.
3. Difficulty in recovery of water soluble solvents.
4. Difficulty in separation, i.e. formation of two phases when polar solvents are used.
5. Difficulty in crystal formation or no crystal formation.
6. Secondary reaction during isolation and purification steps.
7. Oiling out or tar formation.
8. Formation of emulsions

Solutions

Problems associated with isolation and purification, particulary reducing the quantity of solvent can be overcome by adjusting the pH to neutral, followed by the washing step. This would reduce the problem involved.

Recovery of water soluble solvents and materials from aqueous solution could be attempted by salting out with sodium chloride/potassium carbonate, etc. In case where polar solvents are used for reaction, the removal of solvent by distilling it prior to the extraction step could minimise the difficulty in separation.

Problems associated with crystallisation could be corrected by:

1. Seeding the material with pure crystals (a few crystals of pure compound are added and mixture is left for crystallisation) and then slowly stirring the material to induce crystallisation.
2. Cooling of the material: This is particularly useful in case of low melting aroma chemicals. This may require slow cooling along with seeding to bring about crystallisation.
3. The oiling out or formation of tar: This could be avoided by slowly mixing the material which needs to be crystallised along with seeding with pure crystals. In case crystallisation does not proceed even after taking this course of action, cooling to lower temperature may initiate crystallisation.
4. The formation of emulsion could be rectified by adding more solvent or water so as to bring about difference in density of two layers. A little quantity of scavenging chemicals may also be added to break the emulsions, provided these chemicals do not react with the product to be separated.
5. In case of difficulty in fractional distillation, particularly high molecular weight, high boiling aroma chemicals, molecular distillation has to be adopted.
6. Column chromatography separation gives pure component as compared to other techniques used but its speed and capacity to process the material, limits its use if large quantum of material are to be separated.

Among the various techniques used for isolation and purification of speciality aroma chemicals, the choice of technology depends upon the properties of the chemical to be isolated and impurities associated with it. Materials which are heat sensitive, get polymerised on heating. For such materials, column chromatography is a good choice. For aroma specialities having very high molecular weight, molecular distillation is a preferred technique.

TOXICITY OF FRAGRANCES AND FLAVOURS

Few would want to live in a world without the smell of flowers. Products containing scents are a part of daily life. The majority of cosmetics, toiletries and household and laundry products contain fragrances. In addition, there is exposure to fragrance from products that are used to scent the air, such as air-fresheners and scented burning sticks. Research indicates the sense of smell impacts not only psychological, but physical health, as well.

Perfumes and fragrances are a very big business, running to very many billions of dollars in the world. Related industries such as chemical companies supply the chemicals the fragrances are made from. Most fragrance chemicals are synthesised from petroleum products. Some companies formulate fragrances and flavours for other companies.

Industries add fragrance to personal care, personal hygiene and household products to have greater impact on the user. The food industry is also a large user of flavours or aroma chemicals. Flavour/ fragrance chemicals are also in heavy use by the tobacco industry as additives to cigarettes to enhance flavour, especially in the lower tar and nicotine brands. The sense of smell is the least understood of the senses and often considered the lesser important one. Yet it is the basis of a multi-billion dollar industry.

Initially perfumes and fragrance materials came from plant or animal sources. First fragrance that was dominated by the use of synthetic aldehydes, called floral aldehydes was introduced.

After World War II there was an explosion of new synthetics. With the advent of gas chromatography and mass spectrometry, analysis of a fragrance — both natural and synthetic — was possible and copies of expensive, exclusive fragrances were now available at a fraction of the cost. Chemical fragrances are present in most laundry detergents, fabric softeners, anti-cling products, dish-washing liquids, disinfectants, soaps, shampoos and other hair products, deodourants, cosmetics, suntan/sunscreen lotions, after-shaves, colognes, incenses, analgesic creams and lip balms. There is exposure large from flavours in foods and beverages, as well. Considering the tremendous use and exposure, there is limited information available related to health effects of flavours and fragrances. With increased usage and exposure, problems have emerged regarding fragrances. There are concerns for both those that use scented products and those exposed from others use.

With this increased usage and exposure, there are increased anecdotal and clinical accounts of fragranced products causing, triggering, and exacerbating health conditions. Further concerns relate to the bio-accumulation of fragrance chemicals in human tissue and the long-term impact. In addition, there are environmental concerns as fragranced products add to both air and water pollution. Fragrance is increasingly cited as a trigger in health conditions such as asthma, allergies and migraine headaches. In addition, some fragrance materials have been found to accumulate in adipose tissue and are present in breast milk. Other materials are suspected of being hormone disrupters. There are environmental concerns as well, as fragrances are volatile compounds, which add to both indoor and outdoor air pollution. Synthetic musk compounds are persistent in the environment and contaminate waterways and aquatic wildlife. Perfume today is not made from flowers, but mostly from chemicals. More than 4000 chemicals are used in fragrances. Of these, 95 per cent are made from petroleum.

Chemistry

Fragrance chemistry is an extremely complex science and art. It is highly specialised field and there is limited information available outside of the fragrance industry. There are over 5000 chemicals and materials used in the fragrance industry. A fragrance formula may contain as few as 10 or as many as several hundred. One fragrance is reported to have 600 different ingredients.

Many things have to be considered when formulating a fragrance. Compatibility of materials used has to be taken into account. The material that is being fragranced also plays an important role, as products which have extremes in pH are difficult to perfume. Once the physical aspects of the perfuming process are worked out, the resulting scent has to be aesthetically pleasing. Safety of fragrance materials is also of concern. Entry points for fragrance chemicals into the body include the skin, the lungs, ingestion, and olfactory pathways. Fragrance materials are volatile by nature and play a role in the chemistry of indoor air. Concern for safety and health effects of the chemicals used in fragrances extends beyond the user.

Fragrances, by design, get into the air. In order to detect an odour, molecules of that substance must be airborne. Fragrances are complex mixtures of volatile organic compounds (VOCs) formulated to have a specific odour. Once in the air, they break down, mix with other pollutants, and form new compounds that are often more irritating or allergenic than the original substance. VOCs are associated with exacerbating respiratory diseases, such as asthma.

Toxic Effects on Human Body and Surroundings

Exposure to scented products can cause exhaustion, weakness, 'hay fever' symptoms, dizziness, difficulty concentrating, headaches, rashes, swollen lymph glands, muscle aches and spasms, heart palpitations, nausea, stomach cramps, vomiting, asthma attacks (inability to breathe), neuromotor dysfunction, seizures, and loss of consciousness. MCS (multiple chemical sensitivities) is caused by overexposure to toxic chemicals. The toxicity of fragrance materials on the human and animal body are discussed below:

Skin

Fragrances have been long recognised as skin allergens and irritants. The skin is an entry point for materials into the body. Once entry has been gained, there is potential for systemic effects. Fragrance ingredients can be irritants, allergens, photo sensitisers, photo toxins, and they can have other negative effects on the skin. Airborne contact dermatitis occurs when dermatitis develops from contact with fragrance materials in the air.

Respiratory

Fragrances can induce or worsen respiratory problems. There are increasing anecdotal and clinical accounts of fragrance triggering and exacerbating respiratory problems. Fragrances are thought to trigger asthma and other respiratory conditions due to their irritant effect. It has also been found that skin contact may play a role in respiratory sensitisation.

Neurological

Fragrance can impact the brain and nervous system. Some of these effects are immediate and transitory, while other can be long-term. Olfactory pathways provide the most direct connection to the brain of any senses and also provide a means of toxic materials entering the brain. Acetylethyltetramethyltetraline (AETT) and musk ambrette, two materials in common use for decades, were found to be neurotoxic.

Systemic effects

Fragrances can enter the body through numerous routes such as skin absorption, inhalation, ingestion and olfactory pathways. Once inside the body, the materials can impact any organ or system.

Safrole occurs naturally in some essential oils and in sassafras roots was listed as reasonably anticipated to be a human carcinogen and causes liver tumours. Coumarin is widely used in fragrances and there was some evidence of it being a carcinogen associated with an increase in lung, liver and renal tumours. Methyl eugenol is a common fragrance/flavour material and occurs naturally in spices and some essential oils and clear evidence of its carcinogenic activity has been found. Musk xylene was found carcinogenic.

In single large doses 6-Acetyl-1, 1, 2, 4, 4, 7-hexamethyltetraline (AHTN) caused liver toxicity and organ discolouration. Similar, but less prominent, effects were also observed with hexahydro-hexamethyl cyclopenta (γ)-2-benzopyran (HHCB). Both AHTN and HHCB are synthetic musk compounds, which are widely used at relatively high levels. Both of these materials are common in laundry products, which involve skin contact over large, often occluded areas.

Other areas of concern are the potential for fragrance chemicals to impact the reproductive system, foetal development and infant breast-feeding. Synthetic musk chemicals are known to bio-accumulate in human tissue and are present in breast milk.

Effect on Waterways and Wildlife

Most soaps, shampoos and other bathing products contain fragrance. In addition, fragrance is added to most household cleaners and laundry products. A large portion of these materials end up in waste-water. Most waste-water treatment methods do not remove fragrance compounds. These materials end up in streams and rivers from discharge of water from sewage treatment.

Fragrance musks are ubiquitous, persistent, bio-accumulative pollutants that are sometimes highly toxic; amino musk transformation products are toxicologically significant. Musk compounds tend to accumulate and break down slowly. They persist in the aquatic environment and accumulate in the fatty tissue of aquatic wildlife. Shellfish and fish have measurable levels of synthetic musk compounds in their tissues. These materials can be considered 'persistent organic pollutants'.

Toxicity of Some Common Products We Use

Here below is considered many day-to-day products which contain toxic fragrance and flavours.

Camphor

Camphor burning is a part of religious worship in India. Camphor is burnt in almost all the temples and in houses during worshipping. Most of the places of worship, either in the temple or in the houses, do not have proper ventilation for the vapours to escape. Camphor is also used in the preparation of ointments and balms for relief of pain, cough and cold. It is also used in the manufacture of perfume, shaving cream, nail enamel, fabric softener, dish-washer detergent, nail colour, stick-up air-freshener, etc.

The dangers of the camphor are: it is a local irritant, it acts as central nervous system stimulant, is readily absorbed through body tissues; it is irritant to eyes, nose and throat; its usage or inhalation of its vapour leads to dizziness, confusion, nausea, twitching muscles and convulsions.

In many temples in India, burning of camphor is banned and this non-usage is slowly catching up.

Scented sticks

In India, it is customary to burn incense sticks during worshipping. Almost all Hindus invariably practice this without knowing the danger involved in this. The perfumes that are used are narcotic, sensitiser, local anesthetic, CNS depressant, irritation to the mouth, throat, eyes, skin, lungs, and GI tract, causing nausea and abdominal pain. It may cause kidney damage.

95 per cent of chemicals used in fragrances are synthetic compounds derived from petroleum. They include benzene derivatives, aldehydes and many other known toxics and sensitisers—capable of causing cancer, birth defects, central nervous system disorders and allergic reactions. Central nervous system disorders (brain and spine) include multiple sclerosis, Parkinson's disease, Alzheimer's disease, and sudden Infant death syndrome.

Incense sticks contain phthalates to reduce fast evaporation and to provide anti-cracking and penetrating properties to the coatings. Phthalates have been connected to birth defects in humans, being anti-andraogeonic, suppressing hormones involved in male sexual development.

Burning of scented sticks leads to heavy concentrations of CO in air, which causes headache, mental dullness, dizziness, weakness, nausea, heart disease, and death, in high doses. Burning also results in the release of carbon particles into air, along with tar, which are highly injurious to health.

Air-fresheners

Many of the air-fresheners sold in the market contains *p*-dichlorobenzene (PDCB) used in the cars, living rooms and also to de-odourise bathrooms and toilets. The chemicals in the air-fresheners stick to the clothes and do not wash out easily. PDCB is a known carcinogenic. Certain air-fresheners also contain solvents like acetone which has the following toxicity: inhalation can cause dryness of the mouth and throat; dizziness, nausea, lack of co-ordination, slurred speech, drowsiness, and, in severe exposures, coma. It acts primarily as a central nervous system (CNS) depressant. The words 'air-freshener' suggests that such products would improve air quality. In actuality, the opposite is true.

Aerosol hair-sprays

As with many aerosol cosmetic and household products, the flammability of most aerosol hair-sprays is attributable to the use of hydrocarbon propellants in combination with SD alcohol 40 solvent. This mixture has been widely used to replace chlorofluorocarbons (CFCs), which were banned from aerosol propellant use, because of environmental concerns. Another problem can occur with aerosol sprays for powders: if they are inhaled, they can cause lung damage.

Cosmetics

Cosmetics includes:
1. Skin care creams, lotions, powders.
2. Perfume, cologne, toilet water.
3. Make-up (lipstick, foundation, blush).
4. Nail polish, polish remover, cuticle softener.
5. Hair colouring preparations.
6. Deodourants.
7. Shaving cream, aftershave, skin conditioner.
8. Shampoos (except dandruff shampoos).
9. Bath oil and bubble bath.
10. Mouthwash and toothpaste.

The use of the following ingredients for use in cosmetics, are either restricted or prohibited by regulation because of the dangers they impose:
1. Bithionol.
2. Mercury compounds.
3. Vinyl chloride.
4. Halogenated salicylanilides.
5. Zirconium complexes in aerosol cosmetics.
6. Chloroform.
7. Methylene chloride.
8. Chlorofluorocarbon propellants.
9. Hexachlorophene.
10. Methyl methacrylate monomer in nail products.

Of 138 compounds used in cosmetics that are most frequently involved in adverse reactions, five chemicals (alpha-terpineol, benzyl acetate, benzyl alcohol, limonene and linalool) are among the 20 most commonly used in the 31 fragrance products.

Alpha-terpineol

Used in the manufacture of perfume, cologne, laundry detergent, bleach powder, laundry bleach, fabric softener, stick-up air-freshener, vaseline lotion, cologne, soap, hair-spray, after-shave, roll-on deodourant.

Highly irritating to mucous membranes, aspiration into the lungs can produce pneumonitis or even fatal edema. Can also cause excitement, ataxia (loss of muscular co-ordination), hypothermia, CNS and respiratory depression and headache. Prevent repeated or prolonged skin contact.

Benzyl acetate

Used in the manufacture of perfume, cologne, shampoo, fabric softener, stick-up air-freshener, dish-washing liquid and detergent, soap, hair-spray, bleach, aftershave, deodourants. Carcinogenic (linked to pancreatic cancer); form vapours irritating to eyes and respiratory passages, exciting cough. It can be absorbed through the skin causing systemic effects.

Benzyl alcohol

Used in the manufacture of: perfume, cologne, soap, shampoo, nail enamel remover, air-freshener, laundry bleach and detergent, vaseline lotion, deodorants, fabric softener. Irritating to the upper respiratory tract, headache, nausea, vomiting, dizziness, drop in blood pressure, CNS depression, and death in severe cases due to respiratory failure.

Linaloöl

Used in the manufacture of perfume, cologne, bar soap, shampoo, hand lotion, nails enamel remover, hairspray, laundry detergent, dish-washing liquid, vaseline lotion, air-fresheners, bleach powder, fabric softener, shaving cream, after-shave, solid deodourant.

Narcotic, respiratory disturbances, attracts bees. In animal tests: ataxic gait, reduced spontaneous motor activity and depression, development of respiratory disturbances leading to death, depressed frog-heart activity. It causes CNS disorder.

Limonene

Limonene used in perfume, cologne, disinfectant spray, bar soap, shaving cream, deodourants, nail colour and remover, fabric softener, dish-washing liquid, air-fresheners, after-shave, bleach, paint and varnish remover. Limonene is carcinogenic. With skin or eyes, it is an irritant and sensitiser.

Musks

Musks are ubiquitous, persistent, bio-accumulative pollutants that are sometimes highly toxic; amino musk transformation products are toxicologically significant. Synthetic musks comprise a series of structurally similar chemicals (which emulate the odour but not the structure of the expensive, natural product from the Asian musk deer) used in a broad spectrum of fragranced consumer items, both as fragrance and as fixative. Included are the older, synthetic nitro musks (e.g. ambrette, musk ketone, musk xylene, and the lesser known musks moskene and tibetene) and a variety of newer, synthetic polycyclic musks that are best known by their individual trade names or acronyms.

The polycyclic musks (substituted indanes and tetralins are the major musks used today, accounting for almost two-thirds of worldwide production) and especially the inexpensive nitro musks (nitrated aromatics accounting for about one-third of worldwide production) are used in nearly every commercial fragrance formulation (cosmetics, detergents, toiletries) and most other personal care products with fragrance; they are also used as food additives and in cigarettes and fish baits.

Musks are refractory to biodegradation and therefore can bioconcentrate/bioaccumulate. Concern has been expressed regarding developmental toxicity in aquatic organisms also. Musk ambrette (2,6-dinitro-3-methoxy-4-tert-butyl toluene) may play a role in damaging the nervous system.

Food products

Charred carbohydrate is injurious to health if it is consumed and coffee seed is one such example. In the preparation of instant coffee charred soyabean is used to provide thickening effect to the coffee. They are carcinogenic. The alcoholic beverage 'rum' contains a colour made out of charred sugar, which is carcinogenic. The flavouring agent used is a combination of ethyl acetate and ethyl butyrate. Ethyl acetate is toxic, narcotic, irritating to the eyes and respiratory tract, may cause headache and narcosis (stupor), defatting effect on skin and may cause drying and cracking, may cause anaemia with leukocytosis and damage to liver and kidneys.

Alcohol in the liquor, namely ethyl alcohol, is also toxic. It causes fatigue; is irritating to eyes and upper respiratory tract even in low concentrations, ingestion and inhalation of ethanol vapours can have the following effects: an initial stimulatory effect followed by drowsiness, impaired vision, ataxia, stupor. It causes CNS disorder.

Vinegar which is used to provide sour taste contains acetic acid which may damage the kidney. In pickles commercially produced acetic acid is used to acidify the pickle.

Laundry products and cleaners

The following common fragrance chemicals are used in laundry products and cleaners. While this is not a complete listing of the fragrance chemicals used, it includes the more common ones:

Alpha terpineol, agrumen aldehyde light-4, allyl cyclohexane propionate, alpha pinene, amyl cinnamic aldehyde, amyl salicylate, benzoin resinoid 80 per cent in DEP, benzyl acetate, benzyl alcohol, benzyl benzoate, benzyl salicylate, beta pinene, cedarleaf, cedarwood terpenes, cinnamic alcohol, *cis*-3-hexenyl tiglate, citral, citrathal, citronella, citronello, civet artificial, clary sage-western, clove stem oil, coumarin, decyl aldehyde, diethylphthalate, dihydro myrocenol, dipropylene glycol, dodecalactone, ethylene brassylate, eucalyptol, eucalyptus, eugenol, fixateur, frutene, galaxolide 50 per cent, galbanum 50 per cent, geraniol, geranium, bourbon oil, geranyl nitrile, hexyl cinnamic aldehyde, hydroxycitronellal, indol, intreleven aldehyde, ionone, gamma methyl, ionone methyl, isobornyl aceate, isocyclo citral, isoeugeno, labdanum resin, laevo menthone, lavandin, lavender, lavol, lemon cold pressed, lemongrass, linaloöl, linalyl acetate, LRG 201, methyl beta naphthyl ketone, methyl cedrylone, methyl nonyl acetaldehyde, methyl dihydro jasmonate, methyl salicylate, moskene, musk xylol, myrcenyl acetate crude, nerol, nonalactone, oakmoss, octyl aldehyde, olibanum resinoid 80 per cent, opoponax oleo resin 70 per cent, orange oil cold pressed, orange phase oil, orange terpenes, parahydroxy phenyl butanone, para tertiary bucinal, patchouli, peppermint RP, peru balsam, petitgrain, phenyl ethyl alcohol, pine oil, rose otto synthetic, rosemary, spearmint natural, spruce, terpineol, terpinolene, terpinyl acetate, 4-tertiary butyl cyclohexyl acetate, tetrahydro linaloöl, tonalid, thyme white oil, trichloromethyl phenyl carbinyl acetate, vanillin, vertivert, vertivert acetate, and ylang ylang.

Toxic Properties of Raw Fragrance Materials

These are the characteristics of materials used in the formulation of fragranced products and flavours and not necessarily that of finished products.

Materials that are possible carcinogens (usually based on animal studies)

4-hydroxybutanoic acid lactone, DL-isoleucine, L-leucine, Dl-valine, benzyl acetate, butylated hydroxytoluene (BHT), coumarin, ethyl vinyl ketone, eugenol, polysorbate 80 and quinoline.

Materials that are considered toxic

(R)-(+)-pulegone, 1,2-ethanedithiol, 1-butanethiol, 1-decanol, 1-furfurylpyrrole, 1-methyl-1,4-cyclohexadiene, 1-octen-3-ol, -phenyl-1-propanol, 2,4-hexadienal (sorbaldehyde), 2,4-xylenol, 2,5-dimethylfuran, 2,5-xylenol, 2,6-diisopropylphenol, 2,6-dimethylpyridine, 2,6-xylenol, 2-acetyl-5 methylfuran, 2-ethylbutyric acid, 2-isopropylphenol, 2-methoxy-4-propylphenol, 2-methyl-3-buten-2 ol,

2-methyl-3-furanthiol, 2-methylfuran, 2-naphthalenethiol, 2-propylphenol, 2-thienyl disulphide, 3,4-xylenol, 3,7-dimethyl-6 octenoic acid, 3-Acetyl-pyridine, 3-penten-2-one, 4-methyl-5 vinylthiasole, 4-methylpentanoic acid, 4-methylthiazole, 4-pentenoic acid, 4-propylphenol, 4-vinylphenol, 5-ethyl-2-methylpyridine, α-methylbensyl alcohol, α-terpineol, *m*-cresol, *o*-cresol, *p*-cresol, *trans, trans*-2,4-heptadienal, *trans*-2-heptenal, *trans*-2-hexenal, allyl butyrate, allyl cyclohexanepropionate, allyl disulphide, allyl isothiocyanate, allyl isovalerate, ally phenoxyacetate, ammonium sulfide, benzenethiol, benzothiazole, benzyl acetate, benzyl acetate natural, benzyl mercaptan, birch oil sweet, butylamine. butyric acid, butyric acid natural, caffeine, cassia oil, citronellal, coumarin, diacetyl, dimethyl disulphide, formic acid, furfural, furfuryl alcohol, glutaric dialdehyde, *o*-guaiacol, heptyl alcohol, hexanoic acid, hexanoic acid natural, indole, isobutyric acid, isobutyric acid natural, isoquinoline, isovaleric acid, methyl propyl disulphied, methyl salicylate, nonyl alcohol, origanum oil, phenethyl alcohol, phenethyl alcohol natural, phenethylamine, phenol, piperidine piperine, propionic acid, pyrazine-ethanethiol, pyrrolidine, quinine, monohydro-chloride dihydrate, quinoline, resorcinol, salicylaldehyde, styrene oxide, styrene, trimethylamine, undecylenic acid, and valeric acid.

Materials that target the nerves

1-octanol, 1-propanol, 2,6-dimethyl 1-4-heptanol, 2,6-dimethyl-4-heptanone, 2-butanone, 2-pentanone, 3-acetylpyridine, 4-methyl-2-pentanone, *d*-camphor, *m*-cresol, *o*-cresol, *p*-cresol, *p*-cymene, amyl alcohol, amyl formate, benzaldehyde, benzenethiol, benzyl acetate natural, benzyl alcohol, biphenyl, butyl acetate, butyl alcohol, butyl propionate, diethyl phthalate, dimethyl phthalate, ethyl 3-methyl-3 phenyl-glycidate, mixture of isomers, ethyl alcohol, 190 proof non-denatured, ethyl formate natural, eugenol, furfural isoamyl acetate, isoamyl alcohol, isophorone, isopropyl alcohol, maltol, 1 wt. per cent solution in benzyl alcohol, phenethyl alcohol, phenethylamine, phenol, quinine, monohydrochloride dihydrate, resorcinol, salicylaldehyde, salicylic acid, and styrene oxide.

Materials that target the lungs

m-Cresol, *o*-cresol, *p*-cresol, amyl alcohol, amyl formate, butylated hydroxylamine (BHT), ethyl vinyl ketone, and eugenol.

Materials that readily absorb through the skin

(IS)-(-)-α-Pinene, 2,4-hexadienal, 2,4,-xylenol, 5-xylenol, 2,6-xylenol, 2-ethylbutyric acid, 2-mehoxy-4-propylphenol, 3,4-xylenol, 3,7-dimethyl-6-octenoic acid, 3-penten-2-one, 4-methyl-3-penten-2-one, 5-ethyl-2-methylpyridine, α-phellanderene, *m*-cresol, *o*-cresol, *p*-cresol, *trans, trans*-2,4-heptadienal, *trans*-2-heptenal, *trans*-2-hexenal, ammonium sulphide, 20 wt., per cent solution in water, benzenethiol, butyric acid, butyric acid, natural, dimethyl phthalate, *p*-cresol, *trans*-2,4-heptadienal, *trans*-2-hexenal, ally butyrate, allyl heptanoate, allyl hexanoate, allyl heptanoate, allyl hexanoate, allyl isothiocyanate, allyl phenoxyacetate, phenol, piperidine, propionic acid, pyridine, quinoline, salicylaldehyde, styrene, and undecylenic acid.

Materials that target the liver

1-Octanol natural, 1-propanol, 2-ethylhexanoic acid, acetic acid, biphenyl, butylated hydroxyanisole (BHA), coumarin, ethyl alcohol, 190 proof, non-de-natured, furfural, quinoline, and sassafras oil.

Materials that are sensitisers

β-Ionone, (R)-(+)-limonene, 1-phenyl-1,2-propanedione, 2-phenethyl isothiocyanate, 4-vinylphenol, 10 wt. per cent solution in propylene glycol α-ionone, *dl*-menthol, 1-menthol, acetaldehyde, anise oil, azodi-carbonamide, bay oil, benzaldehyde, benzoic acid, benzylideneacetone, (*trans*-4-phenyl-3-buten-2-one), butylated hydroxyanisole, butyraldehyde, cassia oil, cinnamon bark oil, cinnamon leaf oil, ceylon, citral, mixture of *cis* and *trans*, citronellal, dihydro-β-ionone, eugenol, (4-allylguaiacol, 4-allyl-2-methoxyphenol), furfural, (2-furaldehyde, purified), glutaric dialdehyde, 50 wt. per cent solution in water, methyl benzoate, phenethylamine, phenyl salicylate, phenylacetaldehyde, propyl gallate, quinine, monohydrochloride dihydrate, and styrene oxide.

Materials that target the kidneys

(R)-(+)-Limonene, 1-methyl-1,4-cyclo:exadiene, 1-octanol, (alcohol C–8, octyl alcohol), 2,6-dimethyl-4-heptanol, 2,6-dimethyl-4-heptanone, (diisobutyl ketone), 2-ethyl-1-hexanol, α-methylbenzyl alcohol, (styralyl alcohol), *m*-cresol, *o*-cresol, *p*-cresol, acetaldehyde, acetic acid, acetone, acetone natural, benzenethiol, benzyl acetate natural, birch oil, sweet di(ethylene glycol) ethyl ether, diphenyl ether, ethyl acetate, eugenol, (4-allylguaiacol, 4-allyl-2-methoxyphenol), fumaric acid, isophorone, isopropyl alcohol, methyl acetate, methyl anthranilate natural, (methyl-2-aminobenzonate), phenol, pyridine, pyroligneous acid, and salicylaldehyde.

Constraints and Opportunities

Global changes occurring due to eroding forest cover has led to increased environmental awareness, among people. This, in turn, has led to a change in consumer perception and redefining of priorities to save the eco-system and reemphasise the need to encourage use of forest-land plant-based products. God almighty has blessed India with different types of soils and climates that supports growth of a variety of plants, 18,000 native species are found in India of which 1300 species on the last count contain aromas. In spite of its rich natural forest vegetation and a home of many exotic natural plants, India cultivates only limited items of commercial value. There is a great scope for commercial cultivation of several aromatic crops in India as there is always a market demand for new and specific aroma ingredients for development of new exotic fragrances.

Although fragrance usage is on an increase, the availability of quality plant oils for fragrance creation is not sufficient to keep pace with the demand generated. Plant cultivation largely depends on climatic conditions. Yields vary, year after year. Availability differs season to season. Unpredictable quality and odour profile is common. Price fluctuation is rampant. Supply and demand is rarely even. Advent of biotechnology and modern farming techniques has, to an extent, insulated plant cultivation from the vagaries of nature, but this is far too less to make a significant difference on the industry dependence on nature.

Aromatic crop cultivation freshens up the polluted atmosphere and is a renewable resource in the ecosystem. The crops are useful even after the extraction of available essential oil, as they can be converted into artificial board for carpentry, used as fodder for animals, or decomposed to get bio-fertilisers. Essential oil bearing crop cultivation and processing is labour-intensive, generating good employment opportunities.

Steps needed for success

Even today, essential oils are extracted in India in an unorganised manner. This industry can grow only by following scientific means and methods of propagation and extraction. Systematic exploitation of aromatic plants by Indian industry can bring great economic advantage to our country, as more and more aromatic plants are brought under use. Setting up of small-scale essential oil extraction and processing units can provide ample employment opportunities for rural youth. Once these units come into operation, local farmers can be motivated for large-scale cultivation of selected aromatic crops, according to the prevalent agro-climatic conditions. During the initial stages, raw material requirement of these industries can be met either through collection from wild habitats or through intercropping cultivation in agricultural farms. Either way, it will provide employment to millions from the farming communities. Value addition through post-harvest technology can also generate further agricultural income and employment opportunities.

Conservation of aromatic plants by promoting sustainable genetic management schemes at the community level is necessary for equitable distribution of acquired benefits and to improve livelihoods of the rural poor. This can be achieved only if proper training for cultivation, primary processing, grading, packaging, storage and marketing are provided to rural cultivators. In addition, bio-partnership, networking and providing access to information between the prime stakeholders (local communities, R & D scientists and industry) is necessary.

Generating a strong database on genetic resources of aromatic plants and creation of protectorates/biosphere reserves to conserve the genetic stock of endangered species (in situ conservation) is essential. Sufficient quantity of quality seed and planting material of aromatic plants for cultivators should be made available. Newer agro-techniques and technology should be developed, assessed and refined for large-scale cultivation to maintain sustainability and competitive advantage.

Tissue culture transplantation techniques need to be adopted for species whose propagation through seeding is not easy. Analytical laboratories for testing and maintaining quality controls should be established. Utmost priority is to be given to develop skilled manpower to handle all aspects of aromatic plants through intensive training programmes.

Evolving a long-term human resource development strategy for continuous improvement in competence and skills should ensure upgradation of the technical knowledge for field personnel. India's agro-climatic conditions provide an ideal habitat for the natural growth of a variety of aromatic plants and herbs. The climatic diversity also offers large opportunities for domestication of many herbs that are in short supply and have to be imported. This will not only supplement internal demand, but also save substantial foreign exchange.

The fact that derivatives of aromatic plants are nonnarcotic without noticeable side effects, even if used for a prolonged time in permissible doses, fuels its demand around the world. Interestingly, 30 per cent of the ingredients prohibited by IFRA on grounds of safety or otherwise are naturals. Cultivation, processing and use of aromatic plants are a great potential for employment generation in rural areas. Our tilt and liking towards synthetic aroma chemicals is slowly destroying nature's gift of aromatic plant species used for fragrance creation in ancient India and which grew abundantly in our forests.

Another reason for the disappearance of many plant species is our ignorance with regard to its identity and use. In our ignorance, many useful species are treated as useless weeds and destroyed with no scope for regeneration.

In spite of our country's innumerable benefits, there exist many constraints, which are responsible for impeding the growth of this industry. These include:

1. Inequitable trade practices that allow only a very small amount of profit to percolate down to the collectors, cultivators and harvesters of aromatic plants.
2. Inadequate government funding and prioritisation.
3. Insufficient information sharing and coordination among stakeholders.

4. Poor mechanism to improve resource conservation, livelihood security in rural and marginal communities; lack of coordination of any holistic research programme.

5. Weak linkages between stakeholders, right from production to consumption value chain.

Challenge to India

India is no exception to the global phenomenon of environmental problems and depletion of natural plant resources. However, the rich diversity in aromatic plants that nature has provided India needs to be exploited judiciously, without disturbing the ecological balance. Resources need to be harnessed for economic development, and, at the same time, their regeneration, preservation and propagation has to be maintained for sustenance.

The restoration and preservation of our biological heritage is a challenge not only to our planners, administrators, scientists, industrialist, entrepreneurs and farmers, but also to common individuals and citizens at large. Efforts to coordinate development of quality planting material, encouraging commercial cultivation, value addition through processing, liaison with industries and trade, including export, is necessary to boost India's economy and our standard of living.

India, the land of opportunities, is projected to be one of the world's largest economies in terms of GDP, and purchasing power parity. The Indian population of over one billion in this millennium, will be extremely young, with 70 per cent under 34 years of age, unlike in the developed countries. It is up to all of us to grab this opportunity and regain our pre-eminent position as world-leader in the natural fragrance industry, as in ancient times, or rest satisfied by becoming the world's largest consumer of imported fragrances and fragranced products.

Chapter 5

Production of Essential Oils

INTRODUCTION

The majority of essential oils have always been obtained by steam distillation or, in the more general sense, by hydrodistillation. The practical problems connected with distillation of aromatic plants are, therefore, of utmost importance to the actual producer of essential oils.

This chapter will be divided into two parts, the first dealing with the fundamental or theoretical principles underlying all distillation processes, and the second treating more specifically the practical aspects of distillation as applied directly in the essential oil industry.

THEORIES OF DISTILLATION

Essential, volatile or ethereal oils are mixtures composed of volatile, liquid and solid compounds which vary widely in regard to their composition and boiling points. Every substance with a determinable boiling point is volatile and possesses a definite vapour pressure, which depends upon the prevailing temperature and which is very low in the case of very high boiling substances. Hence, the intensity of an odour may be considered, to a certain extent and with many exceptions, as a manifestation of the volatility (boiling point and vapour pressure) of the substance which emits the odour.

Distillation may be defined as 'the separation of the components of a mixture of two or more liquids by virtue of the difference in their vapour pressure'. The process of distillation is obviously of considerable importance to the essential oil producer. There are two general types to be considered:

1. Distillation of mixtures of liquids which are not miscible and hence form two phases. Practically, this applies to the rectification and fractionation of essential oils with, steam and, what is much more important, to the isolation of volatile oils from aromatic plants with steam. Distillation with steam may also be called hydrodistillation, which general term implies that distillation may be carried out either by boiling the plant material or the essential oil with water and creating the necessary steam within the still or by introducing into the retort live steam generated in a separate steam boiler.

2. Distillation of liquids which are completely miscible in each other and therefore form only one phase. Practically, this applies to the rectification and separation of an essential oil into several fractions (fractionation), without the use of steam.

The difference between the behaviour of single-phase mixtures and two phase mixtures can best be understood by considering what happens when a liquid vapourises, especially on boiling. Let us consider first the case of a pure liquid in a closed container. At a given, fixed temperature, the average energy of the molecules is fixed. The molecules are in constant and completely random motion. Any molecule in the main body of the liquid can travel only a short distance before it comes under the influence of other molecules at which moment its direction of motion is changed. Any molecule in the surface layer, however, which happens to be moving in a direction away from the main body of the liquid can escape into the space above the liquid, thus becoming a vapour molecule. Now, the vapour molecules, too are in constant motion, the speed of the molecules of any kind being determined solely by the prevailing temperature. Any vapour molecule hitting the liquid surface has a chance of being captured by the liquid—in other words of being reliquefied (condensed). As the temperature is raised the number of vapour molecules increases. Obviously the chances of a molecule returning into the liquid also increase, so that after a short time the number of molecules vapourising in a unit of time exactly equals the number condensing (being reliquefied) in the same time. Thus, there arises a condition of dynamic equilibrium, with the total number of molecules in the vapour state remaining constant. If the space filled with saturated vapours is opened, vapour escapes and will be replaced by the same number of molecules, i.e. by the same quantity of vapour newly developed from the liquid mass. This applies not only to liquids but to solids, because, as pointed out above, every substance with a determinable boiling point is volatile.

Let us now suppose that, still at constant temperature, a second liquid, completely miscible with the first one, is added. Since the two liquids form a single phase, the surface of the liquid mixture consists only partially of molecules of the first kind. The number of molecules of the first kind escaping into the vapour space per unit time must certainly depend on the number present in the surface layer and will, therefore, be smaller now than it was for the pure liquid. However, the molecules being completely miscible, the total number returning from the vapour to the liquid will not immediately be changed. Since the total amount of surface is unchanged and since now more molecules of the first kind are condensing than are being vapourised, temporarily the equilibrium originally established will be disturbed. This process continues until a new equilibrium is established, when these rates again become equal and this in turn causes a decrease in the number of molecules of the first kind present in the vapour phase at any one time. Exactly the same law applies to the second component of the mixture. In general, the number of molecules of any component of a homogeneous mixture present in the vapour phase will thus be smaller than the number present in the same vapour space if the pure liquid is involved. The fraction of the surface occupied by either liquid is, of course, proportional to its relative amount and consequently the extent to which the rate of vapourisation decreases will depend on the composition of the liquid. The vapour composition of a one phase mixture will, therefore, be determined at any fixed temperature by the composition of the liquid.

Boiling point may be defined as 'the temperature at which, under atmospheric or any other specified pressure, a liquid is transformed into a vapour, i.e. the temperature at which the vapour pressure of the liquid equals the pressure of the surrounding gas or vapour'. When distilling at atmospheric pressure, this vapour pressure corresponds to the weight of a mercury column of 760 mm in height. Any reduction of the pressure above a liquid causes a lowering of the boiling point, any increase of pressure results in a higher boiling point. A liquid consisting of several constituents, completely miscible in one another and possessing different boiling points, in most cases (except the so-called 'constant boiling mixtures') does not have a uniform boiling point but a boiling range. As the lower boiling constituents vapourise or distil off, the boiling temperature of the liquid rises and finally approaches that of the highest boiling constituent.

Next, let us consider the effect of adding to a pure liquid in equilibrium with its vapour a second liquid which is completely immiscible with the first one. This brings us to a discussion of the distillation of heterogeneous liquids, as in the case of essential oil distillation with steam or boiling water (hydrodistillation).

To facilitate visualisation, imagine that the two media are kept well stirred, so that the percentage of each liquid present remains the same in all parts of the mixture, including the surface. Such mixing has little effect on the ultimate result. Again, the rate of vapourisation decreases, because the number of molecules of the first liquid in the surface layer is decreased. In this case, however, the liquids are not miscible and the vapour molecules can only be condensed when they strike a molecule of their own kind, so that the rate of condensation will also be decreased. Now, the rate of vapourisation and the rate of condensation both depend upon the percentage of molecules of the first kind present on the surface. These rates will be affected equally and there will be no change in the number of vapour molecules of the first component present. Applying the same reasoning to the case of the other component leads to the same conclusion. We thus arrive at the important law that the total number of molecules present in the vapour space above a two-phase liquid mixture at any given temperature equal to the sum of the numbers of molecules so present if either liquid were dealt with alone. Furthermore, since the relative amounts of the two liquids present have not in any way entered our reasoning, this conclusion must be true regardless of the relative amounts so long as both liquids are present. In other words, in the case of a two-phase (heterogeneous) liquid the composition of the mixed vapour, at a given temperature, does not depend upon the composition of the liquid.

A system of water and essential oil forms a two-phase liquid; therefore, this type of distillation is of primary importance to the essential oil producer. Let us then consider further the results of the above reasoning for our case. The pressure exerted by a vapour, whether it consists of one or several kinds of molecules, is a manifestation of the constant bombardment by the rapidly moving vapour molecules hitting the walls enclosing the vapour. Pressure measures a force acting on a unit area and this force, in the case of a vapour, results from the vapour molecules striking the wall and rebounding. The total pressure exerted will be equal to the pressure expended by one molecule multiplied by the number of molecules hitting a unit area of the wall in a unit of time. The kinetic energy expended by one molecule will depend on the temperature, but the number of collisions with the wall will depend on the number of molecules, of whatever kind, present in the vapour space. In other words, the pressure will depend on the concentration of the molecules or, stated differently, on the concentration of the vapour.

Now, it has been shown that in the case of a two-phase liquid the total number of molecules present in the vapour phase in equilibrium with it is greater than the number which would be present if either pure liquid were present alone at the same temperature. Hence, the pressure exerted by the vapour mixture will be greater than that exerted by either pure vapour alone. In the distillation of volatile oils with steam or boiling water (hydrodistillation), the pressure in the vapour space is maintained constant, either by connecting the vapour space with the atmosphere or by suitable controls to maintain a reduced or elevated pressure. For definiteness we shall consider an operation at atmospheric pressure. If pure water is heated in a still, it will begin to boil (or in other words, the pressure of its vapour will equal that of the atmosphere), when its temperature has reached 100°C (212°F). Let us suppose that an oil insoluble in water is introduced into the still along with the water. If permitted to do so, the pressure in the vapour space would increase as previously shown. But in our case the vapour space is connected to the atmosphere; therefore, the pressure will be reduced to atmospheric pressure, which can be accomplished only by automatic lowering of the temperature. When the temperature of a liquid is lowered, the tendency of the liquid molecules to go into the vapour phase also decreases, thus decreasing the concentration of the molecules in the vapour and consequently the vapour pressure. Hence, the temperature will be lowered to a value such that the total pressure exerted by the vapour mixture is again equal to the operating pressure (atmospheric pressure in our case). Thus the boiling temperature for any two-phase liquid will always be lower than the boiling point of either of the pure liquids at the same total pressure. For example, water (boiling at 100°C) and benzene (boiling at 80°C) present two such insoluble liquids when a mixture of the two is brought to a boil at atmospheric pressure (760 mm), it vapourises (distills) constantly at 69°C so long as both constituents remain, present in the liquid mixture. The moment either of the two constituents, is completely vapourised (distilled off), the temperature rises to the boiling point of the remaining constituent. Such conditions prevail with all volatile substances, provided they are insoluble in water or only very slightly soluble and are not chemically reacted upon by water. When brought to boiling together with water, they vapourise at a temperature below that of boiling water and also below those of the boiling points of the pure compounds insoluble in water.

In the preceding discussion we emphasised repeatedly that the vapour in equilibrium with a two-phase liquid consists of two kinds of molecules. The total pressure exerted by such a mixture is due, therefore, to the sum of the pressures of each kind of molecule alone. The pressure exerted by either of the pure vapours at the same temperature would be the vapour pressure of that pure component, while the total vapour pressure of the mixture is thus equal to the sum of the partial vapour pressures. By partial pressure we mean the vapour pressure of any one component in a mixed vapour. Obviously for such two-phase liquid systems the partial pressure and vapour pressure of any component are the same. The simple rule of the additivity of partial pressures affords a ready means of estimating the temperature at which any particular steam distillation (hydrodistillation) will occur. The vapour pressures of the two pure components are simply tabulated at a series of temperatures. The operating temperature will then be that temperature at which the sum of the two vapour pressures equals the operating pressure, in the above cited example the atmospheric pressure. In that case, the vapour pressure of water at 69°C is 225 mm, the vapour pressure of benzene 535 mm, added together 760 mm. This condition permits the combined vapours of the constituents to overcome the (normal) atmospheric pressure; in other words, the mixture starts to boil at 69°C under normal atmospheric pressure. In order to effect the boiling of a volatile compound insoluble in water, it remains immaterial whether the substance in question is brought to a boil with water or whether live steam is injected into the liquid or finely powdered substance. It is the steam (water vapours — whence the term hydrodistillation) that causes the boiling (distillation, in our case) of the compound insoluble in water, at a temperature below the boiling point of the compound itself and below that of water.

The composition of the vapour formed from a two-phase liquid mixture depends on the partial vapour pressures of the pure constituents. Thus, if the vapour pressure of component A is high and that of B low, the mixed vapour will consist very largely of component A. The ratio between the weights of component A and B will be given by the ratio of their vapour pressures multiplied by the ratio of their molecular weights. As pointed out, boiling will take place only when the sum of the partial pressures exerted by the components is equal to the pressure maintained in the vapour space; therefore, a heterogeneous (two-phase) liquid boils or distills at a temperature which, at the same total pressure, always lies below the boiling point of the lowest boiling constituent, so long as the latter remains in the mixture. It is for this reason primarily that hydrodistillation has been used for such a long time and so generally in the isolation of essential oils from aromatic plants. By vapourising (boiling) mixtures of water and essential oils (also from plant material), the temperature will always be maintained lower than the boiling point of water at the same total pressure and, in this way, damage and decomposition of the essential oils by overheating are prevented. The fact that the vapour pressures of most essential oils are low relative to the vapour pressures of water at corresponding temperatures accounts for the fact that the ratio of water to essential oil in the condensate is relatively high. It will make no fundamental difference in the behaviour of the mixture whether or not a steam distillation is carried out in the presence of a liquid water phase, but it does influence certain practical aspects of the process, as will be indicated latter in this chapter.

In order to isolate an essential oil from an aromatic plant, the material, in actual practice, is packed into a still, a sufficient quantity of water added and brought to a boil or live steam is injected into the plant charge. Due to the influence of hot water and steam, the essential oil will be freed from the oil glands in the plant tissue. The still, therefore, will contain a mixture of two liquids, viz. hot water and volatile oil which are not mutually soluble or only very slightly so. Gradually the liquid in the still is brought to a boil, the vapour mixture then consisting of water vapours (steam) and oil vapours. This vapour mixture passes through a connecting tube into a condenser, where it is reliquefied (condensed) by external cooling, usually with cold water. From the condenser the distillate flows into a receiver (separator), where the oil separates automatically from the distillation water. In the course of distillation it is necessary continuously to replace the water evaporating from the still or to inject a sufficient quantity of live steam to vapourise all the volatile oil contained in the plant material or present in the still. When the last traces of volatile oil have been recovered, only pure water will distil over; and distillation is completed.

As said, the composition of the distillate from a mixture of two insoluble liquids — in other words, the weight quantities of the two substance — depends primarily upon their boiling points or upon their vapour pressures at the temperature of distillation. If, for example, we distil a water insoluble compound with a boiling point of only 50°C, the distillate will consist of a certain volume of water and a larger volume of the water insoluble compound. If, on the other hand, a water insoluble compound with a boiling point of 300°C is hydrodistilled, the distillate will contain mostly water and very little of the high boiling substance. Thus, in the distillation of a water insoluble volatile compound, the percentage of the latter in the distillate decreases with rising boiling point of the compound. This decrease, however, is not uniform with all substances. Some substances with similar boiling points will occur in the distillate in different proportions; others with a marked differential in their boiling points may accumulate in the distillate in almost the same proportions. Deviations of this sort are caused primarily by the chemical constitutions and reactivity of the various essential oil components. As explained above, the quantitative composition of the distillate (condensate) can be calculated in advance when hydrodistilling chemically uniform, water insoluble substances. The rule underlying hydrodistillation of essential oils or volatile substances in general may be expressed as follows:

The ratio between the weights of the two vapour components and therefore of the two liquids in the distillate (condensate), is expressed by the ratio of their partial vapour pressures multiplied by the ratio of their molecular weight.

$$\frac{W_{H_2O}}{W_{oil}} = \frac{P_{H_2O}}{P_{oil}} \times \frac{M_{H_2O}}{M_{oil}}$$

where, W_{H_2O} = weight of water in the condensate.

W_{oil} = weight of oil in the condensate.

P_{H_2O} = vapour pressure of water at still temperature.

P_{oil} = vapour pressure of oil at still temperature.

M_{H_2O} = molecular weight of water (= 18).

M_{oil} = molecular weight of oil (assuming that this constant may be determined as an average figure).

Essential oils are not chemically pure substances but consist of several, often many, compounds possessing different chemical and physical properties. The boiling points of the volatile oil components range in most cases from 150° to 300°C at 760 mm pressure. According to the preponderance of lower or higher boiling constituents we speak of a low boiling or of a high boiling oil. Distillation of an essential oil reveals its higher or lower volatility to a very marked degree if the oil is in free, direct contact with the boiling water or with the passing steam: in the early stages of distillation the lower boiling component, distil over; the higher boiling ones pass over later.

Let us now study hydrodistillation of a volatile oil with a very simple example: peppermint oil is placed into a glass flask and live steam is introduced into the oil. The external pressure and temperature, in this case, remain immaterial, so long as at least a portion of water remains in steam form. The steam then causes the peppermint oil to form vapours, to vapourise, each steam bubble presenting to the vapourised oil an empty space into which the oil immediately sends vapour molecules. Every volume unit of steam will be filled with an equal volume of oil vapours, rise to the top of the flask and enter the condenser, where steam and oil vapours are condensed. The hydrodistillation of any essential oil is based upon this simple principle which, however, does not fully apply to the oils when they are still enclosed within the plant tissue. There the steam must exert yet another action of considerable influence, i.e. it must transmit heat. Unlike a liquid, the rigid plant matter is not able to conduct the heat from the still walls to all parts of the plant charge.

The heat is actually transmitted by water, either as boiling water when distilling immersed plant material or as water vapours when distilling plants by blowing live steam into the charge. Also, the volatile oils occur in special oil glands, sacks or intracellular spaces of the plant tissue; hence the oils must be freed, prior to distillation, by breaking down the plant tissue and by opening the oil glands as much as possible, so that their volatile content can be readily attacked and vapourised by the passing steam. In unreduced, whole plant material, the oil must be freed during distillation by the force of hydrodiffusion, a very important feature which will be discussed later in more detail.

Let us now return to the more theoretical aspects of hydrodistillation. In steam distillation it is frequently possible to change materially the ratio of water to oil in the condensate by changing the operating pressure. As pointed out earlier, this ratio is determined by the relationship:

$$\frac{W_{H_2O}}{W_{oil}} = \frac{P_{H_2O}}{P_{oil}} \times \frac{M_{H_2O}}{M_{oil}}$$

In any hydrodistillation using saturated steam, the sum of P_{H_2O} and P_{oil} will equal the operating pressure and the still temperature will automatically adjust itself until this condition is met. As the operating pressure is lowered below atmospheric pressure, the temperature of the operation will decrease. In general, the vapour pressure of water decreases much more slowly with the temperature than does the vapour pressure of an essential oil, so that the weight ratio of water to oil increases. Conversely, this ratio decreases with increasing temperature. Data for a typical case are given in Table 5.1.

These data demonstrate that operation at reduced pressure results in a lower operating temperature, but also requires the use of more steam per weight unit of citronellal recovered. Operation at elevated pressure (use of high-pressure steam in the still), on the other hand, permits a considerable saving in the amount of steam required per weight unit of oil, but also involves a higher operating temperature. Provided that the higher temperature does not damage the oil, there is evidently some advantage to be gained by the use of high-pressure steam.

Table 5.1. Effect of operating pressure on water to oil ratio in steam distillation of citronellal.

Total Pressure mm Hg	Temperatrue °C	Vapour pressure mm Hg		Molal ratio water/citronellal	Weight ratio
		Water	Citronellal		
152.2	60	149.5	2.66	56.2	6.6
238.5	70	233.8	4.70	49.8	5.9
263.7	80	355.5	8.20	43.3	5.1
540.0	90	526.0	14.00	37.6	4.4
782.5	100	760.0	22.50	33.8	3.9
1109.1	110	1075.0	34.10	31.5	3.7

Up to this point our discussion has dealt entirely with the use of saturated steam. It is also possible 0—indeed, in some cases advantageous—to distil essential oils by using superheated steam. Pressure and temperature of superheated steam are no longer mutually dependent. Thus, it is feasible to use superheated steam at a fixed pressure and at any desired temperature above the boiling point at that pressure. The temperature at which such a distillation is carried out can thus be raised without increasing the concentration (partial pressure) of the steam. Since the temperature alone determines the vapour pressure and consequently the partial pressure of the volatile oil, distillation with superheated steam results in a lower ratio of water to oil, accomplishing a further saving in the amount of steam used. In the above cited case of water and citronellal mixtures the steam would normally be saturated at 90°C. If superheated to 100°C at a pressure of 526 mm and then used in the distillation, the molal ratio of water to citronellal is reduced to 23.3 (weight ratio = 1.72), the total operating pressure then being 548.5 mm. By increasing the pressure of the superheated steam any ratio between this and 33.8 (corresponding to the use of saturated steam at 100°C) can be obtained.

Two features affecting the use of superheated steam should be pointed out. First, in order to obtain the above cited advantage of superheated steam the still must be completely free of water. When superheated, steam comes into contact with water it immediately vapourises some of the water, being itself cooled in the process and being reconverted into saturated steam. If the quantity of water present is small, it will be vapourised quickly and the process will continue as with superheated steam after the water has been evaporated. Second, the temperature of superheated steam is independent of the pressure; hence the characteristic safeguard against overheating common with saturated steam operation no longer remains operative. The temperature of the charge will reach that of the superheated steam; therefore, the latter temperature must be controlled carefully in order to avoid damage to the essential oil. Also, since there is no water present in the still, the plant charge tends to dry out during distillation with superheated steam and the forces of hydrodiffusion can no longer play their part. This causes a slowing down in the rate of recovery of essential oil and in extreme cases may stop it entirely, long before the recovery is complete; in other words, the yield of essential oil will be subnormal. For all these reasons superheated steam distillation may be undertaken only with caution.

It should be mentioned in this connection that for distillation any hot gas (air, flue gas, etc.) could be used in place of steam but, since these gases are not condensable, the size of the cooler required would be so great as to be impracticable.

Let us now again study the behaviour of mixtures of liquids which form a single liquid phase. These considerations apply particularly to the fractionation of essential oils after they have been isolated from the plant material. As has already been pointed out, all liquids have a tendency to change to vapours, the extent of this tendency depending on the temperature at which the liquid is maintained. This tendency to vapourise may be gauged by the vapour pressure of the liquid. In general, the components of the liquid mixture will have different vapour pressures at any particular temperature. When such a mixture is vapourised, the component with the greater vapour pressure (the more volatile component) consequently tends to concentrate in the vapour phase, while the less volatile component will be correspondingly concentrated in the liquid phase. This condition holds for all mixtures of liquids which are soluble in one another and which do not form constant boiling mixtures. Liquid mixtures which form constant boiling mixtures behave somewhat differently and will not be discussed here. The tendency of the more volatile liquid to concentrate in the vapour phase can be observed very readily by reference to the accompanying Fig. 5.1.

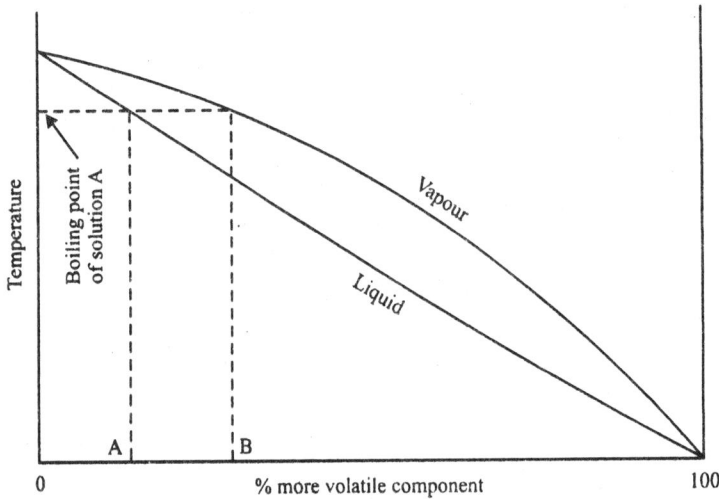

Fig. 5.1. Typical boiling point and vapour-liquid equilibrium diagram for a single-phase binary mixture at constant pressure.

In this diagram the composition of the liquid mixture and its boiling temperature have been plotted. The lower of the two curves represents the relationship between the boiling point of any mixture of these two components and its composition. The upper curve represents the composition of the vapour which is formed from any liquid mixture at its boiling point. Proceeding along a vertical line in the region below the lower curve may be said to correspond to heating a mixture of fixed composition without vapourisation. At the temperature corresponding to the point at which this vertical path intersects the lower curve, this particular mixture will begin to vapourise and the vapours arising first will have a composition represented by the intersection of a horizontal line through the boiling point of this mixture with the upper curve. In the particular case illustrated, a liquid containing A per cent of the more volatile constituent would produce an initial vapour containing a percentage of the more volatile constituent represented by point B. The vapour produced is thereby enriched with the more volatile constituents. If the distillation is continued without adding liquid to the still, the liquid in the still will become progressively poorer in the more volatile constituents. Furthermore, on condensing and then redistilling the vapour produced, a further enrichment in the more volatile constituents will be achieved. Theoretically, then, it appears possible to obtain a vapour consisting entirely of the more volatile components by a suitable number of redistillations. An effect corresponding to a series of redistillations can be produced in a fractionating column such as that shown in Fig. 5.2.

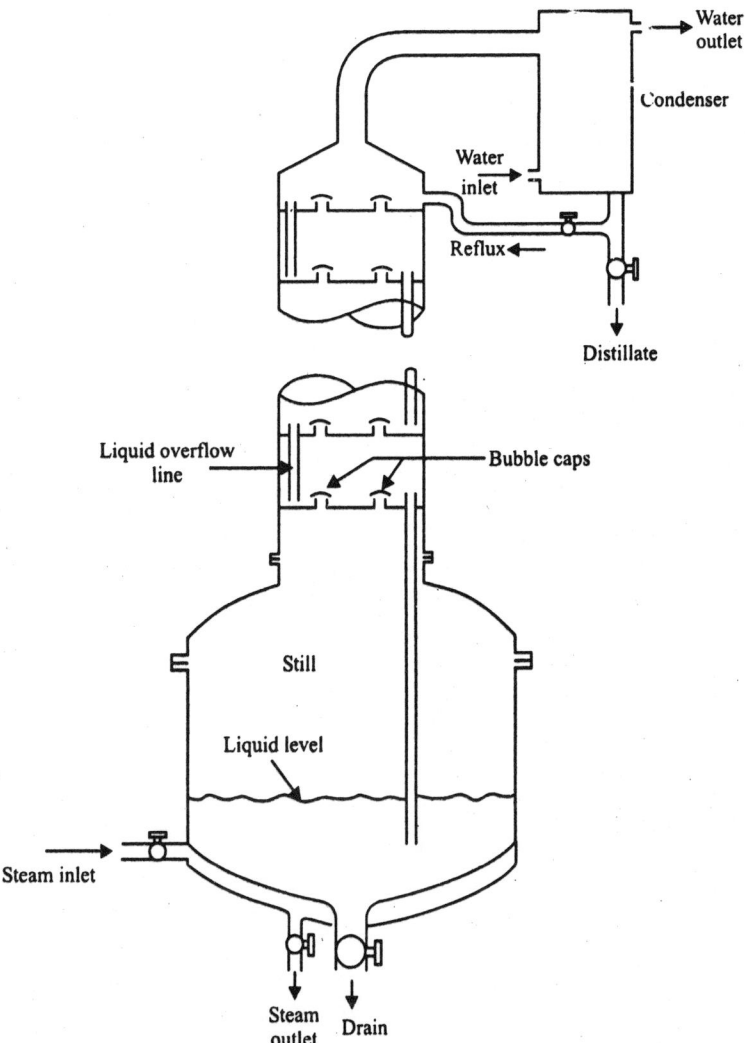

Fig. 5.2. Still with fractionating column. Schematic diagram showing essential parts and typical arrangement.

In this type of system the vapours rising from the still, as always partially enriched with the more volatile component, are essentially condensed and redistilled on the first section above the still. The vapours rising from this section are again condensed and redistilled in the next higher section, this process continuing to the top of the fractionation tower. Such equipment, then, permits obtaining a final distillate which contains a higher percentage of the more volatile components of the mixture than the original material—this, too, in a single piece of equipment. Heat is supplied to such a fractionating system in the still only.

On the plates in the tower above the still the heat liberated by condensation of the vapours furnishes in turn the heat necessary to revapourise the material. Of course, the entire system must be insulated thoroughly in order to prevent excessive condensation of vapours due to the heat losses from the tower. In actual operation, such a tower would ordinarily be run by returning part of the condensate at the top to the top plate as reflux.

The greater the ratio of reflux to product, the more complete will be the separation of the more volatile from the less volatile components. A system of this kind can be operated at any desired pressure either above or below normal atmospheric pressure. In the final purification of many essential oils (not hydrodistillation), the operation must proceed at very low pressures in order to avoid overheating and consequent destruction of the material. The number of plates required in the fractionation tower is determined largely by two factors:

1. The relative volatility of the components of the mixture.
2. The extent of separation required or desired.

Whenever one component is much more volatile than the other, only a few plates will be necessary to give a high degree of separation, but when the volatilities are more nearly equal, the number of plates must be greatly increased. A rough estimate of the relative volatilities can be drawn from the boiling points at atmospheric pressure of the components of the mixture. There exist quite satisfactory methods for calculating the number of plates required for any particular separation. Details of these methods go beyond the scope of this work.

The above considerations show that some separation of the components of a mixture of mutually soluble constituents (such as essential oils) can be achieved simply by vapourising the mixture and condensing the vapours. Usually, however, this separation will be relatively small and it will be necessary to resort either to redistillation of the condensate or to the use of fractionating towers as indicated.

In order to consider in more detail the behaviour of mixtures of soluble liquids, let us take the case of a mixture of only two constituents. The same principles apply to more complex mixtures, but will be easier to follow in the simpler case. In single-phase mixtures the tendency of either component to vapourise will depend on the temperature of the mixture and on its composition. In the simplest case, the partial pressure of one constituent will be given by the expression

$$p_1 = P_1 \times N_1 \qquad\qquad ... (5.1)$$

in which

p_1 = partial pressure of constituent 1
P_1 = vapour pressure of pure constituent 1 at the temperature of the liquid
N_1 = mol fraction of constituent 1.

$$N_1 = \cfrac{\dfrac{w_1}{M_1}}{\dfrac{w_1}{M_1} + \dfrac{w_2}{M_2}} \qquad\qquad ... (5.2)$$

w_1 = weight of constituent 1 in mixture.
w_2 = weight of constituent 2 in mixture.
M_1 = molecular weight of constituent 1.
M_2 = molecular weight of constituent 2.

The relationship between the partial pressures of the constituents, total pressure of the mixture (which is equal to the sum of the partial pressure) and the composition of the mixture for a fixed temperature is shown in Fig. 5.3. Systems which follow this rule are ideal systems and are said to obey Raoult's law (Equation 5.1 above).

In the more general case, the relationships between these variables are not as simple and can be determined only by experimental methods. A typical case is shown in Fig. 5.4.

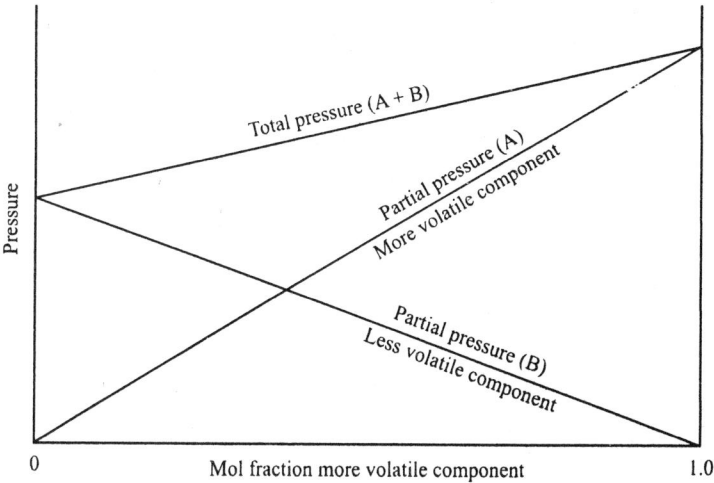

Fig. 5.3. Partial and total pressure curves at constant temperatures for a single-phase binary mixture obeying Raoult's law.

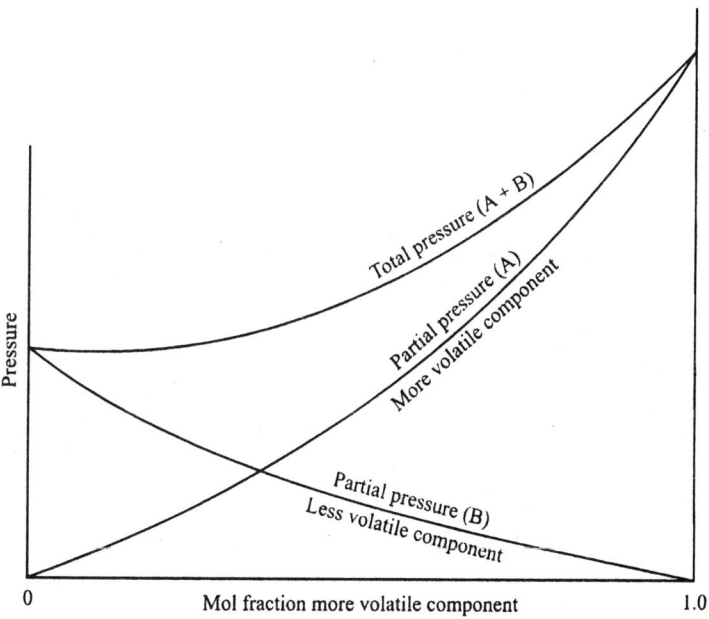

Fig. 5.4. Partial and total pressure curves at constant temperature for a single-phase binary mixture showing one type of deviation from Raoult's law.

Since most distillations are conducted at constant pressure rather than at constant temperature, and since the boiling point of a mixture at a fixed pressure varies with the composition, a somewhat more useful diagram for purposes of analysing distillation problems is shown in Fig. 5.5.

This diagram represents the composition of the vapour corresponding to the composition of the equilibrium liquid mixture at a constant total pressure. Both compositions are expressed in terms of the percentage of the more volatile constituent and obviously the vapour is always richer in this component than is the liquid from which it originated. Thus, the vapour in equilibrium with a liquid of composition A would have the composition B. If this vapour were entirely condensed, the resulting liquid would have this same composition B and, if redistilled, would give an equilibrium vapour, further enriched and having composition C. This is essentially the process which takes place in a fractionation column. The mechanism which accomplishes separation in this type of equipment is evident. The effects of changing reflux ratio and other variables cannot be discussed here in detail.

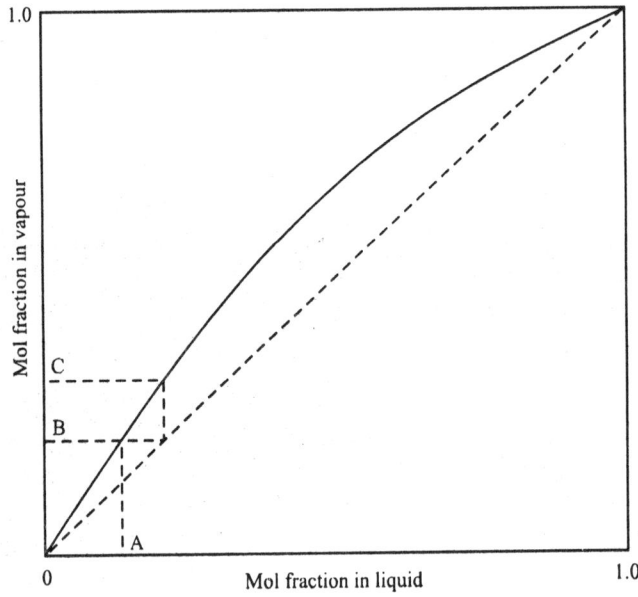

Fig. 5.5. Vapour-liquid equilibrium diagram at constant temperature for a single-phase binary mixture (All compositions expressed in terms of the more volatile constituent).

Although a fractionating tower consisting of separate plates as shown in Fig. 5.2 has been used as an example, an equally satisfactory tower for most purposes column of an open column filled with a suitable packing material. This material can take almost any conceivable shape, but should be characterised by low density (weight per unit volume of the packing), relatively large amount of open space and a large surface area. For example, crushed rock can be used as packing, but because of its high density and low percentage of open space would not be very efficient.

Table 5.2. Pressure equivalents.

Lb. per sq. in.	Kg per sq. cm	Mm of mercury	Atmosphere
1	0.0703	51.7	0.0680
2	0.141	103.4	0.1361
3	0.211	155.1	0.2041
4	0.271	206.8	0.2722
5	0.352	258.5	0.3402
10	0.703	517.0	0.6804
14.7	1.033	760.0	1.000

(Contd ...)

Lb. per sq. in.	Kg per sq. cm	Mm of mercury	Atmosphere
20	1.407	1034	1.361
25	1.756	1293	1.701
30	2.109	1551	2.041
35	2.461	1810	2.381
40	2.812	2068	2.722
45	3.164	2327	3.062
50	3.515	2585	3.402
60	4.218	3102	4.082
70	4.921	3619	4.763
80	5.623	4136	5.443
90	6.327	4653	6.124
100	7.027	5170	6.804

In the distillation of single-phase mixtures, it should be kept in mind that changing the pressure in the still has only a minor effect on the overall operation. Since in the distillation of essential oils the principal reason for ever operating at pressures other than atmospheric is to lower the distillation temperature, the pressure will usually vary between atmospheric and some lower pressure, thus limiting the possible variations in pressure. The efficiency of any particular piece of equipment may be changed slightly by operating at different pressures, but the net result will be practically unaffected. This holds true particularly in the case of mixtures such as those encountered in the purification and fractionation of essential oils.

PRACTICE OF DISTILLATION

Having indicated briefly the general principles of distillation of homogeneous and heterogeneous systems, we shall devote the second part of this section to a discussion of the practical distillation problems and techniques peculiar to the essential oil industry.

Treatment of the Plant Material

Comminution of the plant material

The chief application of distillation is in the initial isolation of essential oils from the aromatic plant material. This process involves the handling of predominantly solid products and the preparation of the material must therefore, be carried carefully if the most efficient and complete recovery of the valuable essential oils is to be assured. The essential oils are enclosed in 'oil glands', 'veins', 'oil sacks', or 'glandular hairs' of the aromatic plants. If the plant material were left intact, the oils could be removed (vapourised) by the steam only after they had passed through the plant tissues to an exposed surface. This can be accomplished only by hydrodiffusion, a mechanism which will later be shown to play a very important part in plant distillation. Diffusion is always a slow process and if the plants or parts of plants were left intact, the rate of recovery of oil would be determined entirely by the rate of diffusion. Consequently, before distillation, the plant material must be disintegrated to some extent. This disintegration process, commonly termed comminution, results in exposing directly as many oil glands as is practically possible. It always reduces the thickness of material through which diffusion must occur, greatly increasing the rate or speed of vapourisation and distillation of the essential oils. Even in comminuted plant material, only a portion of the oil is freed, the balance remaining enclosed or being tightly covered by comminuted plant particles. All actually exposed volatile oil will soon be entrained by passing steam and carried away from the plants.

The extent of comminution required varies with the nature of the plant material. Flowers, leaves and other thin and nonfibrous parts of the plant can be distilled without comminution. The cell walls in these parts are in most cases sufficiently thin and permeable to permit rapid removal of the oil. Seeds (fruits), on the other hand, must be thoroughly crushed in order to rupture as many of the cell walls as possible, to render the oil easily accessible to the passing steam. Roots, stalks and all woody material should be cut into short lengths in order to expose a great number of oil glands.

Seeds can best be crushed by passing them through smooth rolls. These rolls should be arranged so that the distance between them can be varied. The width of this space will determine the extent of crushing obtained. A similar effect can be achieved by regulating the flow of the material upon the distributor above the rolls. If the rolls operate at different speeds, the crushing action is supplemented by a usually advantageous shearing action. Each roll should also be equipped with a scraping device, called a 'doctor blade', which serves to keep it free of adhering crushed material.

Roots and stalks can best be handled in a hay or ensilage cutter or similar device. This action simply reduces the long natural parts of the plant to short lengths which are more readily handled in the distillation proper and, above all, assures a more uniform and compact charge in the still. Otherwise the live steam would find ready passages through the wide interspaces of uncut roots or stalk material and escape without coming in close contact with all plant particles. The result, especially in the case of steam distillation, would be a very inferior yield of oil. Woody parts may be sawed into small pieces or chipped mechanically.

The principal purpose of comminution being to render the essential oils more readily removable by the passing steam, it is evident that once the plant material has been crushed or reduced in size it must be distilled immediately. Otherwise, the essential oils, being somewhat volatile, will partly evaporate, with two adverse effects: first, the total yield of oil will be reduced by an amount equal to the extent to which evaporation has occurred; second, the composition of the oil will change, thereby affecting its odour. This second effect results from the fact that the essential oils are mixtures of several, often numerous, compounds, the more volatile components evaporating to a greater extent than the higher boiling and less volatile ones. In the case of crushed caraway seed, for example, the evaporation loss consists mainly of limonene, which is lower boiling than carvone; the oil distilled from crushed seed which has been left in contact with open air for some time will, therefore, possess a somewhat higher specific gravity. The extent of these oil losses by evaporation can be demonstrated easily by crushing a small quantity of caraway seed, weighing it on an analytical balance, airing it for a few minutes and checking the weight. Smith reported a loss of 0.5 per cent which he can attributed entirely to evaporation of oil, not of moisture, because air-dried seed was used in the experiment. It is, therefore, imperative that comminution be carried out immediately before the product is charged into the still if highest yields and best quality oils are to be obtained.

After the plant materials have been properly prepared for distillation, they are packed into the still and distillation can be started. Methods of charging and the construction of the still itself will be discussed after the general distillation methods have been presented.

Storage of the plant material

The storage of plant material before comminution also offers some hazard in the way of ultimate loss of volatile oil. The situation here is not quite so serious as in the case of comminuted material and, therefore, if a delay in the distilling of the plant material cannot be avoided, it should be stored in its natural condition. Gradual evaporation results in some loss under these circumstances, the major sources of loss being represented by oxidation and resinification of the essential oils. If the plant material must be stored before processing, it should be kept in a dry atmosphere at a low temperature and in a room free from air circulation — if possible in an air-conditioned storehouse. All such losses are obviously avoided if the plants are processed immediately.

Loss of essential oil in the plant material prior to distillation

The volatile oil enclosed in the plant tissue is usually in one way or another affected by the drying of the plant material after the harvest. This effect has been studied and the findings are interesting.

Some fresh plants or parts, with a high water content (e.g. roses, tansy, calamus root) lose much of their essential oil by air drying; others very little. This loss is caused by evaporation, oxidation, resinification and other chemical actions. Contrary to expectation, evaporation here seems to play a subordinate role to oxidation and resinification. Indeed, actual evaporation of the volatile oil through the walls of the plant tissue cannot take place readily because the oil must first be brought to the surface through hydrodiffusion, with water or plant moisture acting as a carrying medium. Thin-walled flowers and leaves present no obstacle to the forces of diffusion and in most cases evaporation will affect the more water-soluble constituents of a volatile oil rather than the low boiling terpenes. It has been shown that by field drying and stacking of citronella grass or lemon grass prior to distillation the total acetylisable constituents of the oil decreased considerably with time after cutting. Since losses of acetylisable constituents were sufficient to account for most of the decrease in yield of oil, various scientists concluded that the major factor leading to a loss of oil was oxidation. Evaporation of whole oil accounted for the additional loss. With both grasses it can be concluded that, for the best results, field drying, with or without subsequent stacking should not be practiced.

Distillation experiments seldom give reliable data on the loss of volatile oil by evaporation during plant drying. The reason is simply that distillation of plant material with a high water content usually leaves doubt as to its completeness. Peppermint offers a classical example in this respect. Formerly it was assumed that its oil content increases during the drying of the cut herb, but systematic distillation experiments proved the fallacy of this assumption. Fresh peppermint herb, like most plants or plant parts with a high moisture content, simply cannot be exhausted completely by distillation or only with great difficulty and after long hours of distillation. By distilling one portion of peppermint herb in the fresh state right after the harvest and the other portion in wilted, almost dry ('clover dry') condition and by calculating the yields upon 100 kg of fresh herb, it has been shown that the fresh herb contains a little more, possibly much more, oil than the dried herb, but it is very difficult to exhaust the fresh herb completely by distillation.

The loss of oil during the period of wilting and drying of the plant material is much greater than the loss occurring during storage of the plant material after it has been dried. This may be explained by the fact that, during the first stages of wilting and drying, the plant retains a large amount of moisture in the cells, which by diffusion carries the oil to the surface and aids in its vapourisation. Once the moisture has disappeared and the plant has become air dried, hydrodiffusion can no longer take place. Any loss of oil during storage of the air dried plant material depends upon several factors — condition of the material, method and length of storing and the chemical composition of the oil. As a rule, but with many exceptions, flowers, leaves and herbs do not endure prolonged storing, whereas seeds, bark, roots and wood, by their very nature, retain their volatile oils much longer. Method of storing (packing tightly in sacks or bales or spreading on the floor and heaping loosely) plays an important role in this respect. Air currents and extreme variations in moisture content of the atmosphere favour oil evaporation, resinification and, particularly, oxidation. It is possible to keep many types of plant materials for a long period, provided they are stored at sufficiently low temperature and in an air-conditioned room. Under such conditions, caraway seed does not lose volatile oil even over a period of six months. In isolated cases, plant materials — guaiac wood and sandalwood, for example — retain their essential oil for many years, even though exposed to considerable variations of weather.

It has been found that the greatest loss of volatile oil by evaporation and oxidation occurs in comminuting the plant material prior to distillation, especially if this is done in rapidly rotating grinders and mills. The extent of loss depends upon the speed of air circulation in the system, the degree of heat development in the material and the composition of the volatile oil (its boiling range and resistance to oxidation).

Change in the physico-chemical properties of essential oils during plant drying

Essential oils distilled either from fresh or from dried plant parts show wide variations in physico-chemical properties and chemical composition. With many oils it seems advisable, therefore, to state whether they were distilled from fresh, wilted or air-dried plant material. This is especially true of flowers, leaves, herbs and roots, which in the fresh state contain much moisture. Peppermint oil, for example, displays marked variations in its properties.

Oil from fresh herb, according to Smith, had a specific gravity of 0.908, that from clover dried herb a gravity of 0.912. The term 'clover dried' means that the stalks are still flexible but the leaves dry. A series of interesting distillation experiments were carried out are:

Angelica root oil

From fresh angelica roots: d_{15}^{15} 0.857 to 0.866

From dried angelica roots: d_{15}^{15} 0.876 to 0.902

The specific gravity of angelica root oil increases in proportion to the length of time the roots have been stored.

Lovage root oil

From fresh lovage roots: d_{15}^{15} 1.002 to 1.035

From dried lovage roots: d_{15}^{15} 1.039 to 1.040

Fresh and dried lovage roots exhibit a difference in behaviour during distillation. During the distillation of dried lovage root, a yellow, gluey, resinous mass appears together with the oil, especially toward the end of distillation. This mass is largely dissolved in the oil; part of it separates in the condenser pipes and in the Florentine flask. Fresh lovage roots do not yield this resin and wilted roots in only a small amount. Oil of lovage from fresh roots, when rectified, is entirely volatile; the oil from dried roots upon rectification leaves in the still considerable quantities of a high boiling residue, which cannot be redistilled with water or steam.

Calamus root oil

From fresh calamus roots: d_{15}^{15} 0.962 to 0.968; α_D +20° to +31°

From dried calamus roots: d_{15}^{15} 0.963 to 0.978; α_D + 15° to +20°

The oil from the fresh roots is more soluble in 70 per cent alcohol than is the oil from the dried roots. The solubility of the oil decreases with ageing (storing) of the root.

Estragon oil

From fresh estragon herb: d_{15}^{15} 0.918 to 0.934; α_D +2° to +4°

From dried estragon herb: d_{15}^{15} 0.890 to 0.923; α_D +5° to +8°

An interesting observation have been reported on the resinification of volatile oils in oils in spice plants. Whether the formation of these so-called resins is caused by the polymerisation of homogeneous compounds or the addition reactions of heterogeneous compounds, by oxidation or other forms of conversion of volatile compounds, is not entirely clear.

Natural (not rectified) peppermint oil distilled from fresh herb is more soluble in 70 per cent alcohol than is the oil distilled from dried herb, but the solubility decreases after a few months. If oil from fresh herb is rectified, it resinifies again, whereas oil from dried herb, when rectified, retains its original solubility.

Certain constituents of peppermint oil, including possibly menthofurane, seem to resinify during the drying of the herb.

During wilting and drying, the cell membranes gradually break down and the liquids are free to penetrate from cell to cell, giving rise to the formation of new volatile compounds, e.g. by glycoside splitting. A typical example is found in bitter almond oil, which develops in the course of brief storing of crushed and moistened almond or apricot kernels. In the live fruit, the enzyme (emulson) cannot contact the glucoside (amygdalin) in aqueous solution; but it can readily do so in the crushed and wetted kernels. Analogous reactions and cleavages undoubtedly take place in many other cases. Fresh orris roots, for example, possess a rather disagreeable 'green' and 'herby' odour; whereas the dried roots, upon ageing, develop a faint violet odour. Freshly harvested patchouli leaves are almost odourless; the well-known typical patchouli odour develops only on drying and curing. Vanilla beans constitute another example, the fresh pods resembling to some degree our common garden beans. The odour of grass is very different from that of hay, which develops its typical coumarin note only during the drying process. A phenomenon not yet explained is the disappearance of geraniol in dried roses, while the content of phenylethyl alcohol seems to increase.

General Methods of Distillation

No investigation has yet been undertaken of the process by which steam actually isolates the essential oil from aromatic plants. It is commonly assumed that the steam penetrates the plant tissue and vapourises all volatile substances. If this were true, the isolation of oil from plants by hydrodistillation would appear to be a rather simple process, merely requiring a sufficient quantity of steam. However, such is not the case. In fact, hydrodistillation of plants involves several physico-chemical processes which will be discussed later.

There has developed in the essential oil industry a terminology which distinguishes three types of hydrodistillation. These are referred to respectively as:

1. Water distillation;
2. Water and steam distillation.
3. Direct steam distillation.

The above terms have become established in the essential oil industry and will, therefore, be retained in our discussion.

In order to avoid needles repetition, their significance will be indicated at this point. All three methods are subject to the same general theoretical considerations.

Water distillation

When this method is employed, the material to be distilled comes in direct contact with boiling water. It may float on the water or be completely immersed, depending upon its specific gravity and the quantity of material handled per charge. The water is boiled by application of heat by any of the usual methods that is direct fire, steam jacket, closed steam coil or in a few cases, open or perforated steam coil. The characteristic feature of this method lies in the direct contact it affords between boiling water and plant material. Some plant materials (e.g. powdered almonds, rose petals and orange blossoms) must be distilled while fully immersed and moving freely in boiling water, because on distillation with injected live steam (direct steam distillation) these materials agglutinate and form large compact lumps, through which the steam cannot penetrate.

Water and steam distillation

When this second common method of distillation is used, the plant material is supported on a perforated grid or screen inserted some distance above the bottom of the still. The lower part of the still is filled with water, to a level somewhat below this grid. The water may be heated by any of the methods previously mentioned. Saturated, in this case, wet, steam of low pressure rises through the plant material. The typical features of this method are: first, that the steam is always fully saturated, wet and never superheated; second, that the plant material is in contact with steam only and not with boiling water.

Steam distillation

The third method, known as steam distillation or direct steam distillation, resembles the preceding one except that no water is kept in the bottom of the still. Live steam, saturated or superheated and frequently at pressures higher than atmospheric, is introduced through open or perforated steam coils below the charge and proceeds upward through the charge above the supporting grid.

In so far as the distillation process itself is concerned and from the purely theoretical point of view, there should be no fundamental difference between these three methods. There exist, however, certain variations in practice and in the practical results obtained, which in some cases are considerable; they depend on the method employed, because of certain reactions which occur during distillation.

The principal effects accompanying hydrodistillation are:

1. Diffusion of essential oils and hot water through the plant membranes, whence the term hydrodiffusion.
2. Hydrolysis of certain components of the essential oils.
3. Decomposition occasioned by heat.

These effects will be considered in order.

Effects of hydrodiffusion in plant distillation

Even after the plant material has been carefully prepared by proper comminution, only part of the essential oil is present on the surfaces of the material and immediately available for vapourisation by steam. The remainder of the oil arrives at the surface only after diffusing through at least a thin layer of plant tissue.

The term diffusion, as used in this connection, implies the mutual penetration of different substances until an equilibrium is established within the system. Such diffusion is caused by the live force of molecules. Where two substances are not separated by a wall (diaphragm), the term 'free diffusion' is applied, whereas diffusion through a permeable membrane is called osmosis. The diaphragm may be permeable by only one substance or all.

The distillation of plant material is connected with processes of diffusion and principally of osmosis. In the steam distillation of plant material the steam does not actually penetrate the dry cell membranes. This can easily be proved by distilling plants with superheated (dry) steam. The plant charge, in this case, finally dries out completely and yields the retained volatile oil only when saturated (moist) steam is applied, after superheated (dry) steam no longer vapourises the oil. Thus, dry plant material can be exhausted with dry steam only when all of the volatile oil has first been freed from the oil bearing cells by previous very thorough comminution of the plants.

Entirely different conditions obtain if the plant tissue is soaked with water. The exchange of vapours within the tissue of living plants is based primarily upon their permeability while in swollen condition. Microscopic studies have led some to believe that the walls of normal plant cells are almost impermeable for volatile oils. According to Smith only limited osmosis of volatile oil can take place at ordinary temperatures. This may easily be proved by soaking uncomminuted dried spices (such as cinnamon or cloves) in cold water for a day or two, then pouring off and distilling the water. The yield of oil, if any, will be negligible, all the oil being retained within the plant tissue. If, on the other hand, the spices (or other plant material) are first sufficiently powdered so that the cell walls are broken and the oil liberated, the water poured off contains considerable quantities of essential oil. Distillation offers better conditions for the osmosis of oil, because the higher temperature and the movement of water, caused by temperature and pressure fluctuations within the still, accelerate the forces of diffusion to such a point that all the volatile oil contained within the plant tissue can be collected. The effect of a higher temperature may easily be demonstrated by repeating the above described experiments, but by soaking the spices in hot, instead of cold water. The hot water will extract much larger quantities of oil.

Smith describes the process of hydrodiffusion, in the case of plant distillation, as follows: At the temperature of boiling water a part of the volatile oil dissolves in the water present within the glands. This oil-in-water solution permeates, by osmosis, through the swollen membranes and finally reaches the outer surface, where the oil is vapourised by passing steam. Replacing this vapourised oil, additional quantities of oil go into solution and, as such, permeate the cell membranes while water enters. This process continues until all volatile substances are diffused from the oil glands and are vapourised by the passing steam.

The speed of oil vapourisation in hydrodistillation of plant material is influenced not so much by the volatility of the oil components (or in other words by the differential in their boiling points), as by their degree of solubility in water). If Smith's assumption is correct the higher boiling, but more water-soluble, constituents of an oil enclosed within the plant tissue should distil before the lower boiling, but less water-soluble, constituents. That this actually takes place can be demonstrated by steam distilling comminuted and uncomminuted caraway seed. Uncomminuted (whole) caraway seed will first yield the higher boiling, but more water-soluble, carvone and only later the lower boiling, but less water-soluble, limonene. With crushed seed the opposite is true: the first fraction consists of limonene, the following of carvone. The fact that occasionally the final fraction may contain some limonene only goes to show that, as a result of incomplete comminution, the forces of hydrodiffusion come into play anew. Distillation of uncrushed caraway seed requires almost twice as much time as that of crushed. This well-known fact applies to distillation of all seed material. The explanation is simply that hydrodiffusion acts only slowly and requires time in the distillation of uncrushed seeds, all volatile oil enclosed within the plant tissue must first be brought to the surface of the seeds by hydrodiffusion.

It is a well-known fact, borne out by experience, that comminution (crushing) of seed material increases the yield of oil. This, however, does not imply that uncomminuted plant material always gives a very low oil yield. Smith whole (uncrushed) caraway seed should be soaked in tepid water until it became swollen and distilled it with direct, saturated steam at pressure of 5 atmospheres in a well-insulated still. A very slightly lower yield of oil can be obtained by distilling crushed caraway seed. This small loss consisted exclusively of carvone, which had been resinified during the longer hours of distillation required for uncrushed, thoroughly wetted seed. Such soaking, steeping or macerating of plant material was frequently resorted to in the old days of small-scale distillation, when saturated steam of high pressure, generated in a separate steam boiler, was not yet available. In fact, steeping in water as a preliminary process should not be condemned in the case of seed material containing relatively low boiling volatile oils—caraway, fennel, coriander seed, for example. Obviously this process requires more steam, fuel, time and equipment, but the oil yield will be about normal, provided distillation has been carefully carried through. It should be borne in mind, however, that saturated steam of low pressure, if not properly employed, may easily result in a thorough wetting of the plant charge and that this factor becomes much more troublesome with a comminuted charge than with an uncomminuted one. Smith performed experiments in point with dill, ajowan and fennel seed, as well as with cloves and clove stems. His results again prove that, in the case of uncomminuted material, the oil constituents vapourise according to the degree of their solubility in water and not in the sequence of their boiling points: carvone distils before limonene in the case of dill seed; thymol before pinene, dipentene and *p*-cymene in the case of ajowan seed; anethole before fenchone in the case of fennel seed; methyl amyl ketone before eugenol and caryophyllene in the case of cloves; eugenol before caryophyllene in the case of clove stems. In experiments conducted by Smith, the distillation of uncomminuted material required twice as many hours as that of comminuted material and the yield of oil was slightly and in some cases considerably, lower.

The presence of some water is distinctly beneficial in that it increases the rate of removal of essential oils by distillation and it would appear, from this fact alone, that water distillation or water and steam distillation should be preferred to steam distillation. However, the maximum temperature that can be obtained with water distillation and water and steam distillation, is limited entirely by the operating pressure in the still, which in ordinary operation equals atmospheric pressure. A complete summary of the advantages and disadvantages of the three methods of distillation will be given after the other factors affecting distillation have been discussed. It should be remembered, too, that all essential oils are soluble in hot water to at least a slight degree; therefore, the amount of water present will determine the extent to which the yield of oil will be decreased as a result of the retention (by water in the still) of oil or certain constituents of the oil. This factor is of special importance in water distillation, since all of the essential oil must first go through the water solution stage and the water in the still will always be very nearly saturated with oil, especially with the more water-soluble constituents of an oil — with phenylethyl alcohol for example, in the case of rose distillation. The situation is not quite so serious in the case of water and steam distillation because a little of the oil dissolves in the still water only as a result of drainage from the still charge which is mechanically separated from the still water. The extent of this drainage will depend upon the amount of condensation taking place within the plant charge and especially along the still walls, but it can be kept at a minimum by suitable insulation of the still.

Effect of hydrolysis in plant distillation

The second effect accompanying distillation of plant material is hydrolysis. Hydrolysis in our case can be defined as a chemical reaction between water and certain constituents of the essential oils. These natural products consist partly and in some instances largely, of esters, which are compounds of organic acids and alcohols. In the presence of water, and particularly at elevated temperatures, the esters tend to react with the water to form the parent acids and alcohols. Two characteristic features are important in determining the effect of these reactions during distillation. In the first place, the reactions are not complete in either direction. Starting with the ester and hot water, only a part of the ester will react, so that when equilibrium is reached there will be present in the system esters, water, alcohols and acids. Similarly, if only alcohols and acids had been present at the start, all four constituents would be present when equilibrium is established.

The relationship between the concentrations of the various constituents at equilibrium may be written as:

$$K = \frac{(alcohol) \times (acid)}{(ester) \times (water)}$$

in which

K	=	a constant value at any fixed temperature.
(alcohol)	=	molal concentration of alcohol at equilibrium.
(acid)	=	molal concentration of acid at equilibrium.
(ester)	=	molal concentration of ester at equilibrium.
(water)	=	molal concentration of water at equilibrium.

Consequently, if the amount of water and hence its concentration, is large, the amounts of alcohol and acid will also be large and hydrolysis will proceed to a considerable extent. As a result, the yield of essential oil will be correspondingly decreased. This result is one of the principle disadvantages of water distillations since the amount of water present is always large and hydrolysis relatively extensive. In the case of water and steam distillation, the degree of hydrolysis is much less; it is even less with steam distillation, particularly with slightly superheated (dry) steam. As second important characteristic of hydrolysis reactions in the disdillation of essential oils, it should be noted that hydrolysis proceeds at a measurable rate. The fact that these reactions are not infinitely rapid means that the extent to which they proceed will depend upon the time of contact between oil and water; this holds particularly true for short periods of contact. This is another obvious disadvantage of water distillation, since the oil and water have a maximum time of contact under the conditions there employed.

Effect of heat in plant distillation

The third important effect accompanying distillation is the influence of temperature on essential oils. The pressure of distillation (atmospheric, excess or reduced) can be selected at will, but the temperature of the steam/vapour mixture rising through the charge in the still varies and fluctuates in the course of the operation. It is lowest at the beginning because the lowest boiling constituents of the volatile substances, freed by comminution of the plant material, vapourise first. As the higher boiling constituents begin to predominate in the vapours and as the quantity of oil vapours *per se* in the steam/vapour mixture decreases, the temperature gradually rises, until it reaches that of saturated steam at the given pressure. Practically all constituents of essential oils are somewhat unstable at high temperatures. In order to obtain the best quality of oil, it is, therefore, necessary to insure that during distillation the essential oils (or the plant material) are maintained at low temperature or, at worst, that they be kept at a high temperature for as short a time as possible. So far as operating temperature is concerned, there is really little choice between the three commonly used methods of distillation. In the case of water distillation or water and steam distillation, the temperature is determined entirely by the operating pressure. If the still is open to the atmosphere — the usual procedure — the temperature will be at or slightly below, 100°C (212°F). If a valve is inserted between the still and condenser and if the apparatus is sufficiently strong to withstand the pressure, the still can be operated at pressures above atmospheric and at temperatures correspondingly above 100°C. In the case of steam distillation, the operating temperature will be at, slightly below or above 100°C, even at atmospheric pressure, depending on whether low pressure saturated or superheated steam is used. Any of the methods may be operated at temperatures below 100°C by use of suitable pressures below atmospheric.

Thus, although the three processes of diffusion, hydrolysis and thermal decomposition have been considered independently, it must be remembered that in practice all three occur simultaneously and hence they will frequently affect one another. This holds particularly true of the effect of temperature. The rate of diffusion usually will be increased by higher temperatures. The solubility of the essential oils in water— an important factor, as indicated above — in most cases also increases with higher temperatures. The same holds true of both the rate and extent of hydrolysis. Since the products of hydrolysis are in general more water soluble, they will also affect the diffusion process. Hence, a complete analysis of the various processes incidental to distillation offers a difficult problem. In general, observance of the following principles leads to the best yields and to a high quality of essential oil: (i) maintenance of as low a temperature as is feasible, not forgetting, however, that the rate of production will be determined by the temperature; (ii) in the case of steam distillation, use of as little water as possible in direct contact with plant material, but keeping in mind that some water should be present in order to promote diffusion; and (iii) thorough comminution of plant material before distillation and very careful, uniform packing of the still charge, remembering, however, that in all but water distillation excessive comminution will result in channeling of steam through the mass of plant material, thus reducing efficiency because of poor contact between steam and charge.

A brief résumé of the advantages and disadvantages of the three distillation methods in the light of the above discussion will be helpful and is presented in Table 5.3. For small-scale installations, particularly in portable units, water distillation or water and steam distillation offers the advantage of simplicity of equipment. The latter method is rapidly superseding water distillation (except in a few special cases) because of the better quality and yield of oil and higher rate of vapourisation, i.e. speedier distillation.

For larger and fixed installations, steam distillation unquestionably offers the most advantages. In such plants the necessary control can be readily installed and under these conditions the quality, yield and rate of oil are superior. Also, as a result of possibility of temperature control, the method is more adaptable. Plant materials containing either low or high boiling oils can be handled in the same equipment with equal ease. Because of the auxiliary equipment required steam distillation cannot be recommended for all distillation. It is especially impracticable for the small producer in the field. Whenever conditions permit the construction of a suitably located, modern plant to process raw material from a large area, such distillery should be equipped to carry on direct steam distillation.

Before closing the general discussion of the three principal distillation methods, it should be mentioned briefly that the three principal distillation methods mentioned above each method can be modified by changing the pressure in the still. Accordingly, distillation can be carried out:

    (a) At reduced pressure.
    (b) At atmospheric pressure.
    (c) At excess pressure.

The effect of these variations may be observed in the ratio of distillation (condensed) water to volatile oil. Any type of distillation carried out below the prevailing atmospheric pressure (usually with the aid of a vacuum pump) falls into class (a). Characteristic of distillation at reduced pressure is a low distillation temperature which has its limit only in the temperature of the cooling water and the efficiency of the condenser. The outstanding advantage of this form of distillation consists in the absence of the decomposition products resulting from heat. On the other hand, the vapourisation capacity of high boiling substances, especially of those somewhat soluble in water, is considerably reduced.

Table 5.3. Advantages and disadvantages of three distillation methods.

	A. Water distillation	B. Water and steam distillation	C. Steam distillation
Type of still	Simple, low priced, portable stills; easily installed in the producing regions	Somewhat more complicated and higher priced than A. The smaller type is also movable and may be installed in the field	If well constructed, usually more solid and durable than A and B. Possibility of large size for large-scale distillation
Type of plant material	Most advantageous for certain materials, especially when finely powdered; also for flowers which easily lump with direct steam. Not well adapted for materials containing saponifiable, water-soluble or high boiling constituents	Well suited for herb and leaf material	Suited for any charge except finely powdered material through which the steam forms channels ('rat holes'). Especially well suited for seed, root and wood materials containing high boiling oils
Mode of comminu-tion	Best results with finely powdered materials	Plant material must be uniformly but not too finely comminuted. Granulation gives best results with seeds and roots	Similar to B
Mode of charging	Material must be completely covered by water	Material must be evenly charged into the still	Similar to B. Proper charging is very important; otherwise the steam channels through the plant material and low yield results
Diffusion conditions	Good, if material is properly charged and moves freely in the boiling water	Good	Good, if steam is slightly wet. Distillation with superheated steam or high pressure steam dries out the plant material, prevents diffusion and causes a low yield of oil. Such distillation must, therefore, be followed with wet steam
Steam pressure within the still	Usually about pressure atmospheric	Usually about atmospheric	Can be modified (high or low pressure steam), according to the plant material
Temperature within the still	About 100°C. Care must be exercised not to 'burn' the plant material by contact with overheated still walls. Vapourised water must be continuously replaced	About 100°C	Can be modified (saturated or superheated steam), according to the plant material

(Contd ...)

	A. Water distillation	B. Water and steam distillation	C. Steam distillation
Hydrolysis of oil constituents	Conditions usually unfavourable. High rate of ester hydrolysis	Hydrolysis fairly low, provided no excessive wetting of the plant charge by prolonged distillation and steam condensation within the still takes place	Conditions good, hydrolysis usually slight
Conditions within the plant charge	Good, if plant material is kept covered with water and moves freely in it	Good, if material is properly comminuted and charged. Prolonged distillation causes excessive wetting by steam condensation and lumping of the charge. Stills should be well insulated	Conditions good, if plant material is properly charged. Prolonged distillation with wet steam, causes excessive steam condensation within the still and lumping of the charge
Rate of distillation	Relatively low	Fairly good	High
Yield of oil	In most cases relatively low, due to hydrolysis, also because watersoluble and high boiling oil constituents are retained by residual water in the still	Good, if no excessive wetting and lumping of the plant charge occurs. This would prevent steam from penetrating the charge thoroughly and result in abnormally low oil yield	Good, if plant material is properly comminuted, evenly charged and distillation properly conducted. Lumping of the charge or steam channelling might cause an abnormally low yield of oil
Quality of oil	Depends upon careful operation; 'burning' of plant charge must be avoided, especially when distilling with direct fire	Usually good	Good, if operation properly conducted all around
Distillation water	Distillation water in some cases must be redistilled or more conveniently returned into the still during distillation (cohobation). Distillation waters contain products of hydrolysis	If properly separated, the distillation water can be discarded in many cases	Similar to B

By inserting a valve into the gooseneck of the retort and by partly closing this valve during distillation, it is possible to throttle the outflow of the steam/oil vapours and to increase the pressure within the still. Such distillation at excess pressure (0.5 to 1.0 atmospheres excess pressure or 1.5 to 2.0 atmospheres absolute pressure) is occasionally resorted to in the essential oil industry, but its use remains very limited, because of the resulting decomposition of many oil constituents.

Equipment for Distillation of Aromatic Plants

The equipment required for carrying on distillation of plant materials depends upon the size of the operation and the type of distillation to be used. There are, however, three main parts which, in varying size, form the base for all three types of hydrodistillation. A fourth part is necessary for any method of heating the still other than by direct fire. The three universally employed parts are:

1. The retort or still proper.

2. The condenser.

3. The receiver for the condensate.

The fourth part consists of a boiler generating steam. The latter is necessary for the process which is called steam distillation, since direct live steam, often slightly superheated, is required and this can be produced only in a separate steam boiler. In the case of water distillation or water and steam distillation, the still may be heated by direct fire but even here heating is frequently and indeed preferably, accomplished by steam jacketing the retort or by means of closed (or occasionally open) steam coils. A separate steam boiler becomes indispensable, also, if anyone of the latter heating methods or a combination of them, is used. These four parts of the distillation equipment will be considered in order.

Retort

The retort or still proper, commonly also called 'tank', serves primarily as a container for the plant material and as a vessel in which the water and/or steam contacts the plant material and vapourises its essential oil. In its simplest form the retort may consist merely of a cylindrical container or tank, with a diameter equal to or slightly less than its height and equipped with a removable cover which can be clamped upon the cylindrical section. On or near the top of the cylindrical section a pipe (gooseneck) is attached for leading the vapours to the condenser. For water distillation this simple equipment is sufficient, since water and charge can be introduced, the cover put in place and a fire simply built under the retort. For water and steam distillation a grid or false bottom is inserted sufficiently far above the real bottom of the still so that boiling water and plant material (the latter supported by the grid) do not come in contact.

The water is brought to a boil either by a steam jacket or through a closed steam coil or in simpler apparatus by a fire directly beneath the still. In the case of direct steam distillation the grid may be closer to the real bottom. Here live steam is introduced through a steam line, usually a perforated coil or cross below the false bottom. Such a simple retort, while entirely adequate, would be inconvenient to use because of the difficulty of removing the spent plant material. Figure 5.6 shows a drawing of this type of retort.

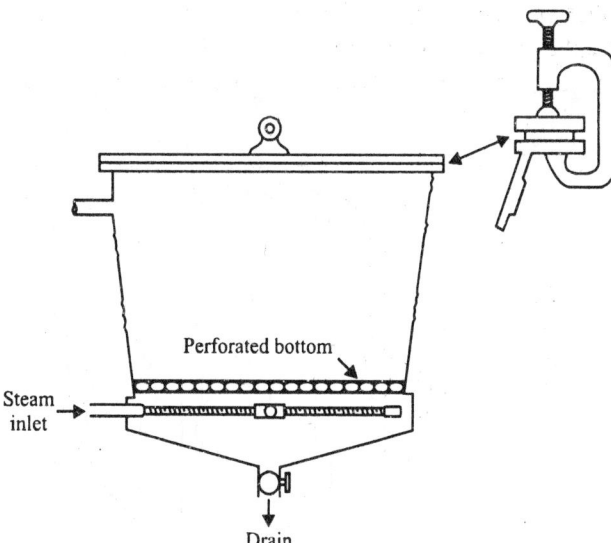

Fig. 5.6. Galvanised iron retort for steam distillation.

The cylindrical section, slightly tapered to facilitate application of the support rings, can be made of 14–20 gauge galvanised sheet metal depending on the size of the retort. For larger sizes, heavier metal (smaller gauge number) should be used. This is bent to shape, soldered steam tight and the circular bottom soldered on. Support rings, their number depending on the size of the retort, are fastened outside and around the cylinder at 2 or 2½ ft intervals, always with one at the top and one at the bottom, of the section. Except for the top ring, these may be strap metal or angle iron and in any case about 2 inches wide. The top support ring should be of 3 inches angle iron, to form a suitable contact surface for the cover. Just below the top support ring a 6 to 8 inches length of pipe is soldered to the side of the retort, to serve as a connection to the condenser. Frequently the gooseneck leads from the centre of a convex or spherical top cover to the condenser, but the gooseneck should never be high, as it would then act as a sort of reflux condenser. Any unavoidable vertical section of the gooseneck must be well insulated. This connecting pipe should be at least 4 inches in diameter and, if the rate of distillation is to be very rapid, may be even wider. Finally, just below the grid supporting the plant charge a steam inlet line, a 1 inch pipe, enters through the side of the retort. The distance between the bottom of the retort and the steam pipe must be large enough to permit any water condensing within the retort to accumulate at the bottom without contacting the steam pipe. To insure adequate steam distribution, the steam pipe inside of the retort should be arranged in the form of a coil or of a cross, as shown in Fig. 5.7 with small holes, about 1 inch in diameter, drilled in the top of each arm throughout its length. The total surface of these small holes should not be larger than the orifice of the coil or of the arms on the cross, as otherwise the steam will escape from the first holes without reaching the entire length of the coil or cross. In other words, the steam should be injected into the retort in such a way that it will be evenly distributed on the bottom of the retort and in rising will penetrate the plant charge uniformly. Larger stills are equipped with two steam coils, each with a separate steam valve. Prior to injection, the steam is freed from excess water through a water separator. Years ago, it was customary to equip the steam stills, directly above the bottom, with a closed coil, for heating with indirect steam of high pressure. The idea was to keep the injected direct steam as dry as possible, by heating it through this closed (indirect) steam coil. Such precaution, however, is of doubtful value, because dissolved, nonvolatile extractive matter always drips from the plant charge to the still bottom and is apt to 'burn' and decompose in contact with the very hot indirect steam coil. Vapours of disagreeable odour are thus emitted, which might easily affect the odour of the essential oil in the receiver.

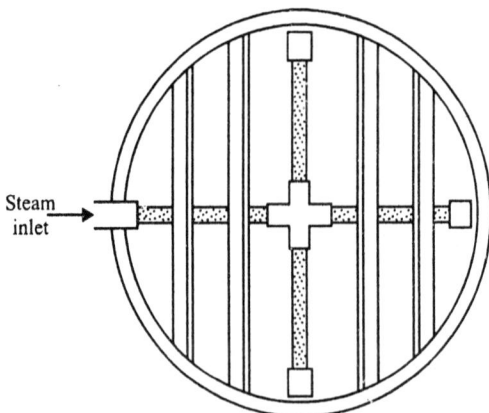

Fig. 5.7. Top view of galvanised iron retort showing crossed tee steam inlet on bottom.

The bottom of the retort is provided with a drain valve sufficiently wide so that any water condensing within the charge and dripping to the bottom can be drawn off in the course of distillation. (This drain valve also serves as an outlet for the wash water, when the still is cleaned.) Otherwise such residual condensed water will accumulate and engulf the steam coil, with the result that the entering live steam will first have to pass through a layer of water, becoming wet in the process. In other words, instead of direct steam distillation we would then have a case of water and steam distillation. Wet steam has a tendency to wet the plant charge and agglutinate it. The advantages of direct steam distillation are thus lost. Whether or not this wetting takes place depends also upon the temperature and pressure. of the injected live steam. At any rate, it is preferable continuously to remove the condensed residual water from the still bottom. The same result can be achieved by an automatic water separator (steam trap) attached to the still bottom. It is constructed in such a way that only water flows from it, but not steam. This steam trap should be installed in plain view so that its proper functioning is assured at all times. Steam traps are apt to lose their efficiency after a certain time and permit unutilised steam to escape; or they do not separate the condensed water effectively and more and more water accumulates within the still. This means an ever-increasing wetting of the plant charge in the still. Such a condition is recognised by a crackling noise and by trembling of the still. If there is no steam trap, a funnel should be attached beneath the outlet at the still bottom and the water thus conducted away. Here, too, the water faucet is regulated in such a way that no unused steam escapes and at the same time, no condensed water accumulates within the still.

This arrangement completes the still proper. Needless to say, all joints must be soldered steam tight, as any steam leak represents loss of essential oil and fuel.

Brief comment should be made about the top of the still and the gooseneck, i.e. the tube connecting the retort with the condenser. The oldfashioned convex or crane-like still heads are becoming obsolete and rare. The top of a modern retort is simply pierced and a pipe inserted to serve as a gooseneck. The perfect still head is short and well insulated; if convex, it curves gradually and tapers, so that it fits into the gooseneck. Any fancy designs, sudden turns, bends or too narrow tubing must be avoided, as these would result in a throttling effect and in back pressure within the still.

The gooseneck also is only slightly curved and, gradually descending, leads from the retort directly into the condenser. It should not ascend, as this would give rise to considerable vapour condensation, the resultant liquid refluxing into the retort. A semicircular gooseneck, such as is sometimes found on old stills, has a purpose only if high boiling and resinous constituents of an essential oil can, by its means, be condensed and returned into the retort. A gooseneck of this type, therefore, may be useful in the rectification of essential oils, but not in the distillation of plant material. In fact, these two operations must never be confused. Ascending and high goosenecks are excusable only if the distillation waters are purposely made to flow automatically back into the retort from the higher placed Florentine flask; but in such a case the gooseneck must be well insulated. It usually is preferable to return the distillation waters into the retort by an injector, which measure makes high goosenecks superfluous. Furthermore, a high gooseneck produces a slight back pressure within the retort; it must, therefore, be amply wide.

The retort cover shown in Figs. 5.7 and 5.8 may be made of sheet metal similar to that used on the retort. It should be strengthened and ringed with strap metal to coincide with the horizontal face of the top angle iron supporting ring on the retort.

Any suitable device for lifting the top may be used. Figure 5.8 illustrates one such device, which can be attached easily. In order to avoid steam leaks between the retort and cover, they must be held tightly together with a suitable gasket, which may conveniently be a single piece of $\frac{1}{2}$ inch to $\frac{5}{8}$ inch soft rope laid all the way around the top angle iron on the retort. Commercial gasket materials (asbestos in rope form) give good service. The top and retort may be held together by external clamps or by bolts and washers, in which case the top angle iron on the retort and the outer ring of the cover must be suitably drilled with holes to accommodate the bolts. For best results bolts should not be more than one foot apart.

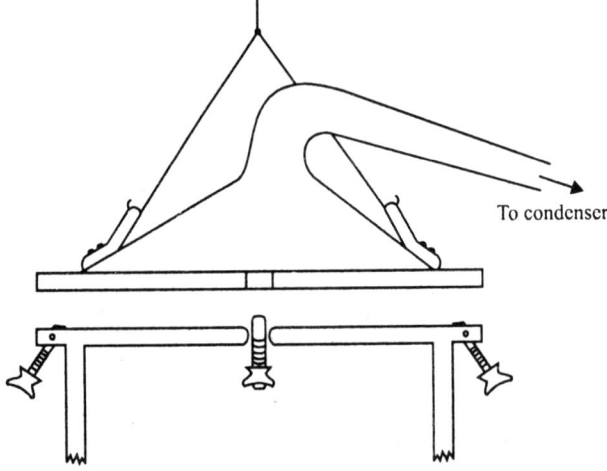

To condenser

Fig. 5.8. Top of retort.

Another device occasionally used for holding the top to the retort consists of a simple water seal or hydraulic joint (Fig. 5.9). It eliminates all clamps and saves a good deal of labour, as the still top is easily hoisted in its place after the still has been charged and can be removed with equal facility.

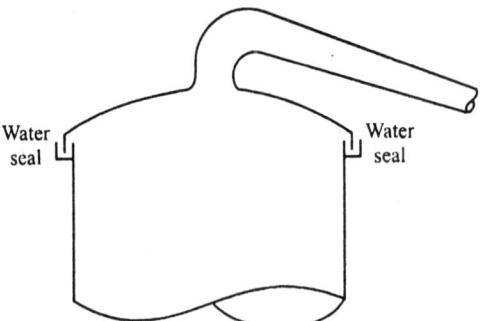

Water seal

Water seal

Fig. 5.9. Hydraulic joints or water seals between still top and retort.

However, the layer of water within the water seal must be sufficiently high to withstand any slight steam pressure developing within the retort; hence a water seal cannot be used when distilling with high-pressure steam. Also, some water evaporates from the seal in the course of the operation, for which reason a water seal is recommended for the distillation of grass or herb material, but not of roots or woods requiring long hours of processing. The false bottom or grid supporting the plant material may be a circular piece of coarse wire mesh, a tray perforated with many narrow slits or a wooden platform made in the form of a lattice. In the distillation of seed material — and, especially of crushed seed — it will be necessary to cover the grid with sack cloth or any other suitable coarse material, to prevent dust and fine particles from falling to the bottom of the retort and clogging the perforations on the steam coil. If the still serves for water and steam distillation, the false bottom should be supported about 2 ft above the bottom of the retort. In the case of direct steam distillation it need be only far enough above the bottom to clear the steam inlet line. Chains or heavy wires attached to three or four equally spaced points around the circumference of the grid may serve as handles so that the plant charge can be easily removed after distillation simply by lifting the grid. If charges in excess of 200 or 300 lb. are to be distilled, it will be convenient to use more than one such section, placing a new one on top of the first layer and continuing the charge above this section. This arrangement prevents excessive packing, assures better steam distribution and facilitates discharging the spent material, in as much as only a fraction of the total charge need be removed at one time. Coarser and specifically lighter material can be packed higher, whereas finer and heavier material should not exceed a certain height.

Retorts serving for water distillation should be wider than they are high, so that the plant charge can be kept shallow, avoiding the pressure caused by the weight of a high charge. This will permit the comminuted plant particles to move freely in the boiling water and assure quicker distillation and a better yield of oil. Retorts serving for water and steam distillation may be of approximately equal height and diameter. Retorts for direct steam distillation should be somewhat higher than they are wide so that the rising steam passes as much plant material as possible. As a rule, the diameter should be 6 to 8 ft at the most; if larger-scale operation requires a larger still capacity it is preferable to increase the height rather than the diameter of the retort. In this case it will be necessary to guard against excessive packing of the charge, which would cause uneven distribution of steam and excessive pressures near the bottom. When calculating the dimensions of a still one should keep in mind not only that some plant materials are very voluminous but also that during distillation the mass often swells and expands by one-third of its original volume. The height of the retort in relation to its width depends upon the porosity of the plant material. A greater height is chosen for voluminous material and shorter stills are preferred for more compact material. Excessive pressure can be avoided by a construction similar to that shown in Fig. 5.10.

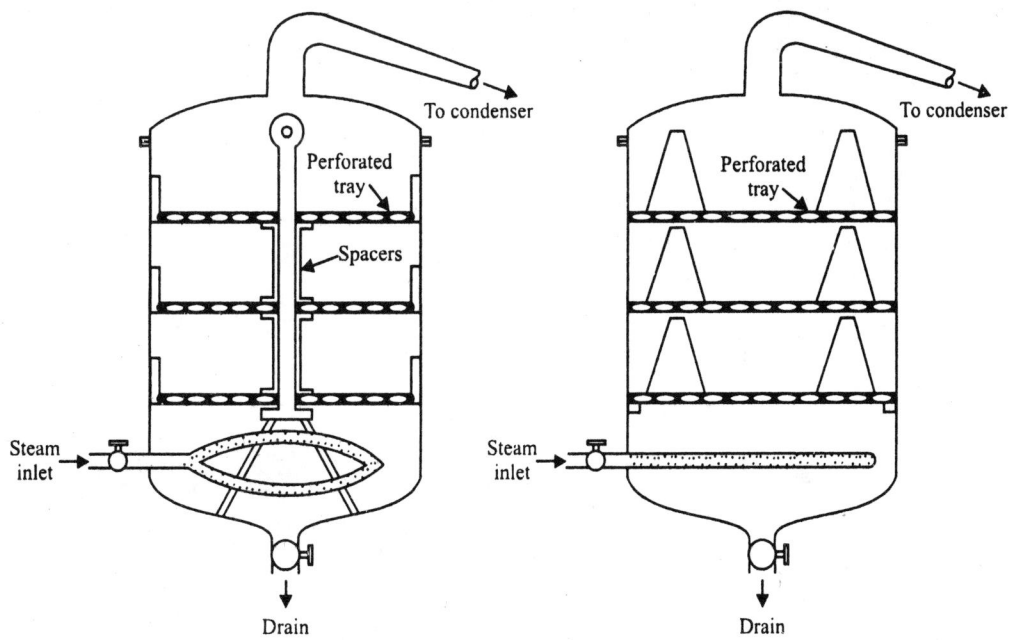

Fig. 5.10. Sketches of two types of multi-tray retorts.

The screen or grid trays may be permanently installed at intervals of 2 to 3 or 3 to 4 ft, according to the size of the retort and each tray must then be filled or emptied individually through the 2 ft or 3 ft manholes. By supporting each section of the charge separately, excessive pressures in any one section are avoided and packing is kept at a minimum. Care must be exercised to fill each tray with only a relatively shallow layer, to insure a uniform distribution of material and, therefore, of the steam. This is particularly true of seed distillation, which requires much more experience and attention than distillation of herbs or leaves. As pointed out above, the trays may also be movable, so that they can be lifted from the retort with chains or strong wire. For best results, the trays should not lie directly on top of the charge of the next lower tray but be separated by a space of 2 ft or more, depending upon the size of the retort. This may be effected in several ways, e.g. by supporting legs or attaching all of the trays to a central vertical shaft on which the trays may be hoisted from the retort after completion of the operation. The principal precaution is to be sure that the steam actually penetrates the plant charge and does not find an easy passage along the side of the still wall. This may be prevented by coiling ropes around the outer edges of the various trays where they touch the wall of the retort. For the same reason, baskets are not generally to be recommended, particularly those with perforated sides, such as wire baskets. The steam always follows the way of least resistance and has a tendency to rise along and through the perforations of the wire meshing, between the walls of the basket and the retort.

Baskets with walls of solid (not perforated) sheet metal and perforated bottoms are preferable (Fig. 5.11). However, these should fit quite tightly into the retort proper, leaving only a very small space between the walls of the basket and the walls of the retort. Even this small space, must be completely sealed with rope, so that the steam does not find an easy way from the still bottom to the top by passing outside the basket. If every precaution is taken, such baskets may be useful for the distillation of herb material; while one batch is being distilled, another basket outside of the still can be charged with plants and hoisted into the retort after the first basket has been lifted out. Also, the exhausted contents of such baskets can easily be dumped on a truck and carried away.

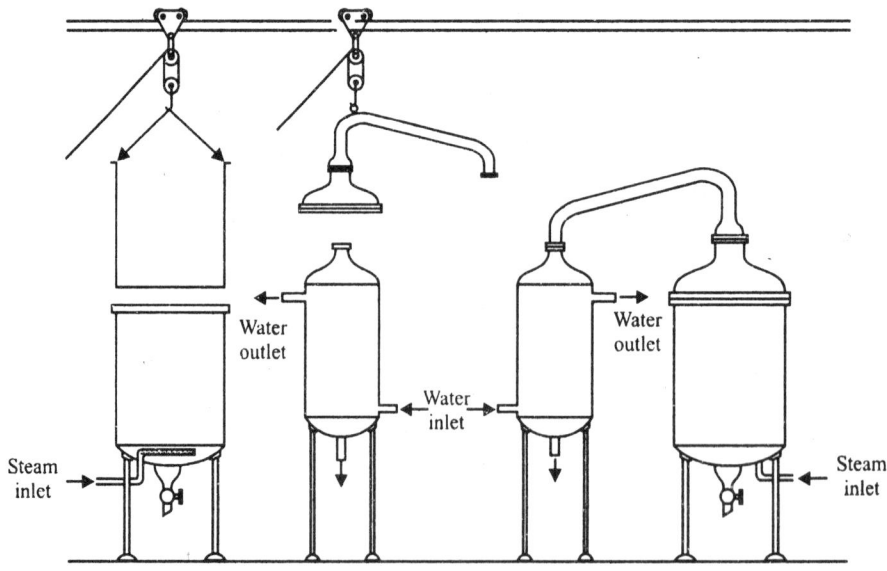

Fig. 5.11. Use of baskets (perforated on bottom) for holding still charge.

In the case of the smaller stills, yet another method of discharging may be found convenient. The entire apparatus may be supported on trunnions located slightly above the middle of the retort. Distillation completed, the retort is disconnected from the condenser and steam line, the top removed and the entire spent charge dumped out by rotating the retort about the trunnions. Figure 5.12 shows a typical arrangement.

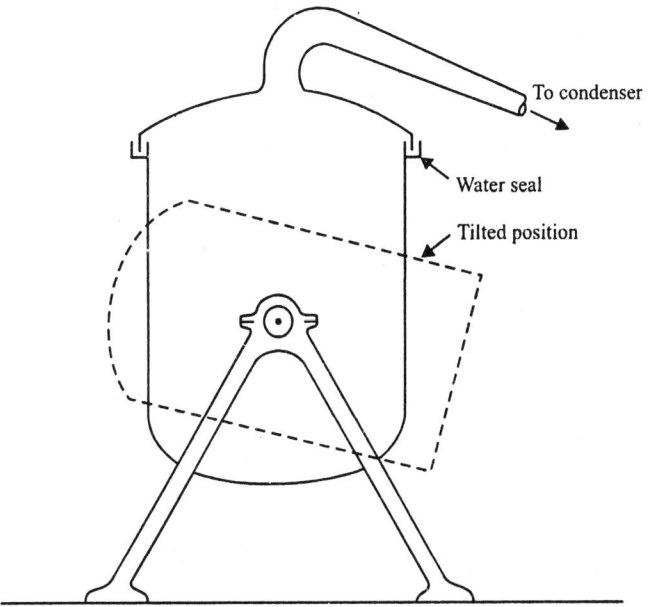

Fig. 5.12. Tilting still on trunnions.

In years past most stills serving in most industry were constructed of copper. This metal has the advantage of durability; copper stills retain a certain value even after being dismantled, as the metal can be reworked. The inside of a copper retort, however, should be heavily tinned (lead-free tin); this is true also (in fact more so) of the gooseneck and condenser. Otherwise the essential oils wall contain copper, imparting to the oils a bluish-green colour which must be removed before the oil is acceptable to the trade. Sheeted aluminium can also be used for the construction of stills, giving satisfactory results except with phenol-containing oils (phenols attack aluminium). Today most retorts serving for large-scale steam distillation of plant material are made of galvanised sheeted iron, which renders good service for our purposes. Tinned copper is still being favoured for equipment used in the water distillation of aromatic plants and for apparatus employed in the redistillation, rectification or fractionation of essential oils. Some retorts in more primitive countries are made of wood; if solidly constructed they cannot be condemned, but should be used always for distillation of only one type of plant material. Wood has a tendency to absorb a little essential oil, which cannot be removed even by the most thorough washing and boiling with lye. Hence, a certain odour always adheres to wooden retorts which might easily spoil the odour of another type of oil, if the latter were distilled in the same wooden retort.

Insulation of the retort

In all cases the retort, including the top, should be well insulated to conserve heat. This holds true particularly of stills exposed to cold air, wind and draft. If insulation is neglected, excessive condensation of steam within the retort will occur as a result of heat losses from its surface. This causes undue wetting of the charge, lumping and agglutinating of the plant particles, excessive steam consumption, prolonged distillation and, usually, an inferior yield of oil. For small portable units, considerable insulation can be afforded by surrounding the retort with a jacket made of wooden planks and held in place by wire. The interspace may be filled with powdered cork or sawdust. Much better insulators are asbestos and magnesia. Either of these can be applied directly to the retort in the form of a very thick paste in water, which dries to a hard adherent layer. Three to six inches of this material will suffice for most economic operation.

A high, grade of insulation of this sort appears particularly important in large installations, where much steam is required. Thus, all heated sections and steam lines should be well insulated to prevent escape of heat, which represents an unnecessary expense. Probably the most effective insulation material is asbestos, which, in the form of bricks or pipe covering, can be suitably fastened to the still and pipes or, in the form of powder, can be made into a thick paste with water. This paste may be applied with a trowel to the parts to be insulated. A paste made from ground kieselguhr, water and animal hair, if available, also serves as insulation. In any case, such an insulating layer should be about 2 inches thick. Following method is suggested for insulating stills and steam pipes:

> 'Fifty litres of calcined kieselguhr, ten litres of gritty ground cork waste and three handfuls of clear pulled pigs' or calves' hair are thoroughly mixed. A thin, hot, stirred soup of rye, wheat or corn flour is added, to make a viscous, stiff mash. Stones of brick size and strength are then formed and dried on the steam boiler or elsewhere. These bricks serve to cover the stills and steam armatures after they have been covered with a viscous flour soup. If necessary, the bricks are held in place by iron straps. The whole cover is smoothed and the joints and grooves are filled with a mash of calcined kieselguhr. Finally, cheap, thin fabric is pasted on top and painted over twice with oil paint.'

Very hot steam pipes are more advantageously covered with asbestos fibre. The joints of the steam armatures, which are best made with flanges, should not be insulated.

Charging of the still

The problems of charging a retort with plant material and of discharging it, are more important than is usually realised and should be attacked by considering the labour involved. Any labour saving device might mean considerable economy in the final calculation. As a rule the plant material should be transported (trucked, hauled, etc.) as near as possible to the still. If the material has to be comminuted, the machines should be located near-by, if possible on a floor or platform above the stills, so that the comminuted material falls or slides by gravity into the retort. The old-fashioned way of charging and discharging with pitchforks and shovels is costly and, although the initial cost is high, a conveyor belt or a small crane, will soon pay for itself and in general speed up the operation.

Condenser

The second major part of the distillation equipment is the condenser. Here again the size and design are variable and several typical cases will be considered. The condenser serves to convert all of the steam and the accompanying oil vapours into liquid. This requires the removal of an amount of heat equivalent to the heat of vapourisation of the vapours plus steam and a small additional amount of heat to cool the condensed material (condensate) to a convenient temperature below its boiling point. The rate at which heat will be removed from the vapours is expressed by

$$q = UA\Delta t$$

in which: q = heat removed per unit time

U = a constant depending on operating conditions

A = the area available for removal of heat

Δt = the temperature difference between the hot vapours and the cooling medium.

The scope of this work does not permit a full discussion of all factors that affect the value of U. Several of them will be considered in the discussion of condenser operation. Probably the most important ones are the rate of flow of the cooling medium (cold water) past the heating surface, the rate of flow of the vapours and the material of which the condenser is constructed. The value of U increases as these factors increase and this fact should always be borne in mind when constructing a condenser. The area available can be made as large or as small as desired, but it is evident from the above relation that the total capacity of a condenser, and therefore of a still, will be directly determined by the area used. The temperature difference can be controlled by the temperature of the cooling medium (hereinafter referred to as water, since water is by far the most commonly used cooling medium) because the temperature of the vapours is fixed within rather narrow limits by the distillation itself. Figure 5.13 shows the simplest type of condenser, now seldom used and described here chiefly for its historic interest.

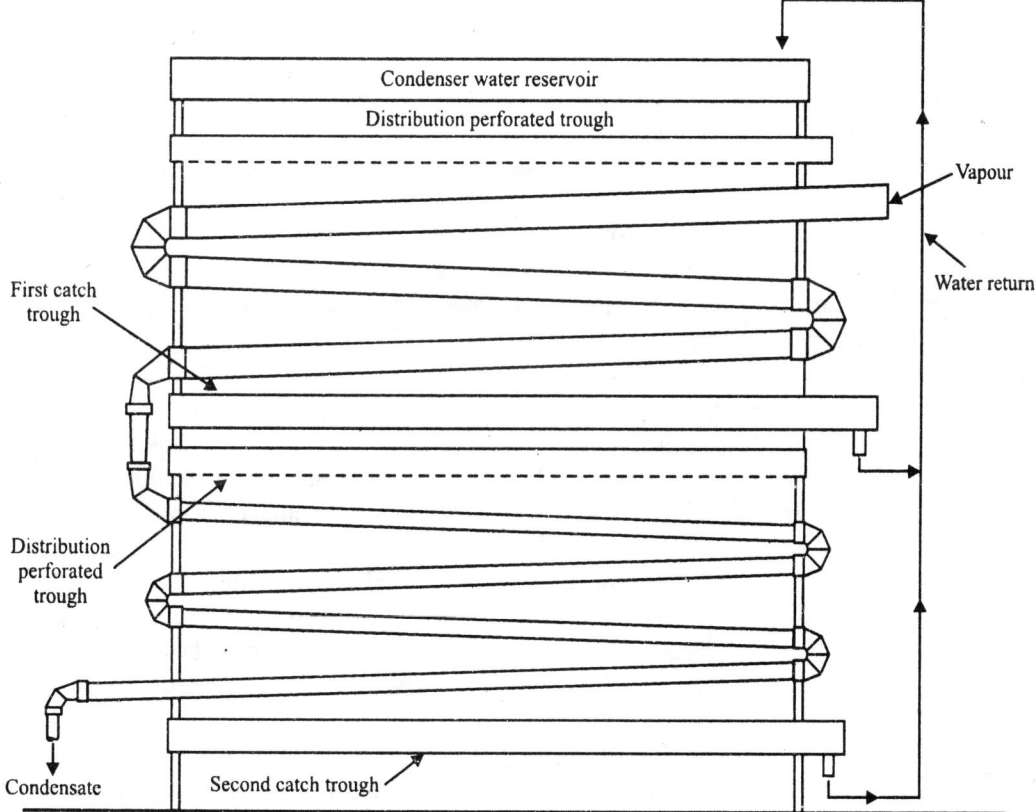

Fig. 5.13. Sketch of an old-fashioned zigzag condenser.

Water is fed to the overhead reservoir from which it flows to a distributor trough which consists simply of a shallow pan with a perforated bottom. This permits the water to trickle over the entire length of the condenser tubes. The water may be caught in an intermediate catch pan, as shown and a second distributor installed to insure efficient condensation. It will be noted that the condenser tubes are all sloped downward slightly, to insure proper drainage of the condensed oil and steam. Also the size of the condenser tubes becomes smaller as the cold end is approached. In order to avoid excessive back pressures being built up in the still, it is necessary to use fairly large tubes to accommodate the vapours immediately after they leave the retort. Since the volume of the vapours and, therefore their velocity, decreases rapidly on cooling, as a result of condensation, the size of the condenser pipes can be reduced proportionately. In Fig. 5.13, for example, the first two tubes may be 4-inch pipe, the next two 3-inch and the remainder 2-inch. A 4-inch pipe coming from the still will accommodate up to 700 lb. per hour of condensate (about 85 gal.), in so far as the development of back pressure is concerned. The length and number of tubes to be used will be determined by the amount of vapour to be condensed. An estimate of the pipe area required can be made by using a value of 40 for the factor U in the above equation. The temperature difference will be equal to the average value of the difference between 212°F (100°C) (the temperature of saturated steam at ordinary pressure) and the temperature of the water in the first and second troughs. For example, if the fresh water in the top trough is 60°F (15.56°C) and the water in the first catch trough is 90°F (32.22°C), the temperature difference to be used would be the mean of (212°–60°F) and (212°–90°F) or 137°F. The value of q, the amount of heat to be removed, can be calculated approximately by multiplying the number of pounds of condensate per hour by 1000. The pipe area required will then be given in square feet. By connecting two or more such zigzag sections in parallel, the same cooling water system can be used for all of them, thus increasing their capacity, conserving height and permitting the use of shorter tubes for a given amount of condensation.

Another very simple and inexpensive type of condenser consists merely of a series of long pipes, usually 2-inch in diameter, laid horizontally in a trough, through which water flows. Four 2-inch pipes will have the same vapour capacity as one 4-inch pipe as given above, but will offer considerably more cooling surface. Since the value of the factor U in both of these cases is somewhat lower, the length of the pipes must be proportionately greater. Again, the pipes should have a definite slope toward the cool end, to insure adequate drainage of the condensate.

The above described methods of condensing vapours, although cheap and entirely satisfactory, lead to rather awkward and bulky construction.

The most commonly used condenser is that in which coils are inserted into a tank supplied with running cold water, which enters from below and flows against the steam and oil vapours. In order to utilise the cooling water more effectively, it is advisable to insert two adjoining coils into one condenser tank. Figure 5.14 shows a coil condenser.

In an even more satisfactory condenser arrangement, advantage is taken of the fact that a more rapid flow of cooling water results in more efficient cooling. The condenser tubes are assembled in a single vertical bundle, the number and length depending on the amount of condensation to be accomplished, in such a way that the vapours to be condensed enter the tubes and cooling water circulates around the tubes. Figure 5.15 shows a typical construction.

Condensers of this type are available ready built from any equipment supply house and should be purchased from such a specialist. The construction of a satisfactory leak-proof tubular condenser presents an exceedingly difficult problem for an unskilled workman. The factor U for such a condenser will usually be about 200; thus, for a given amount of condensation and a given cooling water temperature, only one-fifth of the area required in a zigzag condenser will be required. Tubular condensers should be used in a vertical position with vapours entering the top and condensate leaving the bottom. Connection with the retort must again be of adequate size to avoid excessive back pressure in the still. Tubular condensers not only are more efficient and require much less space than spiral condensers, but they also permit easier and more thorough cleaning. If possible they should be fed with soft water to prevent the formation of scale (incrustation), which reduces the exchange of heat and necessitates frequent cleaning.

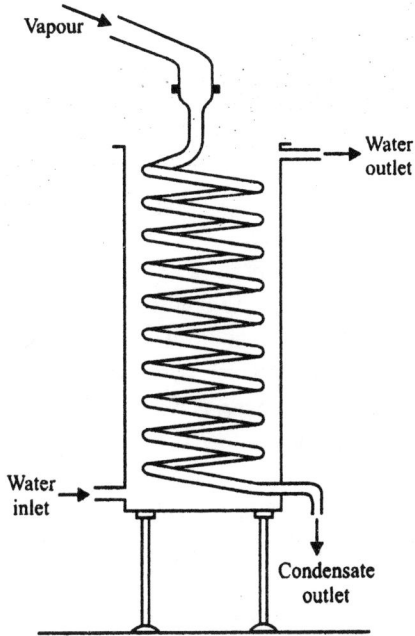

Fig. 5.14. Coil condenser.

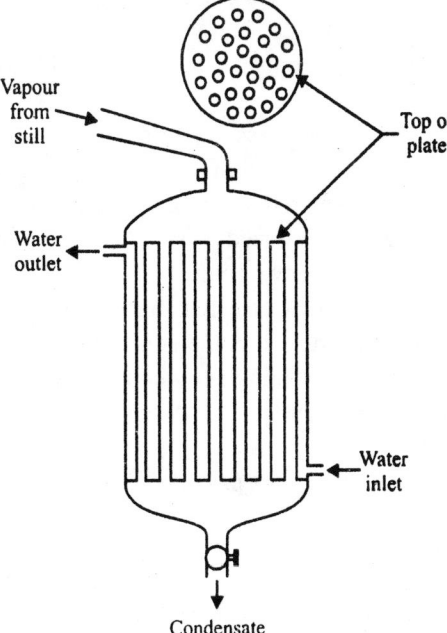

Fig. 5.15. Tubular condenser.

It is always better to construct the condenser a little too large rather than too small. Longer tubes or coils require less cooling water, as the contact with the vapours and with the flowing condensate lasts longer and permits the absorption of more heat, so that the temperature of the condensate at the end more closely approaches that of the inflowing cooling water. At any rate, the condenser surface must be large enough to cool the distillate sufficiently, even at a very high rate (speed) of distillation. Slow distillation has many disadvantages, such as hydrolysis of esters, wetting, agglutination and conglomeration of the plant charge, frequently with a concomitantly low yield of oil.

The cooling water in the condenser tank does not need to be cold from top to bottom; such a condition, on the contrary, is rather a disadvantage, because too rapid and excessive cooling of the steam/vapour mixture causes the distillate to run off the condenser unevenly or jerkily. For this reason, the condenser tank should be fed with only as much cold water as is necessary to condense the vapour mixture and to cool the condensate sufficiently — a factor depending also upon the type of oil produced.

The maximum efficiency of a condenser is attained when the condensate has been cooled to a sufficiently low temperature by heat transfer to the cooling water, which then flows out at a temperature approaching that of the incoming vapours. This effect, however, is rarely achieved. Usually it suffices if the cooling water flows out at a temperature of 80°C (about 175°F) and if the distillate has a temperature of 25° to 30°C (77° to 86°F).

If the ratio between condenser surface and heating surface (in the still) is correctly maintained the condenser will permit rapid distillation. But if the condenser surface is too small — and in many of the small field distilleries this is true — the rate of distillation must be adjusted to the efficiency of the condenser. Distillation must then be slow and this, as pointed out, involves many disadvantages and inadequacies. Otherwise, the vapours blow at high speed through the condenser coils or tube, which are too short for complete condensation of the vapours or for sufficient cooling of the condensate. Considerable oil may then be lost by evaporation.

The condenser tubes or coils must be made of heavily tinned copper, of pure tin, aluminium or stainless steel, if discolouration of the oil by iron or copper is to be prevented. Aluminium, however, cannot be used with oils containing phenols.

If distillation is to be carried out at reduced pressure, the tubes or coils must be made strong enough to support a pressure differential of one atmosphere without letting water seep from the condenser tank into the condenser. This is particularly important in the case of oil distillation (rectification, fractionation) *in vacuo*. Condensers serving for distillation at reduced pressures should also be sufficiently wide to permit an unhindered flow of steam and vapours, as any throttling by too small a diameter increases the pressure within the still — in other words, creates back pressure. As a general principle in the construction of distilling equipment it should be kept in mind that the steam and oil vapours should flow easily and smoothly through the system, without encountering any sharp bends or curves in the tubes.

A wire screen, inserted between condenser and gooseneck, prevents plant particles lifted up by live steam from entering the condenser tubes or coils. As the wire screen may become clogged and would then cause an explosion in the still, the retort should be provided with one or two efficient safety valves.

Oil separator

The third essential part of the distillation equipment consists of the condensate receiver, decanter or oil separator. Its function is to achieve a quick and complete separation of the oil from the condensed water. Since the total volume of water condensed will always be much greater than the quantity of oil, it is necessary to remove the water continuously. The condensate flows from the condenser into the oil separator, where distillation water and volatile oil separate automatically. Many separators are constructed according to the principle of the ancient Florentine flask, hence, are often called Florentine flasks. Volatile oil and water are mutually insoluble; because of the difference in their specific gravities, the two liquids form two separate layers, the usually specifically lighter oil floating on top of the water. Whenever the specific gravity of the oil is greater than 1.0, the oil sinks to the bottom of the separator. The design of the receiver should permit the removal of water whether the oil being distilled is heavier or lighter than water.

Smaller florentine flasks are made of glass, larger separators (about 15 litres and more) of metal— usually tin, tinned copper, aluminium or galvanised iron. For all-around use, heavily tinned copper vessels are most practical. Lead must not be employed, as oils containing free fatty acids would form lead salts, which might cause poisoning if the oil were used internally. Rubber tubing or rubber stoppers cannot be used because rubber, being partly soluble in essential oils, gives to them an objectionable odour. Figure 5.16 shows two oil separators, one for oil lighter than water and one for oil heavier than water.

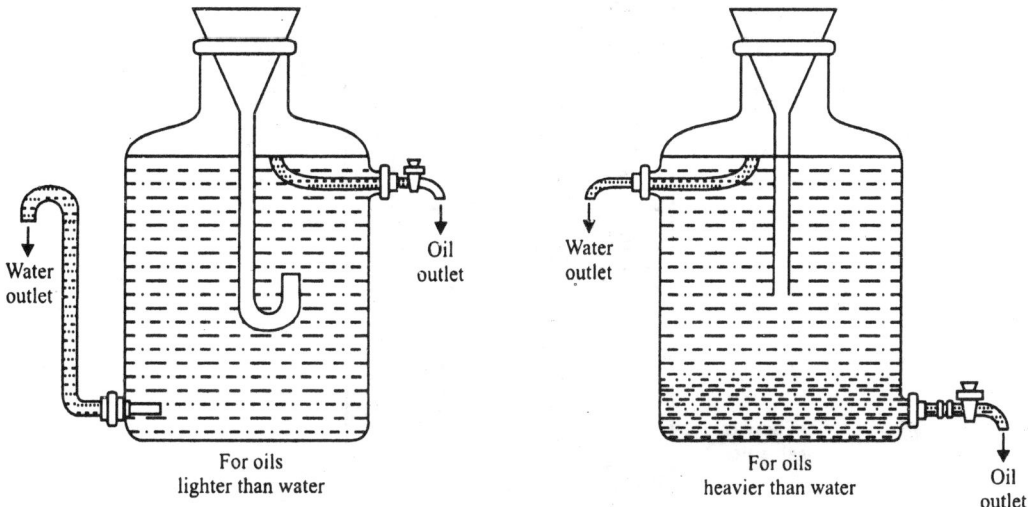

Fig. 5.16. Florentine flasks.

Another and quite satisfactory type of receiver operates according to the following principle:

A cylindrical or rectangular vessel is divided into two chambers by a partition which ends a few inches above the bottom of the vessel. The two chambers are connected with one another. The distillate flows into the first chamber, while the distillation water runs off through a tube on the second chamber. Oil lighter than water collects in the upper part of the first chamber and flows out from there, while oil heavier than water sinks to the bottom of the two chambers and is drawn off from there. Figure 5.17 shows an oil separator of this type.

Oil and water often do not separate immediately in the oil separator, especially if the differential between the specific gravities of water and oil is slight. The distillate must not, therefore, flow too rapidly and any turbulence in the liquids must be avoided; in other words, the separator must be large enough to permit water and oil to separate as completely as possible. Otherwise droplets of oil will be carried away with the outflowing water. A smooth flow of the distillate can be assured by inserting a long stemmed funnel into the separator, the lower outlet of the funnel being turned upward. The distillate streaming from the condenser thus flows first through the funnel, without disturbing the oil layer and the oil droplets rise slowly from the orifice of the funnel toward the oil layer, in which they dissolve. If, on the contrary, the distillate is permitted to run from the condenser directly into the oil layer, the distillation water exerts a dispersing effect on the constituents of the oil having a specific gravity close to that of water: a sort of suspension will result. It should be a general rule to separate the oil layer from the water as quickly as possible and to avoid any agitation of the two media.

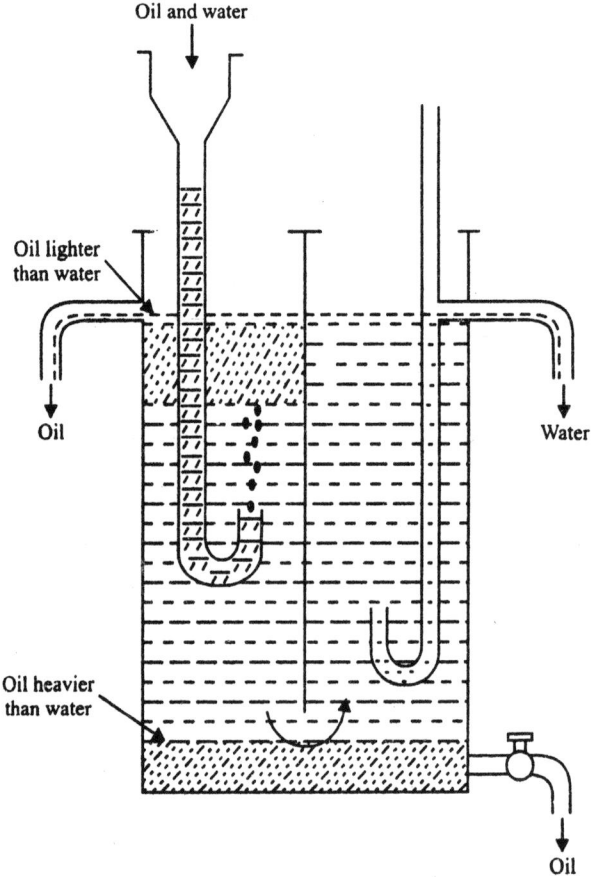

Fig. 5.17. Oil separator for oils lighter and/or heavier than water.

If the single oil separator is not large enough, several should be employed, connected serially, usually in the form of step-like cascades, each of the separators being placed a little lower than the one that precedes it, so that oil and water will separate clearly in the last and lowest vessel. Occasionally, distributing bridges are used, in which the distillate flowing from the condenser is distributed into several oil separators.

Some plant materials yield oils which distil over first in fractions lighter than water and in the later course of distillation, in fractions heavier than water. This is caused by a progressive increase in the specific gravity of the oil fractions. In such cases, two types of oil separators must be employed: the first for separating any oil lighter than water and the second, connected with the first, for separating any oil heavier than water. The same distillate thus flows through both separators or the two-chamber separator described previously can be used to advantage.

The oil and water separator shown in Fig. 5.18 offers the advantage of combining several features in a single unit.

The water outlet is placed as far away from the oil layer as is possible. For oils lighter than water, the oil is drained at A, valves B, C and D are closed; and water is taken off at E through the automatic drain.

For oils heavier than water, the oil is drained at B, valves A, D and E are closed; and water is taken off at C through the automatic drain.

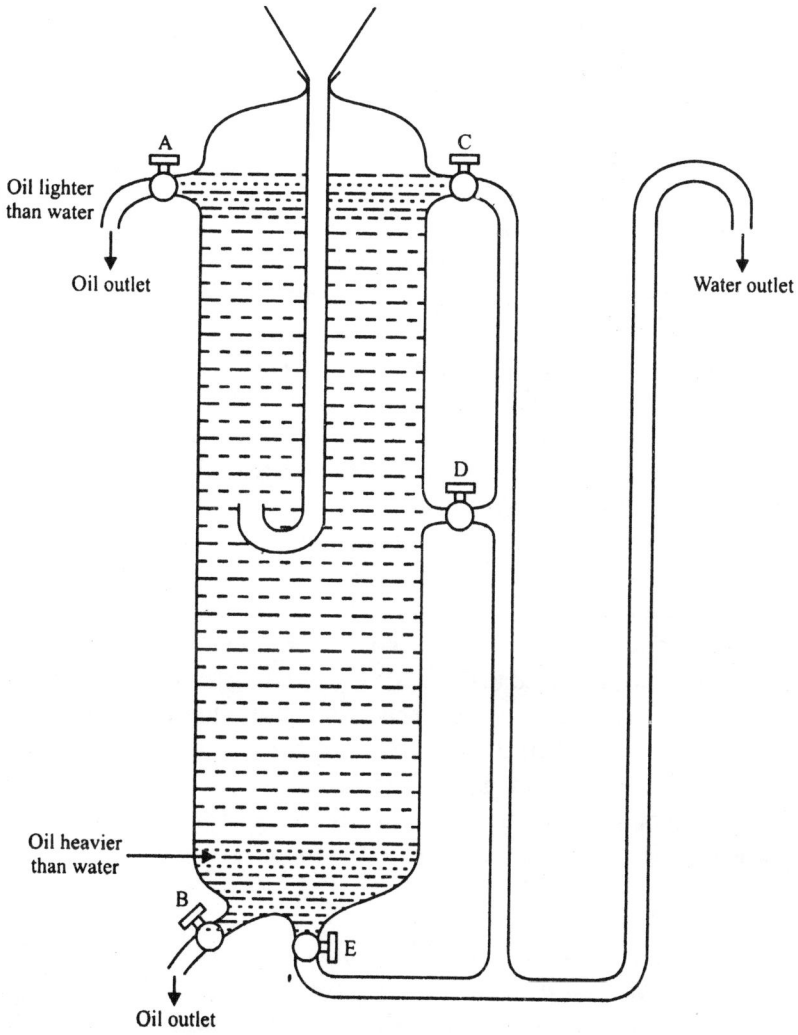

Fig. 5.18. Oils and water separator for oils lighter and/or heavier than water.

For oils separating into two fractions, one heavier and one lighter than water, the lighter oil is taken off at A; the heavier oil is taken off at B; valves C and E are closed; and water is taken off at D through the automatic overflow.

Some oils (e.g. rose oil) deposit separate crystals when cooled below a certain temperature. Such oils are liable to clog the condensers if the distillate flows too cold. In this case it is necessary to let the distillate run tepid by reducing the volume of cooling water entering the condenser tank.

Obviously the separation of two insoluble liquids takes place more quickly and more completely the wider the differential between their specific gravities. Therefore, oils or fractions of oils which have a specific gravity only slightly below that of water do not readily separate from the distillation water at room temperature, but form milky suspensions or emulsions. In such cases, the distillate must be forced to run warmer from the condenser into the Florentine flask, because with rising temperature the specific gravity of the oil decreases relatively more than that of the water. The resulting greater differential in the specific gravity between the oil and water at elevated temperature causes the two layers to separate more readily. If, on the other hand, the specific gravity of an oil at room temperature is slightly higher than that of water (oils heavier than water), the distillate should run as cold as possible. Any increase in the temperature, in this case, would further decrease the already small differential between the specific gravity of the oil and that of the water and separation of the two layers would become even more difficult, if not impossible.

This, however, is the exception. As a general rule and in the case of most essential oils, the temperature of the condensers should be kept as low as possible in order to prevent evaporation and loss of oil.

The separated oil is finally set aside until suspended water droplets and solid or mucilaginous impurities have separated, when it is filtered clear and stored in well-filled, airtight containers in a cool, dark cellar or in an air-conditioned room.

It should be remembered that the condensed water will always be saturated with oil. Discarding this water means a loss in yield of oil. In the case of water distillation or water and steam distillation this condensed water may be used again as the water supply for the next charge of the same type of plant material or the distillation water may be returned into the still and redistilled (cohobated) during distillation. For this purpose the oil separator (Florentine flask) must be installed sufficiently high above the still so that the pressure of the flowing distillation water may overcome the slight pressure usually prevailing within the still. In order to avoid excessive height of the gooseneck, the condenser can be set up side by side with the still, the distillation water then being pumped or injected into the still with a steam injector. This procedure prevents loss of oil, since the oil in the water simply means an additional volatile oil charge to the still. It has been suggested that the condensed water be returned to the steam generating equipment (boiler), but this idea cannot be recommended because of the difficulties encountered with the boiler and also because of the heat in the steam boilers, which would have a deteriorative effect upon the quality of the dissolved oil. In the case of direct steam distillation, the dissolved oil is recovered through redistillation (cohobation) of the distillation water or through extraction with volatile solvents, both of which will be discussed later in more detail.

Steam boilers

Before leaving the subject of equipment, we must make brief mention of the use of auxiliary boilers when water and steam distillation or steam distillation is used. The size of the boiler will depend on the amount of steam required; no generalisation can be made. Because of the danger involved in the operation of a steam boiler, it is recommended that such equipment be purchased from an established dealer in power generation equipment. Briefly, besides the usual fire box and tube heater, the system should include gauges for determining water level and pressure, safety valves to guard against operation at too high pressure, a pump or injector for circulating the water and all necessary piping for the particular operation at hand. The supplier should be consulted before ordering any equipment. All reputable suppliers maintain well-trained engineering staffs for the purpose of analysing customers requirements and advantage should be taken of this service.

There are two types of boiler, viz. the so-called low-pressure boiler, developing 40 to 45 lb. of pressure, as measured at the boiler gauge and the high-pressure boiler, which develops a steam pressure of approximately 100 lb. and more. High-pressure steam is used to attain higher temperatures rather than merely to force the steam through the plant material contained in the retort. Theoretically the temperature of saturated steam is a function of the steam pressure. Steam, as developing from boiling water (pressure at the gauge = 0), has a temperature of 212°F (100°C); at 40 lb. it, has a temperature of 287°F (141.7°C) and at 100 lb., 338°F (170°C). Steam of low pressure and, therefore, of comparatively low temperature, is likely to be recondensed to water in the lower part of the plant charge, whereas steam of higher pressure and temperature penetrates the plant material more effectively and with less condensation in the still. High-pressure boilers are, therefore, more efficient in regard to distillation, shortening its length. On the other and, it is claimed that low-pressure steam, as a rule, yields more alcohol soluble oils, free of bitter resinous matter.

In actual operation low-pressure boilers produce little pressure but a large volume of steam. They are constructed of appropriate gauge sheet metal with cast-iron beads. Even the flues are made of galvanised sheet metal. All of the other boilers are 'high pressure'. It is true that some distillers use 30 to 100 lb. of pressure, but that depends on the steam requirements. Data collected by experts on retort temperatures in the distillation of peppermint oil, show that there exists little difference between the temperature of the trays at 20 lb., and at 80 lb., but the speed with which the distillation takes place is an important factor economically.

The explanation is obvious if one considers that the steam is released into a large retort, not under pressure. There the steam temperature will be reduced to the still temperature immediately without pressure. In some cases, of course, the steam is 'pushed' in so fast that a slight back pressure results, but this will seldom cause more than a 10°F (about 5°C) rise above 212°F (100°C) in the still.

If superheated steam is to be used, a superheater of one form or another must be installed. One method of superheating steam consists of permitting high-pressure, dry saturated steam to expand suddenly to a lower pressure through a well-insulated valve. This will result in a moderate amount of superheating, at least theoretically speaking. A well-designed boiler should produce very nearly saturated steam and the above method will, therefore, result in slight superheating. If the steam as generated is very wet, it will be necessary to do one of two things in order to accomplish superheating. One method consists of installing in the high-pressure line a water separator, which will remove most of the liquid water from the steam. This dried steam may then be expanded as described above to produce superheated steam. An alternative method is to expose the line carrying wet or saturated steam to a temperature sufficiently above the boiling point of water at the steam pressure to permit the extent of superheating desired. This can be accomplished by running the steam line through a region in which the waste gases from the boiler can transfer part of their heat to the steam.

The amount of exposure must be carefully controlled, to avoid excessive superheating. If desired, this heating may also be done in an entirely separate unit and since the stack gases always contain waste heat, this might just as well be recovered. In the installation of superheating equipment, the boiler supplier can again be of great assistance.

Practical Problems Connected with Essential Oil Distillation

At this point it is advisable to devote space to a few practical suggestions for the operation of essential oil stills. Many of the points brought out in the following paragraphs have already been mentioned, but it appears desirable to emphasise them, since failure to adhere to them may well represent the difference between successful and unsuccessful operation. The three general methods of conducting steam distillation will be considered in order.

Water distillation

Let us first consider the operation of a water distillation system. In every method of plant distillation, whether steam distillation, water and steam distillation or water distillation, only those quantities of the essential oil with which the steam comes in direct contact can be vapourised. Any oil held within the plant tissue must first be extracted from the glands and brought to the surface of the plant by osmosis. But the forces of hydrodiffusion work very slowly whenever the distances to be bridged are relatively long. Water distillation necessitates a thorough comminution of the plant material to the smallest possible size; in other words, the reduction must exceed that required for direct steam distillation or water and steam distillation. All interspaces between the plant particles, which in the case of water distillation are filled with water, must be penetrated continuously by rising steam.

The retort is charged with the plant material to be distilled and sufficient water added to fully cover the entire charge, leaving, however, ample vapour space above the charge to avoid boiling over and carrying over of spray into the condenser. After the cover has been fastened tightly — using a suitable gasket between cover and still to avoid loss of vapours at that point — the retort is connected to the condenser and the cooling water permitted to flow through the latter. The fire is then started, if a direct fired still is being used or the steam line opened, if either a steam jacket or steam coils are used for heating. Once the charge has reached its boiling point at the particular pressure used, condensate will begin to issue from the open end of the condenser and should be run directly into the separator, which was previously filled with water. The rate of distillation can be controlled by the intensity of the fire, by the pressure in the steam jacket or by the rate of introduction of steam. With direct fire, special care must be taken to avoid overheating the plant material. As the water and oil evaporate, part of the charge will soon cease to be covered with water and hence no longer will be automatically protected from overheating. It may be advisable to add more water as the distillation proceeds, to prevent any part of the charge from becoming exposed to the full heat of the fire. When a steam jacket or closed steam heating coils are used, there is less danger of overheating unless the water level falls below the top steam coils. Here again the addition of sufficient water will prevent such an undesirable result. With open steam coils this danger is largely avoided, since for every pound of steam injected, a pound of steam condenses as distillation water in the condenser. However, care must be taken to prevent accumulation of condensed water within the retort or the water level will rise gradually to the top. Therefore, the still should be well insulated and not exposed to draft or cold wind. Furthermore, the water charged into the retort at the beginning of the operation should be hot, as cold water would condense too much of the injected live steam.

The rate of distillation must be adjusted to suit the particular equipment and material being distilled. This rate should, of course, be maintined near the maximum in order to obtain the maximum production of oil. There are other, perhaps less apparent, reasons for maintaining a rapid rate of distillation when using water distillation. Principal among these is the fact that only by rapid distillation can the charge be maintained in a sufficiently loose condition to insure thorough penetration of the plant material by the rising steam. Steam which does not contact the charge, for example steam generated at the water surface as in slow distillation, cannot carry any essential oil with it and will be wasted. A lively conduct of distillation prevents to a large extent undesired agglomeration of the plant material and brings about a more effective contact area between charge and steam. This in turn causes not only an increase in the rate of production, but also a better total yield of oil. It is commonly assumed that during water distillation all parts of the plant charge are kept in motion by boiling water. This, however, is only partly true. Steam bubbles form mainly along the closed steam coils, along the heated bottom and walls of the retort and rise to the surface by the shortest way, avoiding any obstacles. Provided the distillation material is charged loosely and remains loose in the boiling waters, the steam bubbles probably will contact all plant particles quite evenly and vapourise their volatile oil. This is the case especially with woody material, but flowers have a tendency to agglutinate under the influence of steam and form large lumps. True, the volatile oil diffuses quite readily from tenderwalled epidermis glands, but when leaves or flowers cling together diffusion is slowed down. Distillation must then be accelerated to a point where all particles of the plant charge are agitated and kept in continuous motion by rising and exploding steam bubbles. The degree of comminution, the weight of the plant charge and the construction of the still should be calculated accordingly. Plant material which contains an essential oil composed of high boiling constituents can be exhausted by water distillation only if comminuted to small particles.

Many years ago distillation was carried out almost exclusively over direct fire, water distillation then being the rule, steam distillation the exception. Experience had been that complete exhaustion of many plant materials could be effected only under great difficulties and after several days of distilling. Extraction of oil of cloves, for instance, seems to have caused a great deal of trouble. Directions dating back to the middle of the last century claim that cloves could be exhausted only by repeated distillation; in other words, the retort had to be opened from time to time, the content stirred and the evaporated water replaced. In the case of cloves this was repeated from three to eight times. Very probably the plant charge relative to the size of the still was much too large and distillation had to be carried out much too slowly with a small fire; otherwise the cloves in the still would have foamed over into the condenser. Small-scale operators, especially field distillers employing directly fired retorts, still commit the mistake of not putting sufficient water into the retort. Ignorant of the simple rules underlying water distillation, they seem to prefer a slow distillation or they are handicapped by too small condensers or by lack of water. Frequently they add to the plant material such a small quantity of water that only the still bottom, which is directly fired, remains covered with water at the end of the operation. This practice is faulty. Plant parts rising above the level of the boiling water in the course of water distillation tend to lump together, to become almost impenetrable for steam, and therefore, not to yield their oil completely. For this reason, the retort should be only partly filled with plant material, which should remain fully immersed in water, even when distillation is completed. Only by following this precaution is it possible to exhaust the plant charge by water distillation, as far as this can be done at all. Water distillation is still quite widely used with portable equipment in primitive countries. There, lack of roads and poor transport facilities prevent hauling of the plant material from outlying growing regions to centrally located distilleries. Therefore, the apparatus must be moved into the growing sections or in other words follow the plant material. Small stills, simple, sturdy and low priced, hence retain the favour of many native producers. Aside from these purely practical conveniences, water distillation possesses one decided advantage. It permits processing of very finely powdered material (root, bark and wood, etc.) or of plant parts which by contact with direct (live) steam would easily agglutinate and form lumps through which the steam cannot penetrate (e.g. roses or orange blossoms). From such an agglutinated mass, live steam vapourises the oil only from the outside and not from the inside. Steam distillation, therefore, would remain incomplete. The nascent steam bubbles attack all parts of the plant charge only if the latter moves loosely and freely in boiling water. As a matter of fact, material which readily agglutinates can be processed only by water distillation.

On the other hand, water distillation suffers from several disadvantages. Whether comminuted or not, the plant material cannot always be completely exhausted. Furthermore, certain esters, linalyl acetate, for example, are partly hydrolysed; other sensitive substances, such as aldehydes, tend to polymerise under the influence of boiling water, etc. Consequently, all other conditions being the same, the quality of product from a rapid distillation will be better, in general, than that of the product from a slow distillation. Water distillation requires a greater number of stills, more space and more fuel. It demands considerable experience and familiarity with the method and its effect, in fact more experience and care than any other form of plant distillation; otherwise the yield of oil will be affected and fall considerably below that obtained by water and steam distillation or by direct steam distillation. Water distillation is the least economical process, water and steam distillation giving, in general, better results in the case of field distillation.

Another peculiarity of water distillation lies in the fact that high boiling and somewhat water-soluble oil constituents cannot be completely vapourised from the large quantities of water which must cover the plant charge in the still or they require so much steam that they can be recovered only partly from the distillation (condensed) water; therefore, the distilled oil will be deficient in regard to these constituents. In other words, distillation remains incomplete. Such compounds are high boiling alcohols (phenylethyl alcohol, cinnamyl alcohol, benzyl alcohol, etc.), phenols (eugenol, etc.), certain nitrogenous substances and some acids. A typical example is orange blossom oil: the methyl anthranilate present in the flowers cannot be completely recovered by distillation, extraction with volatile solvents giving better results. The case is similar with roses: distilled rose oil lacks the somewhat spicy note of the extracted product (concrete or absolute) and contains much less phenylethyl alcohol, because eugenol and phenylethyl alcohol remain in the residual still waters. How much of these high boiling, somewhat water-soluble compounds are actually carried over by distillation depends upon their boiling points, their degrees of solubility in water and the quantity present in the plant material. If the plant charge, despite comminution, contains coarser particles, which during the boiling do not soften and, therefore, are not torn apart, these particles will retain high boiling, water-insoluble oil constituents, because diffusion through the greatly swollen tissue layers acts too slowly. These factors explain why essential oils obtained from the same plant material by water distillation or by steam distillation vary considerably in regard to yield physical properties and chemical composition.

For all these reasons, water distillation is used today in essential oil factories and for large-scale production only in cases where the plant material by its very nature cannot be processed by water and steam distillation or, even better, by direct steam distillation.

For most efficient operation, a modern retort serving for water distillation should be flat and wide, thereby offering a large surface of evaporation. The plant material should be filled in evenly, not higher than 4 inches. Water is then pumped into the still until it stands about 2-inch above the charge. Steam of at least 3 atmospheres absolute pressure, generated in a separate steam boiler, is injected into the steam jacket beneath the still, so that the water in the still is brought to lively boiling and each particle of the plant charge thoroughly and continually agitated. The quantity of the plant charge does not necessarily depend upon the size of the still. A somewhat loose charge contains sufficient interspaces to permit an unhindered penetration by the steam bubbles rising from the still bottom; hence the charge can be higher than 4 inches. If, in addition, the plant material does not agglutinate or lump while softening under the influence of heat, the charge may be considerably higher. However, complete exhaustion is not always assured; in general, good results in the case of water distillation are obtained only if the charge is sufficiently low to permit the rising steam bubbles to overcome the weight of the plant charge. In other words, the steam should continually agitate the plant particles. In this case it is preferable to work without a perforated grid above the bottom of the retort. If, on the other hand, the charge is high, exercising a marked pressure upon the bottom, the insertion of a perforated grid is advisable.

For certain types of plant materials, e.g. roses, orange blossoms and ylang flowers — which can be kept floating in the boiling water by lively steam development, much deeper or spherical stills may be employed. Heating coils (instead of a steam jacket) should be avoided in this case because plant particles easily attach themselves to the coils and may give trouble.

Very finely powdered material — such as almond or apricot kernels — has a tendency to 'burn' in contact with the hot steam jacket; the water in the still should, therefore, be heated, not by indirect steam, but by direct steam, injected through a steam coil within the still. High, cylindrical stills are better adapted to this purpose than wide, flat ones. In this case, the distillation water is collected separately and not pumped back into the still during the process, because too much liquid would accumulate in the still by condensation of the injected live steam. A general rule which applies to all methods of distillation is that each charge should be completed on the same day. The quantity of plant material charged and the rate of distillation must be calculated accordingly. It should be kept in mind that the shorter the distillation, the less the forces causing hydrolysis, decomposition and resinification will come into action. The loss of essential oil arising from these forces may amount to several per cent, as calculated upon the oil. In the case of water distillation, it is not always possible, however, to shorten distillation to a one-day operation.

Figure 5.19 shows a still for water distillation, with automatic return of the distillation water.

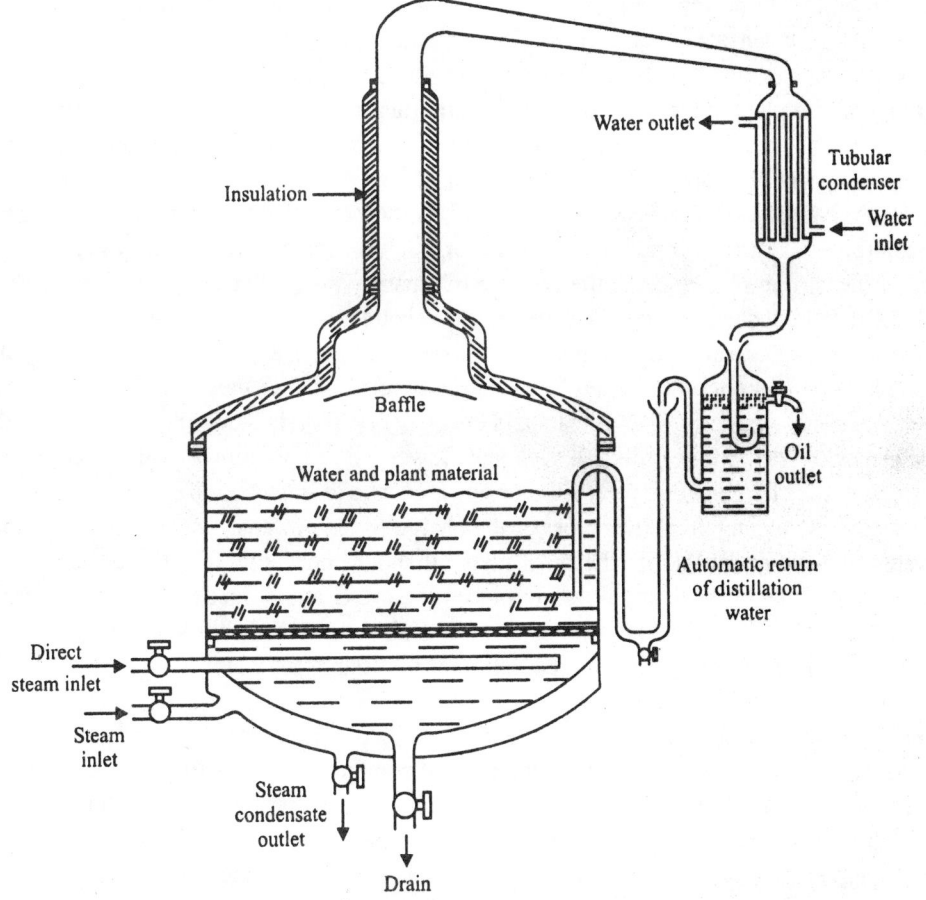

Fig. 5.19. Still for water distillation.

Water and steam distillation

Let us now consider some practical aspects of water and steam distillation, a method which in recent years has become quite popular among small producers using portable distillation equipment that can be moved from field to field, following the harvest. The smaller units are heated by direct fire, the larger ones by a steam jacket a closed steam coil or in rarer cases by open steam coils. When using direct fire, precaution must be taken to insure that only the bottom of the still, the section containing water below the grid which carries the plant charge, is heated. Otherwise, one of the major advantages of water and steam distillation over water distillation, namely, freedom from the danger of overheating the plant material, will be lost. As was stated previously, when this method of distillation is employed the plant charge itself is kept out of contact with boiling water. Hence, if the upper part of the still were exposed to direct fire, the plant material might be dangerously overheated. It is advisable, therefore, to use indirect steam as a source of heat, but not direct fire.

In this type of distillation, observing the precautions mentioned in the last paragraph, steam alone contacts the charge, the steam either being generated from or passing through, water in the still. Thus overheating or drying of the charge is avoided because the temperature cannot rise above that of saturated steam at the pressure prevailing in the still (at atmospheric pressure never above 100°C). Water and steam distillation, therefore, represents a typical case of distillation with saturated low pressure steam. For this reason, the condensate contains fewer decomposition products than that obtained by direct steam distillation with live steam and particularly with high pressure or superheated steam.

Preparation of the plant material is much more important in this method of distillation than in water distillation. Since the steam contacts the material only by rising through it, the plant charge must be so disposed that all parts of it are uniformly contacted, if high yields of oil are to be maintained. This requires that the charge be homogeneous as to size and, furthermore, that the average size of the individual pieces be controlled within rather narrow limits. If, for example, the material is finely ground, it will tend to pack and offer strong resistance to the passage of steam. This in turn may develop steam pressure beneath the charge until such pressure is sufficient to penetrate it. Such penetration, however, will take place at only a few places, releasing the pressure and permitting the steam to escape through only a few passages or channels—sometimes called 'rat holes'. Obviously, under these circumstances most of the plant material is never contacted by the steam and the recovery of oil is incomplete. If, on the other hand, a charge consists of, say, whole stalks, leaves and flowers, there obviously will be some fairly large passages through the charge which offer little or no resistance to the passage of steam. Steam will then escape through these and again permit most of the charge to remain unaffected by it. Therefore, in the case of water and steam distillation, the plant material should not be too finely ground; nor should it contain excessively long stalks or large roots or pieces of bark. Granulation usually gives the best results. Experience alone can determine the optimum size to which the material should be reduced and this will vary from plant to plant. At any rate, the preparation of the charge for water and steam distillation must always be given most careful attention.

Another problem to be considered in water and steam distillation arises from the fact that the charge is cold at the start and that the first steam to enter it will condense, thus wetting the plant material. This wetting will continue until the entire charge reaches the boiling temperature of water at the operating pressure. With certain types of plant materials—for example, leaves or ground seeds, bark, roots, etc. excessive wetting may result in lumping or agglomeration of the charge and, therefore, in a subnormal oil yield. Such wetting, again, may cause channeling of the steam. If a charge tends to agglomerate when wet, it is sometimes advisable to add dried twigs or short small pieces of stalk or any other loose but absolutely neutral material, in limited quantities, so that the charge may be kept porous. To avoid continuation of wetting due to loss of heat by radiation from the walls of the still, the upper part of the retort — in other words, the section housing the charge — should be insulated.

The rate of distillation in the case of water and steam distillation is not as important as in the case of water distillation. It affects only the rate of production but not always the quality or yield of oil. A lively pace of distillation recommends itself, however, in order to prevent excessive wetting of the plant charge and in order to increase the production rate. Regarding oil production per hour, water and steam distillation is less efficient than steam distillation; it approaches that of water distillation.

Compared with water distillation, water and steam distillation has the advantage in that it gives less rise to products of decomposition in the oil (hydrolysis of esters, polymerisation, resinification, etc.). As far as portable stills and small stationary posts are concerned, water and steam distillation is, in most cases, a better method than water distillation: it requires less fuel shorter hours and yields more oil even with a low rate of vapourisation. If, however, a plant material — for instance, roses or orange blossoms — forms lumps under the influence of steam, the interspaces disappear and the steam can no longer penetrate the charge and reach every plant particle. In such cases, water distillation must be resorted to.

The great disadvantage of water and steam distillation, which limits its adaptation, lies in the fact that, as a result of the low pressure of the rising steam, oils of high boiling range require large quantities of steam for complete vapourisation — hence long hours of distillation. In this process much steam condenses in the plant charge, which becomes increasingly wet, agglutinates and will yield its oil only very slowly. As in the case of water distillation, in water and steam distillation the condenser can be installed at such a height that the distillation water flows automatically and continuously back into the still. Or the distillation water may be pumped back or injected into the retort.

After completion of a charge, the water beneath the perforated grid is discarded and replaced with fresh water. It is not advisable to employ the same water for the next charge because some steam always condenses within the plant charge and water-soluble extractive matter from the plant charge accumulates in the water beneath the grid. The repeated use and boiling of the same water may cause the extractive plant matter to decompose and to form volatile products of disagreeable odour, which are liable to impart an objectionable by-note to the volatile oil.

Summarising, it can be said that water and steam distillation must be carried out by observing the following principles: uniform size of the plant particles and sufficiently large interspaces for the rising steam; uniform distribution of the plant material in the retort, so that the change is penetrated evenly and completely by steam. Although the method of direct steam distillation serves for a variety of plant materials, water and steam distillation is suitable only for certain types. It is especially adapted to field distillation in small or medium sized stills.

Water and steam distillation can also be carried out under reduced or increased pressure. Indeed, in some cases, reduced pressure gives excellent results. Figure 5.20 shows a retort for water and steam distillation.

Steam distillation

Live steam, usually of a pressure higher than atmospheric, is generated in a separate steam boiler and injected into the plant charge within the retort. This type of distillation is referred to as direct steam distillation or distillation with live steam or dry steam distillation. Most aromatic plants are distilled today with direct live steam at atmospheric pressure.

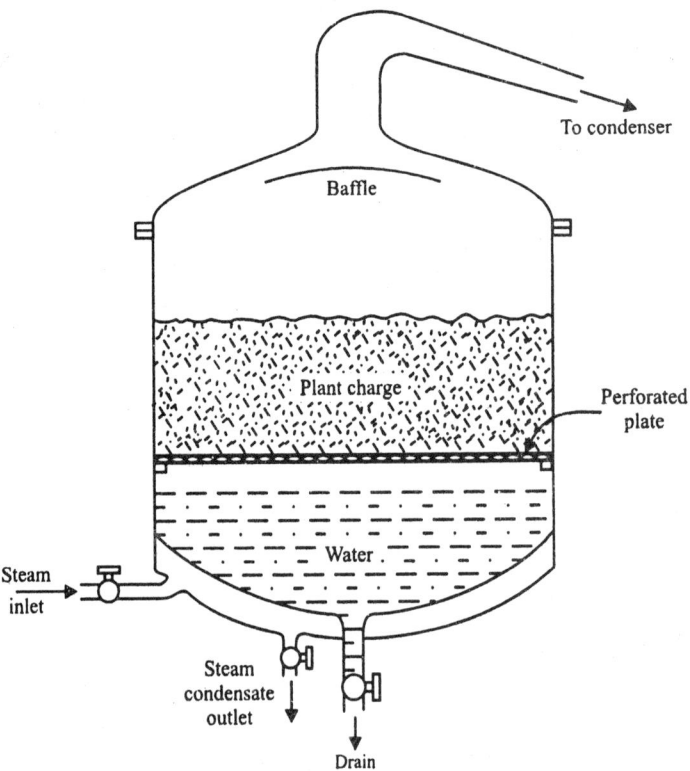

To condenser

Baffle

Plant charge

Perforated plate

Water

Steam inlet

Steam condensate outlet

Drain

Fig. 5.20. Still for water and steam distillation.

The application of steam distillation is subject to exactly the same reservations mentioned in the discussion of water and steam distillation, plus one additional factor. When using steam distillation, it is always possible, after the initial period during which the charge in the retort is warming up and condensation taking place, that the steam may be slightly superheated. Indeed, in some cases the steam may be purposely superheated, as already mentioned, in order to improve the oil to water ratio. Two factors then assume importance. First, the temperature of the charge will no longer be maintained at the boiling point of water, under the operating pressure, but will rise to the temperature of the superheated steam. The operator, therefore, must guard carefully against overheating. Second, superheated steam has a tendency to dry out the charge and reduce the rate of recovery of the essential oil. As was pointed out above, a good part of the oil is vapourised only after diffusing, as an aqueous solution, through the cell membranes to the outside of the plant particles. This diffusion, however, becomes possible only by the presence of a certain amount of hot water and may be stopped altogether or seriously slowed down, when the charge is completely dried. If, therefore, in the case of direct steam distillation, the flow of oil stops prematurely, it may be necessary to continue distillation with saturated (wet) steam for a time, until hydrodiffusion is re-established. After that slightly superheated steam may again be employed.

In general, it can be said that direct steam distillation excels water distillation, as well as water and steam distillation in regard to cost, rate of distillation and capacity of production. As far as the condition of the plant material and the method of charging are concerned, the same principles apply here as to water and steam distillation. Special attention must be paid to the quality of the live steam. The higher the pressure of the steam, the higher is the temperature at which it enters the still; but in this respect the moisture content of the steam plays an important role. Saturated steam usually carries some water in the form of minute droplets, which are condensed by the expanding steam. Hence, the effect of superheating becomes noticeable only if saturated (but dry) steam, of markedly high pressure, is used. The higher the pressure of the steam in the steam boiler, the drier the plant material will remain during distillation. Only the portions of the charge touching the still walls will then become moist through condensation, despite insulation of the still against emanation of heat. In order to limit such loss of heat and consequent excessive lowering of the temperature, the high-pressure steam, before entering the still, is sent through a water separator and partly dried. In this connection, it should also be kept in mind that the different systems of steam boilers generate live steam, containing more or less moisture. In cases of prolonged distillation, considerable quantities of steam are condensed in the plant charge and water accumulates on the bottom of the still. This may give trouble by wetting the lower part of the plant charge. Such condensed water must be drawn off, from time to time, through a stopcock in the still bottom.

Since high-pressure steam causes considerable decomposition, distillation is best started with steam of low pressure, followed by steam of higher pressure toward the end of the operation, when the oil content of the charge has decreased considerably and when chiefly the high boiling constituents of the essential oil remain in the retort. No general rule can be laid down in this respect, as every type of plant material requires a different and specific method of preparation and also of distillation.

End of distillation

As the distillation proceeds and as the oil content of the charge decreases correspondingly, the ratio of water to oil in the condensate will increase, because the steam can no longer contact the oil in the charge efficiently, regardless of the rate of distillation and also because the remaining constituents are mostly high boiling. The operator must then decide at what point it is no longer economical to continue the distillation. Several criteria can be applied here. From a knowledge of the size of the charge and the yield to be expected and from experience or trial distillations in a pilot still, it can quickly be determined whether or not the charge has been nearly exhausted. If yield data on the particular material charged are not available, it usually will suffice to take a small sample of the condensate directly into a test tube or glass cylinder and estimate from this the rate at which oil is being distilled at any particular time. Then, knowing the amount of oil already distilled and calculating the amount that will be distilled in any additional period of time, it can be decided whether distillation should be continued for that period or whether it would be more economical to stop and begin a fresh charge. The value of the product also enters into consideration, since a very valuable oil can be run profitably to a much larger water to oil ratio than can a less valuable oil. Certain oils, e.g. vetiver or angelica root oil — contain their most valuable constituents in the last runs (highest boiling fractions) and in these cases distillation must be prolonged for hours even though almost no oil seems to distil over toward the end of the operation. Otherwise valuable, high boiling constituents will be lacking in the oil. This rule, by the way, applies to all types of distillation.

It should also be kept in mind that the oil to water ratio measured at any time during distillation will always be higher than during any succeeding period, since this ratio decreases as the distillation continues. Experience with the distillation of any particular plant material will enable the operator to evaluate these matters properly, so as to obtain a maximum yield, a maximum rate and a high quality of oil.

Treatment of the volatile oil

The handling of the condensed oil is worthy of brief comment since its quality may deteriorate, particularly if the oil must be stored for some time. Just as the condensed water (distillation water) is always saturated with oil, so the condensed oil will always be saturated with water. There remains also the probability of slow reaction between the oil and water, unless the latter is almost completely removed. The oil can be brightened (cleared of cloudy appearance) by filtering through kieselguhr or magnesium carbonate on filter paper. This procedure removes all small droplets of water which cause the cloudiness, but it does not completely dry the oil. Larger quantities of oil may be filtered through mechanical filters, filter presses or run through high-speed centrifuges.

Treatment of the distillation water

The distillation water flowing off the oil separator (Florentine flask) contains some of the volatile oil in solution or suspension, the quantity depending upon the solubility and specific gravity of the various oil constituents. Considering that the distillate presents a mixture of condensed steam and oil vapours, it is evident that the water phase of the distillate actually represents an aqueous solution of oil, completely saturated at the prevailing temperature. Those oil constituents which are somewhat soluble in water will be partly dissolved in the distillation water and the dissolved portion of this oil will be different in composition from that of the oil separated in the Florentine flask. The latter is usually called main or direct oil, the former water oil. The water-soluble constituents consist mostly of oxygenated compounds and since these compounds possess a higher specific gravity than nonoxygenated compounds (terpenes, sesquiterpenes, etc.), the water oil usually has a higher specific gravity than the main oil. This difference, however, is not always pronounced, because the distillation water contains not only oil in actual solution, but also in suspended (minute droplets) and emulsified form. A more or less milky appearance of the distillation water thus indicates the presence of oil.

Such distillation water cannot be discarded; but must be submitted to further treatment to prevent loss of oil. In the case of water distillation or water and steam distillation, it may be automatically returned into the retort during distillation. For this purpose the Florentine flask must be installed at a sufficient height above the still so that the flow from the flask overcomes the pressure within the still. In the case of steam distillation (with live steam from a separate steam boiler) the distillation water should not be returned into the retort, as too much liquid would condense and accumulate within it and wet the plant charge. The distillation water therefore, is pumped or injected into a separate still for redistillation. The process of recovering the oil from the water by redistillation is commonly called cohobation, the stills serving for this purpose being known as cohobation stills. In its original and stricter sense, the term 'cohobation' implies that the distillation water is used over and over for the distillation of a new plant charge (in the case of water distillation or water and steam distillation), but today cohobation simply means redistillation of the distillation waters.

The distillation waters are redistilled most efficiently in round stills provided with a steam jacket or a closed steam coil. Indirect heating is preferable, because the injection of live steam into the retort would cause too much water to accumulate within the retort and hinder the vapourisation of the oil from the water. In the case of many distillation waters only 10 to 15 per cent need be distilled off to recover most of the oil dissolved or suspended therein. The residual water may be discarded. Occasionally, however, it is necessary to distil off more than half of the quantity of water; in such case, a considerable portion of the oil distilled over will again be dissolved in the distillation water. To shorten the cohobation and increase the quantity of oil in the condensate, the water in the cohobation still is saturated with common, salt (NaCl). This decreases the solubility of the volatile oil in water: the oil distils over more quickly and with a smaller quantity of water. This procedure is recommended particularly where the distillation water contains slightly water-soluble constituents of high boiling point, which cannot be recovered by mere steam distillation. The separation of oil and water by cohobation is based upon the simple principle that a mixture of oil vapours and steam possesses a slightly lower boiling point than pure water vapours (steam) and that the vapour mixture arising contains more oil than the liquid phase. By a reduction of the speed of cohobation, the oil content of the distillate may be increased because the rising steam will be more thoroughly saturated with oil vapours.

The following figures give an idea of the quantities of volatile oils which can be obtained by the cohobation of various distillation waters:

Plant material	Quantity of water oil recovered from 1000 kg of distillation water (grams)
Chamomile flowers	100–120
Coriander seed	625–650
Dill seed	360–450
Fennel seed	175–200
Lavender flowers	150–200
Peppermint herb	400–500
Sage herb	300
Tansy herb	540

Another method of recovering the oil dissolved or suspended in the distillation water consists in saturating the latter first with salt and then extracting the solution with volatile solvents, e.g. highly purified petroleum ether or benzene. This is usually done twice. The drawn off and united solvent solutions are then concentrated in a still by driving off the solvent, first at atmospheric pressure and later *in vacuo*, until every trace of solvent is eliminated from the oil.

Any distillation of aromatic plants, unless conducted at fairly low temperatures, gives rise to products of decomposition in the nonvolatile plant constituents. These products (methyl alcohol, formaldehyde, acetaldehyde, acetone, low fatty acids, nitrogenous compounds, phenols, etc.) are carried into the condensate and present objectionable impurities. Because of their water solubility, they dissolve mainly in the distillation water, since the quantity of water by far exceeds that of oil. Because of the presence of such decomposition products, the crude water oil obtained by cohobation or extraction will in most cases be of dark colour, often of disagreeable odour. It should not be combined with the main oil, as it would spoil the odour and flavour of the latter. It is, therefore, advisable to rectify the crude water oil by fractionation in a good vacuum still.

In many cases the great water solubility of the aforementioned decomposition products serves for the purification of volatile oils: when rectifying (redistilling) an oil by hydrodistillation, the distillation water is then simply discarded.

Disposal of the spent plant material

The disposal of the spent plant material, which represents a rather large bulk, frequently offers an annoying problem. One very economical method of disposal consists in using it as fuel — after air drying, of course, either in the sun or near the still in the case of direct fire stills or near the boiler when a separate steam generator is used. Since the spent material has a rather low fuel value per unit volume, consideration must be given to the construction of a special fuel box. In many cases the spent material may be used effectively as fertiliser. Certain spent plants make an excellent cattle feed; this is particularly true of seeds which contain a high percentage of protein and fatty oil. The drying is done in dehydrating apparatus or by air drying on shelves. When sweetened with molasses, some spent grasses, such as lemongrass, seem to be relished by cattle.

Laboratory trial distillation

No discussion of distillation as used in the essential oil industry would be complete without some consideration of the interpretation to be placed upon the results of laboratory distillations or, as they are frequently called, trial distillations. Since the oil content of plant material to be distilled fluctuates rather widely with such variables as geographical origin, growing conditions, ambient temperature, rainfall, period of harvest, moisture content, etc. it is not usually possible to state any values for the oil content other than by upper and lower limits (which in some cases may be quite widely separated). As already pointed out, handling of the plant material after harvesting and prior to distillation, also has a marked effect on the oil content. As knowledge of the efficiency with which a large scale distillation is being conducted can be obtained only by comparison of the actual yield with the possible yield, it becomes quite important that the latter value be known with some accuracy. The only means of determining this value is to conduct a laboratory distillation using a sample of the plant material to be distilled in the larger scale operation.

The aim of any commercial distillation is, of course, to recover as large a percentage of the valuable oils in as high a state of purity as possible. Only in the laboratory, on a small scale and under carefully controlled conditions, can both of these conditions be met. Therefore, the results of such laboratory distillation may be considered as a standard which the large scale operation should approach as closely as practically possible.

There are two ways of carrying out such trial distillations:

1. On a very small scale in a glass flask.
2. On a larger scale in a pilot still.
1. Numerous method of assaying the contents of essential oil in plant material have been suggested. Many modifications of these methods, all of which aim at a quantitative yield of oil. The best and most commonly used methods is that of Clevenger, which has found official recognition in 'Methods of Analysis'. This method permits assaying quantitatively the content of essential oil in a small amount (50 to 500 gram) of plant material. Although the amount of oil thus obtained is not sufficient to carry out a complete analysis, conclusions regarding its odour and flavour characteristics can be drawn from the small sample. Occasionally, the oil will have to be set aside for several days, until the slightly 'burnt' or 'still' odour of the freshly distilled oil has disappeared.
2. A much more satisfactory method consists in distilling a sample of 20 to 50 lb. of aromatic plant material in a regular 'pilot' still. Such a still, made of tin-lined copper, should be constructed so as to embody all the characteristics of large stills. It should allow for water distillation, water and steam distillation and direct steam distillation. It will thus be possible to find for each new plant material the most appropriate method of distillation, to study, as well as possible, the rate of distillation and the consumption of steam (by measuring the quantity of distillation water) and to determine the maximum yield of oil. Interesting observations regarding the effects of hydrodiffusion can be made. In the case of direct steam distillation the use of high-pressure or superheated steam may be studied. The quantity of oil recovered will be sufficiently large to examine the oil analytically, even to fractionate it. The pilot still should be provided with several trays, in order to find out the most opportune way of charging, if seed materials are to be processed. A small

crusher and hay cutter will permit trying out the effects of comminuting the plant material according to different sizes. Needless to say, the pilot still should be well insulated—in other words it should resemble large stills in every possible way except size.

For all-around operation the pilot still should also be equipped for automatic return of the distillation waters into the still, in the case of water distillation or water and steam distillation, if the return (cohobation) of these waters into the still during operation seems desirable. In the case of direct steam distillation, the distillation water or a small measured part of it is saturated with ordinary salt and three times extracted with low boiling petroleum ether. The drawn off and united petroleum ether extracts are then carefully evaporated on a hot water bath and the residue dried in a desiccator to constant weight. From this small quantity the oil content of the total distillation waters can be calculated. Obviously, the extraction of only a part of the distillation waters gives an exact result only where the total distillation water, after completion of the distillation, have been bulked in a tank. The distillation water should always be processed right after distillation of the plant material, because when exposed to the air for some time it loses oil by evaporation. While a small part of the distillation water is extracted experimentally with a solvent, another part should be steam distilled (cohobated). If cohobation yields no oil, the distillation water will have to be extracted with solvents. Figures 5.21 and 5.22 show the construction of pilot stills which may have a capacity of about 50 gallons.

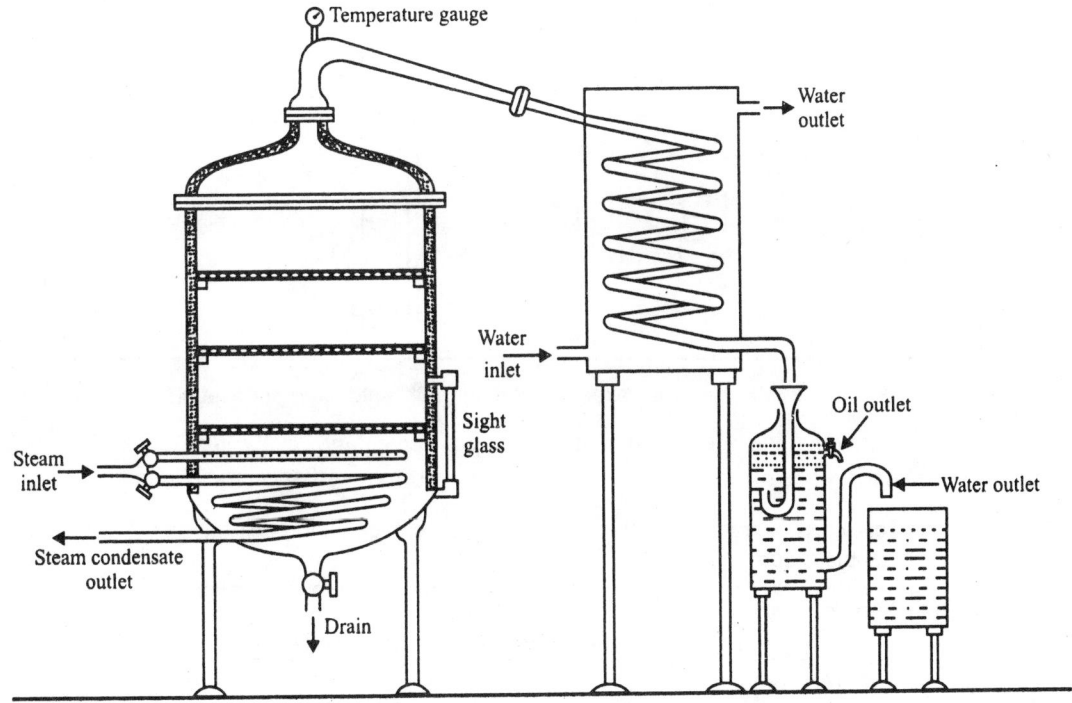

Fig. 5.21. Sketch of an experimental still.

Steam consumption in plant distillation

In the distillation of aromatic plants the distillate (condensed water and oil) usually contains much more water than if the isolated oil itself had been hydrodistilled.

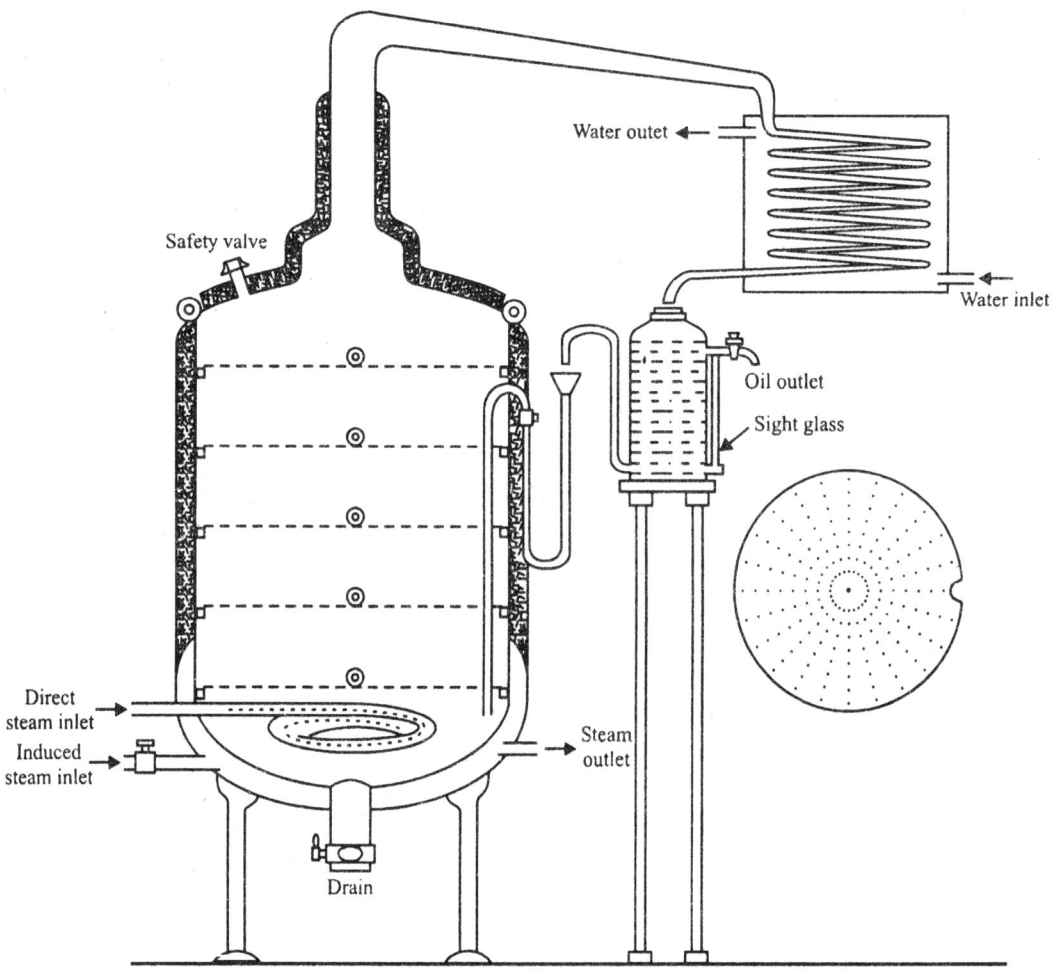

Fig. 5.22. Sketch of an experimental still with automatic cohobation.

Table 5.4 indicates the average oil content, by weight percentage, in the distillates of completed operations based upon years of experience with industrial distillation of aromatic plants:

Table 5.4. Average oil content, by weight percentage, in the distillates of complete operations.

Distillation of plant material; average content of volatile oil in the distillate plant material	% Oil
Ajowan seed	0.77
Angelica seed	0.19
Angelica root, fresh	0.03
Anise seed	0.81 to 1.16
Arnica flowers	0.001
Arnica root, dry	0.06

(Contd ...)

Distillation of plant material; average content of volatile oil in the distillate plant material	% Oil
Bay leaves	0.75 to 0.77
Calamus root, dry	0.23 to 0.24
Calamus root, fresh	0.12
Caraway seed	2.22 to 3.04
Cedar wood	0.97 to 1.41
Celery seed	0.17
Chamomile flowers, dry	0.004 to 0.007
Cinnamon Sri Lanka	0.31 to 0.34
Cloves	0.60 to 0.86
Clove stems	1.03 to 1.52
Coriander seed	0.56 to 0.57
Costus root, dry	0.01
Cubebs	1.2
Cypress	0.12 to 0.2
Elecampane root	0.05
Fennel seed	1.42 to 2.08
Galangal root	0.05 to 0.08
Ginger root	0.28
Juniper berries	0.20
Lovage root, dry	0.05
Lovage root, fresh	0.02
Lovage herb, fresh	0.02
Patchouli leaves	0.12 to 0.13
Peppermint herb, fresh	0.11
Pimenta berries	0.18
Sandalwood, East Indian	0.05 to 0.16
Sandalwood, West Indian	0.23 to 0.34
Savin	0.25 to 0.31
Vetiver root	0.015 to 0.02

Let us now compare these data with those expressing the composition of the condensate resulting from hydrodistillation of some of the pure chemical compounds which occur in volatile oils.

Hydrodistillation of	Content in the distillate (%)	Occurs in
Styrene	57.0	Cinnamon oil
p-Cymene	45.7	Ajowan oil
Pinene	55.6	Ajowan oil
Limonene	40.0	Caraway oil
Dipentene	40.0	Ajowan oil
Linaloöl	18.2	Coriander oil

Menthol	12.0	Peppermint oil
Carvone	9.7	Caraway oil
Anethole	7.1	Anise, fennel and star anise oil
Cinnamaldehyde	3.0	Cinnamon and cassia oil
Eugenol	1.7	Clove, clove stem, pimenta, bay and cinnamon oil
Santalol	0.5	East Indian sandalwood oil

What are the causes of the marked increase in steam consumption during distillation of plant material, as compared with steam consumption during hydrodistillation of essential oils *per se*? Smith found that, in the case of caraway seed distillation, the condensate contains only 2.22 to 3.04 per cent oil, whereas in the case of caraway oil distillation the condensate contains 8.80 to 10.11 per cent of oil. This obviously implies a much greater consumption of steam, in the first case, for the same quantity of oil and longer hours of distillation.

The paucity of oil in the distillation of plant material, is caused by several factors:

1. Many aromatic plants contain a quantity of oil insufficient to saturate the relatively large quantities of steam blowing rapidly through the plant charge. On the other hand, it is not advisable to reduce the speed (rate) of distillation below a certain limit. A high steam velocity causes pressure differentials within the still, which prevent the steam from stagnating in the more densely packed parts of the plant filling. For this reason and in order to increase the efficiency of a still, the operator is always tempted to inject into the still much more steam than is actually required. This results in a large volume of distillation water.

   Example: Let us suppose that a charge of 2000 kg of plant material can be exhausted in 11 hours, if we inject 250 kg/hr steam (250 kg distillation water in 1 hour). If, instead, we inject twice the amount of steam, i.e. 500 kg/hr, the length of distillation will be shortened at best by one-third and in most cases only by one-fourth; but not by one-half, as might be expected.

2. In the course of distillation the oil content of the plant charge decreases gradually and the vapourisation of oil is not stopped abruptly toward the end of the operation. This does not even take place in hydrodistillation of volatile oils *per se* and much less with plant material. Plainly, such a prolongation of the distillation greatly increases the steam consumption and depends also upon the individual operator.

3. While retained in the plant material, the volatile oil may be subjected also to forces of adhesion; this seems true even if small quantities of oil are distributed over large surfaces of comminuted plant particles.

4. The volatile oil is enclosed within the plant tissue and cut off from direct contact with steam by several layers of membrane, often very tough. For this reason most plant materials must be comminuted prior to distillation. Where steam distillation is practiced, this process of comminuting (grinding, pounding, milling, crushing, rasping) should not be carried too far (certainly not to the point of reducing the material to the size of flour particles), because the interspaces within the plant charge would then become too small. The rising steam must have sufficient space to penetrate all parts of the charge uniformly. Very small interspaces necessitate a slow, ineffective distillation, because any increase in pressure would cause the steam to break channels ('rat holes') through the plant charge or to hurl parts into the gooseneck and condenser. In other words, too finely powdered material is not penetrated evenly by steam and cannot be completely exhausted by steam distillation.

If, on the other hand, the plant material is not powdered, but granulated, only a portion of the oil is freed and another portion remains enclosed within the oil glands in the plant tissue. When crushing plant material, such as seed, a portion of the freed volatile oil will be covered again by crushed plant particles. The distillation of excessively crushed seed material, if not properly conducted, may, therefore, require longer hours than that of torn or slightly milled seed, provided the quantity of injected steam is the same.

If the plant material is distilled in uncomminuted condition — as with herbs and leaves and most flowers — the oil remains enclosed within the plant tissue. Hacking with an axe or machete or cutting in a hay cutter offers an advantage only in that the material can be packed into the still more uniformly; the steam then penetrates the charge more evenly, but very few oil glands will actually be broken up. Since the steam can vapourise only those volatile substances which it touches directly and will not affect the oil enclosed within the plant tissue, the oil must first be dissolved by hot (liquid) water and carried, by diffusion, through the swollen cell walls toward the outside. Hydrodiffusion, however, requires much more time than vapourisation, which takes place almost immediately, because all the enclosed volatile oil must be brought to the surface and that is a slow process. This fact is primarily responsible for the paucity of oil in the condensate and for the relatively long duration of distillation in the case of uncomminuted leaves and herbs possessing a tough fibre.

5. If the plant material is comminuted prior to distillation, very high boiling or practically nonvolatile substances, such as resins, paraffins, waxes, fatty oils (contained in other cells or glands), mix with and dissolve in the freed volatile oil, thereby substantially lowering its vapour pressure and reducing its rate of vapourisation. This occurs particularly in the case of seeds, most of which contain large quantities of fatty oils. The following content of fat and fatty oil (ether extract) in seeds from which the volatile oil had first been removed by steam distillation:

Seeds	Fatty oil (%)
Ajowan	33.20
Anise	18.59
Caraway	16.06
Celery	31.32
Coriander	26.40
Fennel	16.71

Assuming that air-dried caraway seed, such as is used for distillation, contains about 15 per cent moisture and 5.5 per cent volatile oil, we arrive at a ratio of 5.5 per cent volatile oil to 12.8 per cent of fatty oil in the seed. For practical distillation, this implies that 5.5 per cent volatile oil must be vapourised from 12.8 parts of fatty, nonvolatile oil. In other words, it is necessary to distil a mixture of fatty oil and volatile oil, which holds 30 per cent of volatile substances in solution. Assuming a content of 5.0 per cent volatile oil in fennel seed, 3.0 per cent of volatile oil in anise seed, 3.5 per cent in ajowan seed, 2.5 per cent in celery seed and 1.0 per cent in coriander seed, we find that we would have to distil:

Ajowan oil mixture containing	11.5% volatile oil*
Anise oil mixture containing	16.0% volatile oil
Caraway oil mixture containing	30.0% volatile oil
Celery oil mixture containing	9.7% volatile oil
Coriander oil mixture containing	4.2% volatile oil
Fennel oil mixture containing	27% volatile oil

*In all cases a 15 per cent moisture content of the seed is assumed.

Such relatively large quantities of fatty, nonvolatile oils are well capable of reducing the vapour pressure and thereby the rate of vapourisation of the volatile oils dissolved in these fatty oils.

Other reasons aside, it is thus practically impossible, when distilling seed with steam or boiling water, to saturate the steam completely with oil vapours, even when packing the plant charge very high in the still. The oil vapour phase in this mixture will always remain unsaturated; the more the content of fat in the seed exceeds that of volatile oil, the less the steam will be saturated with volatile oil vapours. This theoretical consideration confirms practical experience in the case of seed distillation. In actual practice, therefore, distillation of seed material can seldom if ever be completed, because the fatty oil tends to retain small quantities of volatile oil. It becomes necessary, therefore, to halt distillation, since the small recovery of oil no longer warrants the increasing consumption of steam and labour.

6. The steam consumption is influenced further by the moisture content of the plant material, particularly in the case of herbs; grasses and roots, which are processed either in the fresh succulent or semidry or dry, condition. When distilling peppermint herbs with live steam, for instance, the following quantities of steam will be consumed, the steam consumption being measured by the quantity of distillation water in the condensate:

   Fresh herb requires 250 to 350 kg of steam per kilogram of oil.
   Semidried herb requires 60 to 80 kg of steam per kilogram of oil.
   Air-dried herb requires 30 to 40 kg of steam per kilogram of oil.

These figures, are evidently relative, as actual steam consumption depends upon the type of the still, the quality of the steam, the way of packing and the experience of the operator.

Because of its high moisture content, fresh peppermint herb, when distilled, has a tendency to lump (agglutinate) and to prevent a uniform penetration by the steam. The volatile oil is, therefore, released from the fresh herb only very slowly.

Taking the above figures of steam consumption as a basis, the steam/oil vapour mixture (in other words, the condensate) will contain the following quantities of volatile oil:

Fresh herb	0.3 to 0.4% peppermint oil
Semidried herb	1.2 to 1.6% peppermint oil
Air-dried herb	2.5 to 3.0% peppermint oil

The oil content in the condensate is not uniform from the beginning to the end of distillation, but amounts in the beginning to a multiple of the average oil content. In the case of air-dried peppermint herb, the condensate contains in the beginning about 8 per cent of oil, which decreases gradually toward the end until it amounts to only 0.004 per cent. For practical reasons distillation should then be stopped. As mentioned previously, certain plants contain volatile oils, the most valuable parts of which are very high boiling. When applying saturated steam of atmospheric pressure only, distillation must then be continued for very long periods, although only small quantities of oil are recovered toward the end. If this is not done the high boiling constituents are lacking in the oil and the oil is of inferior quality. In such cases it will be advantageous to speed up and complete the operation by injecting slightly superheated steam toward the end.

Rate of distillation

The ratio between quantity of distillation (condensed) water and time (in other words, the quantity of water distilled over per hour) may be designated as rate (force or speed) of distillation. It must be regulated according to the diameter of the still and the size of the interspaces within the plant charge (degree of comminution). If the velocity of the rising steam is too low, the steam will stagnate in the denser portions of the charge and complete exhaustion by distillation will be impossible. If, on the other hand, the velocity is too high, the steam may break through the charge, form steam channels ('rat holes') and even hurl plant particles into the condenser, partly clogging it. By collecting the distillation water running off the condenser from time to time and over a period of some minutes and then weighing it, the rate of distillation can be controlled. For practical purposes the volatile oil may be ignored. The quantity of distillation water collected during these few minutes is calculated in terms of kilogram/hr per sq. m. (See example below.) This figure is then compared with the optimum rate of distillation, as established by trial distillation or by experience with the plant material in question (and taking into consideration its degree of comminution). The steam velocity in the actual operation may be regulated accordingly.

Example

If we obtain in one minute 8 kg of distillation water and if the smallest area covered by the charge on the perforated grid in a cylindrical still is 1.2 sq. m., the rate of distillation will be:

$$\frac{8 \times 60}{1.2} = 400 \text{ kg/hr per sq. m.}$$

Once the average oil content of the mixed vapours (steam plus oil vapours) has been established for a certain type of plant material and a certain degree of comminution and once the most favourable rate of distillation is known, the amount of steam necessary for complete exhaustion of a plant charge can be calculated and the steam supply adjusted accordingly. By weighing the quantity of distillation water from time to time, by converting the figures to the total length of distillation and by relating this to the quantity of oil expected the operation may thus be regulated according to optimum conditions. Let us suppose, for example, that 1000 kg of coriander seed must be distilled and that the seed, according to assay, contains 0.8 per cent of oil, in other words that the 1000 kg of coriander seed contain 8 kg of oil. We know from experience or from trial distillations that the average oil content of the vapour mixture (condensate) in the case of coriander seed distillation is 0.5 per cent. Therefore, 1600 kg of steam are required to distil over 8 kg of coriander seed oil. If we work with a distillation rate of 200 kg/hr, i.e. 200 kg distillation water per hour, the charge should be exhausted in 8 hours. In order to shorten the time of distillation, the rate of distillation must be increased. However, in this case attention must be paid to the fact that, on increasing the speed of distillation, the average oil content of the vapour mixture decreases to a certain extent, because the quicker the steam penetrates the plant charge the less it has occasion to become saturated with oil vapours. In other words, much more steam will be consumed than is calculated theoretically.

Pressure differential within the still

The velocity of steam flow is caused by differences in pressure. In the case of plant distillation with live steam, which in the boiler is usually at a pressure above atmospheric, the plant charge in the retort prevents the injected steam from expanding immediately and completely. For this reason, the steam pressure cannot fall immediately to the level of the atmospheric pressure. Thus, there arises a certain excess pressure beneath the charge in the retort; but a gradual equalisation with the atmospheric pressure takes place toward the top of the still. The degree of this excess pressure is a function of the force (speed) of distillation and of the interspaces within the plant charge. According to the height of the charge or the number of layers, this excess pressure can be increased by 0.3 atmospheres and, in some cases, even more. But if the pressure exceeds a certain limit (which depends upon the type and height of the plant charge), the steam forms fine, often scarcely visible channels through a powdered charge, whereas coarser masses are torn apart or even hurled into the gooseneck of the still. An excess pressure ('back pressure') within the retort may be caused also by a gooseneck or condenser pipes too narrow for the volume of steam injected into the still or by sharp bends in the pipes. Irregular heating of the boiler and variations in the steam consumption (such as are occasioned by the turning on and turning off of neighbouring stills) may cause the pressure in a steam generator to undergo continuous fluctuations. High-pressure steam has a tendency to blow into a still somewhat jerkily, giving rise to pressure variations even within the retort. Such fluctuations, however, are by no means harmful; on the contrary, they may exert a beneficial influence, as far as the yield of oil is concerned, by forcing the injected steam to loosen and penetrate the more densely packed portions of the plant charge, where the steam would otherwise stagnate.

Pressure differential inside and outside of the oil glands

As it rises through the plant charge, the steam at first vapourises all the freed volatile oil which by comminution of the plant material is within reach of the passing steam. Saturated steam (not superheated!) will at the same time condense a certain quantity of water within the retort. Consequently, the temperature of high pressure steam will be reduced to that of saturated steam, in other words, to the boiling point of the water/oil mixture. It must be remembered that this boiling point is slightly lower than that of the saturated steam. As the volatile oil vapourises from the plant material, the temperature of the steam rises again to that of pure saturated steam, at the pressure prevailing in the charge. If the plant charge is somewhat tightly packed, the temperature of the steam will show a certain range from the bottom to the top of the charge. This differential in temperature depends upon the force of distillation and the drop in the steam pressure from the lower to the upper section of the retort; in other words, the lowest part of the charge will have the highest and the upper part the lowest, temperature. Gradually the temperature of the steam equalises itself throughout the charge and, despite poor heat conduction, will prevail, even inside of all plant particles. As has been said, the boiling point of a water/oil mixture is somewhat lower than that of steam alone, the total vapour pressure a little higher. Since the temperature inside and outside of the plant particles has become equalised, a certain excess pressure will develop within those oil glands which still contain volatile oil and water enclosed. This pressure differential inside and outside of the oil glands probably has some influence upon the vapourisation of the volatile oil through the cell walls. A sufficiently large pressure differential may well cause some cell membranes to burst (provided they are not too thick and strong) or at least to expand the cell walls, to enlarge the pores and to loosen agglomerated particles of the charge, thus opening new passages for the steam. The more the pressure differential is reduced, the more it loses its significance as a loosening agent; but it remains important for the isolation of oil, in so far as it supports the forces of hydrodiffusion. The pressure differential inside and outside of the oil glands is more effective when first heating the retort and toward the end of distillation, provided temperature and pressure fluctuations actually occur inside of the still. A pressure differential, however, can be created only if water is present in liquid form or by partial condensation of steam when first heating the retort: the water thus formed will penetrate the plant tissue and seep also into the oil glands.

In the hydrodistillation of plant material at reduced pressure, the pressure differential inside and outside of the oil glands exerts itself to a marked degree only with low boiling substances. In the case of distillation above atmospheric pressure, however, the pressure differential assumes considerable importance.

Effect of moisture and heat upon the plant tissue

Any plant material serving for distillation contains a certain quantity of moisture, even air-dried material retaining 10 to 20 per cent of water. If saturated steam of atmospheric pressure is injected into the plant charge, condensation of steam will take place until the temperature of the still content has risen to that of the steam. Heat in conjunction with moisture soon causes the plant tissues to swell, the cells and pores to enlarge and the total volume to expand. Completely swollen seed material, for example, may have expanded by one fourth of its original volume. In actual distillation, this loosening of the plant material may, however, be partly counteracted by the weight and pressure of the softened plant charge.

An actual bursting of the plant membranes by the action of steam takes place probably to a limited extent only. The hot steam undoubtedly exerts a certain preparatory effect important for the vapourisation of the enclosed volatile oil, but the action of steam *per se* is not sufficient to liberate that part of the oil which remains protected by resistant cell membranes.

Influence of the distillation method on the quality of the volatile oils

The quality, as well as the physico-chemical properties, of a volatile oil are greatly influenced by the condition of the plant material (age, dried or fresh) and by the way distillation is carried out. Many factors enter the picture, viz. the method of distillation (water distillation, water and steam distillation and steam distillation), the degree of comminution of the plant material, the quantity of the plant charge, the length of distillation, the pressure applied, the quality of the steam; the treatment of the distillation waters, whether the oil of cohobation is added to the main oil or not, etc.

The effects of water distillation and steam distillation differ considerably, in that high boiling constituents of the volatile oil are recovered only incompletely in the case of water distillation, if the plant material is insufficiently comminuted. Even leaf material yields volatile compounds of high boiling point only incompletely by water distillation. It has been reported that patchouli leaves yielded 3.27 per cent of volatile oil on steam distillation and only 2.98 per cent on water distillation. The latter oil contained only a small quantity of the high boiling constituents, which incidentally possess also a high specific gravity and a high odour and fixation value. Oil constituents which are slightly soluble in water, phenols and certain alcohols and acids for example, are retained in the water, with the result that water distillation and steam distillation yield different types of oil if the plant material contains only small quantities of oil.

General difficulties in distillation

Essential oils consist of volatile compounds which are more or less sensitive to the influence of heat. It is doubtful, therefore, that all the volatile constituents present in the living plants can be isolated as such by distillation. In addition, distillation of certain plant materials is connected with difficulties of hydrodiffusion. The oil in part resinifies and in part remains in the plant tissue. Hence every type of plant material requires a particular method of distillation.

Because of these difficulties and because of the high cost of distillation in certain cases (through excessive steam and fuel consumption), it has been suggested that such materials be extracted with volatile solvents and the concentrated extracts steam distilled. The oils obtained usually contain small quantities of resinous and waxy matter; such oils may be soluble in a certain volume of dilute alcohol, but the solutions often become turbid when more of the dilute alcohol is added.

Hydrodistillation of Plant Material at High and at Reduced Pressure and with Superheated Steam

Steam distillation of plant material at high pressure

Certain plant materials—orris root, sandalwood, cloves, caraway seed, pine needles, for example—are occasionally distilled with steam of a pressure higher than atmospheric, in order to obtain a more favourable ratio of oil water in the distillate, i.e. to shorten the length of distillation and to increase the total yield of oil. Purely physical considerations, a discussion of which would lead too far, show that a substantial gain can be achieved only with a pressure of several atmospheres within the retort. This, however, usually causes such profound decomposition of the plant material and of the volatile oil that the method cannot generally be applied in practice.

The actual pressure within the retort, when using high pressure steam of four atmospheres as measured in the steam boiler, is certainly less than one atmosphere above normal atmospheric pressure. If, notwithstanding, such modest excess pressure leads to favourable results — primarily to a shortening of the distillation process — the explanation must be sought in other, perhaps purely mechanical factors. If the steam were throttled by a valve in the gooseneck and the pressure thus increased, a manometer would indicate continuous pressure fluctuations within the still. These fluctuations prevent the steam from stagnating in the too densely packed portions of the plant charge and seem to loosen all parts of the charge. This is particularly true of direct steam distillation and, to a certain extent, also of water and steam distillation, if the plant material has been packed high and not sufficiently uniformly or tightly. Water distillation, on the other hand, does not seem to be affected by excess pressure. The effect of high pressure appears to be more pronounced when the plant material has been charged improperly into the still and when a less efficient distillation, at atmospheric pressure, has been carried out previously.

The use of high-pressure steam for the rectification of volatile oils *per se* is not advisable, nor is it necessary, because for this purpose superheated steam gives better results. Nor should it be made a general practice to distil plant material with high-pressure steam, as this will increase the quantity of decomposition products in the plant material and in the oil, the degree of decomposition being influenced by the height of the pressure applied, the resulting rise of the temperature and the length of distillation. Ordinary steam distillation, even at atmospheric pressure, affects some of the constituents of the essential oil and of the plant material itself (the latter being even more sensitive to high pressure steam than the oils). The nonvolatile plant matter may thus undergo more or less profound decomposition, with accompanying formation of undesirable volatile substances, which may considerably impair the colour and odour of the oil. The distillate may become so much contaminated with foreign matter that even rectification no longer yields a normal oil. For all these reasons distillation with high pressure steam is not recommended, if the operation aims at obtaining a volatile oil containing delicate constituents. It may, however, be advantageous in some cases, where the distillate is to be further processed — as with oil of camphor and steam distilled pine (stump) oil.

Water distillation of plant material at high pressure

It is not advisable to employ this method, because the resulting higher temperature gives rise to decomposition products which impart a disagreeable 'burnt' odour to the oil. Neither there is any appreciable gain in the ratio of oil to water in the distillate, except perhaps in cases, where previous distillation under atmospheric pressure has been carried out inefficiently.

Steam distillation of plant material at reduced pressure

This method may be subdivided into two types, viz. (i) steam distillation at slightly reduced pressure, and (ii) vacuum steam distillation at such a low pressure that the temperature remains just enough above that of the cooling water to permit sufficient condensation of the steam/oil vapours.

1. It is a known fact that a pressure reduction within the still often shortens the length of distillation. Even a slight reduction may shorten the duration to only one-half the time required for steam

distilling at atmospheric pressure. It has been found that this effect is caused by fluctuations in the steam/oil vapour pressure which, as in the case of distillation at high pressure, exert a continuous loosening effect upon the plant charge.

2. The principal advantage of steam distillation of plant material *in vacuo* consists in the pure odour of the volatile oil thereby obtained. It will be free from any off-odour caused by decomposition, which accompanies most oils distilled above 70°C.

If the hydrodistillation *in vacuo* is not carried out with steam generated by boiling the water within the still (water distillation or water and steam distillation) but by steam generated in a separate steam boiler, a distillation with superheated steam at reduced pressure will result. Even high boiling constituents of the volatile oil will then readily distil over; a previously air-dried plant charge, under these circumstances, may, however, gradually dry out until the volatile oil enclosed within the oil glands can no longer be vapourised, because the forces of hydrodiffusion no longer play their important role. It will then become necessary to apply saturated steam at atmospheric pressure, so that steam condensation within the plant charge again forms (liquid) water, which will permit the forces of hydrodiffusion to act anew.

When hydrodistilling at reduced pressure it is preferable to employ spiral condensers rather than tubular ones, because the former can be tightened better. The surface of condensation should be about five times larger than when distilling at atmospheric pressure. This increase is necessary for several reasons: (i) The differential in the temperature of steam and cooling water is much smaller at reduced pressure. The rate of condensation, therefore, decreases; and (ii) The volume of a given quantity (weight) of steam is much larger at reduced, than at atmospheric, pressure. For instance the volume of 1 kg of steam at the following pressures is:

Millimetre pressure	Cubic metres
760	1.650
380	3.150
150	7.650
76	14.530

The velocity at which the steam enters the condenser will affect the transfer of heat to the cooling surface. Therefore, depending on other variables, an appropriately designed condenser (as to type, length, etc.) will have to be employed. Too long a condenser being impractical, several spiral condensers connected with a T tube may be installed side by side. Since an efficient vacuum pump creates a higher vacuum than is actually required for the distillation of plant material, the pressure within the still should be regulated by a valve permitting enough air to enter the still to sustain the desired pressure. The pressure should be measured by two manometers, one reaching into the receiver and one directly into the retort.

Steam distillation of plant material *in vacuo* is limited in application by the fact that cooling and condensation of the vapours become increasingly difficult as the pressure and temperature of distillation are lowered. The general application of hydrodistillation *in vacuo* to plant material is restricted by another factor. With lowered pressure in the still, the partial pressure of the oil vapours decreases relatively more than that of the water vapours (steam); hence, the ratio of the volatile oil in the distillate is smaller than when distilling at atmospheric pressure. In other words, more steam will be consumed when, hydrodistilling a certain quantity of oil *in vacuo* than the atmospheric pressure. This lower rate of vapourisation of the volatile oil particularly pronounced in the case of water distillation of plant material containing high boiling and partly water soluble constituents. In this case, a multiple volume of steam (as compared with distillation at atmospheric pressure) is often required to attain the same yield of oil. Any increased steam consumption also results in higher working cost, since much more distillation water must be redistilled or extracted.

When processing of plant material by water and steam distillation is practiced at reduced pressure, variations in the still may cause loosening of the plant charge, so the rising steam is better saturated with oil vapours. This factor occasionally results in a lower consumption of steam than when working at atmospheric pressure. The most suitable method of distilling plant material at reduced pressure is with water and steam, provided the nature of the plant material permits its application. In general, it can be said that steam distillation of aromatic plants, under reduced pressure, remains very limited in practice.

Water distillation of plant material at reduced pressure

According to established thermodynamic principles and to the explanation given in the preceding pages, hydrodistillation at reduced pressure has the effect that, with equal quantities of condensate, the steam volume in the distilling space and therefore the steam velocity, will increase enormously as the pressure in the still is reduced. For example, a given quantity (weight) of totally saturated steam and benzaldehyde vapour fills a certain volume at atmospheric pressure (760 mm); at 76 mm. pressure the volume will be approximately ten times larger, at 31 mm approximately twenty-four times larger than that occupied under atmospheric pressure. The velocity under which the vapour mixture rushes through the condenser increases in the same ratio. Hence water distillation of plants at reduced pressure is connected with certain inconveniences with which the operator should be familiar.

Any increase in the speed of distillation affects the purity of the distillate because minute plant particles are carried over mechanically. As a precaution against this, speed must be moderated as much as possible; flat, wide, rather than tall, stills should be selected for this purpose. It should also be borne in mind that the steam is to some extent throttled in the gooseneck (the narrowest part of the still). This may result in a slight back pressure within the retort, relative to the pressure in the receiver, which differential might easily amount to 10 mm.

It is, therefore, advisable to adjust the speed of distillation to the temperature prevailing within the retort. This will prevent a rise in the distillation temperature above a desired point.

The great advantage of water distillation of plant material at reduced pressure lies in the fact that it can be carried out at relatively low temperatures, e.g. at 50°C—which reduces decomposition of the essential oil. It is not advisable to operate at lower temperatures, because the oil vapours can then no longer be sufficiently condensed and considerable losses of oil might occur. Furthermore, higher boiling, slightly water-soluble compounds are retained partially in the plant material and in the water and the oil will be deficient in these constituents. This phenomenon, already discussed under water distillation of plants at atmospheric pressure, is even more pronounced in its effects when reduced pressure is employed. This very factor limits the application of water distillation *in vacuo* to only a few plant materials.

Temperatures of only 30° to 50°C and the presence of water offer favourable conditions for fermentation of the plant material, for which reason distillation of this type should not last longer than a few hours. The oils obtained by this method will never possess a 'still' or 'burnt' odour, but rather a slight 'fermented' one.

Superheated vapours

As was pointed out in the theoretical part of this chapter, a vapour is saturated so long as it remains in contact with the liquid from which it originates. Saturated vapours possess characteristic properties by which they differ sharply from vapours separated from their liquid sources. The slightest cooling of a saturated vapour causes partial condensation, the slightest heating results in increased vapourisation. So long as it remains in contact with its liquid, a saturated vapour is seldom absolutely dry; usually it contains admixed particles of the liquid in the form of spray. Moderate vapourising, even evaporating of the liquid phase, carries microscopically small droplets upward into the vapour space. Vigorous boiling ejects larger quantities from the turbulent liquid; these are kept suspended by the flow of vapours or they drop back into the boiling liquid, to be replaced by new ones. Very wet vapours are more or less hazy. The transparency of a vapour, however, merely proves that it does not contain larger quantities of the liquid phase; it does not prove that the vapour is absolutely free of liquid, since minute droplets floating in the clear vapours are invisible to the eye. Their actual presence in the vapours is proved by the fact that the condensate of plant materials or of volatile oils is usually contaminated with dust or with nonvolatile coloured substances.

Let us assume that we continue to heat and vapourise a liquid at constant external pressure to the point where the last molecule of the liquid phase is transformed into vapour. At this very moment the vapours are still saturated, dry saturated. Further heating no longer induces the formation of vapours, it only increases the temperature of the formed vapours, with a resulting expansion of their volume. The vapours then become superheated. Thus, superheated vapours possess a higher temperature, a larger volume and a lower density than saturated vapours at the same pressure. Superheating of a vapour may also be interpreted as a heating beyond the point of saturation. Saturated vapours, as compared with superheated vapours at the same pressure, therefore, contain a maximum of mass, as well as the highest specific gravity and the lowest specific volume (the specific volume being the reciprocal value of the specific gravity). When comparing the two types of vapours at the same temperature, superheated vapours possess a lower pressure than saturated vapours.

A saturated vapour exerts the maximum pressure at the given temperature. Cooling merely lowers the temperature of superheated vapours, without causing condensation (as would be the case with saturated vapours). Only by further cooling, to and below the point of saturation, will a portion of the vapour be condensed. The moment a superheated vapour is brought into contact with the liquid phase from which it originated, vapourising will take place, until the saturation point is reached once more. The superheated vapour thus passes into a saturated vapour.

Distillation of plant material with superheated steam

Relative to its weight, superheated steam can vapourise and entrain more volatile substances than saturated steam. In practice, steam may be superheated by passing it through fire tubes in a boiler—in other words, through a superheater. This superheated steam, mixed with high-pressure and saturated steam, is then injected into the any oil remaining within the plant tissue can no longer reach the outside by hydrodiffusion, as there is no longer any water present or available; distillation will therefore be incomplete and the yield of oil subnormal, unless saturated steam of low pressure is injected after the application of high-pressure or superheated steam.

There are a few cases in which distillation with superheated steam becomes advantageous, e.g. with plants that contain much moisture (60 to 80 per cent) and are difficult to dry. If such material is distilled with low-pressure saturated steam, the high moisture content of the charge will cause much steam condensation: the plant charge lumps and is difficult to exhaust. This can be prevented by applying superheated steam, a smaller or larger portion of the water within the plant charge then vapourising while hydrodiffusion still functions.

In general, it can be said that plant material containing low boiling essential oils is preferably distilled with low-pressure steam, whereas high-temperature steam recommends itself for the distillation of high boiling oils.

Field Distillation of Plant Material

In primitive countries, where aromatic plants grow wild or are cultivated by natives as patch crops, essential oils are obtained by a form of distillation which may most appropriately be termed field distillation. Lack of roads prevents transport of the plant material to centrally located larger distilleries and the distillation equipment has to follow the plant material into the interior of the growing region. Small portable or movable stills must be used; but they serve only for a certain time of the year and remain unused for the remainder of the time. They must, therefore, be low priced, sturdy, simple, easy to transport and to install in the fields and simple to operate. In many cases this type of distillation is old; it has developed along purely empirical lines as an 'art' inherited through generations. One should not summarily condemn this industry as antiquated and too primitive, however, because, in many instances and in view of the circumstances, a change to more modern and more expensive equipment is difficult, if not impossible. Indeed, such a change in some cases, might be for the worse, so far as prices of the oils, particularly, are concerned. On the other hand, this method of operation is frequently faulty, although it could be improved readily by only a few slight modifications.

Distillation may be carried out either by heating the still with direct fire or by steam generated in a separate small steam boiler. The former is simply an example of water distillation or a water and steam distillation. Direct steam distillation, in this case, represents a stage in the transition to larger distilleries, because steam distillation is economical only if the steam generator is connected with several stills.

Despite the often primitive apparatus, the quality of oil resulting from water distillation in some instances has been good. However, the yield of oil in field distillation is often far below that obtained by water distillation on a large scale in more modern factories. The principal reason is probably that the small distillers do not always observe the fundamental rules of efficient water distillation, i.e. a small plant charge and a quick distillation. Most small operators are inclined to charge their retorts as high as possible in order to utilise them fully; furthermore, the speed of distillation is usually limited by too small a condenser. Also, in primitive operation the plant material is seldom comminuted, although a thorough comminution is the case of water distillation is often of prime importance for a normal yield of oil.

The following cases of actual distillation in the field will prove to what degree the yield, as well as the quality, of an essential oil depends upon the method of distillation. They also show that in many countries production of essential oils remains utterly primitive and that the introduction of better methods would result in a considerable improvement in the yield and quality of the oils.

Distillation of lavender in France

Years ago lavender oil used to be produced in Southern France in numerous small distillation posts, distributed throughout the growing regions of the Départements Basses-Alpes, Drome, Vaucluse, Alpes-Maritimes and Var. These posts consisted of old-fashioned direct fire stills holding about 60 kg of plants and 60 litres of water. An operation was completed after about 15 litres of distillation water had been collected. The action of the boiling water upon linalyl acetate, the main constituent of lavender oil, resulted in considerable hydrolysis of this ester and the lavender oils obtained by this method were relatively low in esters. The introduction of water and steam distillation, in which the plant material is packed on a perforated grid above the boiling water, resulted in a marked increase of the ester content. This effect was even more pronounced when Schimmel and Company showed by systematic experiments in their modern distillery in Barrême (B.A.) that oils containing 50 per cent and more of esters could be obtained by rapid distillation with direct steam.

Distillation of petitgrain oil in Paraguay

Similar conditions prevail in regard to the distillation of petitgrain oil in Paraguay. There, too, the leaf material is charged into primitive field stills and, during distillation, is partly submerged in boiling water. As a result, linalyl acetate, the main constituent of petitgrain oil, is partly hydrolysed. For this reason, principally, the bulk of Paraguay petitgrain oil has an ester content averaging from 43 to 54 per cent only, whereas experiments with direct steam distillation in modern stills have proved that oils containing up to 80 per cent ester can be produced without too much difficulty.

Distillation of linaloe wood in Mexico

The distillation of linaloe wood in Mexico furnishes proof that the yield and quality (physico-chemical properties and chemical composition) of an essential oil depend a great deal upon the method of distillation.

The trunks and branches of the felled trees are reduced to chips with axes and machetes. The chips are then charged into galvanised iron retorts 1.10 m wide and 2 m high. In past years water was added to the chips and distillation of each batch carried out for about 18 to 20 hours the heat being supplied by an open fire beneath the still. Distillation of linaloe wood in past years was thus a typical case of water distillation. The yield of oil then varied from only 0.6 to 1.0 per cent, seldom exceeding 2 per cent. This low yield was undoubtedly the result of insufficient reduction of the wood material and in general of water distillation which in this case should not be applied.

In order to prove this contention, a company imported Mexican linaloe logs to Europe and submitted the mechanically and properly comminuted material to direct steam distillation by modern methods. Yields ranging from 6.0 to 11.0 per cent of oil were obtained. The resulting oils differed considerably from the Mexican distilled oil. The latter contained more Linaloöl, the Schimmel oil more of the high boiling constituents. Evidently in Mexico the wood was not sufficiently comminuted, with the result that little oil was liberated from the oil glands. The old Mexican method of distillation seemed to depend primarily upon the forces of hydrodiffusion, which means that the more water-soluble oil constituents—such as linaloöl—were freed from the wood, while the water-insoluble compounds remained and partly resinified during the long hours of distillation.

On investigating the linaloe oil producing regions in Mexico it was observed that the method of distillation has been improved considerably. Today the stills are equipped with a perforated tin plate, 60 cm from the bottom of the still, the perforated plate supporting the chipped wood material. The section below the plate contains water which does not come in contact with the charge. Thus we have here a typical case of water and steam distillation, the water being heated with an open fire beneath the still. As a result of this method of distillation, the yield of oil today ranges from about 2.2 to 2.6 per cent for chips and from about 3.5 to 4.4 per cent of oil from sawdust. Each operation now requires 8 to 9 hours of distillation. Each charge consists of 230 kg of wood material. In the states of Puebla and Guerrero, it is customary to reduce the linaloe wood into chips, while the producers in the state of Colima reduce the wood into coarse saw dust and thereby obtain a considerably higher yield.

Distillation of cassia leaves and twigs in China

Large quantities of cassia oil are produced yearly in the south Chinese provinces of Kwangsi and Kwangtung. The stills used by the natives are of antiquated Chinese design. Their principal fault lies in the loose connection of the joining parts and in the insufficient condensers. A charge consists of about 60 kg of cassia leaves and twigs and approximately 180 litres of water, which is brought to a boil by an open fire beneath the retort. Distillation of one batch lasts about 2½ hours. The condensate is collected in a series of pots, arranged in the form of cascades. Cassia oil is heavier than water. The yield of oil from leaves alone averages 0.10 to 0.13 per cent and that from a mixture of 70 per cent leaves and 30 per cent twigs 0.15 to 0.17 per cent.

Because of insufficient cooling in the condenser, the distillate usually runs quite warm, if not hot and therefore a part of the oil remains emulsified or suspended in the water. The milky distillation water is added to the next batch of plant material, a procedure which entails a certain loss of oil by evaporation and particularly by resinification. The principal cause of the subnormal yield of oil lies in the use of water distillation in the case of cassia leaves or, more exactly, in the faulty method of carrying it out. Cassia leaves possess a leathery consistency, remaining tough even in boiling water and, therefore, if not sufficiently comminuted, cannot be completely exhausted by mere water distillation.

In order to study the problem by practical experiments, a Company imported dried cassia leaves and twigs from China and submitted them to distillation tests in modern direct steam stills. The leaves yielded 0.7 to 0.8 per cent of oil, the twigs 0.2 per cent. These percentages are much higher than those obtained by the native Chinese distillers. True, the plant material arriving in Europe had lost considerable weight from drying; the Chinese producers use fresher leaves and twigs. Assuming the loss of moisture through drying to be about 50 per cent of the original plant weight, the yields of oil, as calculated upon the fresh plant material would, therefore, be as follows:

Fresh leaves, distilled in Europe	0.35 to 0.40%
70% fresh leaves plus 30% fresh twigs, distilled in Europe	0.31 to 0.34%
Fresh leaves, distilled in China	0.10 to 0.13%
70% fresh leaves plus 30% fresh twigs, distilled in China	0.15 to 0.17%

This differential in yield is actually even greater, because as a result of the long transport and desiccation, a part of the cinnamic aldehyde, the main constituent of cassia oil, had been oxidised.

These experiments prove that the native distillation of cassia oil is carried out in such a primitive and faulty way that quantities of oil amounting to about twice the actual production per year are lost in the residual plant material. The use of water distillation is not the only cause of this waste. Another reason for the subnormal oil yield obtained by the Chinese distillers, appears to be this:

Because of insufficient condensation of the steam/oil vapours, distillation must be carried out very slowly. The motion of the plant charge in the boiling water is, therefore, correspondingly slow and the water between the agglutinating leaves cannot circulate sufficiently. The volatile oil, which diffuses from the leaves into the boiling water partly dissolves therein and remains, in part, suspended between the agglutinated leaves, without being vapourised by contacting steam bubbles. In other words, presence of the liberated, but not vapourised, oil inhibits further diffusion of oil from the leaves. Evidently, the forces of diffusion can come into play only where there exists a differential in concentration. In other words, the quicker the oil solution is removed from the surface of the leaves and the quicker the oil is vapourised, the more forcibly diffusion acts. Otherwise an equilibrium in the charge will result and the distillate will contain very little oil, in spite of the fact that considerable quantities of oil are still retained in the leaves. This also explains the relatively short length of distillation in the native cassia stills; the distillers simply stop the operation when they no longer see oil distilling over. It should not be surprising at all that the admixture of twigs to the leaves increases the oil yield, although the actual oil content of twigs amounts to only one-quarter that of the leaves. By the addition of twigs the charge simply becomes looser and the interspaces between the leaves larger. The boiling water, even though moving slowly, can then penetrate the interspaces much better and carry away the oil as it diffuses from the leaves; the oil is thus conducted toward the surface and vapourised.

Rectification and Fractionation of Essential Oils

Many essential oils, when distilled from the plant material, are contaminated with volatile products arising from the decomposition of complex plant substances, under the influence of hot water or steam. This takes place especially in the case of water distillation in directly fired stills if, through carelessness, the plant charge 'burns' on contact with the retort walls touched by the fire. 'Some of these decomposition products are gaseous, e.g. hydrogen sulphide and ammonia; others — such as methylalcohol, acetaldehyde, acetone and acetic acid — are very soluble in water. Therefore, they occur mainly in the distillation water and accumulate in the water oil when cohobating the distillation waters. For this reason the water oil usually possesses a rather disagreeable odour and should not be mixed with the main oil without previous careful purification.

Occasionally the main oil, too, contains as normal constituents substances of somewhat objectionable odour, e.g. certain aldehydes or sulphur compounds. In order to improve the odour of such oils they must be freed from these undesirable compounds by redistillation. This applies also to crude oils possessing too dark a colour, which is often due to the presence of metals or to fine plant dust carried over by the steam, especially when the live steam enters the still too forcefully or too rapidly. When the steam is injected more slowly, the plant charge becomes somewhat wet by steam condensation and the dust particles are retained by the plant material.

Redistillation of a volatile oil does not necessarily bring about an improvement in its quality; in fact, in some cases the contrary may be true. This is particularly so with oils possessing easily saponifiable esters, such as bergamot or lavender oil. Linalyl acetate, the main constituent of these oils, is hydrolised by boiling with water or by rectification with live steam, the freed acetic acid causing further hydrolysis.

For the redistillation of a volatile oil two general methods are employed, viz. rectification and fractionation, both of which will be described in more detail. Rectification aims at the separation of volatile and nonvolatile compounds if a lighter coloured oil is desired; the colouring matter remains as residue in the still. This may be achieved by dry distillation *in vacuo* or by hydrodistillation (with live steam or by boiling with water). Hydrodistillation can also be carried out at reduced pressure.

Fractionation of fractional distillation

It aims at separating the volatile oil into various fractions, according to their boiling points and odour. In most cases this is achieved by dry distillation *in vacuo*. A volatile oil should never be fractionated at atmospheric pressure, because the high temperatures involved cause decomposition and resinification, the distillate then possessing an odour and physico-chemical properties quite different from those of the original oil. The boiling temperature can be considerably lowered by distilling the volatile oil at greatly reduced pressure, a process also referred to as dry distillation *in vacuo*. Decomposition of the oil is thus reduced to a minimum.

Rectification of essential oils

Rectification with water vapours (steam) is the older of the two methods. Retorts employed for this purpose are usually spherical, made of copper, heavily lined with tin and heated with a steam jacket. To prevent colouring of the oil by contact with metal, the gooseneck and condenser should be made of pure tin or of heavily tinned copper. Condenser and oil separator should be installed at such a height that, if it seems desirable, the distillation water can return automatically into the retort during distillation. Water is poured into the retort to a level of about 4 or 5 inches above the steam jacket and the oil added. Some oils—peppermint and caraway seed oil, etc. easily assume a disagreeable by-odour when coming in contact with the hot still walls. This by-odour, known as 'still odour', may be partly avoided by covering the steam jacket or the steam coils with sufficient water before starting the operation. The water level must be retained throughout the distillation. Flat-bottomed steam jackets are, therefore, preferable for the rectification of volatile oils. A steam coil, provided with many small holes and inserted close to the bottom of the retort, serves for direct heating with live steam (if this modification is preferred) and also for steaming out (cleaning) the still after completion of the operation. Steaming out is usually preceded by a washing with hot water, soap or alkali solution or with volatile solvents.

The speed of rectification is influenced by several factors. If the distillation waters should return automatically into the retort, the speed might be limited by excess pressure developing within the retort; in fact, this might altogether prevent the distillation water from returning automatically into the retort. If the distillate should be absolutely colourless, rectification must be carried out very slowly; otherwise very fine droplets, often invisible in the vapours, are carried into the condenser and oil separator and colour the distillate.

As has been said, some crude volatile oils contain compounds of objectionable odour, which are often more soluble in water than the main constituents. This fact can be taken advantage of by rectifying the volatile oils through hydrodistillation: the distillation water containing most of these objectionable compounds is not returned to the retort, but the water distilling off must be replaced by fresh water; or, instead of heating indirectly, direct live steam may be injected into the oil charge. In the latter case only sufficient water to cover the steam coil need be charged into the retort. However, the danger of oil droplets being carried over mechanically becomes somewhat greater as the live steam entering the retort has a tendency to whirl the oil upward. A short rectification column may be of service in this respect. When rectifying a volatile oil with direct live steam at atmospheric pressure (in other words, with low-pressure steam), some steam will be condensed to water continuously within the retort. The distillation water, in this case, cannot be returned into the retort, but must be cohobated in another apparatus or extracted with volatile solvents. Actually, rectification of a volatile oil with direct steam of low pressure has all the characteristics of a water distillation, because steam continuously separates water as condensate within the retort. If, however, high-pressure live steam (10 atmospheres for instance) is injected into a well-insulated still, condensation of water may be prevented, provided the steam has been carefully dried prior to its entering the still. The distillation then becomes a superheated steam process, because saturated high-pressure steam, on expansion, changes into superheated steam. In other words, distillation of a volatile oil purely by live steam is not practicable. It turns either into a distillation with superheated steam or into a water distillation, the latter with the modification that there will be only a little water within the retort.

The quantity of oil to be charged into a rectifying still depends upon the final purpose of the rectification. If the oil is only to be decolourised, very little oil need be let into the retort, the vapourising oil being replaced continuously as new oil is pumped in. This method offers the advantage that the contact of oil and steam is shortened to a minimum, only a small quantity of oil being in the retort at one time. A prolonged contact of volatile oil with boiling water or steam at atmospheric pressure is likely to cause considerable decomposition, resinification and chemical action, such as hydrolysis of esters, etc.

As has been explained, rectification aims also at freeing the oil from disagreeable by-odours. If these impurities possess a low boiling point — in other words, if they boil below the main portion of the oil — they can be removed in the foreruns of the distillate. Foreruns are then separated so long as they exhibit the objectionable odour. Since a forerun usually amounts to only a small percentage of the total oil, it should be distilled off very slowly. The total amount of oil charged in the still, however, must always be so measured that it can be processed within one day. In order to utilise the capacity of a small still to the fullest, rectification is best carried out with direct live steam; otherwise a part of the retort must be occupied by the water necessary for distillation. After the forerun has distilled over, the speed or rate of distillation may be increased to whatever degree condenser capacity and purity of the distillate will permit.

If the volatile oil to be rectified contains impurities boiling higher than the main part of the oil, the main run should be distilled off slowly, as this will permit better separation and a diminution of the last runs. The speed of distillation may be increased when the last runs containing the impurities start to distil over. To achieve a more complete separation of the foreruns and last runs, a fractionation column may be used and, if necessary, a dephlegmator above the column. Such a dephlegmator causes partial condensation, which affects the higher boiling constituents more than the lower. It thus becomes possible to reduce the quantity of the forerun and to increase the quantity of the main run. As was explained under 'theories of distillation', rectification columns are equipped with perforated trays, often with Raschig rings or porcelain balls. Columns filled with rings or balls have a practical advantage over columns equipped with bell or sieve plates, in that the former retain less condensed liquid and therefore, exert less pressure upon the vapours in the still.

The composition of the condensate, i.e. the average oil content of the steam and vapour mixture, depends primarily upon the boiling point or the vapour pressure of the oil constituents. The lower the normal boiling point — in other words, the higher the vapour pressure of the oil constituents at the prevailing temperature of distillation — the greater will be the ratio of oil in the condensate. The average oil content of the steam and vapour mixture in the distillation of oil is much larger than it is in the distillation of plant material.

Fractionation of Essential Oils

We shall now proceed to a description of the fractionation, which is carried out at reduced pressure (partial vacuum) and usually by distilling the oil alone, without leading water into the retort or injecting live steam into the oil. This process of dry distillation *in vacuo* is widely applied in the essential oil industry today. By its means pressure can be so far lowered that temperature has no longer any marked influence upon quality. The pressure should not be higher than 5 to 10 mm Mercury (Hg) as measured in the still above the boiling liquid. How far the temperature of some oil constituents can be reduced is shown by this example: linaloöl, the main constituent of linaloe oil, boils at a temperature of 198°C at atmospheric pressure (760 mm.) and at:

$$105.4°C \text{ at } 30 \text{ mm pressure}$$
$$97.2°C \text{ at } 20 \text{ mm pressure}$$
$$84.4°C \text{ at } 10 \text{ mm pressure}$$
$$72.8°C \text{ at } 5 \text{ mm pressure}$$

In practice, any further lowering of the pressure requires that distillation be carried out very slowly; it also necessitates an efficient vacuum still, absolutely airtight joints and an effective condenser, so that the low boiling constituents of the volatile oil may be recovered and not lost in the vacuum pump. In the case of almost every vacuum distillation, small quantities of vapours escape into the pumps, especially if the vacuum still is not absolutely tight. The air leaking into the still has a tendency to carry along some volatile oil vapours that may not always be condensed in the condensers. It is advisable, therefore, to insert an absorption vessel, filled with neutral substance which absorbs the vapours, between the oil receiver and the vacuum pump.

In order to distil over the highest boiling oil constituents *in vacuo*, temperatures of 150° to 200°C are often necessary. Such temperatures can be obtained by the use of an oil bath which surrounds the lower part of the retort; in a corresponding steam jacket very high pressure or superheated steam would be required. The oil bath offers the advantage that the heat transmission between the two liquids is more gradual than that between superheated steam and volatile oil. Under these circumstances hydrocarbons possessing boiling points up to 300°C (at atmospheric pressure) can be distilled off, provided any condensation of oil vapours along the upper walls of the retort is prevented by good insulation.

Between the pressure in the receiver and that within the retort there exists always a differential of a few millimetres. If the pressure in the closed receiver is 1 to 2 mm, the pressure in the vacuum still itself (retort) will be about 5 mm, provided the vapour development remains moderate. The faster the distillation, the lower will be the performance of the vacuum pump; the narrower the condenser tubes, the greater will be this pressure differential.

The stills serving for vacuum distillation of volatile oils are spherical, sufficiently strong to withstand at least atmospheric pressure, made of copper and heavily tinned on the inside, with gooseneck, condenser tubes and oil receivers also tinned. A small and strong glass window permits watching of the boiling liquid within the retort. All joints must be absolutely airtight. A jacket around the lower half of the retort forms an oil bath or a steam bath for heating with high-pressure steam (for at least 75 lb. jacket working pressure). A column directly above the still, equipped with plates or filled with Raschig rings or with other packing materials, provides for better fractionation of the boiling liquid. The oil receiver consists of two closed, strong vessels with vertical glass tubes, through which the level of the liquid within each receiver can be gauged. These receivers are tightly connected with the condenser outlet through a three-way stopcock, which permits one receiver to remain *under vacuo* and to collect the fraction distilling over at a given temperature, while the other receiver may be opened to draw off the previous fraction. Pressure manometers on the retort and on the oil receivers indicate the pressure within the retort and within the oil receivers. One thermometer held by a nipple reaches within the retort and ends above the boiling liquid, whereas another thermometer registers the temperature on top of and inside of the fractionation column. An airtight suction line connects the receivers with the vacuum pump which should be of high efficiency. The still shown in Fig. 5.23 serves for the dry (without direct steam) vacuum distillation (fractionation or rectification) of essential oils. Heating is achieved by a steam jacket (or oil bath if so desired). The rectification column can be by-passed. Provision is also made for the rectification or fractionation of essential oils by the use of direct steam at atmospheric pressure. In this case, the distillation waters may be automatically returned to the still (cohobated). The same still may be used for the preparation of terpeneless oils.

Inadequacies of hydrodistillation

A comparative summary of the advantages and disadvantages associated with hydrodistillation of volatile oils and with dry distillation *in vacuo* would reveal, an almost general superiority of hydrodistillation over the latter method. Depending upon the nature of the compound to be vapourised, it is possible to adjust the temperature of hydrodistillation to any desired level.

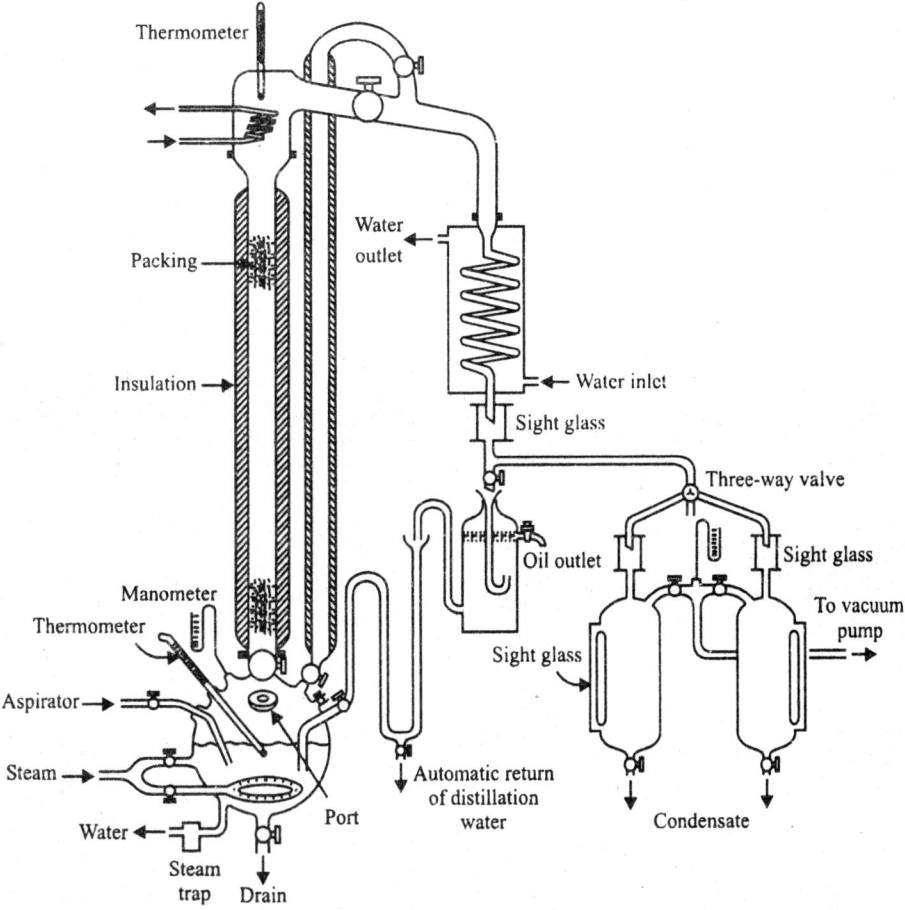

Fig. 5.23. Dual-purpose essential oil still.

The use of dry vacuum distillation remains limited, because high boiling compounds decompose below their boiling points, even *in vacuo*. Vacuum distillation with superheated steam is more advantageous in this respect. On the other hand, the use of hydrodistillation is restricted for several reasons:

1. As in the case of dry vacuum distillation, the compound to be vapourised should be distilled in liquid form or should at least melt below the temperature of distillation. However, solid compounds and even those with very high boiling points, can be vapourised by steam, provided they are reduced to a moderately small size. Comminuted particles should be properly packed on perforated grids within the retort, so that the rising steam penetrates the mass uniformly, just as with plant material.

2. Hydrodistillation cannot be applied to substances which, even at low temperatures, react with water or are hydrolysed by water (esters, etc.).

3. Solubility in water, as well as decomposition by water, may, under certain circumstances, present an insurmountable obstacle to the use of hydrodistillation. This is particularly so if the compound to be distilled is high boiling (aside from being water soluble) or, in the case of plant distillation, if the plant material contains only very small quantities of the water-soluble constituent. Solubility

in water lowers the vapour pressure of the compound and reduces its capability for vapourisation; in other words, relatively much more steam will be required to vapourise the same quantity of oil. Since this lowering of the vapour pressure depends upon the quantity of water present, water soluble and high boiling compounds or corresponding plant matter should be distilled with steam and not with boiling water. For instance, if it were practically possible to distil rose flowers with steam, the phenyl ethyl alcohol would probably not be retained by the flowers or by the residual still waters.

Solubility in water not only reduces the rate of evaporation, it also impedes the separation of the oil from the distillate. For this very reason the aroma of many flowers cannot be isolated by distillation. Any odouriferous compound is also volatile; any compound which, of itself, dissipates vapours into the air should yield the same, if not a larger quantity to steam and particularly at a temperature of distillation higher than that of the air. The difficulty is only that the small quantity of volatile substances cannot be isolated from the large volume of distillation waters.

Hydrodistillation of Essential Oils at High and at Reduced Pressure and with Superheated Steam

Water distillation of essential oils at reduced pressure

This type of distillation is used to prevent decomposition of the volatile oil, because by its use even easily hydrolysed esters are retained intact. With certain oils the method gives most favourable results.

On the other hand, it should be kept in mind that the rate of vapourisation of water-soluble and high boiling constituents decreases as their boiling point and degree of water solubility increase. Stated differently, in the water distillation of essential oils at reduced pressure, the ratio of oil to water in the distillate is even more unfavourable than when water distillation of the same products at atmospheric pressure is practiced, because any lowering in the external pressure reduces the vapour pressure of all high boiling compounds relatively much more than that of water (steam). Also, the differential between the temperature of distillation and that of the cooling water in this case is slight; therefore, considerable oil losses may be caused by evaporation, particularly when the temperature differential is still further reduced by any excessive and unnecessary lowering of the distillation pressure. The same conditions prevail here as with hydrodistillation of plant materials at reduced pressure.

To achieve a high rate of distillation when hydrodistilling volatile oils at reduced pressure, the empty space above the liquid in the vacuum still should be kept sufficiently large to permit the still content to boil without foaming into the condenser. In addition, the condenser surface must be larger (about five times larger than that required for distillation at atmospheric pressure). In the case of vacuum distillation, the efficiency of the condenser is considerably reduced by the high speed at which the steam and oil vapours rush through the tubes and also by the fact that with lower temperatures of distillation the capacity of heat absorption by the cooling water diminishes.

In general, it can be stated that hydrodistillation at reduced pressure is especially suitable for the .rectification of liquids that possess medium volatility and do not withstand heating, as well as for the purification of high boiling mixtures which are to be freed from lower boiling impurities. The method can also be used for removing traces of a solvent from an extract. Hydrodistillation can be conducted at as low a temperature and pressure as the temperature and the efficiency of the condenser permit.

Water distillation of essential oils at high pressure

Pressure within the retort can be increased by inserting a throttling valve into the tube (gooseneck) connecting the retort with the condenser. When operating at a pressure above atmospheric, the unfilled space in the retort above the charge should be sufficient to prevent foaming over of the still content. The use of live steam is preferable, because refilling the still with water during the operation offers some difficulties. When heat is first applied to the retort, no excess pressure must be applied until all air has escaped from the still.

Water distillation of volatile oils at high pressure is useful for certain purposes—for instance, for the hydrolysis of esters, if so desired. This modification, however, by no means represents a general method of rectification. Relative to the steam pressure, the vapour pressure of higher boiling oil constituents increases more as the temperature rises; thus the ratio of oil in the distillate will be more favourable. However, from this angle and from the practical point of view, water distillation at high pressure is not as effective as distillation with superheated steam, because the latter method vapourises more oil without necessitating the high pressure of the former method.

Distillation of essential oils with superheated steam

This occurs when the steam in the steam/vapour mixture rising from the oil is superheated. As was stated previously, this condition of the water component in the steam/vapour mixture is of great importance for the vapourisation of oil. The same unit space occupied by a mixture of oil vapours and steam will contain relatively a much smaller quantity of steam, in a superheated state, than it would contain of saturated steam.

In actual practice, steam can be superheated by two methods:
1. By superheating within the retort: The volatile oil is poured into the retort (without addition of water) and through a steam jacket or closed steam coil or oil bath, heated above the boiling point of water at the corresponding pressure. If saturated but dry steam is injected into the oil and thoroughly distributed, the steam will be superheated in the hot oil layer.
2. By superheating outside of the retort: The steam is superheated in a special oven before it enters the retort and, as such is injected into the oil, which does not have to be specially heated.

A combination of the two methods increases effectiveness of each. The stills serving for distillation of volatile oils with superheated steam should be constructed high with a small diameter; they should be well insulated and provided with a steam jacket and a many-coiled perforated steam pipe. These precautions permit the injected steam to assume the temperature of the heated oil and to become thoroughly saturated with its vapours. When a distillate of high purity is desired, the force of distillation should be moderate — in other words, the quantity of the injected steam should be reduced. This is especially important in the case of vacuum distillation with superheated steam. A reduction in the rate of the injected steam also permits a more thorough saturation of the steam with oil vapours.

In general, it can be stated that distillation with superheated steam is particularly valuable in the case of those volatile oils or oil constituents which are partly soluble in water, because only a small quantity of water (steam) is required and this stays in contact with the oil to be vapourised. The vapourising liquid, therefore, acts like a water-insoluble compound. The method is well adapted to the distillation and purification of benzyl alcohol, cinnamic alcohol; phenyl ethyl alcohol, etc. in other words, to all high boiling and chemically stable compounds which contain higher boiling impurities.

Distillation of essential oils with superheated steam at reduced pressure

In the above described process, the steam can be superheated inside or outside of the still. An important modification, however, consists in connecting the retort and the closed oil/water separator (receiver) with a vacuum pump so that the oil vapourises in the retort at reduced pressure. By this means it is possible to regulate the temperature of the oil vapours at will. According to the chosen temperature, the vapours will be more or less superheated which means a more favourable ratio of oil in the distillate than is the case when the oil is merely steam distilled without superheating. For example, by heating the oil charge in the retort indirectly with steam of 10 atmospheres pressure, by injecting dry live steam of high pressure very slowly into the oil at the same time and by carefully adjusting the vacuum pump and the direct steam inlet to a distillation pressure of 30 to 40 mm at a temperature of about 160°C within the retort, even high boiling compounds such as glycerine, palmitic and oleic acid will distil over in ample quantities. For the vapourisation of high boiling substances, this method therefore exceeds even dry vacuum distillation in efficiency. As for every type of hydrodistillation *in vacuo,* it is necessary to provide for sufficiently large condensers and to inject the direct steam very slowly into the oil charge, so that no foaming takes place and the distillate will not be contaminated with impurities mechanically carried over.

NATURAL FLOWER OILS

As already stated in the section on 'distillation' most essential oils are today isolated from the respective plants or parts of plants in which they occur, by the process of distillation. A few essential oils, i.e. those present in the peels of citrus fruit—can be and in large part are, obtained by cold pressing, which yields products of superior quality.

In the discussion of distillation it was emphasised that the process of distillation suffers from several inadequacies: the relatively long action of steam or boiling water on the plant material affects some of the more delicate constituents of the oil deleteriously; hydrolysis, polymerisation and resinification may and do take place; high boiling constituents, especially if somewhat soluble in water, are not carried over by steam and are therefore lacking in the distilled oil. Other constituents dissolve partly in the distillation water and cannot readily be recovered. As a result of all these factors, a distilled oil does not always represent the natural oil as it originally occurred in the plan.

A few types of flowers— and this is the case with some very delicate ones— yield no direct oil at all on distillation. The oil is either destroyed by the action of steam or the minute quantities of oil actually distilling over are 'lost' in the large volume of distillation water from which the oil cannot be recovered. This applies to jasmine, tuberose, violet, jonquil, narcissus, mimosa, acacia, gardenia, hyacinth and a few others. When hydrodistilled, these flowers yield either practically no oil or in such low yield or of such inferior quality, that for all purposes it is useless. Therefore, flowers of this type must be processed by methods other than distillation.

This fact was recognised empirically hundreds of years ago when such flowers were treated by maceration in cold or hot fat, which process yielded fragrant pomades. From this primitive beginning there developed in the Grasse region of Southern France, in the course of many years, a highly specialised industry, employing the processes of maceration and of *enfleurage* and, for the last forty years, the modern process of cold extraction with volatile solvents. Despite similar, but much less important developments in other parts of the world (Bulgaria, Egypt, Algeria, Sicily, Calabria, Madagascar, etc.), Grasse has remained the centre of this picturesque and charming industry, which today supplies the perfume manufacturers with a great variety of highly prized so-called 'natural flower oil'. Representing the authentic scents as exhaled by the flowers, these flower oils are the finest and most delicate ingredients at the disposal of the modern perfumer, enabling him to create masterpieces of his art by skilful application and blending.

The term 'natural flower oil', as used today commercially, does not include the distilled essential oils; it applies only to flower oils obtained by the methods of *enfleurage*, maceration and extraction with volatile solvents, which will be described later in detail. A few oils, e.g. those derived from rose petals and from the blossoms of the sour (bitter) orange tree — can be isolated either by distillation or by extraction. The oils are then called essential oils and natural flower oils, respectively, the latter reproducing and representing the original scent of the flowers in a more complete way. It is principally the elaborate apparatus required and the higher cost of manufacturing which prevent a more general adaptation of the process of extraction.

EXTRACTION WITH COLD FAT (*ENFLEURAGE*)

In the Grasse region of Southern France, flowers were processed by this method long before the modern method of extraction with volatile solvents was introduced. Generations ago Grasse, an ancient hill town located on the southern slopes of the Alpes-Maritimes and facing the Mediterranean, became the centre of extensive flower plantations and subsequently, of the French perfume industry. Grasse, like few places in the world, is favoured by a mild climate, southern exposure and protection against north winds. There the cultivation of flowers for the extraction of their scent became a highly specialised agricultural occupation, passed down from generation to generation.

In the early days of perfumery, flower scents were extracted with fats and the alcoholic washings of the perfumed fats represented the so-called floral *extraits*. These, blended with certain distilled essential oils and tinctures, constituted the old-style perfumes. In the course of years this simple beginning led to our modern perfume industry with its wealth and variety of raw materials.

Despite the introduction of the modern process of extraction with volatile solvents, the old-fashioned method of *enfleurage* as passed on from father to son and perfected in the course of generations, still plays an important role. Enfleurage on a large scale is today carried out only in the Grasse region, with the possible exception of isolated instances in India where the process has remained primitive.

The principles of *enfleurage* are simple. Certain flowers (e.g. tuberose and jasmine) continue the physiological activities of developing and giving off perfume even after picking. Every jasmine and tuberose flower resembles, so to speak, a tiny factory continually emitting minute quantities of perfume. This phenomenon was first studied by Passy and later by Hesse. Fat possesses a high power of absorption and if brought in contact with fragrant flowers readily absorbs the perfume emitted. This principle, methodically applied on a large scale, constitutes *enfleurage*. During the entire period of harvest, which lasts from eight to ten weeks, batches of freshly picked flowers are strewn over the surface of a specially prepared fat base (corps), left there (for 24 hours in the case of jasmine and longer in the case of tuberose) and then replaced by fresh flowers. At the end of the harvest the fat, which is not renewed during the process, has become quite saturated with flower oil. The latter is finally extracted from the fat with alcohol and then isolated.

Preparation of the Fat Corps

The success of *enfleurage* depends to a great extent upon the quality of the fat base employed. Utmost care must be exercised when preparing the corps. It must be practically odourless and of proper consistency. If the corps is too hard, the blossoms will not have sufficient contact with the fat, curtailing its power of absorption and resulting in a subnormal yield of flower oil. On the other hand, if too soft, the corps has a tendency to engulf the flowers so that the exhausted ones are difficult to remove and retain adhering fat, which entails considerable shrinkage and loss of corps. The consistency of the corps must, therefore, be such that it offers a semihard surface from which the exhausted flowers can easily be removed. Since the whole process of *enfleurage* is carried out in cool cellars, every manufacturer must prepare his corps according to the temperature prevailing in his cellars during the months of the flower harvest. Many years of experience have proved that a mixture of one part of highly purified tallow and two parts of lard are eminently suitable for *enfleurage*. This mixture assures a suitable consistency of the corps in conjunction with high power of absorption. Series of experiments were carried out with various mixtures of vegetable fats, especially hardened vegetable fats which do not easily turn rancid.

Experiments were also done with all kinds of antioxidants and glycoside splitting compounds, incorporating them into the corps before *enfleurage*. The result was a variety of interesting qualities and widely different yields of floral oils, but the highest quality of floral oils most true to nature resulted from the old-fashioned mixture of lard and tallow.

Mineral oils, too, have been suggested as bases for *enfleurage* work and on a limited scale have been practically employed; but they offer no real advantage because their power of absorption is very small as compared with that of animal fats. Furthermore, it is exceedingly difficult to extract and isolate small quantities of absorbed flower oils from the mineral oils with alcohol or by other means.

Many other substances have been suggested as bases for *enfleurage* and have been patented for this purpose, but none so far has attained any wide commercial application. For instance, according to French Patent essential oils and natural flower oils are extracted by treatment of the plant material with esters of polyhydric aliphatic alcohols, containing at the most six carbon atoms, with fatty acids of high molecular weight, as obtained by oxidation of paraffin hydrocarbons of high molecular weight. Thus ester of glycol, glycerol, erythritol, mannitol, hexitol or trimethylolpropane may be used.

The fat corps is prepared in the Grasse factories during the winter months when they are not busy with the processing of flower crops. The crude pieces of tallow and lard, mostly of French and Italian origin, are purified according to a tedious old-fashioned method. The crude fats are carefully cleaned by hand, all adhering particles of skin and blood vessels removed, then crushed mechanically and finally beaten in a current of cold water. After all impurities have been removed, the fat is melted gently on a steam bath. Small quantities of benzoin (0.6 per cent) and alum (0.15 to 0.30 per cent) are then added. This preservation is very important, as otherwise the corps will turn rancid during the hot summer months. While benzoin acts as a preservative, the adding of alum causes impurities to coagulate during the heating; when rising to the surface they can be skimmed off with a spoon. The warm fat is filtered through cloth, then left to cool and stand, so that any water may separate.

During the past years chemistry has made great progress in regard to antioxidants for fats and oil, several of which could undoubtedly be used for preservation of the *enfleurage* corps employed in the Grasse region. The fat corps thus prepared is white, of smooth, absolutely uniform consistency, free of water and practically odourless. If well prepared and properly stored, it will resist rancidity for several years. Some manufacturers also add small quantities of orange flower or rose water when preparing the corps. This seems to be done for the sake of convention. Such additions somewhat shade the odour of the finished product by imparting a slight orange blossom or rose note.

Enfleurage and *Défleurage*

Every *enfleurage* building is equipped with thousands of so-called chassis, which serve as vehicles for holding the fat corps during the process. A chassis consists of a rectangular wooden frame 2-inch high, about 20-inch long and about 16-inch wide. The frame holds a glass plate upon both sides of which the fat corps is applied with a spatula at the beginning of the *enfleurage* process. When piled one above the other the chassis form airtight compartments with a layer of fat on the upper and lower side of each glass plate.

Every morning during the harvest the freshly picked flowers arrive and having first been cleaned of impurities, such as leaves and stalks, are then strewn by hand on top of the fat layer of each glass plate. Blossoms wet from dew or rain must never be employed, as any trace of moisture would turn the corps rancid. The *chassis* are then piled up and left in the cellars for 24 hours or longer, depending upon the type of flowers. The latter rest in direct contact with one fat layer (the lower one), which acts as a direct solvent, whereas the other fat layer (beneath the glass plate of the chassis above) absorbs only the volatile perfume given off by the flowers.

After 24 hours the flowers have emitted most of their oil and start to wither, developing an objectionable odour. They must then be removed from the corps, which process, despite all efforts to introduce labour-saving devices, is still done by hand. The careful removal of the flowers (*défleurage*) is almost more important than charging the corps on the chassis with fresh flowers (*enfleurage*) and, therefore, the women doing this work must be experienced and skilled. Most of the exhausted flowers will fall from the fat layer on the chassis glass plate when the *chassis* is struck lightly against the working table, but since it is necessary to remove every single flower and every particle of the flowers, the women use tweezers for this delicate operation. Immediately following *défleurage*, that is, every 24-hour the chassis are recharged with fresh flowers. For this purpose the chassis are turned over and the fat layer, which in the previous operation formed the top (ceiling) of the small chamber, is now directly charged with flowers. In the case of jasmine, the entire *enfleurage* process lasts about 70 days; daily the exhausted flowers are removed and the chassis recharged with fresh ones.

During the height of the harvest large quantities of flowers arrive every morning, which necessitates certain modifications in the process. Complications result from the fact that at the beginning and at the end of the harvest the quantities of flowers are very limited and, therefore, it is practically impossible to charge the *chassis* each day of the flower harvest with the same amount of flowers.

At the beginning of, and several times during the harvest, the fat on the chassis is scratched over with metal combs and tiny furrows are drawn in order to change and increase the surface of absorption.

At the end of the harvest the fat is relatively saturated with flower oil and possesses their typical fragrance. The perfumed fat must then be removed from the glass plates between the *chassis*. For this purpose it is scraped off with a spatula and then carefully melted and bulked in closed containers. The final product is called *pomade* (*pomade de jasmin, pomade de tubéreuse, pomade de violet*, etc.), the most highly saturated pomade being, because the *corps* on the chassis has been treated with fresh flowers 36 times during the whole process of *enfleurage*. At the beginning of the harvest every chassis is charged with about 360 grams of fat corps on each side of the glass plate, in other words, with 720 grams per chassis. Every kilogram of fat corps should be in contact with about 2.5 kg (preferably with 3.0 kg) of jasmine flowers for the entire period of *enfleurage*, which lasts from 8 to 10 weeks. The quantities differ somewhat in the case of other flowers.

At the end of the *enfleurage*, the fat corps has lost about 10 per cent of its weight because of various manipulations. In other words, the total yield of the fragrant is about 10 per cent less than the fat corps originally applied to the *chassis*. Most of this loss is caused by fat adhering to the exhausted flowers when they are removed (*défleurage*) every 24-hour.

Alcoholic *Extraits*

In the early days of perfumery, the fragment *pomades* were employed directly; later they were extracted with high proof alcohol, the alcohol dissolving the natural flower oil from the pomade. These alcoholic washings are called 'extrait no. 36' when made from 'pomade no. 36'; they reproduce the natural flower perfume to a remarkable degree.

Since no heat is applied during the process of *enfleurage* and during the washing of the pomades with alcohol, the *extraits* contain the natural flower oil as emitted by the living flowers. The only disadvantage exists possibly in a slight fatty 'by-note' which can be eliminated to a certain extent by freezing and filtering the alcoholic washings. This slight fatty 'by-note' is not always objectionable, as it imparts a certain roundness and fixation value to the finished perfumes, especially in conjunction with synthetic aromatics.

In order to prepare the *extraits*, the *pomades* are usually processed during the winter months when the factories are not busy with other work. For this purpose the *pomades* are charged into so-called *batteuses* (Fig. 5.24), closed copper vessels heavily tinned inside and equipped with strong stirrers around a vertical shaft. Several *batteuses* are arranged in batteries, the stirrers of each battery being driven by a powerful motor. The work, which goes on for several months, is carried out in cool cellars in order to prevent loss of alcohol by evaporation. Each batch of *pomade* is stirred for several days, the usual process of methodical extraction being applied. The alcohol employed in the process travels from one batch of *pomade* to the next (constituting in turn the third, second and first washings of successive batches), until it becomes enriched with flower oil and is drawn off as the alcoholic *extrait*. For the last washing, fresh alcohol is used, which also, in its turn, becomes gradually enriched by the continuous process just described. When extended to a fourth and fifth washing, this method extracts the *pomades* so efficiently that the exhausted fat is quite odourless. Being useless for new *enfleurage* it is usually employed for the making of soap.

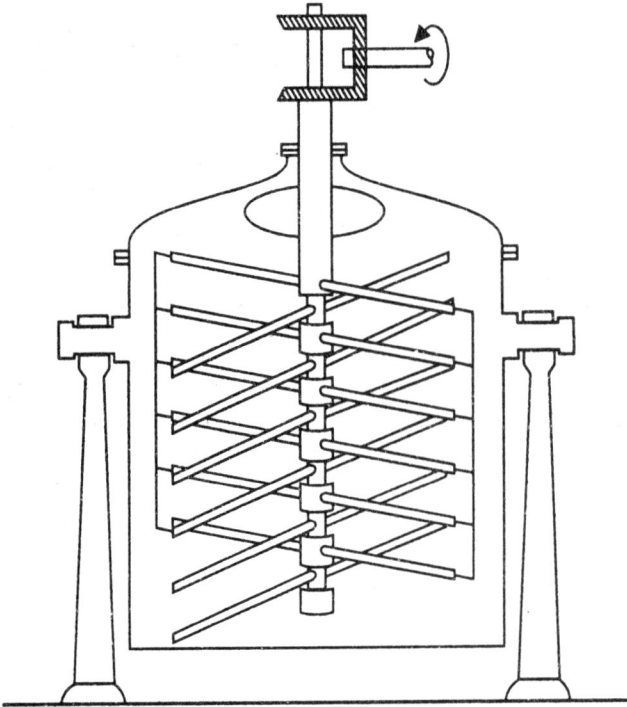

Fig. 5.24. Sketch of a *Batteuse* for the extraction of flower concretes with alcohol. (The agitation is in counter-rotary motion.)

The fully circulated washing called 'extrait no. 36' is run through a refrigerator and cooled to well below freezing temperature, if possible to −15°C. Most of the fat dissolved in the strong alcohol separates.

The cold alcoholic solution is then filtered, also at low temperatures. The quantity of alcohol to be employed for the washing of each batch of *pomade* is calculated with a view to obtaining, finally, 1 kg of *extrait* per kilogram of *pomade*. Obviously some alcohol is lost by evaporation during the process of stirring.

The purified *extraits* reproduce the perfume of the living flowers remarkably well. During past these *extraits* were widely employed as bases of the classical French perfumes and several conservative houses still continue this practice. Some of the well-known French perfumes undoubtedly owe their success partly to a high content of *extraits*. The washing of the *pomades* is carried out not only by the factories in Grasse but in some instances also by perfume manufacturers in Paris, London, Berlin and New York who possess the necessary *batteuses* and freezing apparatus.

Absolutes of *Enfleurage*

As mentioned previously, an *extrait* contains not only the natural flower oil, but also a small quantity (about 1 per cent) of alcohol soluble fat, dissolved from the corps, which cannot be eliminated, even by cooling the *extrait* far below 0°C. When concentrating the extrait by distilling off the alcohol, the content of natural flower oil and fat increases correspondingly. Complete concentration in a vacuum still at low temperature results in a concentrated flower oil, free from alcohol, the so-called absolute of *enfleurage*.

The crude absolutes of enfleurage are usually of dark colour and, because of their fat content, of a semisolid consistency. Lighter coloured products of more liquid consistency can be obtained by certain methods of purification whereby more fat is eliminated. Further elimination of fat and purification increases the price of the final absolute. Every manufacturer has his own standards in this respect.

These so-called absolutes of *enfleurage*, absolutes of *pomade*, concentrates of *pomade* or liquid concretes were widely employed before the introduction of the more modern process of extraction with volatile solvents. Even today these absolutes of *enfleurage* find favour with some perfumers because of their lower price. Experts, however, claim that the absolutes of *enfleurage* when redissolved in alcohol are somewhat inferior to the original alcoholic extracts. Apparently during the process of concentration certain constituents of the natural flower oil, especially the most volatile and delicate ones are lost.
A characteristic of absolutes of *enfleurage* is that they have a slight but noticeable 'by-note' of vanillin quite alien to the true flower perfume. This note originates from the minute quantities of benzoin incorporated into the fat corps for protection against rancidity. Soluble in alcohol, the benzoin dissolves when the *pomades* are extracted with alcohol and upon concentration it accumulates in the absolute.

Absolutes of *Chassis*

When describing the process of *enfleurage* it was mentioned that the flowers are removed from the fat corps on the *chassis* every 24 hours. These flowers are not thrown away because they still contain that part of the natural perfume which was not absorbed by the fat. It must be borne in mind that the perfume or essential oil of the flowers consists not only of volatile constituents, but also of compounds of higher boiling range which are not so readily released by the flowers. The actual conditions are probably much more complicated and many physiological processes take place, which so far have not yet been fully elucidated.

The part of the natural flower oil which is retained by the flowers after removal from the *chassis* (*défleurage*) can be extracted from these partly exhausted flowers with a volatile solvent-petroleum ether, for instance. Concentration of the solution results in a solid mass. (This product must not be confused with the concretes and absolutes obtained by extracting fresh flowers directly with volatile solvents.) The solid mass thus obtained contains a certain percentage of fat originating from the corps with which the flowers were in contact during the process of *enfleurage*; it is purified and made alcohol soluble by eliminating most of the fats at low temperature. The final so-called absolute of *chassis*, a viscous, alcohol-soluble oil, possesses an odour differing somewhat from that of the absolute of *enfleurage*.

Absolute of *enfleurage* and absolute of *chassis* logically supplement one another because each represents only part of the total natural flower oil present in the living flowers. Yet, they are usually marketed separately, perhaps because the absolute of *chassis* is lower priced than the absolute of *enfleurage*.

Absolutes of *chassis* give excellent results in perfume blends, especially in conjunction with synthetic aromatics, the harsh notes of which are thereby softened and blended.

EXTRACTION WITH HOT FAT (MACERATION)

As explained, certain flowers, e.g. jasmine and tuberose — give their greatest yield of flower oil upon extraction with cold fat (*enfleurage*) because their physiological activities continue for 24 hours and longer after harvesting. During this period, the fat on the chassis absorbs the perfume emitted by these flowers.

However, the physiological activities of other flowers — roses orange blossoms acacia and mimosa, for instance — are stopped by picking. When extracted or distilled, they yield, therefore, only as much oil as is contained in the flowers at that moment. Since no further oil develops in these flowers, the long and rather complicated method of *enfleurage* would prove ineffective. Hence, other methods must be resorted to, whereby a medium actually penetrates the plant tissues and dissolves all flower oil present in the oil glands.

Various scientists studied methods of distillation, cold *enfleurage*, maceration with hot fat and extraction with volatile solvents as applied to various flowers and the effect upon the yield of flower oils. Applying *enfleurage* to orange blossoms, for instance it was found that this method yields only one-fifteenth of the amount of volatile oil obtained by steam distillation. Hesse thereby confirmed what had been known empirically in Grasse for generations.

Generations before the modern process of extraction with volatile solvents had been introduced (probably even in classical times), the perfumes of roses, orange blossoms, violets, acacia, mimosa and others had been obtained by treating the flowers with hot fat. The principle is simple:

The flowers are extracted by immersion in hot fat. In other words, the same batch of hot fat is systematically treated with several batches of fresh flowers until the fat becomes quite saturated with flower perfume. The exhausted flowers are removed and the fragrant fat, called *Pomade d'Orange*, *Pomade de Rose*, etc. is sold as such or the *pomade* may be treated further by washing it with strong alcohol, exactly as with jasmine or tuberose *pomades*, obtained by cold *enfleurage*. The alcoholic extraits (*Extrait d'Orange, Extrait de Rose*, etc.) may be marketed as such or they are concentrated *in vacuo*, giving thereby the corresponding absolutes of *pomade*.

The process of maceration, therefore, is somewhat analogous to that of *enfleurage*, with the fundamental differences that, in the case of maceration, hot fat is employed and that the actual macerating of the flowers in the hot fat is done quickly.

Maceration was an important process before the introduction of the more modern method of extraction with volatile solvents. During past orange blossoms, if not distilled, were treated by maceration; acacia blossoms, which do not lend themselves to steam distillation, had to be processed exclusively by maceration. Similarly, roses were macerated in Southern France because French roses, unlike Bulgarian roses, give only a very low yield of oil upon distillation. However, today, the process of maceration with hot fat is employed very little. Its products, especially those from orange blossoms, find application only in a few old-fashioned perfume formulas. Otherwise the concretes and absolutes made by volatile solvent extraction have almost completely replaced the former extraits and absolutes of maceration.

For completeness, however, a brief description of the way this old-fashioned process is carried out is give below:

As solvent a highly purified fat base is employed. It should be prepared most carefully and in the same way as described under *enfleurage*.

A batch of 80 kg of corps is heated to about 80°C and at that temperature macerated with charges of 20 kg of fresh flowers each time. This is repeated unit 1 kg of corps has been treated with about 2 to 2½ kg of flowers. Every extraction lasts about one-half hour, at 80°C, when the mass is left standing for about an hour during which it cools but continues macerating the flowers. The mass is then reheated, melted and strained through metal sieves and filter bags, whereby the exhausted flowers are eliminated. Since they retain some adhering fat, they are, while in the sieves, treated with scalding water, which liquefies the fat. The water easily separates from the fat layer. In order to remove all adhering fat, the flowers are finally packed between filter cloth, placed in a hydraulic press and submitted to pressure ranging up to about 3750 lb. per sq. inch. Scalding water is thrown on the filter bags during the process so that any fat still retained by the flowers is melted and expressed. Expressed fat and water again separate easily. Instead of hydraulic presses, some manufacturers employ centrifuges for removing the exhausted flowers from the fat corps.

The method of maceration is rather cumbersome but it served its purpose in the old days when no better process was available. Its products (*extraits* and absolutes of maceration) often show a fatty 'by-note' which originates from the fat corps and modifies the character of the original flower perfume. A further disadvantage consists in the fact that, on account of this fat content, absolutes of maceration easily turn rancid, thereby developing a sharp, disagreeable note. Because of their high alcohol content, the extraits are better protected against rancidity and spoilage in general.

EXTRACTION WITH VOLATILE SOLVENTS

The principle of extraction with volatile solvents is simple: fresh flowers are charged into specially constructed extractors and extracted systematically at room temperature, with a carefully purified solvent, usually petroleum ether. The solvent penetrates the flowers and dissolves the natural flower perfume together with some waxes and albuminous and colouring matter. The solution is subsequently pumped into an evaporator and concentrated at a low temperature. After the solvent is completely driven off *in vacuo*, the concentrated flower oil is obtained. Thus the temperature applied during the entire process is kept at a minimum; live steam, as in the case of distillation, does not exert its action upon the delicate constituents of the flower oils. Compared with distilled oils the extracted flower oils, therefore, more truly represent the natural perfume as originally present in the flowers.

Despite this obvious advantage the volatile solvent process cannot entirely replace steam distillation, which remains the principal method of isolating essential oils. Steam distillation, in most cases, is a simpler process: by employing portable direct fire stills, distillation can be carried out even in remote and primitive parts of the world, whereas solvent extraction necessitates complicated and expensive apparatus and a crew of well trained workers. Running expenses are comparatively high; a mistake in operation can be costly; the unavoidable loss of solvent, of which large quantities are employed during the process, is an important factor in the price calculation of natural flower oils. Extraction with solvents can, therefore, be applied advantageously only to the higher priced materials, particularly the flowers. A loss of 10 litres of solvent per 100 kg of flower charge remains rather insignificant in the calculation of absolute of jasmine which is normally valued at several hundred rupees; but with low-priced oils such as rosemary or eucalyptus, ranging normally the loss of a few litres of solvent would make extraction prohibitive.

All extracted flower oils are of more or less dark colour because they contain much of the natural plant pigments which are not volatile. Steam distilled oils, on the other hand, are in most cases of light colour. Furthermore, they usually are soluble even in dilute alcohol, while extracted oils require 95 per cent alcohol for complete solution.

Despite these drawbacks, the products of extraction possess one supreme advantage, i.e. their true-to-nature odour. In addition, certain types of flowers, e.g. jasmine, tuberose, jonquil, hyacinth, acacia, mimosa and violet — do not yield their volatile oil on steam distillation and must, therefore, be extracted with solvents.

Selection of the Solvent

The most important factor for the success of the extraction process is the quality of the solvent employed. The ideal solvent should possess several properties:

1. It should completely and quickly dissolve all the odouriferous principles of the flower, yet as little as possible of such inert matter as waxes, pigments, albuminous compounds, etc. In other words, the solvent should be selective.
2. It should possess a sufficiently low boiling point to permit its being easily removed (distilled off), without resorting to higher temperatures; yet, the boiling point should not be too low, as this would involve considerable solvent loss by evaporation in the warm climate.
3. The solvent must not dissolve water since the water present in the flowers would dissolve and accumulate in the solvent.
4. The solvent must be chemically inert, i.e. not react with the constituents of the flower oil.
5. The solvent should have a uniform boiling point; when evaporated it must not leave any residue. The slightest traces of high boiling compounds, upon evaporation of the solvent, would, accumulate and remain in the flower oil and completely spoil its odour. It should be borne in mind that the yield of flower oil is generally very small and that large quantities of solvent are required to cover the flower material in the extractors. In the case of petroleum ether, for instance, even traces of high boiling impurities are apt to impart to the concretes and absolutes an objectionable off-odour of kerosene, which cannot be eliminated without doing considerable harm to the delicate flower oil.
6. The solvent should be low-priced and, if possible, nonflammable.

The ideal solvent which, would fulfil all these requirements does not exist. Considering every feature, highly purified petroleum ether appears to be the most suitable one, with benzene (benzol) ranking next.

Mixed solvents form a fascinating problem which so far has been little touched, but which promises quite interesting results. As compared with straight solvents, mixed solvents can either reduce or increase their dissolving power. Much experimental work along these lines has still to be undertaken.

Petroleum ether

Crude petroleum on fractional distillation yields a number of hydrocarbon fractions of different boiling ranges which find certain industrial applications. The fractions, boiling range 30°–70°C, commercially called petroleum ether, consist of saturated paraffins, viz. mainly pentane and hexane. Because of their chemical inertness and complete volatility, these fractions are particularly suited for flower extraction. A further advantage lies in their selective power of dissolving: they yield products which contain relatively little wax, albuminous and colouring matter, but correspondingly more of the odouriferous compounds. Certain American petroleums are best suited for our purpose, because they consist mostly of inert, saturated paraffins, whereas Galician, Rumanian, Russian or 'cracked petroleum' contain derivatives of benzene and naphthene, as well as unsaturated olefinic compounds, the latter being chemically active and liable to polymerisation. They may thus form high boiling compounds of objectionable kerosene odour, especially on prolonged use of the solvent.

The petroleum ether must be free from sulphur and nitrogenous compounds. It is purified by washing in turn with strong sulphuric acid, water, hot dilute sodium hydroxide solution, water and then drying. Smith recommended repeated washing with sulphuric acid mono hydrate, followed by washing with alkaline potassium permanganate solution and drying. He found the hexane fraction of petroleum ether, boiling range 65°–70°C, of great advantage in extraction work because solutes remain in their normal molecular state; unstable compounds stay unchanged and no addition compounds are formed.

When testing petroleum ether for use in extraction work, special attention must be paid to the presence (absence) of a nonvolatile residue. For this purpose a sample of 50 cc. should be evaporated in a glass or porcelain dish at a temperature not exceeding 40°C. After complete evaporation the glass dish should show no residual odour whatsoever, but especially no odour indicating the presence of kerosene or sulphur compounds. A similar test can be carried out by permitting the solvent to evaporate on a clean filter paper at room temperature. The petroleum ether is usually prepared by submitting petroleum fractions to slow and repeated rectification in special stills provided with high fractionation columns and dephlegmators. As a rule, a small quantity (about 5 per cent) of odourless paraffin or fat is added to the gasoline in the still so that higher boiling compounds are retained and prevented from distilling over. According to the quality of the gasoline employed, 20 to 40 per cent remains as residue in the still, while 60 to 80 per cent represents the final *coeur* (heart) of petroleum ether suitable for extraction. Its boiling point should not be higher than 75°C.

Although petroleum ether, is the best solvent found so far for flower extraction, it possesses some inherent disadvantages—for example, relatively high solvent losses in the course of the extraction process. These losses are due primarily to evaporation of the low boiling, almost gaseous, fractions. Furthermore, petroleum ether is readily inflammable and dangerous to work with.

Benzene (benzol)

Benzene ranks next to petroleum ether as a solvent for the extraction of flowers. It is a coal-tar product made by treating and purifying coal-tar naphtha with sulphuric acid and subsequently with sodium hydroxide. The fractions below 130°C contain the lower benzene hydrocarbons which are composed mainly of benzene (C_6H_6), toluene and other homologues. The industrial 'benzol' often contains pyridine, carbon disulphide and thiophene which must be removed by treatment with concentrated sulphuric acid, water and caustic soda solutions. Further fractionation eliminates most of the higher boiling homologues but complete purification is obtained only by repeated crystallisation. Thus, pure benzene, melting point 5.5°C, is obtained, the higher homologues remaining liquid and being separated by vacuum filtration or other method.

Crystallisable benzene is of such purity that 95 to 98 per cent of it distils within 1 per cent of the theoretical boiling point 80.1°C. This uniform boiling point is of great advantage in extraction work, also because solvent losses are reduced. Yet, 80.1°C is a relatively high boiling point, which makes it rather difficult to remove the last traces of solvent from the concentrated flower oil.

A further drawback of benzene in flower extraction work lies in its high dissolving power. It dissolves not only the odouriferous principles but also much wax, albuminous and colouring matter, so that the final flower oils extracted with benzene are dark, highly viscous, often almost solid masses, which can be purified only under considerable difficulties and by special processes.

Compared with petroleum ether, benzene usually gives much higher yields of concretes, due to the higher amount of inert wax, albuminous and colouring matter present. As far as the actual odouriferous principles are concerned, the yields obtained by benzene or petroleum ether are usually quite similar.

Summarising, it can be stated that petroleum ether is preferred for extracting the more expensive flowers, while benzene serves in the case of lower priced plant material such as oak moss and labdanum, where the presence of colouring matter is not considered of too great a disadvantage.

Alcohol

Alcohol cannot be used for the extraction of fresh flowers because it dissolves the water contained in them and becomes increasingly more dilute. With some flowers (tuberoses, for example) alcohol develops a most disagreeable odour; from others (jasmine, for example) it extracts dark, solid masses which possess an odour similar to molasses.

High-proof alcohol—in some instances dilute alcohol—is widely employed, however, for the extraction of dried plant materials, leaves, barks roots and especially gums, from which alcoholic tinctures are obtained. These tinctures find wide application in pharmacy and perfumery.

Concentration of these tinctures, usually by driving off the alcohol in a vacuum still, results in the so-called oleoresins and resinoids. These products are usually viscous, often almost solid, masses of dark colour, representing the concentrated odouriferous principles, plus the alcohol soluble resins, colouring matter, etc. contained in the original plant material. Resinoids of olibanum, myrrh, opopanax, benzoin, etc. are widely employed in perfumery, oleoresins of vanilla, ginger root, capsicum, celery seed, etc. in the flavouring of all kinds of food products and beverages.

Apparatus of Extraction

General arrangement

The extraction buildings of the Grasse region are usually of light masonry, one-storied, painted in light colours. The flat roof serves as a shallow water tank, insulating the building against sunheat and providing the condensers in the building below with water. The steam boilers are housed separately, at a safe distance from the main building, in order to exclude any danger of fire. The employment of volatile, highly inflammable petroleum ether or benzene also necessitates that all electric motors and switches be explosion proof or be housed outside of the extraction building. The reserve solvent which is not in circulation must be stored in fireproof cellars, separate from the buildings.

The extraction building is equipped with one or two stills or columns for fractionating the solvent, a few batteries for extracting the flowers and stills for concentrating the flower oil solutions. The batteries are of different size, so that they can be used according to the quantity of available flower material, which varies according to weather conditions and with the progressing harvest.

Construction of apparatus

Until some years ago the extractors and stills were constructed of copper, because this metal retains its value after scrapping the apparatus and the pliable copper can be hammered and repairs are easily made.

Lately, however, the extractors are constructed more often of heavily tinned sheet iron which is much cheaper and, therefore offers the advantage of lower investment and quicker amortisation.

The apparatus must be of solid construction to stand wear and tear; all extractor pipes and valves should be within easy reach to save time and exclude mistakes on the part of the operators. Pipes and valves must be sufficiently wide to prevent formation of pressure by air and petroleum ether vapours, one of the principal causes for loss of the solvent in vapour phase. Large diameters also permit quicker flow of solvent and solutions to and from the apparatus and considerably speed up operation. Pumping of solvents and solutes is done by air pressure created by air compressors.

The extractors are mounted on elevated metal platforms along the inside walls of the building. The platform runs even with the ground outside of the building, so that the arriving flower material may be charged directly into the extractors and the exhausted flowers discharged with equal ease.

Loss of solvent during the operation presents one of the most serious problems. These losses are usually caused by incomplete distillation of the solvent from the exhausted flowers, by insufficient condensation in the condensers or by too narrow pipes and valves creating pressure and blowing off a mixture of air and solvent vapour. To avoid this as much as possible the whole system of extractors, evaporators and solvent tanks is arranged as a closed circle, with only one outlet where escaping solvent vapours can be condensed. An efficient, rather small sized apparatus has been developed in which solvent vapours are absorbed by activated carbon and recovered by blowing live steam through the saturated carbon. A current of hot air then reactivates the carbon. The apparatus is simple and permits considerable economy in factories where large amounts of solvent are in circulation.

Description of extraction batteries

A battery usually consists of three or four extractors, four or five metal tanks holding solvent and solutions and an evaporator for concentrating the flower oil solutions. There exist two types of extractors, viz. the stationary and the rotatory types. Some factories employ both, but only one type can be used in the same battery.

The stationary extractors usually have a capacity of 1200 litres, holding about 135 kg of jasmine flowers or 180 kg of rose flowers. From 400 to 450 litres of solvent are required for extracting 100 kg of flowers. Losses of petroleum ether may range from 12 to 14 litres for 100 kg of flowers treated, but the loss can be considerably reduced with the solvent recovery apparatus described above.

The stationary extractors are cylindrical, standing vertical. In the interior they should be provided with several perforated metal grids arranged horizontally around a vertical central support shaft. The flowers are charged upon these grids, thus spreading loosely over a larger surface and preventing lumping. The solvent can thus penetrate the mass freely and uniformly. After the flowers have been charged into the extractor, the metal cover on top is closed tightly with clamps.

Extraction is carried out methodically by successive washings whereby each batch of flowers is treated three times with solvent. A third washing is used as second washing for the next flower batch, then as first washing and is finally pumped into the evaporator for concentration. The solvent distilled off is used as fresh solvent for a third washing which serves again as second of the next flower batch, etc. A fourth extraction, in most cases, yields at best only small quantities of waxes and other inert substances. The actual flower oil is contained in the first and second washings, while the third one serves merely to wash down parts of the second washing still adhering to the flower material. There exist, however, cases of emergency, especially during the height of the harvest, when great quantities of flowers arrive and must be worked up quickly in order to avoid fermentation. In such cases the third washing is often eliminated altogether, in order to save time. Just how to proceed requires experience and good judgement on that of the factory manager.

After third washing the flowers are practically exhausted and can be discharged. However, they still contain a considerable amount of adhering solvent which, before discharging the flowers from the extractor, must be recovered by steam distillation, i.e. by simply blowing live steam through the mass. Water and solvent, after condensation, separate automatically in a specially constructed Florentine flask.

The first washing requires about 45 minutes the second 35 minutes the third 25 minutes. For drawing off the solutions and pumping in the next washing, 5 to 10 minutes must be allowed for each operation. Including 90 minute of steam distillation for recovering the solvent still adhering to the exhausted flowers, complete extraction of one batch of flowers requires about 4½ to 5 hours. However, no strict rules can be laid down, as every flower type requires a different method of working and every manufacturer follows his own ideas. Figure 5.25 shows a schematic diagram of a system for extraction of flower material with volatile solvents.

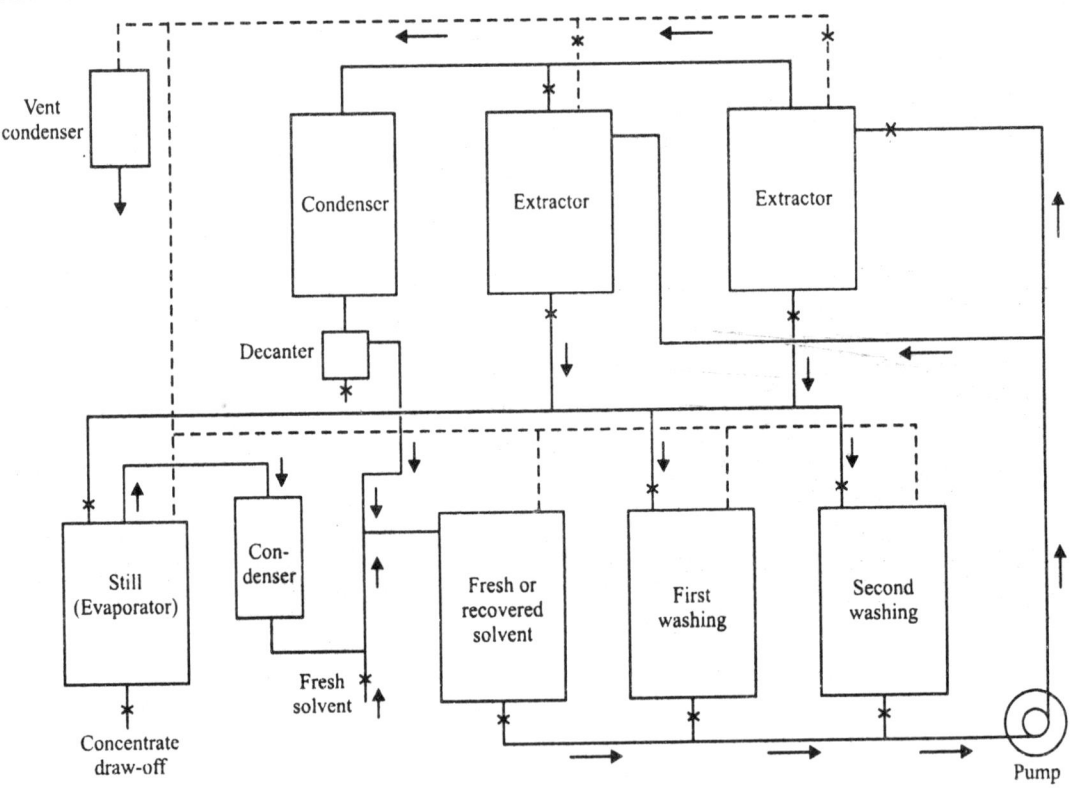

Fig. 5.25. Schematic diagram of an extraction system (extraction with volatile solvents).

Rotatory extractors

A rotatory extraction apparatus is adopted by many factories. In modified and improved form the apparatus represents a simple, solid and moderately priced piece of machinery.

The latest model (Fig. 5.26) consists of a heavily tinned iron drum rotating around a horizontal axle. Four perforated metal partitions, rectangularly and horizontally arranged around the central axle, divide the interior into four compartments into which the flowers are charged through four manholes. While the whole system rotates slowly, the flower material moves, tumbles and dips into the solvent lying on the bottom of the extractor. The liquid seeps through the perforations and drips back to the bottom when one compartment is lifted out of the solvent in the continuous movement of the whole drum. Thus, the solvent does not fill the extractor but only the lowest part, the flowers dipping slowly and continuously into the solvent and rising again in the rotatory movement.

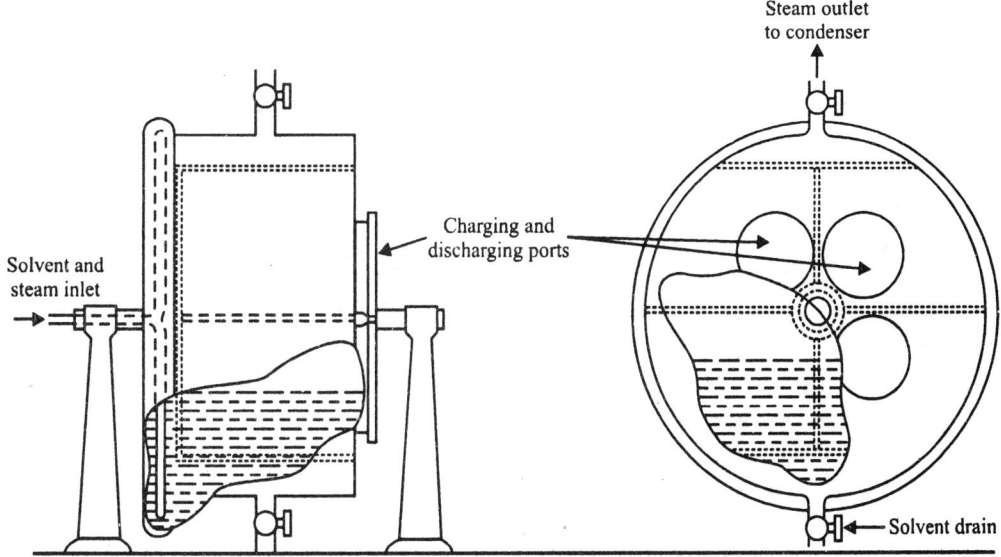

Fig. 5.26. Rotary extractor, Garnier type.

Three successive washings are usually made, carried out similarly to the systematic extraction method described under stationary apparatus. The first, i.e. the most saturated washing, is then pumped into the evaporator and concentrated by distilling off the solvent. After the third washing has been drawn off the exhausted flower material, live steam is blown into the extractor to distil over and recover the petroleum ether still adhering to the extracted flowers.

The advantages of the rotatory extractors as compared with stationary apparatus are evident. Through the movement of the flower material in the solvent, its action becomes more penetrating and more effective, resulting in a somewhat higher yield figured as concrete, it is about 8 per cent higher in the case of the rotatory apparatus. Since the solvent covers only the bottom of the rotating drum and not the whole flower material, as in the stationary apparatus, much less solvent is in circulation and, therefore, evaporation losses are reduced. Only 160 to 170 litres are required in the rotatory apparatus to extract 100 kg of flowers. The loss of solvent for 100 kg of flowers is less than in stationary extractors; it may be 8 to 12 litres but can be reduced by using the previously described solvent recovery apparatus. One rotatory extractor does the work of three or four stationary extractors arranged in one battery. Although superior in many ways the rotatory extractors suffer from several disadvantages and cannot altogether replace the stationary type; for example, the latter is better adapted to voluminous plant material, such as lavender, which cannot be so easily charged and discharged through the manholes of the rotating drum.

Concentration of solutions

The first, i.e. the most concentrated, washing is filtered through a fine screen and pumped into the so-called evaporator in which the greater part of the solvent is driven (distilled) off. These evaporators are of varying construction, representing basically a modified water or steam bath. In other words, the heating is done by indirect steam blown into a steam jacket beneath the still. The solvent, however, should not be completely driven off in this operation. Most manufacturers stop operation when the temperature in the still (evaporator) reaches about 60°C, because any higher temperature at atmospheric pressure would be harmful to the delicate flower perfume. The first washing contains, of course, only a small percentage of flower oil. Therefore, concentrating of this washing in the evaporator means driving off 90–95 per cent of the solvent. (The recovered solvent serves as fresh solvent for a third washing.) The concentrated solution remaining in the evaporators is permitted to cool, is filtered, then transferred to a special, smaller vacuum still and there completely concentrated *in vacuo*.

Final concentration

Vacuum stills (Fig. 5.27) of small capacity (50 to 100 litres) serve for this purpose. The final concentration represents a most delicate operation and requires much experience and constant attention on the part of the operator. The concentrating has to be done at as low a temperature as possible, yet any trace of solvent must be eliminated. Every manufacturer has his own, often secret, methods of purification. The completely concentrated and, purified products represent the so-called floral concretes, which contain the odouriferous principles of the natural flower perfume, plus a considerable amount of plant waxes, albuminous material and colour pigments. The concretes are, therefore, usually of solid consistency and only partly soluble in 95 per cent alcohol.

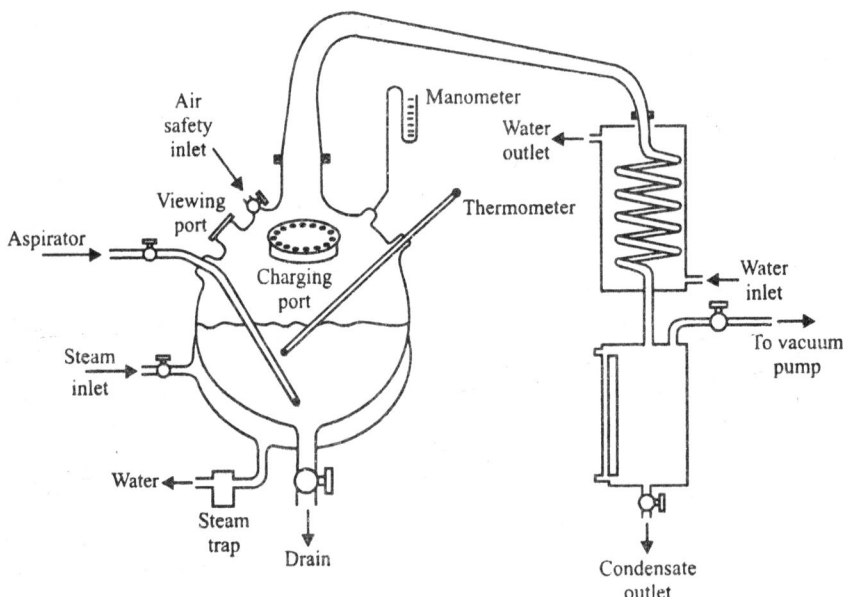

Fig. 5.27. Vacuum still for the final concentration of natural flower oils (removal of last traces of solvent).

Concrete flower oils

Although these insoluble concretes are more difficult to work with, some perfumers prefer them to the alcohol soluble absolutes, which are obtained by precipitating and eliminating the insoluble waxes with strong alcohol and concentrating the filtered alcoholic solutions. Distilling off the alcohol from the solutions when making these absolutes undoubtedly entails the loss of some of the most volatile and delicate constituents of the natural flower oil. It is often claimed that an alcoholic washing of a concrete is superior and more true to nature than a simple alcoholic solution of the corresponding absolute. On the other hand, the processing of concretes requires special equipment and considerable time; therefore, the absolutes represent a more convenient form of flower oils than the concretes.

Conversion of concretes into absolutes

The alcohol soluble absolutes are prepared from the concretes by the following general method:

The concrete is either thoroughly rubbed down in a large mortar with a quantity of high-proof alcohol or, as some manufacturers prefer, melted and dissolved in warm alcohol. Subsequently eight to ten times the amount of alcohol is added and the mass stirred for a prolonged period in *batteuses*, as described under *enfleurage*. Usually five to six washings of the concrete are made in a systematic way, i.e. a third washing serves as a second one for a following batch of concrete; the second is used as first for a batch of new concrete the first washing consequently representing the most concentrated solution. After standing and drawing off the clear solution from the alcohol insoluble waxes, the first washing is then thoroughly cooled in a refrigerator or in a special room, at temperatures ranging from –20° to –25°C, when more wax precipitates and is filtered off in the cold. The resulting clear solution can be used as such in alcoholic perfumes.

Most perfume houses have neither the time nor the facilities to carry out their own washing of concretes and prefer using alcohol soluble floral oils. For those, the manufacturers in Grasse offer the so-called liquid absolutes as the most concentrated and convenient form of floral oils. These liquid absolutes of extraction are obtained by carefully concentrating the first alcoholic washing of the corresponding concrete at low temperature in a good vacuum still. This process of concentrating involves a loss of several litres of alcohol per kilogram of absolute.

The absolutes are usually viscous oils with a more or less pronounced colour, according to the degree of final purification (for which each manufacturer employs his own process). The absolutes are soluble in high-proof alcohol and represent the most concentrated form of natural flower oils used in practical perfume work. However, they must not be confused with the actual volatile flower oil in the scientific sense. The absolutes usually contain from 50 to 80 per cent of alcohol soluble waxes and only 20 to 25 per cent volatile oil, which can be isolated from the absolute by steam distillation. However, these volatile oils from the absolutes are not offered on the market because of their excessively high price and because they completely lack the high fixation value of an absolute, which is due to the presence of alcohol soluble natural waxes, etc. in the absolute.

Thus, it might be worthwhile to review briefly the advantages and disadvantages of the various methods of manufacturing natural flower oils.

1. *Steam distillation*: Of flowers yields volatile oils—for example oil of neroli bigarade, rose, ylang ylang. Not all types of flowers, however, can be processed by hydro distillation, because boiling water and steam have a deteriorating influence upon the rather delicate odouriferous constituents. The flowers of certain plants yield no oil at all when distilled and hence must be processed by methods other than distillation.

2. *Enfleurage* (extraction with cold fat): This method is carried out only in France, where it is still practiced, but on a much smaller scale than in former years. The method is restricted to those flowers (jasmine, tuberose and a few others) which, after picking, continue their plant physiological activities in forming and emitting perfume. *Enfleurage*, in these cases, gives a much greater yield of flower oil than other methods. Despite this advantage, *enfleurage* has lately been replaced by

extraction with volatile solvents because *enfleurage* is a very delicate and lengthy process, requiring much experience and labour.

3. *Maceration* (extraction with hot fat): This process used to be applied to those flowers which gave a very small yield by distillation or by enfleurage. Maceration, however, has lately been almost entirely superseded by the modern process of extraction with volatile solvents.

4. *Volatile solvent process*: Of general application, this process is today applied to many types of flowers and carried out in several countries. It is technically the most advanced process, yielding concretes and alcohol soluble absolutes, the odour of which truly represents the natural flower oil as it occurs in the living flowers or in the plants.

Evaluation of Natural Flower Oils and Resinoids

The assay of distilled volatile oils has made remarkable progress during the last fifty years, probably because such oils are employed in much larger quantities than natural flower oils obtained by extraction with volatile solvents or by *enfleurage*. Moreover, the pharmaceutical profession, which uses many volatile oils, has always endeavoured to assay carefully any products employed as medicine. Yet it seems strange that so little attention should have been paid to the assay of such highly priced products as extracted flower oils, especially since it is common knowledge that sophistication of concretes and absolutes has become quite frequent, causing considerable loss to the often too credulous buyers. The reason for this neglect may be sought in the unfamiliarity of many users with these highly priced yet somewhat ambiguous products, the quality of which may depend upon many factors—methods of manufacturing, solvents used, degree of concentration, care in purification, etc. No wonder then that definite norms of quality do not yet exist and that the manufacturer may offer various explanations for deviations in his products. Indeed, some manufacturers market their natural flower oils in several grades, according to different degrees of dilution, in order to suit the usage and the purse of the users. Too, they claim that such 'standardisation' will guarantee a uniformity every year which nature alone does not achieve.

Natural flower oils, therefore, have remained strictly articles of confidence and the examination of them is usually carried out by simple olfactory tests. Even such tests, however, require an intimate knowledge of the subject, a well-trained sense of smell and familiarity with manufacturing methods and possible variations in quality, which very few buyers or even perfumers possess. Furthermore, any olfactory test should be based upon the comparison of an offered sample with standard samples of unquestioned purity and, if possible of the same age (such samples, unfortunately, are seldom on hand). It is surprising how the odour character of a natural flower oil may change during the first six months or year after its manufacture. Some odours improve for a certain period and then slowly deteriorate, assuming a somewhat sour or rancid note. Something of a parallel may be drawn with wines of young and older vintage. In view of these facts, it seems highly desirable and timely to establish definite and universal standard methods for the physico-chemical assay of natural flower oils and resinoids from gums, balsams and similar plant material.

The adaptation of routine methods as applied to distilled volatile oils cannot *per se* be extended to extracted flower oils or resinoids, as these products contain large proportions of natural substances which, although olfactorily inert, possess a variety of chemical functions which would make the interpretation of the analysis most difficult, if not outright impossible. Logically, any physico-chemical assay should, therefore, be applied mainly to the odouriferous portions of the extracted flower oils, which are usually identical with the volatile fraction. In other words, the extracted floral oil is steam distilled and the separated volatile portion examined by the usual tests for specific gravity, optical rotation, refractive index, acid number, ester number, ester number after acetylation, content of aldehydes, ketones, phenols, etc. Separation of the two portions by dry distillation at reduced pressure is inadvisable, because of the tendency toward pronounced and often destructive pyrolysis of the higher boiling constituents. Consequently, the method of distillation with steam suggests itself for the separation of volatile and nonvolatile portions.

The first attempts toward establishing such a standard method were made by Walbaum and Rosenthal who described an apparatus for the determination of the content in products distillable with steam from concrete and absolute flower oils. However, the separation of the volatile constituents from the waxes in this apparatus remains incomplete, even after 5 hours of distillation and gives much trouble, such as frothing, etc. Furthermore, live steam at atmospheric pressure causes hydrolysis and other chemical reactions. The method, therefore, can at best give only comparative results as far as the yield of volatile constituents is concerned and only if carried out under absolutely unvarying and most carefully controlled conditions.

There is a more reliable, accurate and practical method, using distillation with superheated steam under reduced pressure. When superheated, dry steam behaves like a gas, follows the gas laws and in the condensate yields a higher ratio of volatile aromatic constituents to carrier steam. Acting solely by its volumetric effect, dry, superheated steam is chemically less active than wet steam. Thus, with superheated steam it becomes possible to distil delicate esters and other compounds which would undergo hydrolysis with wet steam at the temperature of boiling water.

Further progress in the perfection of the assay of natural flower oils can be achieved by examing the content of volatile constituents of concretes and absolutes and also by codistilling these floral products of resinoids, etc. with ethylene glycol in a partial vacuum. Ethylene glycol is a more efficient carrier than steam and the waxes or residues remaining in the distilling flask will be practically devoid of any odouriferous compounds. The application of a partial vacuum reduces the distillation temperature to a degree not harmful to the delicate constituents of the floral oils. Sabetay's method possesses the added advantage of simplicity:

If a concrete or absolute is mixed with glycol and distilled under 8–15 mm pressure at a temperature of 900°–100°C, all of the volatile oil contained in the concrete or absolute can be driven over, separated and measured. For instance, weigh 1–10 grams of the concrete or absolute, add 25 cc. of ethylene glycol and distil at 90°–100°C; from a 50–100 cc. Claisen flask with Vigreux points, fitted with a thermometer, capillary tube and receiver and with a metaillic or oil bath as a source of heat. As a rule, the residue in the flask will have little odour, but, if necessary, 20 cc. more of ethylene glycol can be added and the distillation repeated a second and, possibly, a third time, until the distillate no longer becomes turbid upon addition of water. The combined distillate is diluted with water (or brine), treated with sodium chloride (if brine is not used) and extracted with three 20 cc. portions of a mixture of equal parts of pentane and ether. Dry the combined ether-pentane extracts over anhydrous sodium sulphate, remove most of the solvent by distillation, rinse the residue with pentane into a small Claisen flask with Vigreux points fitted with a capillary tube and heat gently under 50–100 mm pressure to constant weight. The volatile oil thus obtained may then be subjected to the usual physico-chemical tests.

By comparing the figures (yield of volatile oil from the absolute or concrete or resinoid, specific gravity, optical rotation, refractive index, acid and saponification number of the volatile oil) thus obtained with those of absolutely genuine products, conclusions can be drawn as to the purity of the flower oil sample investigated. The method of Sabetay may have to be modified in certain respects and will have to be applied to numerous lots of unquestionably pure natural flower oils before definite standards can be agreed upon by the trade. Naves prefers the use of superheated steam for the isolation of the volatile constituents from natural flower oils rather than codistillation with glycol, as certain constituents are relatively soluble in glycol-water solution.

Interpretation of Analytical Results

Before concluding it might be well to discuss briefly the interpretation of analytical results, as well as the deterioration and possible adulteration of natural flower oils.

If absolutely pure and manufactured according to unvarying methods and from flowers grown in the same geographical location, natural flower oils should be of similar character and show little variation, especially in regard to their content of volatile (distillable) portions and to the physicochemical properties of the volatile constituents. This, however, is not always the case, particularly with *enfleurage* products. The care exercised in the manufacturing process and especially in the final purification of the, product, exerts considerable influence upon its quality. The latter depends primarily upon the ratio between the weight of flowers treated during the entire *enfleurage* season and the weight of fatty vehicle (corps) employed. Thus a jasmine *pomade* will contain more volatile constituents and possess a much stronger odour if 1 kg of natural corps has been treated during the flowering season with 2.5 or 3.0 kg of jasmine flowers rather than only 1.5 kg of flowers. Concretes obtained by extracting the flowers three times with solvent, instead of only twice, will contain more waxes. An absolute obtained by extracting the concrete four or five times with alcohol, instead of only three times, will contain more alcohol soluble waxes and other inert material and correspondingly less volatile, odouriferous material.

Concretes and absolutes usually acquire a reddish colour upon ageing. This colour alteration, noticeable particularly in jasmine and orange flower extracts, may be attributed mainly to the presence of indole. The odour improves, usually, for a few months and assumes a harmonious fullness and depth lacking in the freshly extracted product. After a year or two of stability, depending of course upon proper storage, the product deteriorates gradually, finally acquiring a somewhat acid, rancid note, which is caused by the formation of acetic acid and ethyl acetate. This holds true especially if the product originally contained a small percentage of ethyl alcohol which was not removed during the final concentration. Hence, it is advisable to examine the aqueous phase of the analytical distillate, after extraction with ether, for its acid and ester number.

Pomades and absolutes of *enfleurage* are particularly susceptible to rancidity and development of acidity. In fact, even the freshly prepared absolutes of *enfleurage* show a relatively high acid number (which should not exceed 80), but this is caused by the presence of alcohol soluble free fatty extracted from the fat corps.

Adulteration of Natural Flower Oils

Adulteration of natural flower oils can be carried out in different ways, viz. by substitution with natural flower oils from lower priced geographical sources, by addition of volatile oils or fractions therefrom, aromatic isolates or synthetic aromatics or by dilution with inert materials. Thus, an absolute of jasmine marketed under the label of the Grasse region may contain the Egyptian product, a misrepresentation which, at present, can be detected only by olfactory tests, as we do not yet possess sufficient analytical data to differentiate between the products from these two geographical sources. The addition, to concretes, of exhausted natural flower waxes, obtained is alcohol insoluble residues in the preparation of alcohol soluble absolutes, results in a correspondingly lowered content of distillable volatile portions of the concrete. This can be proved by the above described distillation tests. Determination of the congealing point of the concrete may also give valuable hints in this respect. A dangerous form of adulteration consists in the addition, to concretes or absolutes, of both odourless matters such as exhausted waxes, fats or fatty oils and volatile, odouriferous compounds which occur also in the genuine flower oil, but which can be obtained synthetically or by isolation from lower priced essential oils. Thus benzyl acetate, benzyl alcohol, indole, etc. may be added to jasmine absolute; phenylethyl alcohol, rhodinol, etc. to rose absolute; linaloöl, linaloöl acetate, methyl anthranilate, etc. to orange flower absolute. If cleverly carried out by properly balancing the ratio between odourless nondistillable and odouriferous distillable compounds, such sophistication may give considerable trouble to the analyst, who will have to depend upon olfactory tests — and that, as pointed out, requires a highly trained and experienced sense of smell. Occasionally, natural flower oils are adulterated with odourless solvents such as diethyl phthalate.

When evaluating any natural flower oil, it is always advisable to test first for solvents and for alcohol. Traces of alcohol should not be objectionable as they are difficult to remove in the final purification during the manufacturing process without impairing the quality of the product. However, a flower oil should never contain any solvents like petroleum ether, benzene or, particularly, kerosene, because their presence indicates incomplete purification; they impart to the product an off-note most detrimental to the delicate odour of natural flower oils.

CONCENTRATED, TERPENELESS AND SESQUITERPENELESS ESSENTIAL OILS

Most essential oils consist of mixtures of hydrocarbons (terpenes, sesquiterpenes, etc.), oxygenated compounds (alcohols, esters, ethers, aldehydes, ketones, lactones, phenols, phenol ethers, etc.) and a small percentage of viscid or solid nonvolatile residues (paraffins, waxes, etc.). Of these the oxygenated compounds are the principal odour carriers, although the terpenes and sesquiterpenes, too, contribute in some degree to the total odour and flavour value of the oil. The oxygenated substances possess the added advantage of better solubility in dilute alcohol and with the exception of some aldehydes, of greater stability against oxidising and resinifying influences. Due to their unsaturated character, the terpenes and sesquiterpenes oxidise and resinify easily under the influence of air and light or under improper storing conditions which means spoilage of odour and flavour and lowering of the solubility in alcohol.

For many years, therefore, it has been the endeavor of the essential oil industry to supply the users with concentrated, terpeneless and sesquiterpeneless oils. Such oils consist mainly of oxygenated compounds; they are more soluble, more stable and much stronger in odour, yet retain most of the odour and flavour characteristics of the original oil.

The degree of concentration is automatically limited by the amount of oxygenated compounds present in the natural oil. For example, an orange oil containing only 2 per cent of oxygenated constituents and 98 per cent of terpenes, sesquiterpenes and waxes can, theoretically, be concentrated fifty times at the most, whereas a bergamot oil containing 50 per cent esters, alcohols, lactones, etc. and 50 per cent hydrocarbons can be concentrated only to double strength.

Before discussing in more detail the methods of manufacturing these concentrated, terpeneless and sesquiterpeneless oils, we should point out for clarity's sake that they must not be confused with the so-called isolates or aromatic isolates or commonly but incorrectly called 'synthetics' which are isolated from certain essential oils. For instance, citral can be isolated by fractionation or by chemical means from lemongrass oil, eugenol from clove oil, safrol from sassafras oil or camphor oil fractions, citronellal from citronella oil. These isolates may be converted chemically into other compounds, real synthetics, viz. citral into ionones, eugenol into vanillin, safrol into heliotropin, citronellal into citronellol, citronellyl acetate, hydroxy citronellal or synthetic menthol. Terpeneless and sesquiterpeneless oils have nothing to do with these isolates as the latter consist usually of only one well defined chemical substance, while the former are composed of several, often many, oxygenated compounds as present in the normal essential oil. Because of the different composition, the deterpenation of each essential oil requires a special process. The general method is based upon two principles: (i) removal of the terpenes, sesquiterpenes and paraffins by fractional distillation *in vacuo*, and (ii) by extraction of the more soluble oxygenated compounds with dilute alcohol or other solvents. In many cases, especially with citrus oils, a combination of the two methods may be employed.

The commercial term 'sesquiterpeneless' oils conventionally includes also the terpeneless oils. In some cases, especially when the content of sesquiterpenes in the natural oil is small, the two terms are employed synonymously. The trade designations and the names of the many brands on the market, however, are not always correct from the scientific point of view. It would be more appropriate to name these products 'concentrated oils,' 'terpeneless oils', and 'terpeneless and sesquiterpeneless oils'.

Concentrated oils are those from which only a part of the hydrocarbons have been removed. This can be done by simple fractional distillation *in vacuo*. According to the process applied and the intended concentration, a wide range of concentrated oils, with different properties, may be obtained. Thus, we speak of a twofold lemon or orange oil, a fivefold oil, etc. Terpeneless oils are those from which all or most of the terpenes and waxes have been removed, usually by fractional distillation. Terpeneless and sesquiterpeneless oils are those from which the terpenes, the sesquiterpenes and the waxes have been eliminated. The common manufacturing practice is to distil off *in vacuo* first the terpenes and then to extract the terpeneless oil with dilute alcohol or other solvents, whereby the sesquiterpenes and waxes are eliminated; or, the sesquiterpenes and waxes may be removed by further fractionation of the terpeneless oil *in vacuo*. The resulting terpeneless and sesquiterpeneless oil represents the highest possible concentration of a natural essential oil.

The manufacture of these products requires that the operator be well acquainted with the chemical composition, especially with the boiling ranges of the various terpenes, sesquiterpenes and oxygenated compounds occurring in the natural oil which he expects to concentrate. The boiling range of terpenes varies in most cases from 150° to 180°C at atmospheric pressure; that of sesquiterpenes from 240° to 280°C. The boiling points of most oxygenated compounds (terpene alcohols, aldehydes, esters, etc.) lie between those of the terpenes and sesquiterpenes. Phenols, phenol ethers and a few aromatic aldehydes form an exception, also the sesquiterpene alcohols, esters, etc. their boiling range falling into that of the sesquiterpenes or above. As far as solubility in dilute alcohol is concerned, the terpenes are, in general, only sparingly soluble, the paraffins and sesquiterpenes practically insoluble. The oxygenated compounds, on the other hand, possess in general much better solubility: the alcohols, aldehydes, ketones and phenols are most soluble, the esters and phenol ethers somewhat less soluble.

As pointed out, the terpenes may be removed by fractional distillation of the natural oil under reduced pressure. Most constituents of essential oils being deleteriously affected by heat, the distillation temperature must be kept as low as possible, which can be achieved with the aid of a good vacuum. For best results a well-constructed fractionation still as described in the section on 'distillation of essential oils' should be employed. It must be equipped with an efficient fractionation column.

It should be borne in mind that the terpenes cannot be removed quantitatively from a natural oil by mere fractional distillation; indeed, one of the greatest disadvantages of fractional distillation lies in the incomplete separation of the constituents, especially if their boiling points lie close together. A typical example is lemon oil which, aside from citral, contains also lower boiling aldehydes, such as octyl, nonyl and decyl aldehyde. If natural lemon oil is fractionated at 2 mm pressure, the lower boiling terpenes should come over first and theoretically the terpene fraction should contain no citral. However, even with a very efficient fractionation column, the aldehyde content of the terpene fraction will amount to about 1.0 per cent. The terpene fraction may be refractionated, but it will still retain small quantities of aldehydes; furthermore, repeated heating affects the flavour. Separation of the oxygenated compounds by chemical means is limited to certain cases only.

Repeated fractionation results in several intermediary fractions which consist of terpenes and a slight amount of oxygenated compounds, the latter increasing in proportion as the distillation temperature rises. Fractionation may be conducted in such a way that the residual oil is free from terpenes, but in this case the residual oil will be deprived also of those portions of the oxygenated constituents which have been carried over into the intermediary fractions. In order to recover these compounds, it will be necessary to refractionate the intermediary fractions, but, as said, prolonged heating is likely to have a deleterious effect upon the odour and especially the flavour of the fractions. Fractionation may be controlled by testing each fraction for solubility and for its rotatory power.

The elimination of the sesquiterpenes presents even more difficulties than that of the terpenes. In some cases the sesquiterpenes may be separated from the terpeneless oils by mere fractionation *in vacuo*, provided that the oils are not affected by the relatively high boiling temperature required for the distillation of sesquiterpenes (about $120°$–$140°C$ at 10 mm pressure) and by the partial overheating in the still which easily takes place. A vacuum of 3 to 5 mm. is desirable. In this case, too, the manufacturer must be familiar with the boiling points, at reduced pressure, of the various oil constituents. In some cases the differential in the boiling points of two compounds, as prevailing at atmospheric pressure, does not remain constant at reduced pressures; it may even be reversed. Too, every fraction should be tested for its rotatory power and for solubility in dilute alcohol, the insoluble ones to be rejected as containing mainly sesquiterpenes. Refractionation of the rejected fractions may be necessary. Even at a pressure of only 1 mm, a relatively high temperature is required to distil over the oxygenated compounds, most of them boiling between $90°$–$110°C$. Moreover, the temperature in the still itself will usually be about $10°C$ and even $20°C$ higher than the boiling point of the liquid and intense local heating occurs especially along the walls of the still. All these factors tend to impart to the oil a note which the expert easily recognises as 'distilled' or slightly 'burnt' as it does not occur in natural cold-pressed citrus oils, for example. Furthermore, the influence of heat seems to decompose the so-called 'molecular compounds' which some authorities assume to occur in natural oils. It is a well-known fact that, upon ageing, the odour of a perfume or flavour mixture changes and improves considerably. This may be caused by chemical reactions of functional groups—for example, by the interaction of alcohols and aldehydes which form acetals. Such compounds may exist in the natural oil and be decomposed upon heating and distilling.

Another method of removing the high boiling sesquiterpenes and waxes from the terpeneless oil consists in steam distilling the terpeneless oil at reduced pressure. This process is more gentle than dry distillation *in vacuo* and leaves the high boiling sesquiterpenes and waxes as residues in the still. In this case the distillate should be tested for solubility; any sesquiterpenes distilled over may be removed by treating the fractions with dilute alcohol. This method, however, has the inherent disadvantage that compared with dry vacuum distillation it takes much longer, especially in the case of oils containing a large percentage of high boiling compounds. Also, certain constituents of an oil are liable to dissolve in the distillation water, e.g. phenylethyl alcohol or eugenol. In this case the distillation water has to be returned into the still for cohobation.

In view of these inadequacies, some manufacturers remove all remaining terpenes and sesquiterpenes from concentrated oil by extracting the latter with dilute alcohol. The strength of the alcohol to be employed for this purpose depends primarily upon the solubility of the oxygenated compounds. Thus, the concentrated oil from which most of the terpenes and sesquiterpenes have been eliminated by fractionation *in vacuo* or by steam distillation under reduced pressure is shaken for some time with fifteen to twenty times its volume of dilute alcohol, for instance, with 60 per cent alcohol by volume; or the concentrated oil is first dissolved in the corresponding volume of strong alcohol and then the required amount of distilled water is gradually added with continuous stirring until the desired degree of alcohol dilution is reached. In both cases the turbid mixture should be cooled for a prolonged period and set aside until clarified. Thus, the oxygenated constituents dissolve in the dilute alcohol, while the terpenes and sesquiterpenes remain undissolved and (together with traces of oxygenated compounds) may be separated.

Because of the small differential in the specific gravity of the undissolved parts of the oil and that of the solution, emulsions may form and the separation of the two layers may require some time. In order to break the emulsion, small quantities of low boiling petrol ether are added or the emulsion may be separated by centrifuging. The undissolved oil is repeatedly treated with dilute alcohol in order to extract any quantities of oxygenated compounds which it might still retain.

The clear solution of oxygenated compounds in dilute alcohol is then transferred into a still and the alcohol fractionated off at reduced pressure, until only oil and water remain in the still. The two layers of oil and water can easily be separated. The employment of an efficient condenser will prevent losses of alcohol. The recovered alcohol and the residual water may be used again for treating the next batch of oil. No standard method has been adopted yet for the preparing of terpeneless and sesquiterpeneless oils and every manufacturer uses his own process. It has been found that terpeneless and sesquiterpeneless citrus oils are manufactured in Sicily by first removing the terpenes by fractional distillation. The sesquiterpenes are then eliminated from the terpeneless oil by extracting the oil with dilute alcohol, the strength of which should be somewhat lower than that in which the sesquiterpeneless oils must finally be soluble. The sesquiterpeneless oil is separated from the alcoholic solution by the addition of water or by distilling off the alcohol under reduced pressure. This constitutes the general method described previously and with some modifications it forms, today, the basis of most commercial processes.

A more novel process in which the natural oil is extracted by two solvents which are only partially soluble in one another—for instance, pentane and dilute methyl alcohol. The two solvents are made to flow, according to the countercurrent principle, through a horizontal glass cylinder and the oil is entered in the middle. The terpenes dissolve in the pentane phase, the oxygenated compounds in the methylalcohol phase. After separation of the two phases, the solvents are removed by distillation, only low temperatures being necessary. This, is the principal advantage of their method, aside from the fact that high-grade terpeneless oils are obtained in almost quantitative yield. The principal difficulties of this process lie in the necessity of working with large volumes of solvents, furthermore, in the tendency toward formation of emulsions which, however, might be broken in some cases by the addition of 0.1 per cent of citric or tartaric acid.

After having discussed the various methods of manufacturing terpeneless and sesquiterpeneless oils, it might be advisable to add a few words about their concentration, as there exists a great deal of confusion regarding this point. The price lists and tables on the concentration of terpeneless and sesquiterpeneless oils issued by the various essential oil houses differ widely in regard to their concentration value. Yet, the theoretical concentration could be calculated only from the actual yield of terpeneless or sesquiterpeneless oil as obtained from a given weight of natural oil. However, the actual odour and flavour strength of two oils, although of the same theoretical concentration, may differ, concentration not being necessarily proportionate to odour and flavour strength. Let us assume, for instance, that 100 kg of natural lemon oil are converted into terpeneless oil and that the yield is 8 kg of terpeneless oil containing about 40 to 45 per cent of citral (some citral has been destroyed by distillation and, besides, the oxygenated compounds cannot be completely freed of terpenes). In this case the actual concentration of the oil, but not necessarily of the flavour, is obviously twelve and one-half times.

It is difficult, if not impossible, to indicate general and definite limits for the physico-chemical properties of concentrated, terpeneless and sesquiterpeneless oils because of the fact that these properties depend upon the degree of concentration and upon the relative proportions of oxygenated constituents originally present. Furthermore, every manufacturer has his own standards which are based upon this particular manufacturing process.

On analysing the physico-chemical properties of more than fifty terpeneless and sesquiterpeneless oils, it has been found that the specific gravity affords a valuable clue to the presence of any remaining terpenes. These hydrocarbons possess a low specific gravity and refractive index and their complete removal should raise the specific gravity and refractive index of the terpeneless oil relative to that of the original oil. The determination of the optical rotation, too, provides a good indication regarding the extent to which the terpenes have been eliminated. By far the most important criterion for a terpeneless and sesquiterpene less oil is its solubility in dilute alcohol, 70 per cent ethyl alcohol usually being employed for this purpose. A terpeneless oil should usually be soluble in 3 to 10 volumes of 70 per cent alcohol, while a sesquiterpeneless oil should be more soluble.

Aside from the determination of the physico-chemical properties, it is advisable to test a terpeneless or sesquiterpeneless oil also for its content of oxygenated compounds, especially for alcohols, esters and aldehydes, which can be done by the usual analytical methods. A method of evaluating and examining terpeneless lemon oils which is based on treating the aldehyde-free oil with 51 per cent alcohol to remove all oxygenated compounds and on measuring the quantity of terpenes and sesquiterpenes left. For this purpose, 10 cc. of the oil is first treated with a solution of neutral sodium sulphite which removes the aldehydes. The remaining, unabsorbed oil is shaken with 100 times its volume of 51 per cent alcohol in a separatory funnel, cooled to about –2°C and left for a period of 6 hours or more, until the liquids have completely separated when the lower layer can be removed. After washing the oil layer with a further quantity of 51 per cent alcohol, all undissolved oil is transferred to a burette tube and its volume carefully measured. From this amount the percentage of nonoxygenated constituents of the original oil can be determined. In order to obtain more exact results the terpeneless oil is first fractionated and process applied to both the first and the last fraction. However, this method is not absolutely quantitative, as some terpenes will dissolve in the weak spirit, also because the transfer of the oils from the separatory funnel to the measuring burette always causes some loss.

The main advantage of the terpeneless and especially of the sesquiterpeneless oils consists in their better solubility in dilute alcohol. The employment of these oils, therefore, effects a considerable saving of alcohol in the finished goods; odour and flavour of the oil are better utilised. A further advantage consists in the fact that, by the process of concentration, the oils are also freed of any products of decomposition or resinification which might result from improper handling or ageing of the natural oils. Another merit of the terpeneless and sesquiterpeneless oils lies in, their better stability. While natural citrus oils are apt to resinify, primarily due to polymerisation of certain hydrocarbons, the concentrated oils are much more stable. Thus, they may be employed in powders, for the flavouring of gelatine desserts, for example or for the scenting of bath salts.

The introduction of terpeneless and sesquiterpeneless oils on the market has met with some resistance. Several authorities contend that the elimination of terpenes and sesquiterpenes removes also a part of the characteristic odour and flavour of the natural oil. The application of heat undoubtedly has some effect on the delicate flavouring constituents of the oil and, if improperly prepared, concentrated oils may not display the freshness and bouquet of the original oil. Furthermore, the terpeneless and sesquiterpeneless oils contain a lower proportion of natural fixatives such as waxes and stearoptenes which contribute to the retaining of the flavour on the palate. Weighing the advantages against the disadvantages, the conclusion may be drawn that concentrated, terpeneless and sesquiterpeneless oils have their definite place in many formulas where highest possible concentration, solubility and stability are required, but that they cannot replace the natural oils for all purposes.

EFFICIENCY OF DISTILLATION

Efficient distillation system can be defined as any system capable of extracting and recovering maximum quantity of oil in a shortest possible time utilising minimum steam, will be considered as efficient distillation system.

Extraction of oil is one part of the system and recovery is another. Recovery of oil can be 100 per cent in case there is no escape/conversion of the extracted oil by way of reflux or hydrophyllic effect of poor condensation/separation or otherwise. Further, it should be understood that one particular system may be termed as efficient for one type of herbs but may prove inefficient for another type of herbs. Even the system can behave differently under the varying conditions for any particular oil.

Factors Affecting Efficiency

The factors which affects efficiency of a distillation system can be summarised as under:
1. Nature of herb surface.
2. Quality/quantity of steam.
3. Density of charge.
4. Size of still.
5. Pressure of still.

Nature of herb surface

Herb surface can be divided into three categories:
1. Highly absorptive.
2. Moderately absorptive.
3. Poorly absorptive.

Under the first category, herbs like, lavender and to some extent Russian Mint (EC 41911) are classified which possess thick hairy surfaces. These herbs have considerable absorption power and can absorb plenty of moisture even when in a fresh stage. These type of herbs require no drying or wilting before distillation.

Under the second category, herbs like, M.piperita, M.citrata, M.arvensis, Basil and Geranium fall. These herbs have a flat surface which can be made absorptive by partial drying under sun or shade for one or two days. Partially dried or wilted herbs of this category behave as good as highly absorptive herbs. Herbs of cymbopogan species can also be classified in this category but their oil is not freely available as is the case with other herbs mentioned above.

Under the third category, herbs like, eucalyptus, cinnamon/clove leaf and also citrus leaves are classified which possess flat and smooth surface. The oil is also situated well below the outer surface of the parent herb and is not exposed on the surface of herb.

The absorption capacity of the herb directly affects the formation of heat transfer area which is one of the vital factors for the evaporation of oil. The effective size of oil-water interface, already termed as 'heat transfer area' will be much enhanced if the two liquids tend to intermingle with each other where they meet. In fact, the two mutually insoluble liquids, oil and water, tend to form a heterogeneous mixture when they are in contact on absorptive surfaces.

This can be demonstrated by allowing the spreading areas from a drop of each liquid to meet on a blotting paper: (i) drop of oil (mint) and water spreading on paper, and (ii) the spreading area of oil and water meet and the intermingling of oil and water has created more surface area (Fig. 5.28).

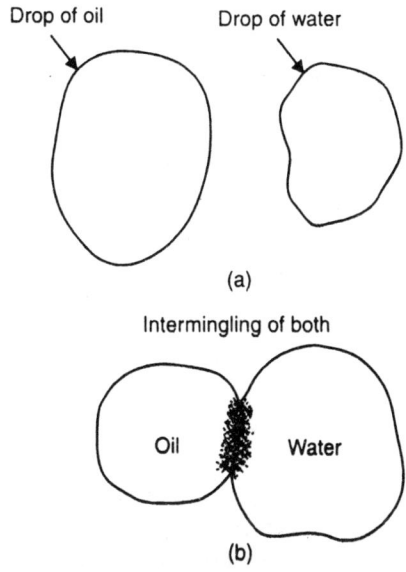

Fig. 5.28. Intermingling of oil and water.

Another example of distillation of fresh mint herb with wet steam will explain the effect of this factor more clearly. When fresh mint leaves are distilled, their surfaces become flooded by liquid from collapsing aqueous plant cells as well as condensation and cloud particles from the steam. The oil glands are also ruptured but the oil floats on the water and no intermingling with it can take place. In such cases, distillation is slow because there is very little surface area to transfer the heat of evaporation. Also the recovery of oil is very poor because of the downward reflux flow is washing the oil to the bottom of the still.

A similar example can be seen when herb is soaked by rain water and then all attempts to distil the oil are prolonged and the resulting yield is also very low.

In all these cases, the absorptive capacity of the herb has been spoiled by the excessive water present on the surface of herb. When distillations of such herbs are over, one can observe a lot of discoloured water at the bottom of stills which reflects towards the inefficiency of the system and shows that some of the oil has gone into it after conversion. Thus, by intermingling of oil and water, more interfaces are created or more surface area is made available for steam to condense and impart its latent heat to the oil for evaporation. Nature of herb surface will determine the effective surface area available as interfaces.

Quality/Quantity of Steam

Steam is required to fulfil the following functions:

1. Provide latent heat of evaporation besides raising the temperature of the mass.

2. Provide necessary current to remove saturated vapours of oil from surface of the herb as soon as these are formed.

3. Assist in moisture balance.

The jobs under 1 and 2 are performed by maintaining proper flow of steam to the still. As the extraction time is directly proportional to the quantity of steam delivered to the still, it is most advisable to maintain a proper rate of supply of steam. Generally, it should not be less than 2 kgs/min/m^2 of cross sectional area of the still at the top. However, the preferred rate of delivery of steam is 3 to 4 kgs/min/m^2. Of equal importance is the need that the steam's upward current through the charge, opposing any downward flow of liquids, dripping or gathering speed/volume from one layer to the other, should be able to neutralise this. This downward dripping, known as 'reflux' can wash down some of the oil to the bottom of the still.

In case the rate of flow of steam is slow, there are ample chances of reflux of internally available water and juices from collapsing aqueous plant cells.

It is usually indicated by an excessive accumulation of discoloured water in the bottom of a still.

This tendency is increased when wet steam from a direct fired still is used to distil non-absorptive herb which has little ability to absorb any moisture. These oils require time to diffuse to the herb surface and cannot be exhausted from the lower levels of charge before the reflux flow gets established. Such non-absorptive herbs can be fresh herbs or rain soaked herbs.

While it will always be necessary to run the steam at a rate sufficient to stop any loss of oil by a downward flow of reflux, it may be advisable to restrict the speed of steam to minimum.

Another function of steam relates to its quality. Steam can be saturated or superheated. A saturated steam carries microscopic particles of liquid water in the form of 'cloud'. Only superheated steam will be without any cloud. General purpose commercial boilers will generate steam with dryness fraction of 0.98 to 0.97 which means that the steam consists of 98 to 97 per cent dry saturated vapours and 2 to 3 per cent of liquid cloud particles. Similarly, a wet steam may carry more liquid particles, say, up to 10 to 15 per cent. When the steam is generated below the still by direct firing, the condition of steam is wet unless proper arrangements of baffles have been provided at the bottom.

In case steam is generated in a separate boiler under pressure, say, up to 70 to 100 psi, while the stills are operating at over 3 to 5 per cent of its own weight of liquid water as it expands on entering the still. Thus the steam will loose all its cloud particles and will behave just as superheated steam or evaporate some more water particles out of the bottom layers of herbs in order to restore the saturation conditions.

Let us discuss why the distiller should have a choice to use either wet, dry or superheated steam as the situation demands. The correct moisture content of steam is very important for the efficient distillation of oil. The optimum level varies considerably with the individual nature and conditions of a herb. The capacity of herb to absorb more moisture will determine which type of steam is best suited.

In practice, there are circumstances in which a herb is too wet to distil effectively. In such cases, it is useful to deliver superheated steam to dry off the plant surfaces to some extent. On the other hand, in case the condition of the herb is absorptive, like, fresh lavender or moderately absorptive, like, wilted mint or basil, the use of slightly wet steam is recommended.

To summarise this, it can be said, while distilling a partially dried mint or basil, one should not expect better results just by passing a steam generated from a separate boiler at 70 to 100 psi or similarly it will be a tough task to distil a fresh mint or basil in a direct fired still producing wet steam.

Absorptive herb	Wet steam
Moderately absorptive herb	Dry steam
Poorly absorptive herb	Wet steam and/or superheated steam

Density of charge

Uniform density of material in the still is always advantageous. When the charge is uniformly packed, there are narrow openings between the plant pieces. Thus, the rate of displacement of steam over the herb surface is fast and chances of channeling are less. Channeling is one of the causes of prolonged distillations and sometimes patches of herb are left unextracted. In case the packing of charge is not uniform, steam will pass through the most convenient route, i.e. path of least resistance.

Even after prolonged distillation the result would be high water/oil ratio and also undistilled patches of herbs where packing is more dense.

In practice it has been found that pack density should be between 300 to 400 kgs/m^3. Another question arises, whether steam should be used to soften the material at the time of packing or not.

Many experiments have been conducted and its has been found that compared to the charge that was packed without steam assistance, the steam pressed charge consumed more steam. It has also been observed that whenever steam is used for packing a charge and the capacity of the boiler is not big enough to supply steam at a desired rate, the distillation is prolonged to 2 to 2.5 hours and the chances of reflux are more.

It is a good practice to pack the material with the assistance of manual labour till the still is filled up to the top. Then steam can be released only for about 10 to 15 minutes prior to closing the lid to compact material further. This is common practice of packing the charge for various mints and basil, semi-dried, adopted by many successful distillation units.

Further, it will be seen that packing more herb inside the still will improve yield by reducing losses of oil due to hydrophillic effect.

Size of still

Before considering the effect of height/diameter of still on the efficiency of distillation, it is worthwhile to consider the hydrophillic effect as applicable to absorptive and non-absorptive type of herbs.

It has been observed that in many cases wet steam from a calendria fitted below the stills achieves better yield in a shorter period than a dry steam from a high pressure boiler. This phenomenon is explained with the help of hydrophillic bonding whereas the liquid cloud particles in wet steam would roll up coatings of oil when they impinge on its exposed surfaces in the still. By rolling up coatings of oil and carrying them further up the still, the cloud particles are assisting the movement of oil through the charge without evaporating the same. Sometimes their rate of movement towards the top is well above the rate of vapourisation of the oil which the steam can achieve. Thus, the oil reaches to the top of charge much faster with wet steam than with dry steam.

These cloud particles coated with film of oil lodge on herb surfaces further up the still and are duly vapourised in the usual way. But those which escape through the top of the charge and go through the condenser/receiver will be far too small to rise through the mother liquor and be caught by any normal separator. These oil coatings will be lost in distillate water and is termed as 'loss due to hydrophillic bonding'.

The extent of loss of oil due to hydrophillic bonding will depend on the following factors:

1. Nature of surface of herb.
2. Height of still.
3. Density of packing.

In the case of absroptive herbs, the cloud particles with coatings of oil will roll up towards the top and get absorbed and even mix up with exposed oil patches near the top layers. So the loss is **negligible**.

However, in case the height of the still is not sufficient to allow these cloud particles to settle on any of the layers some of these will just pass on to the receiver and lost in distillate water. Similarly, uniform density of packing, between 300 and 400 kgs/m³ will also provide more herb surfaces for the above purpose. It has been found that heights below 1.3 metres are not capable of holding most of such particles.

However, in case of nonabsorptive herbs, such as, eucalyptus, the losses due to hydrophillic bonding may be quite serious. Surfaces of such type of herbs are flat and smooth and possess very little capaciy to absorb these cloud particles with roll on coatings of oil. In many cases, the loss is to the extent of 20 to 30 per cent of the recovered oil. It would be considered a good practice in case the stills for such type of herbs are kept above two metres deep and herbs are also properly comminuted. A properly comminuted herb will provide more surface area for absorption and also packing of charge would be more uniform.

Diameter of the still has not much bearing upon the efficiency of distillation till sufficient steam is available to maintain the flow per sq. m. area. Generally it varies from one to two metres.

Pressure of still

Herbs which contain high boiling oils which are chemically stable at higher temperature associated with high pressure distillation, are best distilled under pressure.

When a distillation is carried out under pressure, the following two parameters are affected:

1. Density of steam.
2. Temperature gradient.

Besides the fact that distillation takes place at higher temperature.

These factors do have a bearing on efficiency of distillation:

1. In case the pressure inside the still is raised from one atm. to two atm., the density of the steam or in turn, the mass of steam is raised to 1.5 times. This indicates that 1.5 times more steam is in contact with the charge or the oil receives its latent heat of evaporation at 1.5 times the former rate and boils away faster with no increase in the rate of flow of steam.
2. Similarly, by increasing the pressure inside the still, the temperatures gradient between the general vapour space and the oil's point of evaporation on the herb surface also increases.

These factors helps in reducing the extraction time as the rate of evaporation of oil increases on account of above factors.

Data for a typical case is shown in Table 5.5.

Table 5.5. Effect of operating pressure on water to oil ratio in steam distillation of citronellal.

Total pressure mm Hg	Temperature °C	Vapour pressure mm Hg		Molal ratio water/citronellal	Weight ratio
		Water	Citronellal		
152.2	60	149.5	2.66	56.2	6.6
238.5	70	233.8	4.70	49.2	5.9
263.7	80	355.5	8.20	43.3	5.1
540.0	90	526.0	14.00	37.6	4.4
782.5	100	760.0	22.50	33.8	3.9

These data demonstrate that operation at reduced pressure results in a lower operating temperature, but also requires the use of more steam per weight unit of Citronellal recovered. Operation at elevated pressure (use of high pressure steam in the still), on the other hand, permits a considerable saving in the amount of steam required per weight unit of oil, but also involves a higher operating temperature.

The higher temperatures associated with saturated steam under increased pressures may also accelerate diffusion of the oils to the surface because of the greater molecular activity. The loss of oil due to hydrophillic effect is also reduced as the vapours before entering the condenser, are expanded, thus vapourising the cloud particles (coated with film of oil) which have escaped from the still.

On the other hand, it has been found that the oils of herbs containing linalyl acetate as main ingredient, such as lavender oil, *M.citrata* oil, lanaloe berry oil when distilled under reduced pressure, consists of much higher quantities of linalyl acetate, an ester which apparently is hydrolised in ordinary steam distillation. Similar is the effect of steam distillation of lavender at high altitudes where atmospheric pressure is low.

After evaluating the effect of all these factors on efficiency of distillation, it becomes ample clear that no set rules can be laid down for distillation of a particular herb. Specific trials are to be conducted to arrive at the best possible practice for the most efficient distillation of any herb.

So, an efficient distillation system can be defined as 'a package of practice adopted by an operator for the extraction of oil from a herb after taking into consideration the nature and condition of herb, availability of steam and its quality and utilising the equipment for the maximum recovery of oil in a shortest period.

PRACTICAL DISTILLATION OF HERBS

For the purpose of establishing the most efficient system of distillation for various herbaceous oils, it would be worthwhile to divide these into two categories.

Surface Born Oils

Surface born oils are those which are entirely born on the outer surface of the herb. These oils are secreted in glandular hair reservoirs which are even visible with an ordinary microscope mints, lavender, basils, etc. are typical of this class. Broadly herbs of families, like *Labiatae, Verbenacease, Geraniaceae, Myrterceae* and *Rutaceae* belong to this category.

Some of the herbs under this class, are absorptive by nature while others can be made absorptive by air-drying/wilting in shade. Distillation of these herbs is rather simple operation. Unless the herbs are of highly absorptive type, such as, lavender, it is always advisable to dry the herb under sun for few hours and then under shade for 10–12 hours till at least 50 per cent of the moisture is evaporated. The practice adopted by farmers of Uttar Pradesh can be followed whereas they leave the herb in open field after harvesting for the rest of the day and then collect the same next day morning before the sun rises. Thus leaves get semi-dried and shading of leaves is also avoided.

Too much drying of herb in field or under the sun or at distillation site is also not recommended as it results in losses of oil by evaporation into air which may go up to 20 to 30 per cent. Subsequently, distillation also becomes tough as it becomes impossible to pack the material inside the still uniformly and at the desired density. As a result, possibility of channeling of steam increases, losses due to hydrophillic bonding increases and the time in extracting the oil is prolonged.

Further it should be remembered that the formation of oil in herbs belonging to this category is mostly affected by extrinsic factors, such as, air temperature, relative humidity, cloudiness and rainfall, etc. Moreover, the plant tissue are alive and continue their biological activities to some extent even after a few hours of harvesting the plant. Some metabolic transformations of glycosides takes place during the stage of drying when the plant is under drying stress and hence any loss by evaporation of oil is more than compensated by the gain in oil formation by metabolic transformations.

Both types of stills, i.e. direct fired (fitted with calendria on the bottom) and also fed by a separate oil, are suitable for distilling herbs of this category. For efficient distillation, the following parameters should be maintained:

1. Height of still   > 1.3 metres
2. Density of packing   300 to 350 kgs/m^3
3. Condition of herb   Semi-dried
4. Flow rate of steam   > 120kgs/hr/m^2

Steam should not be used for packing of charge and also the distillation of fresh herb should be avoided (except for lavenders) because of the following reasons:

1. Yields of oil would be low.
2. Steam consumption would be high.
3. Time taken for exhausting would be long.

Further, it would be nearly impossible to distill a fresh herb or rain-soaked herb in a direct fired still which produces wet steam. Distillation of fresh herbs require dry steam or even superheated steam in the beginning to evaporate the extra moisture available on the surface of the herb.

Packing a fresh herb inside the still may also cause tight spots and give rise to channeling.

Moisture balance of still

An operator has to decide on various parameters while planning to distil a herb. Many of the parameters are fixed and once the conditions of charge is decided, he has to decide on the quality and quantity of steam. His decision should be governed by the factor called the 'moisture balance of the still'.

As the moisture is present in both herb as well as steam used for distillation, a balance has to be maintained in order to obtain the best results. In case the quantity of moisture in herb is more, i.e. herb is wet, the quantity of moisture or cloud particles in steam should be quite low, i.e. steam should be dry or superheated. Similarly, in case the moisture in herb is low, i.e. its condition is dry, then the moisture in steam should be high, i.e. wet steam should be used. This adjustment of moisture content in the still is termed as moisture balance of the still and operator has to be conscious of this at all stages. For highly absorptive type of herbs, this balance can be maintained on plus side for better results.

Centre Born Oils

So far we have discussed the distillation of surface born oils which was easier than herbs having centre born oils. Centre born oils are those which are found in schizogenous ducts occurring in the leaves, calyces and stem (e.g. *Lauraceae* and *compositae*) and also oils found in secondary ducts called vittae which are schizogenously formed on the fruits and roots (e.g. *Umbelliferae* and *zingiberaceae*). Thus, oils found in many seeds, root and wood species are classified under these headings. The formation of oil in these materials is least affected by changes in meteorological conditions. Thus, it is possible to store them for certain period depending upon the nature of individual herb.

Centre born oils are secreted deep below the outer surface of the herb and are not exposed on the surface. So, their distillation becomes a two step process:

1. To bring out the oil from centre to the outer surface.
2. To evaporate the oil from the outer surface (as in the case of surface born oils).

Before undertaking the distillation of any centre born oil, the strategy should be defined as to how the oil has to be forced out of its centre, i.e. place of location. An usual process which assist this process of movement is comminution of the herb material. This may best be done by crushing in between rollers so that the material is reduced to flattened surfaces similar to a coin placed under the wheel of a passing train. Similarly, woods can be reduced to chips and some of the seeds/roots can also be pulverised to a coarse size. In many cases the purpose is to break the outer casing only. Hard leaves can also be chopped suitably which will assist in packing charge more uniformly.

Theory of Hydro-Diffusion

It has been noted that distillation of oil bearing seeds proceeds at a much faster rate when seeds are soaked in water prior to distillation.

It was also observed that when uncomminuted seeds were distilled the oxygenated compounds of the oil, which have greater affinity to water but are less volatile, are distilled first. Conversely, when seeds are comminuted, the more volatile hydrocarbons which have low affinity to water comes first.

This can be explained by the fact that while the seeds are comminuted some portion of the oil is secreted and is exposed to steam just like a surface born oil.

It, therefore, seems quite clear that liquid water plays a significant role in bringing deeply secreted oils to the herb surface.

There is no doubt that hot water softens the plants materials and penetrates towards the centre where oil molecules are located. The secreted oil components are presumed to have sufficient affinity for water to enable the diffusion process to set up, by which the oil tends to equalize its concentration by intermingling with water particles and thus diffusion to the surface. The oil diffused to the surface is evaporated and carried away by steam and thus more and more oil diffuses to the surface to be evaporated by steam as a surface born. This process of hydro-diffusion is quite slow and, as such, the distillation time is prolonged.

Unless water distillation is adopted, the process, of comminuting should not be carried too for. In case the material is reduced to fine size, the interspaces within the plant charge would then becomes too small and the rising steam would find it difficult to penetrate all parts of the charge uniformly. Very small interspaces necessitate a slow, ineffective distillation, because any increase in pressure would cause the steam to break in channels through plant charge or to hurl part of the charge into condenser, causing further trouble.

Effects of fatty oils

When a plant material is comminuted, very high boiling or practically non-volatile substances such as, resins, paraffins and waxes, fatty oils (contained in other cells and glands) mix with and dissolve in the freed volatile oil; thereby, substantially lowering its vapour pressure and reducing its rate of vapourisation. This occurs particularly in the case of seeds, most of which contain large quantities of fatty oils. The fatty oil content of some of the seeds are reported as follows:

Seeds	Oil %
Ajowan	33.20
Anise	18.59
Caraway	16.06
Coriander	26.40
Fennel	16.71

Such relatively large quantities of fatty, nonvolatile oils are well capable of reducing the vapour pressure and thereby the rate of vapourisation of the volatile oils dissolved in these fatty oils.

Further, it is suggested to keep the height of still more while distilling centre born oils. These are two reasons to support this view:

1. The rate of diffusion of oil is slow than the rate of evaporation. So, the steam can be enriched with more vapours of oil while passing through layers of plant materials in case they are more in number. This will improve the oil's ratio in distillate which ultimately will affect the extraction time or efficiency of distillation.

2. The surfaces of plant materials under this class are not absorptive and hence any hydrophillic bonded oil with liquid droplets of water will pass through the still untrapped unless the height of charge is sufficient to hold these back.

Effect of quality/quantity of steam

Another most important factor in the distillation of this category of oils is to decide about the quality and quantity of steam to be injected. In this connection, it would be useful to repeat that there are two mechanisms which help in extraction of oil which are given below:

1. Evaporation by steam.
2. Upward movement of oil by hydrophillic bonding.

In case oil is to be extracted by evaporation only then dry steam would be the ideal choice. Steam consumption would be low in comparison to other method but rate of distillation would also be slow. In such cases, only sufficient moisture has to be maintained on the surface of the charge to expedite the diffusion of oil from the inner ducts of the outer surface. For this reason, steam has to be generated at somewhat high pressure in the boiler to enable the steam to expand and loose its moisture while entering into the still. This is termed as 'dry steam distillation'.

Similarly, the other possible way is to utilise the gain by movement of oil by hydrophillic bonding. In that case only wet steam has to be passed. The cloud particles present in the steam would roll on oil coatings to the top of charge where these can be evaporated as surface born oils. As ample moisture is available on the surface, the diffusion is also better. However, the flow of steam has to be kept on the higher side so as to avoid the risk of reflux inside the still. Even the ordinary, direct fired stills fitted with calendria can serve this purpose. The only disadvantage is that consumption of steam is more and whenever the flow of steam is not sufficient, condensation of steam inside the still is so high that it starts washing the charge downwards. This reflux is apparent by accumulation of more discoloured water on the bottom of the still at the end of distillation. This causes loss of oil. This is termed as 'Wet Steam Distillation'. For obtaining best results, while using wet steam, these parameter should be adhered to:

1. Height of still should be around 2 to 2.5 metres.
2. Density of charge should be above 300 kgs/m^3.
3. Flow rate of steam should be 200 kgs/hr/m^2 or more.

Whether distillation is by dry or wet steam, density of packing should be very uniform and there should be narrow interstices between the pieces through which steam can pass. The comminuted material may be in the form of chips, granules or cut leaves but it must not be reduced to a powder form which can coagulate and block the passage of steam. Materials which are in powder form are more suited to fully immersed water distillation. Sometimes distillation of seeds such as dillseeds, coriander pose a problem of channeling of steam when the seeds for 0.5 to 1 hour. It becomes tough for steam to penetrate such a charge and thus distillation time is prolonged. The preferred way of avoiding such a situation is to mix some straw with seeds (outer skin broken) and thus allowing uniform space to penetrate. The early part of the distillation should be run slowly until all the air has been expelled from the hollow straws.

It is worth considering that if flow of steam is 200 kgs/hr/sqm through a well packed charge, the linear speed of the steam through the interstices between the plant pieces is about 14 cm per second. It can easily blow clear passages through charges of fine materials and thus following open passages. Thus, it is advisable to keep the rate of flow of steam just sufficient to avoid 'reflux'. This will lessen the risk of 'rate holes' in the charge. Whenever a material is comminuted certain fines are obtained. The best practice to distil these fines is to mix these into the upper parts of the charge, just below the top layer. These should not be sprayed on the top layer lest these are blown through the condenser and washed into the receiver. The charge should be loaded in the still immediately after the comminution to avoid loss of oil by evaporation which is quite possible as more surfaces containing oil are exposed to air. In case it is not possible to load the charge at once, it should be packed in bags and kept in a cool place where no wind can pass.

Another problem associated with distillation of high boiling oils is the extended distillation times, sometimes running into days. In case wet steam is used containing sufficient moisture to support heat transference and hydro-diffusion after it has filtered through to the top of the tall charge, then, in most of the cases, the lower layers of plant material may become flooded before the oil is extracted. It becomes highly difficult and slow to distil the oil from these layers.

However, this problem can be solved by using superheated steam to reduce the water flooding the herb surfaces. When the distillate ratio returns to normal, the system can be reverted back to saturated steam. Thus use of saturated and superheated steams, alternatively, helps in faster recovery of oil.

WATER DISTILLATION

Water distillation is the most ancient system of distillation of herbs. In modern times this practice is only occasionally adopted. However, there are several plant materials which are unsuited to steam distillation and can only be distilled while immersed in water.

Steam has a tendency to coagulate the petals of flowers, like, rose and neroli, etc. and as such, vapour cannot pass through coagulated mass. Similarly materials which have been finely powdered will also coagulate and form lumps thus giving rise to channeling. Water distillation is the only choice for such materials. Let us consider various factors which affect the vapourisation of oil from the surface of herb when water distillation is adopted.

Effect of Oil's Affinity for Water

Some of the components of the oil have affinity for water. Such compounds, generally oxygenated are water soluble, such as, phenols and phenyl ethyl alcohol in Rosa damascena. Such compounds get dissolved in water and their recovery becomes quite slow as the mixture boils like an azeotropic mixture whereby the proportion of oil in vapours is quite small.

At the end of distillation, these dissolved compounds can be recovered by fractional distillation or in some cases by adding salt and separating on settlement.

In such cases, it is always advisable to reuse the mother liquor left in the still for subsequent distillations.

Effects of Hydrolysis

Another phenomenon accompanying water distillation of plant materials is hydrolysis. Hydrolysis can be defined as a chemical reaction between water and certain constituents of essential oil. In the presence of water, particularly at elevated temperatures, esters tend to react with water to form parent acids and alcohols. In case the amount of water is large, the amounts of alcohols and acid will also be large and hydrolysis will proceed to a greater extent. As a result, yield as well as the quality of essential oil will go down. In case of steam distillation, the degree of hydrolysis is much less. Another important characteristic of hydrolysis reaction is that these are not rapid and hence their degree of reaction depends upon time of contact between oil and water which is much more in the case of water distillations.

Effect of Temperature/Pressure Differential

Another factor which has got considerable bearing on the recovery of essential oil in water distillation is the difference of pressure and temperature on the bottom of the still and the top of herb/water surface. Temperature/pressure on the bottom of still are higher than on the top.

Under such conditions, when the bubble of steam rises from the bottom layer of herb it has a capacity to carry higher proportion of oil's vapour which gradually decreases as it approaches the top. Generally, it does not affect the extraction of oil unless the bubble is exceptionally rich in oil's vapour or the charge has a greater depth. However, in case the bubble is saturated, the decline in pressure and temperature with the rise of bubble is quite sufficient to condense some portion of the oil which was vapourised at a lower level in the still. When the oil is less dense than water, the condensed oil will float on the top surface and will tend to form a film.

Recovery of such lighter oil is always very slow and is a major cause of poor economy in water distillation. The reason for this is simple to understand. The top surface of water in a still is never at boiling temperature and supply of heat to this surface is quite slow. Thus, rate of vapourisation is also slow. As the major part of essential oil recovered by water distillation is vapourised in the form of saturated bubbles of mixed vapours, the proportion of the oil that will condense internally is directly proportional to the depth of the charge. It follows that, when oil is less dense than water, the depth of the charge should be as minimum as possible.

Effect of Turbulence

Immediately after its being vapourised, oil must be liberated from the herb surface. In steam distillation, this is being done by the current provided by steam. This suggests that some kind of turbulence may have some effect on the recovery of oil.

In this connection, the test carried out by Mr. Phillip Capell of Wynyard, Tasmania (Australia) is worth mentioning. Mr. Capell was carrying out trial distillations (water) of fresh Huon fine saw dust. As the supply of steam was very limited, he was getting poor yield. At this stage he installed an agitator in the still and in spite of keeping the same supply of steam, the yield improved. The prime significance of these observations were that, even after the initial use of the propeller had ensured that the whole charge was in motion, an additional increase in agitation greatly improved both yield and speed of recovery. Thus, the liberation of vapourise oil from the surface of the herb is basically a mechanical operation which can be performed much more conveniently with a small amount of mechanical energy than by burning more fuel to generate steam.

As the performance of water distillations are improved by enhancing the turbulence required to scrub vapour bubbles from surfaces of herb, it also tends to cause splashes which can carry fine particles through to the condenser. As such, as a rule, the equipment should be designed to have sufficient head by inserting a 4 to 5 ft long pipe in between the still and the condenser to enable the splashed particles to loose momentum and return back to the still.

Effect of Cohobation

The technique of returning distillate water to mother liquor at the point of steam generations is known as cohobation.

It has a twofold purpose:

1. To maintain the fluid level in steam generator.
2. To minimise the loss of compounds of oil dissolved in distilling water.

However, it should be understood that the loss of only those compounds can be minimised which are soluble in water to a certain extent by adopting cohobation. For example, recovery of phenyl ethyl alcohol and some phenols can be improved while distilling roses.

On the other hand, there are oils which create problem in separation and sometimes even form emulsion with water as being very close in specific gravity. In such cases, the recovery of oil can be increased by adopting a better design of oil separator or by settling the distillate at a certain temperature for 20/24 hours rather than going for cohobation which will prolong the distillation without much gain.

Chapter 6

Supercritical Fluid Extraction Technology for Quality Essential Oils

INTRODUCTION

Solvent extraction is one of the oldest unit operations employed for separating a wide range of products. Even with the introduction of newer techniques for separation over the years, solvent extraction remains one of the most popular techniques used on the industrial scale. More than a century ago Hannay's observation on dissolution power of the supercritical fluid (SCF) added a new dimension to the solvent extraction field by creating the possibility of using SCF as a new solvent medium. However, most of the effort in the direction of commercialising the supercritical fluid extraction (SCFE) process, gained momentum much latter, only after 1960.

Over the last decade supercritical fluid extraction technology (SCFET) has emerged as a superior alternative to the conventional technique of extraction of natural products using organic solvents. There has been a resurgent awareness in industry of potential applications of supercritical fluid processing in many diverse areas, as evident from the successful operation of a large number of supercritical fluid industrial plants all over the world. The process/product areas range over many sectors of industry, e.g. foods, pharmaceuticals, polymers, surfactants, speciality materials, etc.

Although this technology has been commercialised in a number of developed countries, it is yet to find its true potential in India. The main deterrent factor being, comparatively higher capital investment requirement of SCFET. This in turn can be attributed to requirements of high pressure operation and very accurate process control. Furthermore, it is generally perceived that the high costs of SCFE plants now available from the US and European manufacturers is not only due to the above requirements, but also include very high premium based on the novelty of this technology. Thus to make SCFET competitive, it is important to get the required product yield and quality at the lowest unit cost which includes operating costs plus capital investment. Thus indigenous design and manufacture of components will be the key element in commercialisation of SCFET in India. Over the years India has made remarkable progress in science and engineering and presently it can offer quality engineering services at a relatively modest cost as compared to those in developed countries.

In this regard Indian institute of technology (IIT), Mumbai, has developed for the first time in India, total technology for supercritical fluid extraction (SCFE) of natural products. In association with an industrial partner, the above SCFE technology from IIT, Mumbai has presently reached a stage of commercial-scale adaptation.

The most significant consequence of this developmental work is substantial capital cost reduction *vis-à-vis* equivalent imported commercial SCFE plants. In case of extraction of essential oils by SCFE, further optimisation of cost of investment is possible due to requirement of lower extraction pressures (120 Bar max.). Detailed financial analysis has shown that at the reduced capital cost level, achieved by the above effort, the SCFE technology is made truly economically viable under Indian market conditions. SCFE is a two-step process, which uses a dense gas, e.g. carbon dioxide (CO_2) as the solvent, above its critical temperature (31°C and critical pressure (73.8 bar) for extraction. Supercritical fluids have unique gas like properties such as higher diffusivity and lower viscosity, and thus can penetrate better into the pores and matrices of the solid raw material and allow more effective extraction as compared to liquid solvents. The feed, generally ground solid, is charged into the extractor. CO_2 is fed to the extractor through a high pressure pump. The extract laden CO_2 is sent to a separator via a pressure reduction valve. At reduced temperature and pressure conditions the extract precipitates at the bottom of separator. The gaseous CO_2 stream, free of any extract leaving from the separator is recycled back to the extractor.

EMERGING TREND TOWARDS SCFE PRODUCTS

It is very important to note that, although the initial investment for SCFE plant is higher than solvent extraction process, because of many beneficial features of the SCFE technology, the SCFE venture ultimately show a good profitability. The beneficial features are:

1. Low solvent (CO_2) cost compared to conventional solvents like Hexane, alcohol, etc.
2. Lower batch times (2–4 hours, as compared to 10–15 hours in solvent extraction).
3. Higher concentration of active/desirable components in the extract due to better selectivity of SCF solvent.
4. No pollution control related costs, etc.

Secondly, there are a number of practical problems associated with extracts produced by solvent extraction, affecting the actual viability of this conventional technology in present and future times. These include:

1. The demand and acceptability of hexane and other organic solvent extracted products is limited at present and expected to go down further with on coming stringent regulations and consumer awareness regarding suspected carcinogenic effect of the organic solvents as well as their impact on environment.

   Till recently, majority of spice oil and oleoresins were produced by chlorinated solvents, the use of which is now banned. The solvent, most commonly used today is Hexane. However, in USA market, the residual hexane content in the products has to be less than 25 ppm and this limit is expected to go down further. In Japan even 25 ppm hexane in extracts is to be banned, so also in Europe. SCFE has successfully and totally replaced chlorinated solvents in applications like decaffeination of tea and coffee, Hops extraction, etc. Similar trend is observed in other applications using organic solvents as well. The trend is gaining momentum and thus solvent extraction process may be phased out in near future.

2. Public opinion has become sensitive to the use of eco-friendly technologies in food and other similar material processing. An ISO-14002 certificate is becoming important for exports, especially of food products. It ensures that the process used is free of undesirable effluents that are produced at every step, right from raw material to finished product going to the consumer. Thus solvent extraction process is finding it increasingly difficult and costly to satisfy these regulations.

3. The extract undergoes degradation due to high temperature operations involved in steam distillation/ solvent extraction process, affecting the overall quality of the final product.

The effects of above factors are already seen in India with a majority of existing hexane based natural product extraction plants being either operated below optimum capacity or are closed down even though the world demand and consumption of natural extracts is showing a steady and healthy growth.

Thus, for India to gain its rightful leading place in the global natural product market, the industry needs to change over to modern technologies, which can improve the quality and reputation of Indian products.

Supercritical fluid extraction not only takes care of the above difficulties but also offers some additional benefits. The reasons for preferring SCFE process are the following:

Superior Product

1. Undegraded extracts with delicacy and freshness close to natural.
2. High concentration of desired active components.
3. No residual solvent.
4. Longer shelf life and free of biological (microbial) contaminants.

Superior Process

1. Simultaneous fractionation of extract possible to get desired components separated in a single step.
2. Flexible operating conditions for multiple product extraction without need for any hardware modification.
3. Carbon dioxide (CO_2) is used as solvent that is a generally regarded as safe (GRAS) for food products.
4. No effluent generated/truly environment friendly process (ISO 14002).

Considering all the above factors, SCFE is undoubtedly a much superior process than any other solvent extraction or steam distillation process as on today.

Commercial Application Areas

1. Essential oils: flavours and fragrance.
2. Herbal medicines.
3. Bitter from hops.
4. Food colours and preservatives.
5. Tocopherols.
6. Spice oils and oleoresins.
7. Natural pesticides.
8. Decaffeinated coffee and tea.
9. Nicotine/tar free tobacco.
10. Cholesterol free food products.

Economic Feasibility Analysis

As a case study, a detailed feasibility analysis has been carried out for extraction of different essential oils throughout the year, such as sandalwood, cinnamon and clove oil. These three products are considered to be extracted for four months each per year. The multi-product approach is important due to the variation in availability of raw materials as well as demand for the finished product.

Basis of calculations

The SCFE unit is considered to be 100 per cent export oriented unit (EOU). Other considerations are:

Plant configuration	Total of 3 extractors, with 2 extractors operational at a time and the third one out of cycle for feed change
Production	7 days/week, 3 shifts/day
Capacity utilisation	82%
Production days/year	300
The debt to equity ratio	2 : 1
Interest on long-term loan	12.5% p.a.
Working capital	12.5% p.a.
Margin money on working capital	25%
Working capital:	
Raw materials	1.0 month
Utilities, finished product, salaries and overheads and debtors	1.0 month

Summary of feasibility analysis for SCF extraction of essential oils

Case study for extraction of eandalwood, cinnamon and clove oil is shown in Table 6.1.

Table 6.1. Case study for extraction of sandalwood, cinnamon and clove oil.

Extractor capacity (litre)	100 l × 3	200 l × 3	300 l × 3
Plant capacity (feed) (kg per day)	920	1840	2520
SCFE plant cost (FOB basis) (Rs. lakhs)	180	245	330
Total investment including utilities, land, and building, etc. (100% EOU basis) (Rs. Lakhs)	285	384	503
Break even capacity (%)	46.1	35.6	32.7
Internal rate of return (%)	30.3	50.9	59.4
Pay back period (years)	3.3	2.0	1.7
Average cost of processing (excluding the cost of raw material [feed]):			
Variable cost (Rs./kg feed)	18.5	18.1	18.2
Fixed cost (Rs./kg feed)	24.8	15.7	13.2
Specific operating cost (Rs./kg feed)	43.3	33.8	31.4

To sum up traditionally, major exports of natural materials have been in raw form. The natural products industry in India is needed to effectively tap the rapidly growing international market for quality, value added products through the use of contemporary, eco-friendly and world-class technologies like SCFE.

In the past the SCFE technology did not hold much ground in India, due to very high premium charged by the foreign SCFE equipment suppliers, which affected the economic viability. But now IIT, Mumbai has developed world-class SCFE technology in India, to make it cost effective. Thus SCFE, which is a superior technology in all respect is now made truly economically viable. Thus use of conventional technologies like solvent extraction (using hexane or hydro flouro carbons) and steam distillation now, may not be appropriate for the Indian industry. Therefore, adopting SCFE is need of the hour for regaining India's leadership in the world market of value added natural products.

The higher cost of investment of commercial scale SCFE plant does not fit in small scale sector. However, as stated earlier there is urgent need for state-of-the-art technologies such as SCFE so as to be able to meet stringent demands of the global market. Application of cooperative movement as seen in case of milk, sugar industries may be one of the ways to extend the fruits of increased world demand for quality natural products, to the farmers and rural population of India.

AROMATIC OIL DISTILLATION PLANT SELECTING TO GET HIGHEST YIELD AND BEST QUALITY OF OIL

Aromatic oil grasses are unique agricultural products. They contain oil which are natural and aromatic. The aromatic grasses are distilled to recover oil. Good farming of aromatic crops by itself does not ensure good quality or yield of oil. A good distillation plant is essential to get good quality of aromatic oil from aromatic grasses.

Aromatic oils distilled from grasses and leaves are used in perfumery and other industries where quality of oil is of utmost important. It is the quality which gets good price in the market. And the quality of oil depends very much on the distillation process and the plant.

Distillation also assumes importance because substandard distillation will give low yield of oil at higher cost whereas a well designed distilled plant will not only give high quality of oil but also high yield of oil and save on cost of operations day after day.

Process in Brief

The process of distillation is outwardly very simple. It involves passing steam into the still containing grasses or leaves. The steam vapourises volatile oils contained in the grasses or leaves. These volatile oils pass out of the still along with steam. The vapours of steam and oil are condensed to form a mixture of water and oil. This mixture is passed through a separator to get oil. Oil is collected in bottles while water is left out.

Selection of Distillation Plant

The yield and quality of oil depends on 2 main activity, namely plantation and distillation. The plantation relates to soil, water, weather, seasons, etc. The distillation relates to distillation process, type and construction of the plant.

There are 3 most critical equipments of a distillation plant. They are:
1. Steam boiler: To generate required quantity of steam, at correct press and temperature.
2. Vapour condenser: To condense entire steam generated by the boiler.
3. Water cooling system: To cool water heated in the process and to re-circulate the same.

Yield and Quality of Oil

The yield and quality of oil depends upon:
1. The design and efficiency of water boiler.
2. The design and efficiency of condenser.
3. The efficiency of water cooling system.
4. The over all design of stills and other equipments.

The life of plant and the safety of its operations depend upon:
1. The overall design of boiler and other equipment.
2. The quality and thicknesses of materials used for boiler and other equipment.

3. The quality of fabrication.

The reliability and consistency of day-to-day operations depend upon:

1. Proper integration of boiler.
2. The cooling system.

CONCLUSION

1. The distillation plant is generally located in remote farms but have to run everyday just like a small scale process industry.

   The boiler should be made in minimum 8 mm thick material for inner furnace zone. The tube should be in carbon (C) grade conforming to IS-1239. It should not consume more than 250 kg dry wood for 1 ton of grass. It should have proper safety features. It should produce just the right amount of steam otherwise it will effect yield and quality of oil.

   The condenser should be of stainless steel (SS) 304 pipes and 4 mm thick tube plates and with end caps. The stills should be in minute 4 mm thick material with proper design and fabrication.

   The entire plant should be made as per GMP standard.

2. The quality of oil determines its price and acceptability in markets. Hence progressive farmers should strive to get best quality of oil.

3. The yield of oil as well and cost of operations (quantity of fuel per ton of grass) determines the profitability of this project.

4. Progressive farmers and oils processors should ensure that the distillation plant is of proven design and backed by experience, expertise and commitment of the supplier.

5. The distillation plant which gives: (i) best quality of oil, (ii) high yield of oil, (iii) safety of operation, and (iv) long life — IS the best option for farmers.

Chapter 7

Design of Equipments for Essential Oils

INTRODUCTION

The primary objective of design of distillation system is to determine the size and shape of equipment that will perform satisfactorily under varied circumstances of herbs to be distilled.

The selection of distillation equipment will depend upon the size of the operation and the type of distillation to be carried out, i.e. steam distillation, boiler fed or direct fired or water distillation.

Basically there are two types of distillation set ups prevalent in India:

1. Direct fired stills fitted with calendria.
2. Stills fed with steam from a separate boiler.

Recently, as the size of the distilleries is becoming smaller as run by growers and design of calendria has also improved, the tendency is towards setting up direct fired stills.

However, when volume of work is large, it is always advisable to utilise a boiler for raising steam. At the same time, boiler is more useful while distilling herbs containing high boiling oils.

Generally, big distilleries depend upon boilers and also possess 2 to 3 direct fired stills fitted with calendria. These stills are made use of during lean period or when the load is in excess.

Before, the design of equipment is discussed a short note on the system of loading and unloading of stills and moving the spent herb to the desired place would be worth mentioning.

Stills are installed in a battery of 4 to 5 together, leaving a clear space of about 20′ on each side for movement of cart/trolley, etc. It is advisable to install the stills well above the ground with a slope extending up to 3/4th height of the still to facilitate loading of herb. The following advantages are visualised in such a system:

1. Condenser can be kept vertical without raising the height of connecting pipe from still to condenser.
2. Reflex water can be discharged from the bottom at ground level.

Loading of stills is done manually and it is a time consuming job. Arrangements for quick unloading of stills is very much required. The most suitable arrangements for unloading of stills and moving the load of spent herbs to an allotted place, either for composting or burning as fuel after drying, is to have the overhead gantry with trolley and chain pulley block of right capacity.

In case the number of stills are four or more than four, it is advisable to have an electric chain pulley block to facilitate easy and quick lifting of spent herbs. It is not necessary to pack the charge on single grid or set of strings. The charge can be divided into two or three compartments while packing into the stills by placing intermediate grids or strings in between. This will facilitate lifting of spent material in two or three parts causing less load/stress on the overhead system.

The overhead gantry beam is always kept extended by 5 to 6 ft on one side where these loads of spent material can be off loaded on a cart.

Generally a 3-ton capacity chain pulley block is sufficient to use and, in case, stills are of one ton capacity, these can be unloaded in one stroke otherwise, for bigger stills, loading and unloading is done in two steps by dividing the charge in two compartments.

Besides a suitable arrangement for emptying stills and carrying the spent herbs to an allotted place, there are four main parts which form the base for all types of distillations:

1. Still.
2. Condenser.
3. Receiver.
4. Steam generator.
   (a) Boiler.
   (b) Calendria.

Let us discuss these four parts of the distillation equipments in order.

STILL

In the simplest form, the still consists of a cylindrical container or tank with diameter equal to or less than its height. The still is, equipped with an arrangement to lift the cover quickly and conveniently as this is required to be performed after every two hours or so. In some of the cases, such as, stills needed for distillation of seeds/roots, only manhole is provided and cover is not made removable. The height of the still should not be less than 1.5 metres in any case.

Figure 7.1 shows one of the designs of clamping cover with tank with the use of eye bolts and keeping a gasket in between.

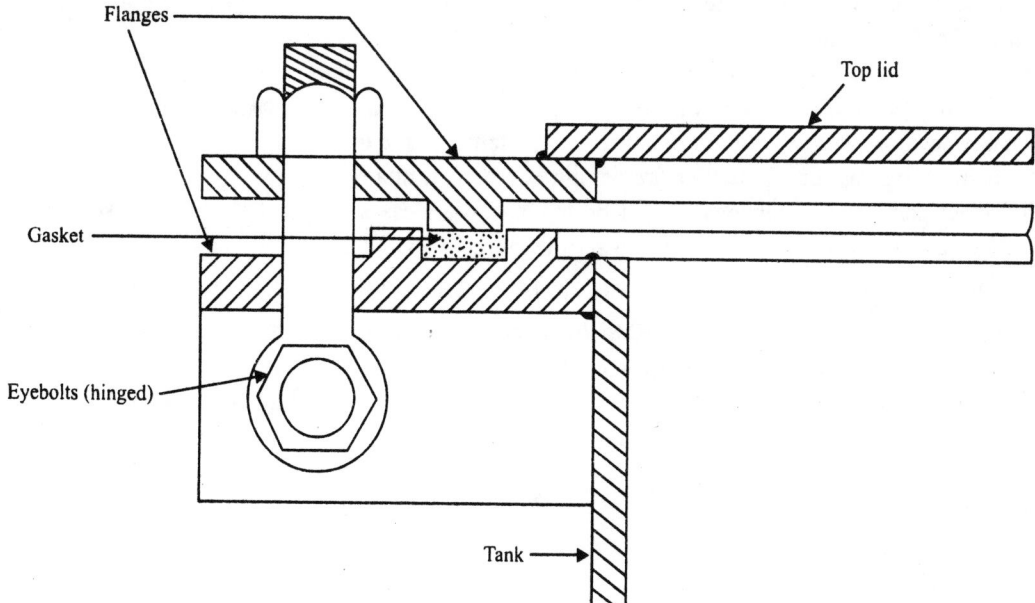

Fig. 7.1. Clamping arrangement of a still.

In many installations, particularly, stills fitted with calendria for generation of steam provision of water seal is made which dispenses with clamping arrangement of the cover. The cylindrical section of the still can be made slightly tapered to facilitate removal of spent plant material.

A false grid or steel frame is placed about 8 to 10 inches above the bottom of tank to support the charge. Below this false grid, either a perforated coil of steam pipes duly connected with steam line, is placed or the cylindrical tank itself is bolted with a calendria having baffles in between for control of splashing of water.

It is advisable to insulate the stills up to the top to conserve heat and minimise condensation of vapours inside the still.

CONDENSER

Condenser is the second major part of distillation equipment. The purpose of condenser is to convert all the steam and accompanying oil vapours into liquid and bring down the temperature of condensed vapours to a desired level. The most commonly used condensers are these in which a bundle of pipes, either straight or zigzag, are placed inside a vessel supplied with running cold water, entering from below and exiting from top. Vapour flows inside the pipes in a countercurrent mode.

Various configuration of pipes are possible and, in fact, are in use. However, condensers with straight vertical tubes have more advantages in comparison to others.

From ten-point of view of efficient heat transfer, it has been found that a more rapid and turbulent flow of cooling water results in more efficient cooling. Similarly, a turbulent flow of vapours inside the tube will also add to this factor. Both these effects can be created in straight tube vertical condensers. These condensers not only offer saving in space but they are more convenient to clean also.

To create turbulence inside the tubes, swirl strips are inserted which help in breaking up the tendency to laminar flow. Similarly, baffles are placed outside the tubes in such a fashion so as to create turbulence in the flow of cooling water.

A condenser should always be designed for an overload so that the temperature of the distillate can be controlled more precisely. A condenser is said to be operating on maximum efficiency when the condensate has been cooled down to a desired temperature and the temperature of cooling water at exit approaching that of the incoming vapours. Usually a temperature of 80°C is attained.

All contact parts of the condenser must be made of stainless steel. To calculate the surface area required for transfer of heat in a condenser, a simple guide to follow is:

$A = 1/K \times$ flow rate of steam (kg/hr/sq.m.) $\times$ top area of still (sq.m.) $A =$ Area in sq. m.

Generally, the value of K varies from 50 to 70 depending upon the design of condenser, temperature and quantity of cooling water available for circulation. Assumptions are made that cooling water is available to the extent of 15 times of distillate flow and temperature of cooling water is about 30°C. The distillate is required to be cooled to a temperature of 40°–45°C.

RECEIVER

The third essential part of distillation equipment consists of a receiver, decanter or oil separator. Its function is to achieve a quick and complete separation of the oil from the condensate water.

In condensate, quantity of water is always much larger. The lighter one floats on the top because of non-solubility as well as the difference in specific gavities. Design of the receiver should permit the removal of water whether oil is heavier or lighter than water.

Oil and water often does not separate immediately in the 'oil separator', especially if the differential between the specific gravities of oil and water is small. The distillate must not, therefore, flow too rapidly and any turbulence in the liquid should be avoided. In other words, separator should be large enough to permit water and oil to separate as completely as possible.

The principle which causes separation of oil and water is the difference in their densities. In this connection, the observations made by Denny are interesting. He has shown that the oils's specific gravity decrease more rapidly than does that of water over any chosen rise in temperature.

Table 7.1 shows the speeds of rise or fall through water of small oil particles at different temperatures.

Table 7.1. Speed of rise or fall through water of small oil particles.

	Speed of particles in mm/min at temperature in °C			
Oil	30°	40°	50°	60°
Lavender	4.5	7.0	12.0	17.0
Peppermint	–	5.2	7.5	11.0
Sandalwood	Fails	Fails	6.0	7.4

For example, take the case of peppermint oil. Small particles of oil rise at a speed of 5.2 mm/min at 40°C while the same rise at 7.5 mm/min at 40°C. This clearly demonstrates the effectiveness of separation of oil from water when temperature of the distillate is more.

Even when the oil's density is quite close to that of water, a large proportion is separated and floats at the top (when oil is lighter than water) very quickly. This should not be taken for granted that separation is complete as there is always a possibility of oil going in distillate water. Most of these losses of oil can be avoided in case necessary steps are taken to ascertain the speed at which smaller particles of oil rise through water at a given temperature.

In the case of peppermint oil we have observed that oil particles rise at a speed of 7.5 mm/min at 50°C, the dimensions of receiver can be chosen so that distillate water passes through it downwards at a speed below 7.5 mm/min.

On the other hand, in case the specific gravity of an oil at room temperature is slightly higher than that of water (oil is heavier than water), the distillate should run as cold as possible.

Figures 7.2 and 7.3 are drawn to suggest some outlines for the basic design of oil separator.

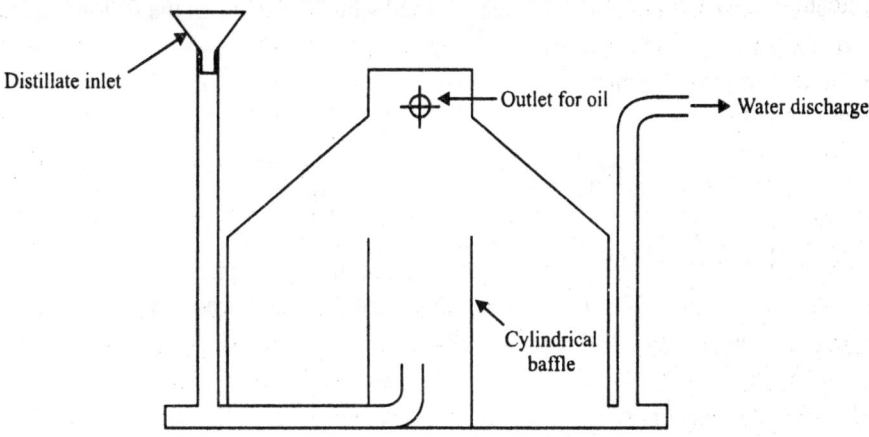

Fig. 7.2. Receiver for oils lighter than water.

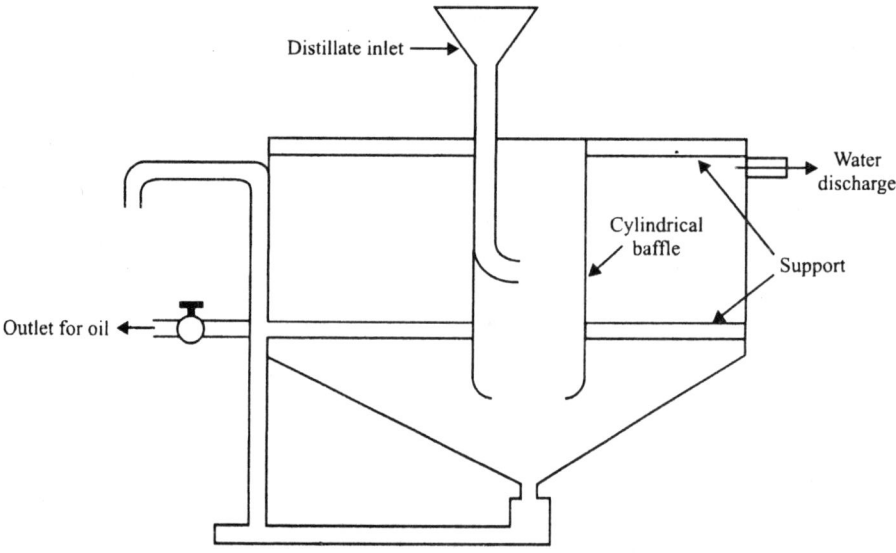

Fig. 7.3. Receiver for oils heavier than water.

Separate designs are suggested depending upon oil is lighter than water or oil is heavier than water. However, for oils which comprise of two parts, one less dense and the other more dense than water, it is suggested to utilise two oil separators in series.

Guenther has suggested to use multiple receivers in series when single is not large enough. Further, it should be remembered that condensate water always carry some dissolved portion of oil. In some cases, this may go up to 20 per cent of the recoverable oil and, hence, should be considered as a potent source for the recovery of oil. Recently efforts are being made to separate the dissolved portion of oil by storing the condensed water and treating it by any solvent or by any other physical means.

STEAM GENERATOR

Steam generator can be either boiler or in case of direct fired stills, 'calendria'. The size of boiler will depend upon steam required. A general guide can be used which is based on the following formula:

$A = \alpha \times n \times s$

A = Sq. m. rating of boiler.

n = No. of stills.

s = Top area of each still in sq. m.

α = Factor depending upon the flow of steam desired, material of construction and efficiency of boiler. Generally, it varies from 4 to 6.

The capacity of the boiler should be calculated based on the assumption that all the stills will be in operation at a time. In actual practice, it is not possible as one or two stills are always being unloaded and refilled. The boiler should be capable of generating steam at 7 kgs/cm^2 (100 psi). Although, it may not be required to produce steam at this pressure but while selecting a equipment it should be done for any eventuality. Generally a pressure of 2 to 3 kgs/cm^2 is maintained.

Wherever it is not feasible to use boiler, as the size of operation is small, steam generation is done below the stills by direct firing and the equipment which performs this function is known as 'calendria'.

It is quite important to have a proper size and design of calendria to obtain as good results as with a steam boiler or in some cases better.

Taking into consideration the basic principles of steam generator, the design of calendria is based on the following factors:

1. Heating surface area.
2. Temperature gradient (between flue gases and water).

As far as temperature gradient is concerned, in a direct fired, two pass system, the maximum possible gradient is attained which is also dependent on rate of firing. From the design point of view, heating surface area is all important for obtaining the desired rate of evaporation inside the still. Other factors which affect the performance are design of furnace and height of chimney. Design of calendria is also important as it also governs the movement of flue gases which is the transferring media of heat.

Figures 7.4 to 7.6 show various ways of designing a 'calendria' or bottom part of direct fired still. A flat surface can generate only 36 to 48 kg of steam per hour per sq.m. of still area. So, it would be impossible to distil any herb efficiently.

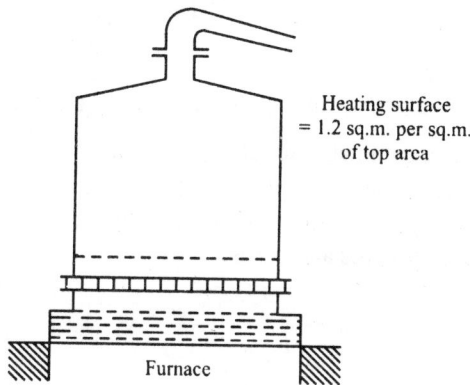

Fig. 7.4. Flat bottom.

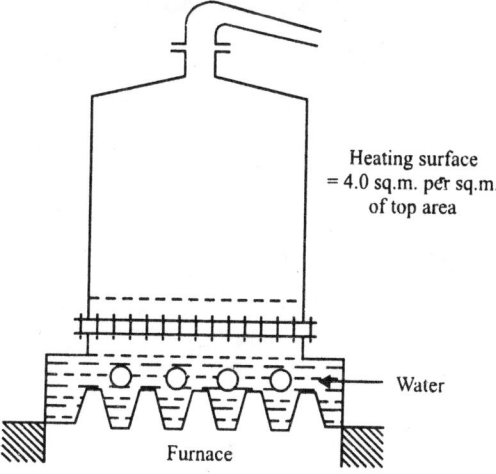

Fig. 7.5. Existing design of calendria having two pass systems.

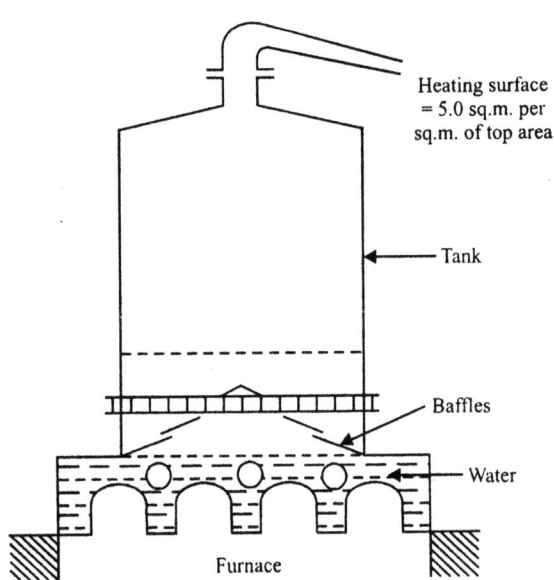

Heating surface
= 5.0 sq.m. per
sq.m. of top area

Tank

Baffles

Water

Furnace

Fig. 7.6. Improved design of calendria with two pass systems + baffles (designed by author).

Calendria with an improved design contains about 5 sq.m. heating surface area and thus can very well generate 150 to 200 kg of steam per hour per sq.m. of still area which is generally desired flow rate of steam for most of the herbs. This improved still was designed in the beginning of 1992 specifically for distillation of semi-absorptive type of herbs and seeds.

Chapter 8

Indian Attars

INTRODUCTION

Attar from the ancient Persian word is transliteration of the Arabic *itr*, meaning 'fragrance', 'scent' or 'essence'. Attar or Otto refers to essential oils obtained by distillation and in particular, that of the rose, an extremely precious perfumery material.

Attar oils are a specific type of fragrance products, first produced by the great Persian Physician Hakim Avicenna, generally regarded as the greatest individual physician who ever lived. The Indian, Chinese and Egyptians knew natural aromatic materials three thousand years ago.

Archaeological evidence shows the earliest inhabitants of the Indian subcontinent held plants in great reverence. But nature worship among primitive people is not unusual. What makes the Indian reverence for plants unique is its unbroken continuity from prehistory to the present day, when plants have long since ceased to be the major source of human food, clothing, and shelter. In time, scented oils were extracted by pressing, pulverising and distilling aromatic vegetal and animal produce. Such processes led to development of the art of alchemy, the earliest indications of which are available from the perfume jars and terracotta containers of the Indus Valley civilisation. That the art has survived centuries and of late, the advent of synthetic perfumes, makes Indian attars so special.

The art of perfumery was practiced in many early civilisations. Persian rulers were known to wear attars more than 5000 years ago. In India, a wide variety of natural aroma products have been traditionally used at home, as well as for worship. Burning of incense is a practice in all temples and home; similarly, sandalwood paste and Holy basil (*Ocimum sanctum*). The *Charaka* treatise emphasises that the sense must be healthy if humans are to experience true well-being, and because ayurveda considers the human body both in its totality as well as in its relation to nature, therefore the garden and its flowers are essential to ayurvedic science. The most obvious sensory satisfaction provided by aromatic plants is the olfactory pleasure they give to human beings. Science of perfumery is one of India's most ancient and venerated crafts, integrated into India's daily life. Scented plants are used to celebrate every aspects of Indian culture, from the ritual to the culinary, from the celibate to the erotic. Scented flowers in India have always been strung into garlands or worn to decorate the hair. *Vedas* mentioned the use of combinations of numerous herbs, twigs, barks and flowers as offering to Gods in *yagnas*.

The use of odour bearing materials such as turmeric and sandalwood oils for imparting fragrance to the human body in the shape of pastes and other preparations is described as common. For instance, the henna paste used by Indian women to colour their hair and to paint the intricate patterns on their skin is the same cooling paste recommended by *ayurveda* as a cure for the skin rashes brought on by summer heat. India has a very old tradition of using natural fragrances (*Attars*). The history of natural attars is very much associated with the history of a city called 'Kannauj', which is situated in Uttar Pradesh, north of India. Attar the centuries old Indian art of blended perfumes, comes redolent with nostalgia when the elegant, dignified, sophisticated, grand and unhurried life-style made people praise the aesthetic subtleties of grace and personal charm.

What is great about Indian perfumes is that they have not been subjected to gender equations as the western ones are made separately for men and women. Attars are like flowers — as old as them, but as fresh as tomorrow dew drops. The story of Indian perfumes is as old as civilisation itself. Whenever Ghalib used to meet his beloved in winters, he purposely smeared his hands and face with attar *hina*. Besides, aromatherapy, a new branch of curing diseases by attars was developed in India long ago. The attars too are known for their medicinal effects. The simplest example of aromatherapy is after *Gill* (sondhi mitti) that has the fresh aroma that emanates from the earth after the first summer shower. Smelling it stops flow of blood through nose owing to intense heat. Sherbet of attar *khus* (sugar syrup flavoured with attar khus) is relished in summers as it provides a cooling effect to the digestive system.

Attar, originally an Indian perfume, has a heritage of multipurpose potency behind it, distilling the unforgettable fragrances of the world being presented in cut glass decanters for you. Now this fragrance is in vogue in the Parisian fashion seminaries especially when a world renowned bewitching model fell for Indian mehndi and attar of late. Stolen from fresh flowers, the fragrances are whisked into glass bottles after a very tedious and long drawn process. A very specific fact about Indian perfumes is that people keep using the same perfume for years together — in fact for the whole life! People using foreign perfumes keep changing one brand to another but sans satisfaction. Maulana Azad was fond of attar *majmua*. The queen of all attars happens to be *ruh gulab*, which was one discovered by Noorjahan, the wife of Mughal emperor, Jahangir. Once while she went for her morning bath, she fond an oily layer over the water kept with rose flowers to cool overnight: *Ruh gulab*, the costliest attar.

'A good perfume is like a good woman! It shouldn't be too blatant it should slowly but surely make way into your mind and then your heart.'

Multipurpose potency of the attars is incredibly vast indeed. Passages in Indian literature are replete with examples of attar being quite an aid to romance. Young men and Gods dreamt of maidens walking in a cloud of jasmine, roses and marigold scents and maidens confiding to their friends about trysts with their lovers, went into raptures over 'his handsome body smeared with sandalwood power'. The real drama still remains in the dab of attar over the jingle of bangles of a Mughal princess or the wick of attar-socked cotton behind the ear of a Mughal noble man. Cleopatra used it, the heady art behind seduction, a symbol of prosperity and culture. In *Aain-e-Akbari*, Abul Fazal, has mentioned about Akbar using the fragrant attar along with the burning of incense sticks daily burnt in gold and silver censers. A princess's toilette was incomplete without incense and attar.

Attar oils are a specific type of fragrance product derived from natural plant extracts. While some varieties are pure oils, which are fragrant enough (such as amber, sandalwood and eucalyptus), others need to be blended with resins or concentrates in natural base or carrier oil. The unique aroma of attar is derived from condensing vapours directly into a base oil of sandalwood (since its own fragrance is easily displaced by other scents).

Moreover, sandalwood oil does not easily turn rancid and serves as a good preservative. Over the centuries, attar perfumes have been used for a variety of purpose ranging from aromatherapy and spiritual healing, to mood enhancement and as emotional adjusters. Since attars do not contain any alcohol, these have found particular favours with Muslims.

A traditional hydro-distillation process manufactures the attars. Copper stills called '*Degs*' are used for distilling floral and herbal materials and have capacities ranging from 10–160 kg. The copper vessel is heated by direct fire and the unique odour of attar is obtained by condensing the vapours into the base materials, mainly sandalwood oil. Sometimes, liquid paraffin is used to make cheaper attars. Distillation is a highly skilled job, as the pressure inside the still has to be matched by the boiling and condensation rate. After the condensation, water layer is separated by separating the condensate in two layers.

TYPES OF ATTARS

Attars can be broadly categorised in three types based on raw materials used. Attars are not only classified according to their contents but also according to the time of the year in which they are to be used:

1. Floral Attars: These are the attars made from single species of flowers such as Gulab (Rose), *Kewra* (Pandanus odaratissium), *Motia* (Jasminium sambal), *Chameli* (Jasminium grandifloram), etc.
2. Herbal and Spicy Attars: These are manufactured from combination of floral, herbal and spicy materials. Musk Amber, Musk Hina Shamama, etc. are some of the popular names.
3. Others: These attars used neither floral nor herbal materials. Attar Mitti (earth) falls under this category and is produced by distillation of backed earth over base material.

The warm notes of the spicy *hina* prepared from musk and saffron have the greatness of smelling different on every skin. It gives a great feeling in winters. Apart from the floral attars, the most remarkable item in the repertoire of traditional Indian perfumery is attar *hina*. The number of raw materials used in its production is very large and varied as their geographic origin, as well as the botanical species. The techniques of distillation are more intricate, while the equipment remains primarily the same. The materials that goes into the production of attar *hina* may be classified into the broad categories: herbals, gums/ resins, species, products of animal origin and flower oils.

The *attar* of *hina*, whose varied shades are also know as *Shamama-ul-amber* is the chief product for which the Indian perfume industry can today be credited with for producing an aroma which is unique to India. With their own secret formulations and recipes, different perfumery houses produce their own specialities in different price ranges. But, one thing is common to all preparations, i.e. in the genealogy of perfumes they fall into one single category, i.e. heavy oriental with spicy, floral, amber and animal notes predominating.

The strength and long lasting qualities of good attar endow it with an attraction that perhaps our modern perfumes do not have.

Let us first understand as to what distinguishes the traditional Indian perfumes from the modern or western style perfumes prevalent the world over. Whereas the modern perfumer makes judicious use of natural essential oils, absolutes and resinoids; the major components of the composition being synthetics and isolates, in the traditional Indian perfumery, only, natural raw materials were used.

APPLICATIONS OF ATTARS

The Indian attars in the past were used by elite class of society particularly kings and queens. Today, people who do not like the presence of alcohol in perfumes use attars as personal perfumes. Attars are also used in some of the traditional Indian edible products. The traditional attars of Indian are rarely found in their pure form today.

They are often adulterated with synthetic chemicals or the base oil, sandalwood, is stretched with liquid paraffin and other substances. In the traditional process various flowers, roots, herbs, spices, etc.

are hydro distilled in copper vessels into a receiving vessel containing sandalwood oil. It means that a certain proportion of flowers or other aromatic plants is put into a copper vessel containing water, sealed and the aromatic vapours produced from a wood or cow dung fire, rises through bamboo pipes and passes into another copper vessel containing sandalwood oil, sitting below the larger distilling one.

There the vapours condense and after days distillation the water and oil separate, allowing most of the aromatic molecules to become adsorbed into the sandalwood oil. The water is decanted off and added back to the distilling vessel for the next day's distillation. The process, in the case of single flowers like rose, jasmin, kewda, night queen, kadam, heena, etc. is repeated for a minimum of 15 days until the sandalwood becomes totally saturated with the perfume of that particular flower. The process for making *hina*, *shamama*, amber, and saffron attar is much more sophisticated and requires numerous other steps; as many as 60 natural ingredients go into their production which takes place over a couple of months.

Ruhs (hydrodistilled oil) are rarely found in pure form today. They are often adulterated with synthetic chemicals. In the traditional process various flowers, roots, herbs, and spices, etc. are hydrodistilled in copper vessels into a receiving vessel. This is similar to the process for attar except that with a ruh the receiving vessel does not contain sandalwood oil (it is, therefore, a pure essence of the flower). A certain proportion of flowers or other aromatic plants are put into a copper vessel containing water, sealed and the aromatic vapours produced from a wood or cow dung fire, rises through bamboo pipes and passes into another copper vessel, sitting below the larger distilling one. Even flowers, which cannot be steam distilled because the higher heat can destroy their highly volatile constituents and pressure of distillation can be done by hydro distillation. *Ruhs* are being prepared in India by this method, are *Bela* (Jasmine sambac), Kewda (Pandanus odaratissimus), Gulab (Rosa damascena) and Khus (Vetiveria ziazaniodes).

The unique odour of attar is obtained by condensing vapours directly into a base oil of sandalwood in a 'receiver'. Sandalwood is used because its own fragrance easily is displaced by other scents and it does not turn rancid. The beauty of using attar oils is that by wearing them you create an aura of tranquillity, confidence and mystery around yourself. Because attars contain no alcohol, the scent 'clings' within one or two feet of your body, in the 'zone of intimacy'.

These attars are the very same fragrances used by women and men of the east for centuries to create a spiritual beauty. These elegant aromas are traced directly to the ancient healers and prophets, who used fragrant oils to enhance moods, adjust emotions and uplift the soul.

There are three important aspects of purchasing and using attar perfumes and essential oils:

1. Quality and purity of the oils.
2. The depth and elegance of scent.
3. Safety in application and use.

The real issue that seems to arise with most customers is whether a product is natural or not. Besides the initial problem that there at present exists no national or international standard as to precisely what constitutes a truly natural substance, many wild claims can be, and often are. But let's look at this complex subject in more details. Some ill-meaning people use the confusion and complexity of natural ingredients to make wild claims in the market place. As a matter of fact, even if one performed expensive analysis, there is no method to distinguish between the chemical structure of a natural or synthetic floral oil. Even if we could agree that natural perfume oil should contain only natural essential oils, determining purity is difficult and expensive.

Determining the purity of attar oil (or any essential oil) presents special problems. Now, some people with very little knowledge or experience may take bottle of an oil look at it or smell it briefly, or see it being sold or carried in a clear bottle and instantly declare that it is synthetic or impure. Watch out for this kind of expert. As a matter of fact, the large testing labs, even, keep most oils in clear bottles. It is known that the biggest determent to delicate oils is oxygen, not sunlight.

Also, many oils actually improve with age. Sandalwood is kept for decades in the Near East, and given by grandmothers to their grandchildren as a treasure. Frankincense, amber, sandal, vetiver and almost all of the resins and barks will improve considerably when aged.

Many people imagine that because an essential oil come from 'nature' or a plant, that it is harmless and safe, and is good for ones health. But the opposite can be dangerously true. Experts also do not advise using essential oils or attars in 'diffuser' type of devices. These can disperse one dram (about one teaspoon) to one half ounce of an oil per hour. While many people feel that diffusing the environment with these mechanical devices is a good thing, experts urge caution.

Traditionally, maybe two drops of an oil is applied to 'punk' stick to make incense, which disperse this in very minuscule amounts for 20 minutes or so. A second reason for blending is that true jasmine, or myrrh, or rose oil in absolute form are not really particularly appealing fragrances. Up to ten thousand pounds of rose petals are 'condensed' into an ounce or less to product attar of rose. Besides being prohibitively expensive for the average consumer, the scent, which result from such high compression, is exaggerated and actually smells little like a rose in a garden. Attar of rose contains a fairly high concentration of various chemicals as its natural composition. It may contain up to 7 or 8 per cent citronellol. The unskilled person may smell even the very highest grades of rose attar, and imagine that it has been cut with citronella oil, when it is a fact, that is the true natural scent of attar of rose. Therefore, some natural perfumes such as Arabian Rose or other similarly name are not strictly speaking only that floral oil. Rather they are blends containing that oil as the primary ingredient, but enhanced in ton and intensity by addition of other oils in various quantities. This blending process really, lies at the heart of all perfumery.

Most perfumes today are mixtures of various chemicals, which are dilute in a type of colourless and odourless alcohol. These chemical mixtures cannot compare in any way with the power and lure of natural perfume oils that for over 1000 years have created such an aura of deep mystery and romance. In fact, regardless of how skilful a synthetic perfume is constructed, it is a kind of miniature chemical toxic pool, which after a brief moment of pleasure, immediately starts to deteriorate.

How many times have you been at a party or gathering, or even at the office, when a woman or man walks in and almost 'knocks you over' with their perfume or cologne? The reason this happens is twofold. First, the alcohol dilutes the molecules of the base scent, and make them lighter, causing them to travel all the way across a room. It is not only unpleasant to force this overpowering scent on everyone in the room, but most people expose to it feel embarrassed for the woman or man wearing such an 'overdose'.

Natural attar floral oils, by contrast, retain their natural heavy molecular structure, and remain close to the person wearing it, within a foot or two, in the 'zone of intimacy', and only send out their elegant, subtle lure, to those within her range of personal intimacy. As a matter of fact, despite the thousands of fragrances in the stores, very few women really know the proper way to select fragrances to maximise their effect on those around them. For example, most women when preparing for a date or an intimate evening select a perfume to wear, but their selection may prove to be disastrous, because they fail to appreciate the effect of the scent.

In the first place, almost all of the commercial alcohol-type perfumes are an irritant to the subtle sense of smell in men and women. So without knowing it, a woman may ruin her entire evening, even a whole relationship, by wearing the wrong fragrance. There are certain fragrances suitable for love and romance, like rose, some suitable to dispel overbearing people, like amber, others work their charm by boosting your mood and banishing depression, like jasmine.

MANUFACTURE OF ATTARS

There are number of methods used to produce attars of the quality and purity. Below is a brief discussion of these methods.

Traditional Degree of Steam Distillation

Attar distillation is different from the steam distillation methods used in Europe and the United States. The manufacture of attars today is done using the original 1,000 years old ancient methods. Large copper stills are used, called *degs*. These stills are heated from below with a direct fire ignited from wood or dung. These stills have a capacity from 22 to 352 pounds of floral material. The lid of the still is made of copper with fittings for connections to receivers, which ultimately hold the extracted oils. The top of the still is filled with plant substance (flowers, petals, leaves, etc.), water is added and the lid is sealed with a mixture of cotton and clay.

The apparatus and equipments used for manufacture of attar are light, flexible and easy to repair with a fair degree of efficiency. The equipments that are used are *Bhapka* or receiver, *chonga* or bamboo condenser, *gachchi* or cooking water tank, traditional *bhatti* or furnace.

The stills held about 10–160 kgs of flowers/various herbs submerged in water. Angling out from the top of the *degs* are bamboo pipes wrapped in twine made of local grasses. These pipes, or *chongas*, connected the *degs* to another long necked copper vessel called a *Bhapka*, which sat in a water-bath below the bigger vessel. This smaller vessel held precious sandalwood oil into which the aromatic vapours produced in the *deg* condensed. The water of distillation that collects below the oils is sometimes recycled. The heating of the still underneath causes a great pressure to build inside the still.

The unique odour of attars is obtained by condensing vapours directly into base oil. The most commonly used base oil is low-grade sandalwood oil, which is contained in the receiver. Liquid paraffin is also sometimes used, mainly for making cheaper *attars*. The receiver is constructed of copper, round in shape, with a long neck. A hollow bamboo pipe wrapped with thin rope for insulation, and pushed inside the condenser joins the still controls the temperature and speed of distillation. The attendants of the still are called *dighaas*. They must use extraordinary skill to maintain the precise temperature for best results with each type of attar. The *dighaas* feel the outside of the containers, and carefully listen for and evaluate sounds within the still. When the desired quantity of vapour have condensed, the *dighaa* wraps a wet cloth around the still, which temporarily halts the distillation process. The receiver is then replaced with a second receiver containing fresh plant material. For the highest grades of attars, this process may be repeated three or more times. The receiver is then allowed to cool and sit. The steam cools, and condenses back into water. The oil floats on top, is then drawn off, filtered and bottled for sale.

There are grades (first, second, and third, etc.) of these types of attars, depending upon the amount of substance used in the distillation process. Once desired concentration has been reached the total distillate is poured into leather bottles for storage. Leather is a choice material as any water still contained in the oil can pass from the porous membrane by osmosis, but no oil will be loss. If there is any unrefined material left in the attar it will settle to the bottom and can be easily removed by filtering. This storage method for the oils has been in existence for centuries and people engaged in the cottage industry of making them are still to be seen in Kannauj today.

But whether the attar is of a single floral note or a complex bouquet consisting of many ingredients, one other distinct advantage of this method of this type of distillation from the fragrance standpoint is that the odour improves with age. Sandalwood is not only an excellent fixative but also a fantastic preservative and if such oils are carefully stored it has been found that like a good wine they improve with age.

Enfleurage

Another method of extraction of attars is called *enfleurage* (French for 'to saturate with perfume scent'). It is common in France, the Middle and Near East and in India. This mode is often called cold rolling in India. A long stone trough is employed, into which a quantity of base or collecting oil is placed inside cheesecloth and rolled up.

This is then submerged in the trough containing the base oil. After a time, usually a day, the attar oils contained within the floral substance mingle with the base oil. This cheesecloth is removed after the first day, and replaced with fresh florals. This procedure is repeated up to thirty or forty times, after which the base oil has become saturated with the desired fragrance.

A low grade of sandalwood and olive oils is commonly used as base oils, because they do not easily turn rancid; and in the case of sandalwood, its own fragrance easily is displaced by other scents. Fatty oils such as peanut, safflower and so forth are unsuitable for this process, as they spoil too easily. In the West and some foreign countries, lard is used as the base oil. The lard is heated to liquefy, and then the process is done the same as above. However, for aromatherapy, especially spiritual applications, oils extracted using lard should not be used.

Hydraulic Expression

Another method, which produces oils of similar quality, is by hydraulic expression. In this method, a large quantity of blossoms leaves or barks is subjected to a great pressure, which squeezes out the essential oil. Both this method and centrifugal extraction can damage the subtle ingredients in the more delicate flower oils. Either of these methods requires a huge quantity of blossoms or other substance to produce a small quantity of oil. Thus, these oils are the most expensive. For examples, first pressing rose oil requires about 20,000 pounds of rose petals to produce one kilogram (2.2 pounds) of true attar of rose oil.

Other Methods

There are several other methods being used in modern times to produce attars or essential oils. One is called centrifugal extraction. The blossoms or other substance are placed in a large cylinder, and caused to rotate or spin at a very high rate of speed. The pressure exerted by gravity as the spinning occurs forces the oil content of the blossoms out. Usually oils extracted by this process are called first-pressing oils, absolutes or concretes. Many delicate petals, such as Gardenia, Jasmine, Lily of the Valley and others, cannot stand the force of this method of extraction.

Oils produced using traditional degree of steam distillation, *enfleurage*, or hydraulic expression are all termed attars. In natural perfumery, it is often the case that several attar oils are blended together to produce a final scent that is pleasant and unique.

One reason for this is that absolutes or concentrated essential oils in their natural state are not only prohibitively expensive, but also often quite irritating to the skin, and if taken internally, can be fatal, even in small doses of less than a teaspoon.

Attar fragrance oils should specifically not be thought of or compared to products sold as 'essential oils'. Well over two hundred fifty oils are sold as essential oils. Attars include some individual essential oils, which are known in their own fight as suitable for fragrance use, such as sandalwood, amber and patchouli. Another difference is that attars can be not on single substance oils, but made from multiple oils, sometimes as many as 30 or 40 blended together from centuries old secret attari family formulas.

QUALITY STANDARD

The quality of attars can be ensured by:

1. Controlling the qualities of raw material, i.e. flowers and base materials like sandalwood oil, etc.
2. Standardisation of process parameters.

The BIS specification is available for the analysis of sandalwood oil. Most of the species which are used in the manufacturing of Indian traditional fragrances, for example, Sugandh Mantri, Sugandh Bala, Kapoor Kachri, Jatamansi, andNagarmotha, etc. have no specification of their quality assessment.

The quality of attars depends upon:

1. The quality of flower.
2. The time duration between the plucking of flower and charging into the stills.
3. The process parameters of distillation.

To survive in the world market of fragrance and flavour, it is necessary that attars should be of standard quality. Therefore, their standardisation is essential to sustain in the world market.

SOURCES OF EQUIPMENT

The equipments which are used in this industry are designed and fabricated in and around Kannauj and Farrukhabad districts of UP by the local fabricator. The equipments are easy to be fabricated and are made of copper. They can be made by any good fabricators after getting designed from any authentic source.

Chapter 9

Examination and Analysis of Essential Oils, Synthetics and Isolates

INTRODUCTION

'The examination and analysis of essential oils, synthetics and isolates' describes the commercial methods of testing and evaluating the raw materials of the essential oil industry. Most of these methods have been used in United States and European countries. They frequently represent standard official procedures or modifications of such procedures. Many highly specialised techniques which are of value in the scientific examination of essential oils have not been included because they are seldom used in a commercial laboratory.

The essential oil chemist works in a highly specialised field requiring careful analytical ability, ingenuity and a highly developed sense of smell and taste. He must always be on the alert for known adulterants and impurities and for new and hitherto untried adulterants. Above all, he must have sufficient chemical background and experience to be able to interpret the results of his analyses.

Crude adulteration of oils has lessened considerably, because of careful analytical control. Seldom does one encounter today the adulteration of lemon oil with turpentine, or the addition of acetanalide to vanillin. However, some adulterations are still in evidence, especially where strict analytical control is not maintained by government agencies and buyers. For example, at a comparatively recent date, the orange oils of French Guinea were so badly adulterated with kerosene and mineral oil fractions that the reputation of this oil suffered; government control entirely checked this gross adulteration. Sri Lanka citronella oils have been adulterated with mineral oil fractions for so long that the trade has almost accepted this as a necessary evil, trying to limit the amount of adulteration rather than to stop it altogether. Such crude adulterations usually offer no problem to the essential oil chemist. A routine analysis easily discloses such falsifying.

A much more dangerous and common type of adulteration is the addition of materials that do not materially affect the physico-chemical properties of an oil. Often materials are added that are normal constituents of the oil: materials that are obtained as by-products, isolates from other oils or synthetics. Such 'sophistication' is much more difficult to detect and often may be suspected but proved only with great difficulty at best. It is in cases such as these that a well-developed sense of smell and taste proves of immense value. Here it is important for the chemist to know what adulterants to expect. Organoleptic tests, in conjunction with physico-chemical analyses, also are of great importance in evaluating the quality of unadulterated oils.

A discussion of the general procedure to be followed in examining an essential oil, isolate or synthetic may prove of value.

A study of the odour and in some cases the flavour, helps materially in detecting adulteration or 'sophistication' and in judging quality. Comparison should be made with an oil of high quality, a 'type' oil of known purity. A drop or two of the oil in question is placed upon a strip of blotting paper; the same amount of the pure 'type' oil is placed upon a second strip; and the two held together at right angles by means of a clip. The odour of the two oils should be studied carefully and compared at intervals. When first on blotters, addition of the more volatile adulterants is often discovered. Solvent 'by-notes' may also be detected in the case of a product obtained by extraction. When the blotters have dried considerably, addition of the less volatile adulterants may often be detected—materials such as cedarwood and heavy camphor oil. The study of the odour and flavour often suggests the presence of adulterants which may be confirmed by special chemical or physical tests. Or adulterants indicated by the analysis may be confirmed by a study of the odour and flavour. Moreover, organoleptic tests are probably the only satisfactory method, thus far developed, of detecting burnt, pyroligneous 'by-notes' resulting from improper distillation and of detecting slight spoilage in certain oils, as for example the citrus oils.

Also of great importance is the determination of the physical and chemical properties of a given oil. The specific gravity, the optical rotation, the solubility in dilute alcohol and the refractive index should be determined for all oils and liquid isolates and synthetics as a matter of routine. Other special tests are also to be carried out, depending upon the material under consideration (e.g. ester content, total alcohol determination, congealing point, evaporation residue). For an optically inactive, crystalline solid, the best criterion of purity lies in the determination of the melting point. Comparing these analytical figures with results of previous analyses and with data, the chemist may obtain an indication of the purity and quality of the oil. Crude adulteration often is discovered at this point.

The relationship between the individual chemical and physical properties is often very revealing. Thus, the addition of orange terpenes to an orange oil will cause a lowering of the specific gravity, refractive index and the evaporation residue, and a corresponding increase in the optical rotation; the addition of turpentine oil will cause a lowering of the optical rotation as well as of the other three properties.

Another factor to be considered is possible sources of adulteration or contamination. Benzaldehyde should be tested for chlorine, since a positive halogen test would indicate manufacture from benzyl chloride or insufficient purification. Low refractive index and specific gravity of a linaloe oil suggest adulteration with ethyl alcohol, a common form of adulteration for this oil.

The value of the relationship between each physical and chemical property and between the analysis and the odour and flavour cannot be stressed too strongly.

The analytical figures obtained in as complex a material as an essential oil seldom represent actual percentages of single constituents. Thus, in the case of an ester determination, all saponifiable material is calculated as a certain ester, regardless of the fact that unquestionably other esters are present or that other constituents are capable of saponification. The figures obtained, however, are no less valuable for practical purposes. Nevertheless, it may be seen that in this field of chemistry it is of utmost importance that a procedure be rigidly followed in order to assure reproducible results that are of practical value.

The main purpose of the following discussion is to help standardise such analytical procedures so that chemists throughout the essential oil industry may obtain results that can be reproduced by other workers in this field as well as by chemists in related industries.

SAMPLING AND STORAGE

It is important that the sample used for analysis be representative of the entire contents of the container. Since most materials encountered by the analyst are homogeneous oils, sampling is not a difficult operation.

However, a few cautions are noted to assure a representative sample. Most essential oils are obtained by steam distillation with subsequent separation of the oil and water layers; therefore, shipments of oil frequently contain water. If the oil has a specific gravity of less than 1.0, the water will be found at the bottom of the drum. It is a wise precaution to test each drum for water by introducing a sampling thief made of a long glass tube with one end slightly constricted. With the other end of the glass tube securely closed (by pressing the thumb over the opening), the thief is introduced into the drum and lowered until the constricted end just touches the bottom of the drum; the thumb is removed to permit the oil and water (if present) to enter the tube; the thumb is replaced and the tube withdrawn (the thief should be held in a vertical position). The oil within the tube is permitted to drain into a flint glass bottle or graduate. Any water, sediment (e.g. dirt and rust) or precipitated waxes are readily discernible. For oils that have a specific gravity greater than 1.0, any water that is present will appear as a supernatant layer. Hence, in introducing the thief, the tube is not closed with the thumb and is lowered into the drum slowly.

The sample in the flint bottle or graduate should receive a cursory examination—colour, clarity, viscosity, the presence or absence of sediments, separated waxes and water, all should be observed and noted; finally the odour of the sample should be studied. Oils stored in drums for long periods will frequently show a slight musty 'by-note' which rapidly disappears; this is a typical 'drum-note' and does not reflect adversely on the quality of the oil. Freshly distilled oils frequently show a slight, sharp empyreumatic or burned note which disappears as the oil is aged. The 'drum-note' and the 'freshly distilled note' should disappear if the oil is permitted to stand in an open graduate overnight. If such notes do not disappear, the oils should be examined more carefully; it may be necessary to aerate the oil to remove persistent 'by-notes'. A small sample of the oil (about 50 cc.) should be treated by bubbling air through the oil for a period of several hours. It may be necessary to warm the air which is bubbled through the oil. Figure 9.1 shows a convenient apparatus for carrying out such aeration. If this treatment yields a satisfactory oil, the contents of the drum may be treated similarly.

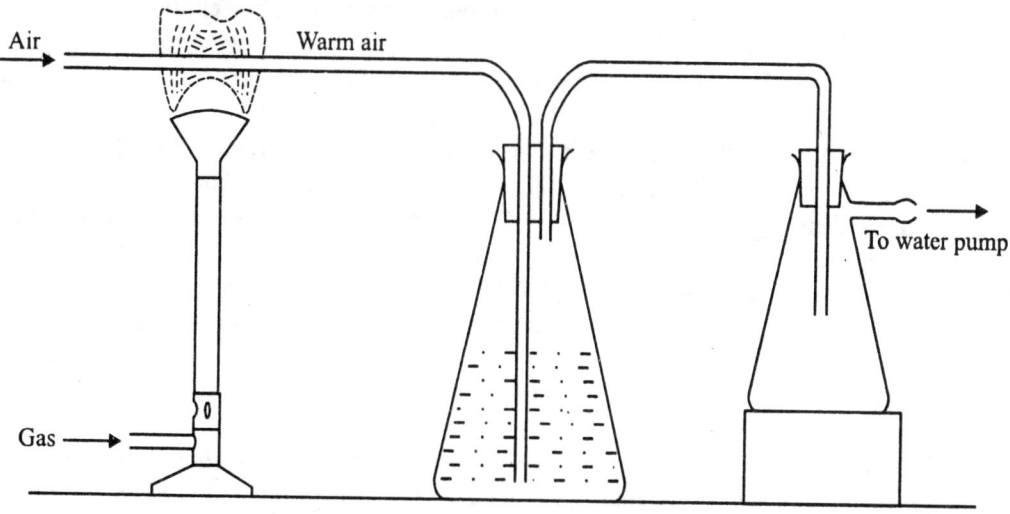

Fig. 9.1. Apparatus for the aeration of essential oils.

Citrus oils frequently deposit large amounts of waxes. These are easily observed by the water testing technique described above. Another indication is the 'feel' of the tube as it hits the bottom of the drum.

If the drum shows no evidence of water or insignificant amounts of water and sediment, the sample drawn may be used for analysis. If water, wax or sediment is present to a large-extent, a fresh sample should be drawn from the supernatant oil.

When the sample is received by the chemist, it should be clarified and freed from sediment and separated waxes by decantation or by filtration if necessary. A small amount of dry sodium chloride placed in the folded filter will frequently aid in removing traces of water and will remove the haze from an oil. Treatment with clay or kieselguhr may be necessary to remove a haze caused by suspended materials. If the oil is very dark in colour owing to the presence of heavy metals or other metallic impurities, the colour may be lightened by shaking with tartaric acid and filtering. The colour and appearance of the oil both before and after treatment should be described in the analytical report, as well as the treatment used.

Because of possible variation in the oils of a shipment of more than one drum, it is best to sample each drum of oil. However, if the oils are to be bulked (e.g. several drums are to be pumped into a tank to yield a uniform lot), an average or representative sample may be made based on the weights of the oil in the individual drums. The odour and general appearance of each drum should be examined before such a sample is made, to prevent the addition of a drum of poor quality to the tank. If this average sample is found to be of inferior quality or shows any abnormalities, then each drum must be re-sampled and examined individually.

Oils that congeal at temperatures normally encountered should be given special attention. These drums should be permitted to stand in a warm place and stirred occasionally (or heated in a steam room if the congealing point is high) until the last trace of solid material is dissolved. Anise oil may be taken as a typical example. During the cold weather a drum may be received in a frozen condition. Upon standing in a warm place, the anethole slowly melts until the drum is half solid, half liquid. The solid settles to the bottom. If a sample of the liquid portion is drawn, it will be deficient in anethole and may fail to meet the official requirements of 'The United States Pharmacopoeia'; such a sample would not be representative of the drum. Synthetics and isolates such as anethole, benzyl benzoate and diphenyl oxide usually require a steam room to melt them completely to assure a representative sample. Upon chilling or long-standing, some oils deposit small amounts of crystalline materials such as menthol, cedrol or camphor; in these cases, the oil should be gently warmed and stirred to redissolve the crystalline material before a sample is drawn.

In sampling materials other than oils, certain precautions should be observed. For resinoids, oleoresins and balsams the drum or can should be stirred well with a flat stick to assure thorough mixing. A sample should not be drawn before the material is uniform. This is of importance for items such as styrax, which usually shows a separation of styrene, polystyrene and water.

The sampling of crude drugs offers considerable difficulties. 'The United States Pharmacopoeia' gives three methods for the sampling of vegetable drugs from original containers to obtain an 'official', representative sample:

1. It is recommended that gross samples of vegetable or animal drugs in which the component parts are 1 cm or less in any dimension, and all powdered or ground drugs, be taken by means of a sampler which removes a core from the top to the bottom of the container, not less than two cores being taken in opposite directions; that when the total weight of the drug to be sampled is less than 100 kg at least 250 grams shall constitute an official sample. When the total weight of the drug to be sampled is in excess of 100 kg, repeated samples shall be taken by the above method, and according to the schedule given below, mixed and quartered, two of the diagonal quarters being rejected, the remaining two quarters being combined and carefully mixed and again subjected

to a quartering process in the same manner until two of the quarters weigh at least 250 grams, which latter quarters shall constitute an official sample.

2. It is recommended that gross samples of vegetable drugs in which the component parts are over 1 cm in any dimension be taken by hand. When the total weight of the drug to be sampled is less than 100 kg, at least 500 grams shall constitute an official sample and this shall be taken from different parts of the containers. When the total weight of the drug to be sampled is in excess of 100 kg, repeated samples shall be taken by the above method and according to the schedule below, mixed and quartered, two of the diagonal quarters being rejected and the remaining two quarters being combined and carefully mixed, and again subjected to a quartering process in the same manner until two of the quarters weigh not less than 500 grams, which latter quarters shall constitute an official sample.

Schedule recommended for sampling	
Number of packages in shipment	Number of packages to be sampled
1 to 10	1 to 3
10 to 25	3 to 4
25 to 50	4 to 6
50 to 75	6 to 8
75 to 100	8 to 10

When over 100, the total number sampled should not be less than 10.

3. When the total weight of a drug to be sampled is less than 10 kg it is recommended that the above methods be followed but that somewhat smaller quantities be withdrawn and in no case should the final official sample weigh less than 125 grams.

The sampling of a pure chemical which is a solid (e.g. vanillin) will now be considered. The well-known method of quartering will assure a representative sample. Most manufacturers give an identifying number to each batch manufactured and consequently it may be assumed that each batch is uniform so that a sample taken at random will be representative of the whole batch.

The final sample should be transferred to a bottle of light-resistant glass (amber, blue or green). The bottle should be well filled to prevent adverse action by the air and well stoppered with a sound cork. Screw caps should be used with caution, since the liners may contaminate the oil. If a screw cap is to be employed it is well to stopper the bottle with a cork before using the screw cap.

If the shipment of oil is to be stored for any appreciable length of time, the precautions noted below should be observed:

1. The oils should be clarified and thoroughly dried.
2. The oils are best stored in glass containers in a cool place protected from light and air. Half filled containers should be avoided. Storage in glass is frequently impractical; if drums or cans must be used, heavily galvanised or heavily tinned iron usually will prove satisfactory. Aluminium and stainless steel can be used with some oils, but not universally.
3. Certain oils are much more susceptible to oxidation and polymerisation than others; oils rich in terpenes (e.g. citrus oils) and oils containing large amounts of aldehydes (e.g. benzaldehyde) are readily affected. Some oils (e.g. vetiver, sandalwood and patchouly) show very good keeping qualities and may actually improve upon ageing.

4. In general, the use of antioxidants for essential oils is not necessary if the oils are properly and carefully stored.

DETAILED ANALYSIS OF ESSENTIAL OILS LEADS TO THE UNDERSTANDING OF THEIR PROPERTIES

Essential oils are valuable natural products used as raw materials in many fields; including perfumes, cosmetics, aromatherapy and phytotherapy, spices, and nutrition. Essential oils are complex mixtures comprised of, in some cases, more than 250 single compounds. Each of these constituents contribute to the beneficial or adverse effects of these essential oils. Therefore, the intimate knowledge of essential oil composition allows for a better and specially directed application. For example, an essential oil with a high content of a relaxant cannot be applied for activating purposes. An essential oil containing furocoumarines cannot be used as perfume material for sunscreens. As a natural product, essential oil composition depends on climate, soil, harvesting time, method of production and similar factors. The different chirality of main constituents governs the uses of essential oils and should be considered as well.

A series of factors influencing the composition of essential oils are discussed under the general topic of cosmetology applications. Because essential oils are naturally occurring fragrance mixtures, the question is, why are fragrances used in cosmetic products? To answer this, we must answer the following:

1. One must not forget that many cosmetic raw materials possess an odour that cannot be described as pleasant, sometimes smelling outright disagreeable. Because of this, one main goal of any fragrance addition to a cosmetic product is to conceal, to mask a bad smell or a malodour inherent to ingredients.

2. The application discipline of a cosmetic product is often increased by a pleasant fragrance. This is beneficial to both partners: the user, who gains efficacy by following the recommended application schedule, and the producer, who can sell more of his product.

3. The germicidal properties of essential oils should be considered. This is especially true in creams. Due to their content of water and organic compounds, they offer excellent growing conditions for bacteria and fungi. Dry powders, on the other hand, offer an unfavourable environment to these organisms. With each finger touch to the cosmetic product in an opened jar, the user inserts about 10,000 new germs. Repeated contamination to the cosmetic product by such a method is a fact. However, fragrance compounds, and particularly those containing terpenic alcohols, do not only support preservatives in their function, but also kill germs, or at least stop their growth. Therefore, the safety for the user as well as the extended usefulness of the cosmetic product is guaranteed.

4. A pleasant fragrance creates or restores the self-confidence of the user. Who does not want to feel clean, good-smelling and therefore, appreciated and attractive?

5. A deliberately chosen fragrance stresses advertising statements (e.g. a fresh odour creates the illusion of an ocean breeze, supporting the feeling of freshness, freedom and cleanliness).

6. Essential oils and single-fragrance compounds are added to a cosmetic product in order to create a characteristic matchless aroma profile.

Aspects of Essential Oils

Essential oils are naturally occurring mixtures of many volatile compounds with the common property of emanating a scent. Some essential oils consist of only a few volatiles while the analysis of others shows more than 200 (e.g. rose oil contains up to 270 single constituents). Each constituent possesses a distinct molecular formula, certain molecular weight (roughly between 100 and 300 amu) and therefore certain physico-chemical properties, like polarity, electron density and optical activity, among others. By means of these properties, fragrances are used in medical and/or cosmetic treatments.

Fragrance compounds can act in a pharmacological capacity beyond their abilities to evoke emotions. Because of their lipophilicy, they penetrate the skin (the absorption through the nasal mucosa is as fast as an intravenous injection) and demonstrate a high affinity to adipose tissues and central nervous system. It is known that they can pass the blood brain barrier due to the discovery of races in brain tissue of animals, as experiments have shown. The staying power of these chemicals can be as high as about 58 hours beyond original exposure. The application of single-fragrance compounds as well as of essential oil has to be done carefully, considering all toxicological and pharmacological data.

Roots of Oil Character

The most important tool for considering the proper application of an essential oil is detailed analysis via a capillary GC. The composition of an essential oil is dependent on such characteristics as the geographic character from which the plant is obtained, seasonal variations and climate, production techniques and purity. Certain geographic places very often bring forth specific species of essential oil, producing plants, therefore, the same plant from different geographic origins produces varying constituents of the essential oil in either the concentration pattern or the lack of certain volatiles. Chamomile oil from Morocco is not the same as the English or German versions, though the material is always obtained from the flowers of *Matricaria chamomilla L. (Matricaria recutita L.)* (Asteraceae).

The GC's of their essential oils are distinctly different from one another. In the essential oil of *Artemisia laciniata* (Asteraceae) from the Himalayan region near Srinagar, Kashmir, altitude is responsible for differences in the composition of oils. The essential oil of a plant grown at an altitude of about 1800 metre above sea level, contains no piperitone, while the essential oil from *Artemisia laciniata* grown in the same region at 2700 metre above sea level shows this terpene ketone as the main compound. The camphor concentration in the first essential oil is about ten times higher than in the second. Artemisia ketone can be found in a range of concentrations between 12 per cent and one per cent. These results, published some years ago by Weyerstahl and his team from the Technical University of Berlin, clearly demonstrate the influence of temperature, total amount of sunhours and UV light on the composition of an essential oil.

Seasonal variations and the time of harvesting also show a great influence on the composition of essential oils. The content of geranial in the essential oil of the flowers of *Dracocephalum moldavica* (lamiaceae), an aromatic plant of Asia and Eastern Europe used for its antibacterial, antiviral, antispasmodic and culinary qualities, increases from about 18 per cent (early flowering stage) to 35 per cent (full senescens stage). The differences in flowering stages also affects the concentration of its corresponding alcohol, geraniol which decreases from about 17 per cent to five per cent respectively. Depending on the length of sunlight (UVB), the concentration of menthol in the essential oil of *Mentha piperita* (lamiaceae) declines from 48 per cent to 10 per cent, while the content of menthofurane rises from 9 per cent to 20 per cent, thus giving evidence of a type of ageing.

Oil composition is also affected by variations in production techniques. Essential oil qualities vary if obtained by hydrodistillation (the plant material is heated in two to three times its weight of water with indirect steam from outside the still) as opposed to steam distillation (the plant material is extracted by direct steam, produced in the still or by indirect steam, produced outside and fed into the still), hydrodiffusion (low-pressure steam [< 0.1 bar] replaces the volatiles from the intact plant material by osmotic action) or CO_2 extraction. For example, as was shown by Boelens some years ago, the chemical composition of the essential oil of the flowers of *Rosa damascena* (rosaceae) is very different depending on the production technique. In an essential oil sample obtained by hydrodistillation, the main compounds are citronellol (30 per cent) and geraniol (18 per cent). In the CO_2 extraction, 2-phenylethanol (67 per cent) was found as the main constituent. The concentration of the very potent trace and character-impact compound β-damascenone is about three times higher in the essential oil obtained by hydrodistillation. The resultant oil varies if the distillation still for the production of the essential oil is totally or partly filled, or if the distillation process is performed in a glassware-equipment or copper still, as has been reported on different composition of geranium oils from *Pelargonium graveolens* (geraniceae) of France's Reunion Islands.

Safety Concerns

An important factor in the industry is the use of solvents and pesticides because developing countries, where environmental considerations still do not play the same role as in the industrialised world, represent about 55 per cent of total global essential oil production. For example, as has been shown by Schilcher and his team at the Free University of Berlin, in 72 samples of approximately 110 commercially available essential oil samples, 34 different essential oil organochlorine pesticide residues were found. DDT, long forbidden in the industrialised world, was located often. Also detected were lindane, α-endosulphane and hexachlorocyclohexane. All of these can create serious health and safety problems if such tainted essential oils are used in cosmetics. Even if the detected amount is too small for a toxic reaction after a single application, the danger of accumulation in adipose tissues exists, especially upon repeated cosmetic and perfume product applications. In nonsense applications such as aromatherapy-massage wherein essential oils are applied on cellulite, the skin often acts as a reservoir for topically applied chemicals.

Life Span of Essential Oils as Perfume Constituents in Cosmetic Products

Perfumed rinse-off products, like shampoos, can be used without a great fear of toxicity. However, this attitude is not valid with regard to creams, lotions, lipsticks, etc. which are used on large skin areas, have a prolonged contact with the skin or are applied to mucus membranes. In all cases, the absorption through the skin has to be considered. Normally, the perfume concentration in most of cosmetic products ranks between 0.5 per cent and 2 per cent, thus being too small for any toxicity risk from essential oil-constituents, with the exception of some more or less toxic terpenic ketones, such as thujone or pulegone. However, none can ignore the cumulative effect of the lipophilic fragrance compounds in adipose tissues (e.g. cutaneous reservoir), diverse organs of the body or its misuse in the form of repeated high-quantity applications. The cosmetic chemist also has to consider biochemical interactions of the essential oil constituents with the skin. This includes oxidations, de-acetalisations and ester cleavages, which often occur on moist skin (e.g. in the axilla), thus furnishing an altered perfume composition. Esteras of the skin cleave phenylethyl acetate to phenyl ethyl alcohol and acetic acid, which may, in some cases, cause skin irritations changing the odour of cosmetic products. Another good example is *d*-limonene, which hardly shows a sensitising capacity. However, because of its easily formed oxidation products, it can be compared to common allergens such as formaldehyde. The volatilities of each single compound in the essential oils is different, thus aiding longer skin contact for low-volatile compounds (e.g. 1 hour after the application of benzyl acetate to the skin, this fragrance compound shows a tripled skin-life over that of limonene and *cis*-jasmone; at times, this can increase up to 20 fold longer). Substances with a somewhat higher toxicity potential should not remain too long on the skin.

Another fact that clearly shows the importance of a detailed analysis of an essential oil sample is the danger of phototoxicity and dermal sensitisation. Furocoumarines are well-known to cause the Berloque-dermatitis, when such a treated skin area is exposed to sunlight. This is also true with cinnamic derivatives, oak moss and balms. The fact that fragrance compounds may, in some cases, cause dermal sensitisation should not discredit their careful use. Sesquiterpene hydrocarbons and cinnamic derivatives are known to possess a high sensitisation potential. Chirality, a molecular property, is frequently encountered in natural products in mono- and sesquiterpene compounds of essential oils. The absorption rate of an enantiomeric pair of such fragrance compounds is different, as has been shown using (+) - and (–) - carvone, or (+) - and (–) - limonene in human experiments. (+) - Carvone and (+) - limonene have been found to have a longer plasma life than their enantiomers, which get metabolised more quickly (on the other hand, the concentration of their corresponding metabolites in the urine is higher).

Thus it is evident that essential oils are mixtures of volatile compounds and not esoteric miracles. Because of the molecular attributes of each single essential oil constituent, the perfumer is able to create perfumes for cosmetic products in safe ways while carefully considering the harmful properties of some fragrance ingredients and using the guidelines of the International fragrance association (IFA). Considering all the aforementioned differences in essential oil composition, it is clear that only a detailed knowledge of the constituents of an essential oil will lead to a proper use in cosmetics by perfumers and cosmetic chemists. However, such a detailed knowledge can only be obtained by means of a carefully performed capillary-GC. Therefore, each essential oil charge should be provided with such a precise chromatogram. A careful quality control testing of each sample, dealing with the residue, authenticity of the main compounds by chiral determination and concentration pattern is a must. Each batch should be labelled properly. Regarding essential oils as harmless because they are natural is as stupid as it is irresponsible.

Chapter 10

Determination of Physical Properties of Essential Oils

INTRODUCTION

The physical properties play an important role in determining the various aspects of essential oils. This chapter discusses the important physical properties of essential oils such as—specific gravity, optical rotation, refractive index, solubility, melting and boiling points, evaporation residue and flash point.

SPECIFIC GRAVITY

Specific gravity is an important criterion of the quality and purity of an essential oil. Of all the physico-chemical properties, the specific gravity has been reported most frequently in the literature. Values for essential oils vary between the limits of 0.696 and 1.188 at 15°C in general, the gravity is less than 1.000. For each individual oil, however, the limits are much narrower and in most cases have been established during the course of years.

The specific gravity of an essential oil at 15°C may be defined as the ratio of the weight of a given volume of oil at 15°C to the weight of an equal volume of water at 15°C. (The density of a liquid is the weight of a unit volume. Thus, density may be expressed in pounds per cubic foot, or more frequently in grams per cubic centimeter. At 3.98°C (the temperature of maximum density for pure water, free from air) 1 cc. of water weighs 0.999973 gram; furthermore, at this temperature 1 ml of water weighs exactly 1 gram. Since the coefficient of expansion of water is small, the density of a liquid expressed in grams per cubic centimeter corresponds closely to the specific gravity. However, the fundamental difference in the two concepts should be thoroughly understood.

For determination of this physical property, accuracy to at least the third decimal place is necessary. Therefore, hydrometers are practically worthless and should not be used. The Mohr-Westphal balance may be used but it has the disadvantage that relatively large amounts of oil are required for a determination. Other types of specific gravity balances have been developed which require less oil and which have proven satisfactory. Pycnometers offer the most convenient and rapid method for determining specific gravities. A conical shaped pycnometer having a volume of about 10 cc. with a ground-in thermometer and a capillary side tube with a ground glass cap proves very satisfactory (Fig. 10.1). This pycnometer is similar to that described in American standards of testing material (ASTM). Designation D 153 with the exception that the capacity is approximately 10 cc. instead of 50 cc. Sprengel or Ostwald tubes give even more accurate results; if desired they may be used. However, a determination cannot be made as rapidly or as conveniently. Cleaning these tubes will prove considerably more difficult and time consuming. A small Sprengel tube or a Gay-Lussac specific gravity bottle having a capacity of about 2 cc. will often prove of value when only small amounts of oil are available. For routine analyses the conical pycnometer as described is recommended.

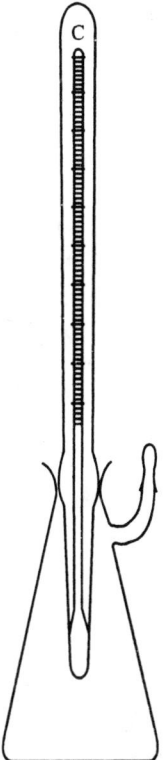

Fig. 10.1. Pycnometer.

Procedure: Clean the pycnometer by filling it with a saturated solution of chromium trioxide in sulphuric acid and allow it to stand for at least 3 hours. Empty the pycnometer and rinse thoroughly with distilled water. Fill the pycnometer with recently boiled distilled water which has been cooled to a temperature of about 12°C and place it in a water bath, previously cooled to 12°C. Permit the temperature to rise slowly to 15°C. Adjust the level of the water to the top of the capillary side arm, removing any excess with a blotter or cloth, and put the ground glass cap in place. Remove the pycnometer from the water bath, dry carefully with a clean cloth, permit it to stand for 30 minutes and weigh accurately. Empty the pycnometer, rinse several times with alcohol and finally with ether. Remove the ether fumes with the aid of an air blast and permit the pycnometer to dry thoroughly. Weigh accurately after standing for 30 minutes. The 'water equivalent' of the pycnometer may be found by subtracting the weight of the empty pycnometer from its weight when full. Fill the clean, dried pycnometer with the oil previously cooled to a temperature of 12°C. Following the same procedure as above, place the pycnometer in a water bath and permit it to warm slowly to 15°C. Adjust the oil to the proper level, put the cap in place, and wipe the pycnometer dry. Accurately weight after 30 minutes. The weight of the oil contained in the pycnometer divided by the water equivalent gives the specific gravity of the oil at 15°C (in air). For a given pycnometer the water equivalent need be determined only once; therefore, it is important that this determination be performed with great care and accuracy.

For scientific work or for cases where the gravity is in question, the determination should be carried out exactly as described above. However, for routine analyses it is permissible to determine the specific gravity of an oil at room temperature compared with water at 15°C and then to reduce this value to a temperature of 15°C by use of a proper correction factor. Numerous workers have determined correction factors for various oils and have recommended a general value from 0.00042 to 0.00084 per degree centigrade.

However, as Bosart pointed out, it would be unsatisfactory to take the average figure obtained from a variety of oils and apply it to a particular oil, all the more so when there is a difference of opinion as to what that figure should be.

In the investigation carried out by Basart the values were obtained which ranged from 0.00070 to 0.00099 per degree for the forty-two essential oils he examined. For synthetics and isolates normally encountered by the essential oil chemist or perfumer, values ranged from 0.00067 to 0.00114 per degree.

Hence, it is unjustifiable to use an average correction factor if accurate data are to be obtained. Variations in specific gravity per degree centigrade for essential oils, isolates and synthetics are given in Tables 10.1 and Table 10.2.

Table 10.1. Variations in specific gravity per degree centigrade for essential oils.

Almond, bitter	0.00089	Linaloe	0.00083
Anise	0.00082	Mace	0.00082
Bay	0.00085	Mirbane	0.00098
Bergamot	0.00081	Orange, sweet	0.00078
Bois de Rose, Brazilian	0.00081	Origanum	0.00076
Cade	0.00074	Palmarosa	0.00073
Camphor	0.00081	Patchouly	0.00073
Cananga	0.00074	Pennyroyal	0.00078
Caraway	0.00078	Peppermint	0.00076
Cassia	0.00081	Petitgrain	0.00081
Cedar wood	0.00071	Pine	0.00079
Citronella, Sri Lanka	0.00081	Rosemary	0.00081
Citronella, Java	0.00093	Sandalwood, East Indian	0.00070
Clove	0.00085	Sassafras, Artificial	0.00087
Eucalyptus (*Eucalyptus globulus*) 70 to 80%	0.00084	Spearmint	0.00079
Geranium, African	0.00076	Spike	0.00082
Geranium, Bourbon	0.00076	Tansy	0.00080
Ho	0.00083	Thyme	0.00079
Lavender	0.00082	Vetiver	0.00071
Lemon	0.00077	Wintergreen (*Gaultheria procumbens*)	0.00099
Lemongrass	0.00079	Ylang Ylang	0.00073

The proper correction is to be added if the temperature, at which the determination was made, is above 15°C; conversely to be subtracted if the temperature is below 15°C. These correction factors may also prove of use for converting specific gravities given in the literature at temperatures other than 15°C when compared with water at 15°C.

Table 10.2. Variations in specific gravity per degree centigrade for isolates and synthetics.

Acetal	0.00103	Dipentene	0.00080
Acetaldehyde	0.00129	Diphenyl methane	0.00078
Acetophenone	0.00086	Diphenyl oxide	0.00085
Allyl alcohol	0.00088	Ethyl acetate	0.00120
Allyl formate	0.00121	Ethyl benzoate	0.00092
n-Amyl acetate	0.00094	Ethyl n-butyrate	0.00103
α-Amyl cinnamic aldehyde	0.00076	Ethyl caproate (tech.)	0.00092
n-Amyl ether	0.00079	Ethyl formate	0.00126
Amyl salicylate	0.00085	Ethyl n-heptoate	0.00089
Anisic aldehyde	0.00085	Ethyl propionate	0.00111
Benzaldehyde	0.00089	Eugenol	0.00087
Benzyl acetate	0.00092	Geraniol	0.00071
Benzyl alcohol	0.00076	Geranyl acetate	0.00085
Benzyl benzoate	0.00081	Glycerol	0.00062
Benzyl ether	0.00079	Heliotropin	0.00093
Bornyl acetate	0.00086	Heptaldehyde	0.00086
Brombenzene	0.00134	Heptyl alcohol	0.00073
Bromstyrene	0.00114	Hydroxycitronellal	0.00077
n-Butyl acetate	0.00102	Ionone	0.00076
n-Butyl benzoate	0.00086	Isoamyl acetate	0.00097
n-Butyl n-Butyrate	0.00093	Isoamyl formate	0.00097
n-Butyl formate	0.00100	Isoeugenol	0.00087
n-Butyl lactate	0.00097	Isopulegol	0.00083
n-Butyl propionate	0.00099	Isosafrole	0.00088
n-Butyl d-Tartrate	0.00091	Lauryl alcohol	0.00067
Butyraldehyde	0.00105	d-Limonene	0.00077
n-Caproic acid	0.00087	Linaloöl	0.00082
n-Caprylic acid	0.00082	Linalyl acetate	0.00084
Carvacrol	0.00076	Methyl acetate	0.00127
Carvone	0.00080	Methyl acetophenone	0.00081
Cinnamic aldehyde	0.00080	Methyl anthranilate	0.00088
Cinnamyl alcohol	0.00074	Methyl benzoate	0.00095
Citral	0.00080	Methyl n-butyrate	0.00107
Citronellal	0.00082	Methyl n-caproate	0.00094
Citronellol	0.00070	Methyl formate	0.00143
p-Cresyl acetate	0.00093	Methyl heptenone	0.00084
p-Cymene	0.00079	Methyl nonyl ketone	0.00076
Decyl alcohol	0.00068	Methyl phenylacetate	0.00093
Diethyl phthalate	0.00084	Methyl phthalate	0.00093

(Contd ...)

Methyl propionate	0.00118	Pinene	0.00082
Methyl salicylate	0.00098	*n*-Propyl acetate	0.00110
Nitrobenzene	0.00098	*n*-Propyl formate	0.00114
Octyl alcohol	0.00068	Rhodinol	0.00071
Phellandrene	0.00078	Safrole	0.00089
Phenyl acetate	0.00098	Salicyl aldehyde	0.00097
Phenylethyl acetate	0.00090	Terpineol	0.00078
Phenylethyl alcohol	0.00074	Terpinyl acetate	0.00082
Phenylpropyl alcohol	0.00073	Valeric acid	0.00091

It is customary to report specific gravities for essential oils at 15°C. For oils that are not liquid at this temperature the specific gravity is conveniently reported at some higher temperature, compared with water at 15°C. Thus, the gravity of rose oils is often reported at 30°C. 'The United States Pharmacopoeia' and 'The National Formulary' specify a temperature of 25°C for most essential oils. 'The British Pharmacopoeia' specifies 15.5°C. In order to convert the specific gravities from 15° to 25°C, the conversion factors given in Table 10.3 may be used. These corrections are to be subtracted from the values determined at 15°C. A more exact determination will result if the water equivalent of the pycnometer at 25°C and the weight of the oil contained in the pycnometer at 25°C are determined by the method described under 'procedure'.

Table 10.3. Factors for conversion of specific gravity from 15° to 25°C.

Oil	Factor	Oil	Factor
Almond, bitter	0.0068	Lavender	0.0067
Anise	0.0060	Lemon	0.0058
Benzaldehyde	0.0069	Methyl salicylate	0.0079
Cajuput	0.0064	Mustard	0.0080
Caraway	0.0057	Nutmeg	0.0065
Cassia, rectified	0.0062	Orange, sweet	0.0057
Chenopodium	0.0063	Peppermint	0.0054
Cinnamic aldehyde	0.0056	Pimenta	0.0068
Clove	0.0065	Rosemary	0.0066
Copaiba	0.0054	Safrole	0.0069
Coriander	0.0067	Sandalwood	0.0047
Cubeb	0.0055	Sassafras	0.0067
Erigeron	0.0062	Savin	0.0058
Eucalyptol	0.0067	Spearmint	0.0062
Eucalyptus (*Eucalyptus globulus*)	0.0063	Sweet birch (*Betula lenta*)	0.0076
Eugenol	0.0066	Thyme	0.0061
Fennel	0.0062	Turpentine	0.0066
Hedeoma	0.0060	Turpentine, rectified	0.0065
Juniper berries	0.0062	Wintergreen (*Gaultheria procumbens*)	0.0076

OPTICAL ROTATION

Most essential oils when placed in a beam of polarised light possess the property of rotating the plane of polarisation to the right (dextrorotatory) or to the left (laevorotatory). The extent of the optical activity of an oil is determined by a polarimeter and is measured in degrees of rotation. Of the numerous types of polarimeters that are available, the most convenient for use with essential oils is probably the half-shadow instrument of the Lippich type.

The angle of rotation is dependent upon the nature of the liquid, the length of the column through which the light passes, the wavelength of the light used, and the temperature. Both the degree of rotation and its direction are important as criteria of purity. In recording rotations it is customary to indicate the direction by the use of a plus sign (+) to indicate dextrorotation (rotation to the right, i.e. clockwise) or a minus sign (−) to indicate laevorotation (rotation to the left, i.e. counterclockwise).

Since the scale reading for an optically active liquid is directly proportional to the length of the transmitting column of liquid, it is necessary to use a standard tube, 100 mm long. If for any reason a longer or shorter tube is used, the rotation should be calculated for a tube of 100 mm and reported as such. Rotations for essential oils given in the literature may be assumed to be for this standard tube unless a different length is specified.

It has become customary in polarimetric work to use sodium light. A suitable source may be obtained by placing large crystals of sodium chloride upon the grid of a Meeker burner or by wrapping a piece of asbestos, previously saturated in a strong salt solution, around the conventional Bunsen burner. By far the most convenient and satisfactory method of maintaining a constant light source is the use of a sodium vapour lamp. Such lamps, designed especially for use with polarimeters, are available.

Although 'The United States Pharmacopoeia' and 'The National Formulary' specify 25°C as the official temperature for all optical rotations, nevertheless, a standard temperature of 20°C is usually adopted for essential oils. For most essential oils the change in optical rotation with temperature variations normally encountered in the laboratory is very small; hence, in routine analyses the readings are usually taken at room temperature. No corrections for temperature variations are made except in the case of citrus oils which contain large amounts of highly active terpenes. The corrections to be used, per degree centigrade, are:

Orange oil	13.2′
Lemon oil	8.2′
Grapefruit oil	13.2′

The proper correction is to be added if the reading is taken at a temperature higher than the desired temperature and, conversely, to be subtracted if the temperature of the reading is lower than the desired temperature.

In scientific work the temperature at which the rotation was determined should be specified. To adjust the temperature to standard, the polarimeter tubes may be immersed in a constant temperature bath. Use may also be made of special water jacketed tubes. All determinations should be carried out in a dark room. Monochromatic sodium light should be employed.

Liquids

The oil or liquid should be free from suspended material. Often oils are hazy owing to the presence of small amounts of water; such an oil should be dried with anhydrous sodium sulphate and filtered before a determination is attempted.

Procedure: Place the 100 mm polarimeter tube containing the oil or liquid under examination in the trough of the instrument between the polariser and analyser. Slowly turn the analyser until both halves of the field, viewed through the telescope, show equal intensities of illumination. At the proper setting, a small rotation to the right or to the left will immediately cause a pronounced inequality in the intensities of illumination of the two halves of the field.

Determine the direction of rotation. If the analyser was turned counterclockwise from the zero position to obtain the final reading, the rotation is laevo (–); if clockwise, dextro (+). Since most instruments are calibrated only to 180°C, some confusion may exist as to the direction of rotation; this is especially true if the liquid is highly optically active. Thus, a reading of +100°C may be reported mistakenly as a reading of –80°C. If any doubt exists in the mind of the chemist, the determination should be repeated using a 50 mm tube. In the example given above, a reading of +50° would be obtained, indicating that the correct value for a 100 mm tube is +100°; the other possible reading with the smaller tube (that is, –130°) corresponds to a value of –260° for a 100 mm tube: so high a value would be most unusual for an essential oil. The optical rotation of an essential oil seldom is greater than ±100°.

After the direction of rotation has been established, carefully readjust the analyser until equal illumination of the two halves of the field is obtained. Adjust the eyepiece of the telescope to give a clear, sharp line between the two halves of the field. Determine the rotation by means of the protractor; read the degrees directly and the minutes with the aid of either of the two fixed verniers; the movable magnifying glasses will aid in obtaining greater accuracy. A second reading should be taken; it should not differ by more than ±5′ from the previous reading.

Some oils are too dark in colour for an accurate determination of the optical rotation when a 100 mm tube is used. In such cases, a 50 mm tube may be employed, or even a 25 mm tube, if necessary. Since the rotation is reported for a 100 mm tube, any experimental error will be multiplied by 2 for a 50 mm tube, and by 4 for a 25 mm tube. Conversely, if a clear, light coloured oil is examined which is only slightly optically active, the use of a longer tube (200 mm) may often prove of advantage; the value to be reported will be found by dividing the observed rotation by 2; any experimental error will also be halved.

Solids

The optical activity of a solid is best determined in solution and expressed as specific rotation. The following formulas may be used:

$$[\alpha]_D t° = \frac{100\alpha}{lpd} \qquad \text{... (10.1)}$$

$$[\alpha]_D t° = \frac{100\alpha}{lc} \qquad \text{... (10.2)}$$

where: $[\alpha]_D t°$ = specific rotation at temperature t°, using sodium light.
 α = observed rotation in degrees of the solution at temperature t°, using sodium light.
 l = length of polarimeter tube in decimeters.
 d = specific gravity of the solution at the temperature t°.
 p = concentration of the solution expressed as the number of grams of active substance in 100 grams of solution.
 c = concentration of solution expressed as the number of grams of active substance in 100 cc. of solution.

Equation (10.2) is more convenient, since it does not require the determination of the specific gravity of the solution.

The experimental value for the specific rotation of a solid is dependent upon the concentration of the solution and upon the particular solvent employed; therefore, the concentration and solvent used should be given when the specific rotation of a solid is reported. The rotation should be determined as soon as possible after the solution has been prepared, so that any change that might result from mutarotation will be minimised.

The use of specific rotation for a complex mixture such as an essential oil is not recommended. For the sake of completeness, the following equation is given:

$$[\alpha]_D t° = \frac{\alpha}{ld} \qquad \qquad ... (10.3)$$

Equation (10.3) applies to optically active liquids.

The symbol $[\alpha]_D t°$ is reserved exclusively for specific rotation; optical rotation determined in a 100 mm tube is indicated by $\alpha_D t°$, the brackets, being omitted. If no temperature is given, it may be assumed that the optical rotation was determined at room temperature.

REFRACTIVE INDEX

When a ray of light passes from a less dense to a more dense medium, it is bent or 'refracted' toward the normal. If e represents the angle of refraction and i the angle of incidence, according to the law of refraction,

$$\frac{\text{Sin } i}{\text{Sin } e} = \frac{N}{n}$$

where n is the index of refraction of the less dense, and N, the index of refraction of the more dense medium.

Refractometers offer a rapid and convenient method for the determination of this physical constant. Of the various types, the Pulfrich or the Abbé refractometer proves very satisfactory. The Abbé type, with a range of 1.3 to 1.7, is recommended for the routine analyses of essential oils, the accuracy of this instrument being sufficient for all practical work. The readings may be made directly from the scale without consulting conversion tables; only one or two drops of the oil are required for a determination; the temperature at which the reading is taken may be adjusted conveniently.

Procedure: Place the instrument in such a position that diffused daylight or some form of artificial light can readily be obtained for illumination. Circulate through the prisms a stream of water at 20°C. Carefully clean the prisms of the instrument with alcohol and then with ether. To charge the instrument, open the double prism by means of the screw head and place a few drops of the sample on the prism, or, if preferred, open the prisms slightly by turning the screw head and pour a few drops of sample into the funnel-shaped aperture between the prisms. Close the prisms firmly by tightening the screw head. Allow the instrument to stand for a few minutes before the reading is made so that the sample and instrument will be at the same temperature. Move the alidade backward or forward until the field of vision is divided into a light and dark portion. The line dividing these portions is the 'border line' and, as a rule, will not be a sharp line but a band of colour. The colours are eliminated by rotating the screw head of the compensator until a sharp, colourless line is obtained. Adjust the border line so that it falls on the point of intersection of the cross hairs. Read the refractive index of the substance directly on the scale of the sector. A second reading should be taken a few minutes later to assure that temperature equilibrium has been attained.

Occasionally, the instrument should be checked by means of the quartz plate that accompanies it, using monobromnaphthalene, or if such a plate is not available, by means of distilled water at 20°C; the refractive index of pure water at this temperature is 1.3330.

Great care should be exercised when determining refractive indexes during hot, humid weather, since moisture in the air may condense on the cooled prisms. This will result in a blurred and indistinct line of separation between the light and dark fields if the oil between the prisms does not dissolve the condensed moisture; if the oil dissolves the moisture, the dividing line will be sharp, but the observed index will be low. It has become the accepted procedure to report refractive indexes for essential oils at 20°C, using a monochromatic sodium light source, unless the material is a solid at that temperature. Thus, in the case of rose oil the refractive index is often given at 30°C, in the case of anethole, at 25°C.

Whenever possible, however, all observations should be made at 20°C. The use of factors to reduce readings to 20°C is not recommended. Various investigators, notably Bosart, have reported the change of refractive index with temperature for numerous oils. According to the findings the values for the fifty-four oils examined lie between the limits of 0.00039 and 0.00049 per degree centigrade and for the forty-seven synthetics and isolates between the limits of 0.00038 and 0.00054. A summary of the findings is given in Table 10.4. and Table 10.5. These tables may be used conveniently to convert values reported in the literature at other than 20°C. If an oil is encountered which is not listed in the table, the use of a correction factor of 0.00045 per degree will give approximately correct results. If the refractive index is reported at a temperature above 20°C, the proper correction must be added; conversely, if reported at below 20°C, the correction must be subtracted.

Table 10.4. Change in refractive index of essential oils.

	Correction per degree		Correction per degree
Almond, bitter	0.00049	Clove	0.00045
Anise	0.00049	Copaiba	0.00040
Bay leaves	0.00047	Coriander	0.00047
Bergamot	0.00044	Erigeron	0.00046
Bois de Rose	0.00044	Eucalyptus (*Eucalyptus globulus*)	0.00044
Cajuput	0.00045	Fennel	0.00047
Camphor, brown, s.g. 0.95–0.97	0.00043	Geranium, African	0.00040
Camphor, s.g. 1.020	0.00044	Geranium, Bourbon	0.00040
Camphor, white	0.00045	Ho	0.00043
Cananga·	0.00041	Lavender	0.00043
Caraway	0.00044	Linaloe	0.00044
Cassia	0.00048	Lemon	0.00046
Cedarwood	0.00040	Lemongrass	0.00044
Cinnamon, Sri Lanka	0.00048	Mace	0.00046
Citronella, Sri Lanka	0.00046	Mawah	0.00041
Citronella, Java	0.00047	Mustard	0.00054

(Contd ...)

	Correction per degree		Correction per degree
Orange, sweet	0.00045	Savin	0.00044
Origanum	0.00042	Spearmint	0.00043
Palmarosa	0.00040	Spike	0.00045
Patchouly	0.00042	Sweet birch (*Betula lenta*)	0.00045
Pennyroyal	0.00042	Tansy	0.00042
Peppermint	0.00040	Thyme, red, 40–45%	0.00044
Petitgrain	0.00044	Turpentine	0.00046
Pimenta	0.00047	Vetiver	0.00039
Pine	0.00042	Wintergreen (*Gaultheria procumbens*)	0.00045
Rosemary	0.00044	Ylang Ylang	0.00042
Sandalwood, E.I.	0.00039		
Sassafras, art	0.00045		

s.g. = specific gravity

Table 10.5. Change in refractive index of synthetics and isolates.

	Correction per degree		Correction per degree
Acetophenone	0.00047	Hydroxycitronellal	0.00040
α-Amyl cinnamic aldehyde	0.00050	Ionone	0.00044
Amyl salicylate	0.00042	Isoeugenol	0.00050
Anisic aldehyde (Aubepine)	0.00046	Isopulegol	0.00045
Benzaldehyde	0.00047	Limonene	0.00045
Benzyl acetate	0.00045	Linaloöl	0.00046
Bornyl acetate	0.00043	Linalyl acetate	0.00043
Bromstyrene	0.00054	Methyl anthranilate	0.00048
Carvacrol, Tech	0.00043	Methyl benzoate	0.00048
Cinnamic alcohol	0.00044	Methyl heptenone	0.00046
Cinnamic aldehyde	0.00052	Methyl phenylacetate	0.00046
Citral	0.00045	Methyl salicylate	0.00047
Citronellal	0.00044	Nitrobenzene (Mirbane oil)	0.00049
Citronellol	0.00040	*o*-Nitrotoluene	0.00048
p-Cresyl acetate	0.00046	Orange terpenes	0.00046
p-Cymene	0.00049	Phenylethyl acetate	0.00046
Diethyl phthalate	0.00041	Phenylethyl alcohol	0.00041
Diphenyl oxide	0.00049	Phenyl methyl carbinyl acetate	0.00046
Eucalyptol	0.00046	Phenylpropyl alcohol	0.00038
Eugenol	0.00046	Rhodinol	0.00040
Geraniol	0.00041	Safrole	0.00045
Geranyl acetate	0.00045	Terpineol	0.00044
Geranyl butyrate	0.00043	Terpinyl acetate	0.00041
Geranyl formate	0.00043		

MOLECULAR REFRACTION

A brief discussion of the fundamental concepts of molecular refraction involved may prove useful.

The index of refraction of a liquid varies with the temperature and with the wavelength of the light. In order to obtain a constant which is independent of the temperatures Gladstone and Dale introduced the use of 'specific refractivity'. Subsequently, Lorentz and Lorenz independently deduced an expression for specific refractivity, based upon the electromagnetic theory of light, which shows considerably less variation than the empirical expression of Gladstone and Dale. In order to compare the refractivities of different liquids, the use of molecular refractivity (molecular refraction) is necessary. This constant is equal to the product of the molecular weight of a substance and its specific refractivity.

Using the Lorentz and Lorenz expression:

$$R = Mr = \left(\frac{n^2 - 1}{n^2 + 2} \right) \left(\frac{M}{d} \right)$$

where, R = the molecular refractivity
  M = the molecular weight
  r = the specific refractivity
  n = observed refractive index at temperature $t°C$
  d = density at temperature $t°C$

The molecular refractivity has been found to be essentially additive. Hence, it is possible to calculate atomic refractivities for the different elements from a series of molecular refractivities of different compounds. By means of these atomic constants, the molecular refractivity of a pure chemical compound can be calculated as the sum of the atomic refractivities.

Investigation has shown, however, that the molecular refractivity is influenced by the presence of double and triple bonds, and also by the constitution of the molecule. Table 10.6 gives values for atomic refractivities for the D-line of the solar spectrum (sodium light), 5893 angstrom units, calculated by different investigators.

By use of these constants it is often possible to establish or confirm the chemical constitution of a pure chemical compound.

Table 10.6. Atomic refractions for the D-line.

	Eisenlohr	*Conrady*	*Brühl-Conrady*
CH_2	4.618	–	–
C	2.418	2.495	2.501
H	1.100	1.051	1.051
O"	2.211	2.281	2.287
O<	1.643	1.679	1.683
O'	1.525	1.517	1.521
Cl	5.967	5.976	5.998
Br	8.865	8.900	8.927
I	13.900	14.120	14.120
Double bond between C-atoms	1.733	1.707	1.707
Triple bond between C-atoms	2.398	–	–

Certain anomalies have been observed. When double bonds are present in a conjugated position, the molecular refractivity will show in general a higher value than one would expect; this is known as optical exaltation. In some cases optical depression is also encountered. It is interesting to note that conjugated double bonds in a ring compound cause no exaltation or depression.

The application of molecular refraction is limited to pure individual chemical compounds; it becomes meaningless when applied to mixtures as complex as essential oils. Nevertheless, this constant has played a very important role in the elucidation of structure in the case of many individual constituents of essential oils after separation and purification.

SOLUBILITY

Solubility in Alcohol

Since most essential oils are only slightly soluble in water and are miscible with absolute alcohol, it is possible to determine the number of volumes of dilute alcohol required for the complete solubility of one volume of oil. The determination of such a solubility is a convenient and rapid aid in the evaluation of quality of an oil. In general, oils rich in oxygenated constituents are more readily soluble in dilute alcohol than oils rich in terpenes.

Adulteration with relatively insoluble material will often greatly affect the solubility. Sometimes an actual separation of the adulterant may be observed. For example, adulteration of citronella oils (which are normally soluble in 80 per cent alcohol) with relatively large amounts of petroleum fractions will result in a poor solubility for the oil in 80 per cent alcohol and an actual separation of oily droplets of the adulterant. However, certain oils will show a normal separation in dilute alcohol. Expressed orange oil, for example, will separate natural waxes in 90 per cent alcohol. In alcohol of lower strength such an oil will separate a terpene fraction in addition to the waxes. Use of this fact sometimes is made in the preparation of terpeneless and sesquiterpeneless oils, concentrates and extracts.

The solubility of an oil may change with age. Polymerisation is usually accompanied with a decrease in solubility; i.e. a stronger alcohol may be required to yield a clear solution. Such polymerisation may be very rapid if the oil contains large amounts of easily resinified terpenes, e.g. juniper berry oil, bay oil. Improper storage may hasten polymerisation; factors such as light, air, heat, and the presence of water, usually exert an unfavourable influence. Occasionally the solubility of an oil improves upon ageing, e.g. oil of anise. This is due to the presence of the difficulty soluble anethole, which yields upon oxidation the readily soluble anisic aldehyde.

Alcohols of the following strengths are customarily used in determining solubilities of essential oils:
50%–60%–70%–80%–90%–95% and occasionally 65% and 75%.
These are volume percentages at 15.56°. In preparing dilute alcohols it is convenient to weigh the alcohol (95 per cent by volume) and the distilled water to give the proper volume percentage. Preparation in this manner is independent of temperature. The strength of the alcohol should be checked by determining the specific gravity at 15.56°C. Final adjustments may be made if necessary (Table 10.7).

Procedure: Introduce exactly 1 cc. of the oil into a 10 cc. glass-stoppered cylinder (calibrated to 0.1 cc.) and add slowly, in small portions, alcohol of proper strength. Shake the cylinder thoroughly after each addition. When a clear solution is first obtained, record the strength and the number of volumes of alcohol required. Continue the additions of alcohol until 10 cc. has been added. If opalescence or cloudiness occurs during these subsequent additions of alcohol, record the point at which this phenomenon occurs. In the event that a clear solution is not obtained at any point during the addition of the alcohol, repeat the determination, using an alcohol of higher strength.

Table 10.7. Preparation of dilute alcohols.

Alcohol (% by volume)	Specific gravity 15.56°C	95% Alcohol by volume (g)	Distilled water (g)
50	0.9342	460	540
60	0.9133	564	436
65	0.9019	619	381
70	0.8899	676	324
75	0.8771	734	266
80	0.8636	796	204
90	0..8336	927	73
95	0.8158	1000	0

Since the solubility is dependent upon the temperature, all determinations should be made at 20°C. It should be noted, however, that 'The United States Pharmacopoeia' and 'The national formulary' specify an official temperature of 25°C for solubilities; 'The British Pharmacopoeia', a temperature of 15.5°C. The proper temperature may be maintained by frequent immersion of the cylinder in a water bath previously adjusted to the desired temperature.

If an oil is not clearly soluble in the dilute alcohols, it is advisable to describe more fully the appearance of the solubility test.

The following terms, which are relative and entirely empirical, are used in the laboratories to describe the appearance of the solution:

Clearly soluble	Opalescent
Slightly hazy	Slightly turbid
Hazy	Turbid
Slightly opalescent	Cloudy

A further term occasionally used is 'fluorescent'.

In the case of turbidity or cloudiness, record any separation of wax or oil that occurs, as well as the period of time required for such separation.

If an oil is soluble in a number of volumes or alcohol which is not a multiple of ½, report the solubility as being between the closest such limits. For example, if 2.7 volumes of 70 per cent alcohol were required to obtain a clear solution, and the solution remained clear upon further additions of 70 per cent alcohol until a total of 10 volumes had been added, the solubility would be recorded as:

'Clearly soluble in 2.5 to 3 volumes of 70 per cent alcohol and more, up to 10 volumes'.

Solubility in Non-alcoholic Media

Several solubility tests have been introduced for the rapid evaluation of oils. The following have proven valuable.

Carbon disulphide solubility for the presence of water

Oils rich in oxygenated constituents frequently contain dissolved water. This is particularly true in the case of oils containing large amounts of phenolic bodies, e.g. oil of bay. Such oils fail to give a clear solution when diluted with an equal volume of carbon disulphide or chloroform. This is the basis of a rapid test to ascertain whether or not an oil has been sufficiently dried.

Potassium hydroxide solubility for phenol-containing oils

Phenolic isolates and synthetics as well as oils consisting almost exclusively of phenolic bodies may be evaluated rapidly by dissolving 2 cc. of the oil in 20 or 25 cc. of a 1 N aqueous solution of potassium hydroxide in a 25 cc. glass-stoppered, graduated cylinder. This test is particularly of value in the case of sweet birch and wintergreen oils. It is well to examine critically the odour of the solution or any insoluble, portion, whereby additions of foreign, odour-bearing substances may be detected.

Upon prolonged standing, the alkaline solution may saponify an ester group, if present. If the products of such a saponification are soluble in the alkaline solution, no separation will be observed, e.g. methyl salicylate. If the products are not completely soluble, a separation may occur, e.g. amyl salicylate. Solutions of the alkali phenolates are frequently good solvents for other compounds; thus terpeneless bay oils containing about 90 per cent eugenol often form clear solutions with a 1 N potassium hydroxide solution.

Sodium bisulphite solubility for aldehyde-containing oils

Oils (such as oil of bitter almond, free from prussic acid) and synthetics (such as benzaldehyde, tolyl aldehyde, cinnamic aldehyde and anisic aldehyde) and isolates (such as citral) may reveal impurities by their incomplete solution in dilute bisulphite solution. This test is usually carried out in a 25 cc. glass-stoppered, graduated cylinder: shake 1 cc. of the oil with 9 cc. of a freshly prepared saturated solution of sodium bisulphite and then add 10 cc. of water with further shaking. The odour of the resulting solution should be carefully examined. Because of the relative insolubility of certain bisulphite addition compounds, no general procedure is satisfactory for all aldehydes. Thus, some must be heated in a beaker of boiling water; and some require a larger amount of water to yield a clear solution. Each chemist soon develops his own techniques in testing these aldehydes; hence, specialised procedures have been omitted here.

CONGEALING POINT

The congealing point (the so-called 'congealing point' of rose oil is not a true congealing point, but is determined by the same method as that used for titer determinations in fixed oils) offers a distinct advantage over the melting point and the titer, in the case of mixtures, such as essential oils (the melting point is usually used for crystalline solids). In determining the congealing point, the oil is supercooled so that, upon congelation, immediate crystallisation with liberation of heat occurs. This results in a rapid rise of temperature, which soon approaches a constant value and remains at this temperature for a period of time. This point is known as the 'congealing point'. With increasing percentage of crystalline material in an oil, the congealing point will approach a maximum (this maximum will be the 'congealing point' of the pure crystalline compound). Hence, this physical property is a good criterion of the percentage of such material. The congealing point is important in the evaluation of anise, sassafras and fennel oils.

Procedure: Place about 10 cc. of the oil in a dry test tube of 18 to 20 mm diameter. Cool in water or in a suitable freezing mixture, the temperature of which should be about 5°C lower than the supposed congealing point of the liquid. To initiate congelation, rub the inner walls of the tube with a thermometer or add a small amount of the substance previously solidified by excessive freezing. The thermometer should be rubbed quickly up and down in the mixture in order to cause a rapid congelation throughout, with its subsequent liberation of heat. The temperature should be read frequently; at first the rise of temperature is rapid, but soon approaches a constant value for a brief interval of time. This value is taken as the congealing point of the oil. The process described above should be repeated several times to assure obtaining the true congealing point.

The thermometer used should be calibrated in 0.1°C units and should be accurately standardised. A thermometer covering the range of –5° to +50°C is satisfactory for most determinations.

Before the oil is tested, it should be thoroughly dried with sodium sulphate, since the presence of small amounts of water will often materially lower the congealing point.

In the case of sassafras oils, it is well to initiate the congelation by the addition of a small piece of solid safrole since sassafras oil can be congealed only with great difficulty if no 'seed' is used.

For a more exact determination of the congealing point, the test tube containing the supercooled oil may be insulated by means of an air jacket. This is frequently of particular importance when determining congealing points which are much below room temperature, as, for example, the congealing point of eucalyptus oils.

Gildemeister and Hoffmann recommend the use of the Beckman apparatus, frequently used for the determination of molecular weights by the lowering of the freezing point. The use of a larger sample (up to 100 cc.) may make the congealing point sharper.

MELTING POINT

The importance of the determination of the melting point of a solid, crystalline material is obvious.

A brief but comprehensive discussion of the determination of melting points has been given from which much of the following is taken:

Procedure: Heat a piece of 15 mm glass tubing in a flame until the glass is soft; then draw out into a thin walled capillary tube about 1 mm in diameter. Cut into lengths of about 6 cm and seal one end in a flame. Powder a small amount of the compound in a polished agate mortar and introduce some of the powder into the capillary tube. Hold the capillary tube vertically and gently rub with a file, which causes the powder to settle to the bottom; pack the material by tapping the tube on the desk. Fasten the tube to the thermometer by means of a rubber and (cut from a piece of rubbing tubing) so that the sample is close to the mercury bulb (Fig. 10.2). Place a heavy white mineral oil in the beaker and heat with a low flame. Clamp a cylindrical metal shield, open at the top and bottom, in the position as shown in Fig. 10.2 in order to protect the flame from drafts. Heat at a rate to cause a rise in temperature of about 1 or 2°C per minute. Stir the oil bath continuously. Note the temperature at which the compound starts to melt and that at which it is entirely liquid; record these values as the melting point range. Note also the temperature recorded by the auxiliary thermometer (t_2); the bulb of this thermometer should be placed midway between the surface of the oil and the top of the mercury thread in t_1. Calculate the stem correction by means of the following equation:

$$\text{Correction} = 0.000154N(t_1 - t_2)$$

where, N =   number of degrees of mercury thread above the level of the oil bath
          t_1 =   observed melting point
          t_2 =   average temperature of the mercury thread

This correction is to be added to the observed melting point.

It is often time saving to run a preliminary melting point, raising the temperature of the bath very rapidly. After the approximate melting point is known, a second determination is carried out raising the temperature rapidly until within 10°C of the approximate value and then proceeding slowly as described above. A fresh sample of the compound should be used for each determination.

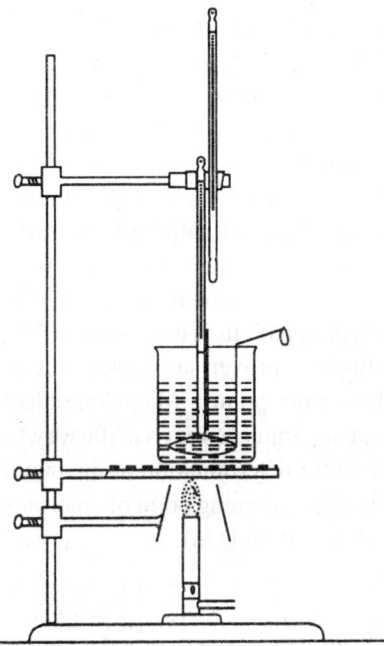

Fig. 10.2. Apparatus for the determination of melting point.

The thermometer should be calibrated by observing the melting points of several pure compounds such as the following:

Melting point of pure compounds

0°C	Ice
53	p-Dichlorobenzene
90	m-Dinitrobenzene
114	Acetanilide
121	Benzoic acid
132	Urea
157	Salicylic acid
187	Hippuric acid
200	Isatin
216	Anthracene
238	Carbanilide
257	Oxanilide
273	Anthraquinone
317	N,N-Diacetylbenzidine

If the same apparatus and thermometer are used in all melting point determinations, it is convenient to prepare a calibration curve. The observed melting point of the standard compound is plotted against the corrected value and a curve is drawn through these points. In subsequent determinations the observed value is projected horizontally to the curve and then vertically down to give the corrected value. Such a calibration curve includes corrections for inaccuracies in the thermometer and stem correction.

The use of short stemmed, standardised Anschütz thermometers eliminates the need for an auxiliary thermometer and subsequent correction for emergent stem.

It is important to record the melting point range of a compound since this is a valuable index of purity. A large majority of pure organic compounds melt within a range of 0.5°C or melt with decomposition over a narrow range of temperature (about 1°C).

When determining the melting point of a solid that readily sublimes, e.g. borneol — certain precautions become necessary. The rate of heating of the oil bath should be increased considerably. The capillary should not be introduced into the hot oil until the temperature is within 10° to 20°C of the expected melting point. The use of a sealed capillary may be necessary, i.e. a capillary that has both ends fused. The use of a Fisher-Johns or similar type apparatus is not recommended for materials that sublime readily. Other types of melting point apparatus have proven satisfactory, e.g. the Fisher-Johns, Thiele and Thiele-Dennis. If a compound has a high melting point a Maquenne block may conveniently be used. It is claimed that the Dennis melting point apparatus is very satisfactory for compounds melting up to 300°C.

Special types have been developed for determination of the melting point of waxes (ASTM melting point apparatus, designation D87), and the softening point of amorphous material (ASTM softening point apparatus [Ring and Ball method], designation D36).

BOILING RANGE

In the case of isolates and synthetics, the determination of the boiling range is an important criterion of purity.

Procedure: Use the apparatus shown in Fig. 10.3. The bulb of the distilling flask should have a capacity of 50 cc. The neck of the flask above the side arm should be as short as possible. The bottom of the flask rests in a circular opening, 2.5 cm in diameter, cut in a square piece of asbestos board having a thickness of about 3 mm; this perforation should be slightly bevelled on the upper edge to make it fit closely to the surface of the flask (This is to prevent upward leakage of hot gases from the flame and subsequent superheating). A wrapping of asbestos paper reaching to a point about 1 cm above the side arm should be used to prevent condensation due to drafts.

Introduce 25 cc. of the sample into the flask by means of a pipette. Add a small clay chip. Insert the thermometer along the central axis of the flask with its bulb slightly below the side tube; attach a light auxiliary thermometer to the main thermometer to correct for stem exposure, the bulb of this second thermometer being placed half way from the cork to the top of the mercury column at the expected reading. (A short-stemmed thermometer of the Anschütz type having the proper range may be used; this will require no correction for stem exposure.) Distil at a uniform rate of about 0.5 cc. per minute until the level of the liquid remaining in the flask falls to the level of the asbestos diaphragm.

Since some time will elapse before the thermometer can acquire the temperature of the vapour, little significance can be attached to readings taken before the end of the first minute after the fall of the first drop of distillate from the side tube. Any readings taken after the liquid falls below the level of the asbestos board will be greatly influenced by superheating. In the case of pure compounds that boil without decomposition, the difference between the first and last significant readings should not amount to more than 1°C. The stem exposure correction may be found by the following formula:

$$\text{Correction} = 0.000154 \, N(t_1 - t_2)$$

where,

N = number of degrees of emergent stem

t_1 = observed temperature of main thermometer

t_2 = temperature of auxiliary thermometer

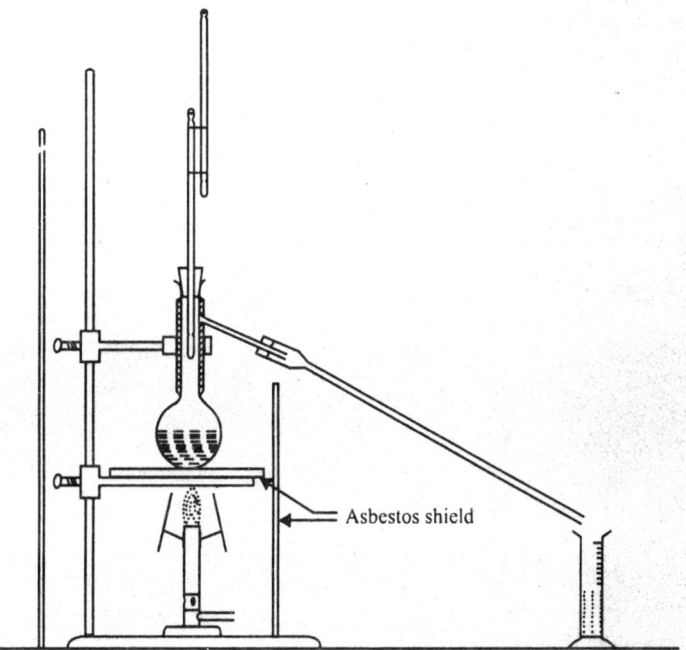

Fig. 10.3. Apparatus for the determination of boiling range.

This correction is to be added. To reduce boiling points taken under pressures between 720 and 780 mm to their approximate values at 760 mm, apply a correction of 0.1°C for every 2.7 mm difference; the correction is to be added if the observed pressure is below 760 mm and to be subtracted if above 760 mm.

The percentage of an essential oil which distils below a given temperature is frequently of importance in evaluating the oil; also, the percentage which distils between certain limits. However, it must be remembered that when fractionating an oil, the quantitative results of different observers will vary greatly; this is due to differences in the types of distilling flasks and condensers employed to the distillation rates and to the degree of superheating of the vapours.

Examination of the various fractions is of great importance; the determination of physical and chemical properties of these fractions and a study of the odour is frequently very revealing. Furthermore, suspected adulterants may be tested for chemically, and if present identified by derivatives.

Only through experience will the chemist know whether or not it is better to distil at atmospheric pressure or under vacuum. In general, for the collection of first fractions it is better to distil at atmospheric pressure. Usually it is more advantageous to separate fractions according to the temperature, measuring the volumes collected; occasionally it is desirable to collect definite amounts, noting the temperatures at which these fractions are obtained.

For fractionations at normal pressure the following technique will generally give satisfactory results. The procedure as described is intended primarily for the distillation of turpentine oil and for the removal and collection of the first 10 per cent of citrus oils.

Procedure: See Fig. 10.4. Place 50 cc. of the oil in a 100 cc. three-bulb Ladenburg flask of approximately the following dimensions: the lower or main bulb 6 cm in diameter, with the smaller condensing bulbs 3.5 cm, 3.0 and 2.5 cm, respectively, in diameter; the distance from the bottom of the flask to the side arm, 20 cm. Support the flask in a hemispherical metal oil bath, 4 inches in diameter, containing a suitable heating medium such as glycerine, cottonseed oil or high boiling mineral oil. Attach a Pyrex straight-tube condenser, 22 inches long, having a water cooled jacket (for oils containing mostly high boiling constituents [such as cassia and bay], use an air-cooled condenser), and fitted with an adapter which is long enough to extend into the graduated cylinder used as a receiver. Use a short-stemmed thermometer of the Anschütz type or a long-stemmed thermometer with an auxiliary thermometer for stem correction. Add a few small clay chips. Heat the bath with a Bunsen burner protected from drafts by a chimney. Fasten a large sheet of asbestos board vertically to act as a shield for the flame, bath and flask. Distil the oil at a uniform rate of 1 drop per second until the required distillate is obtained.

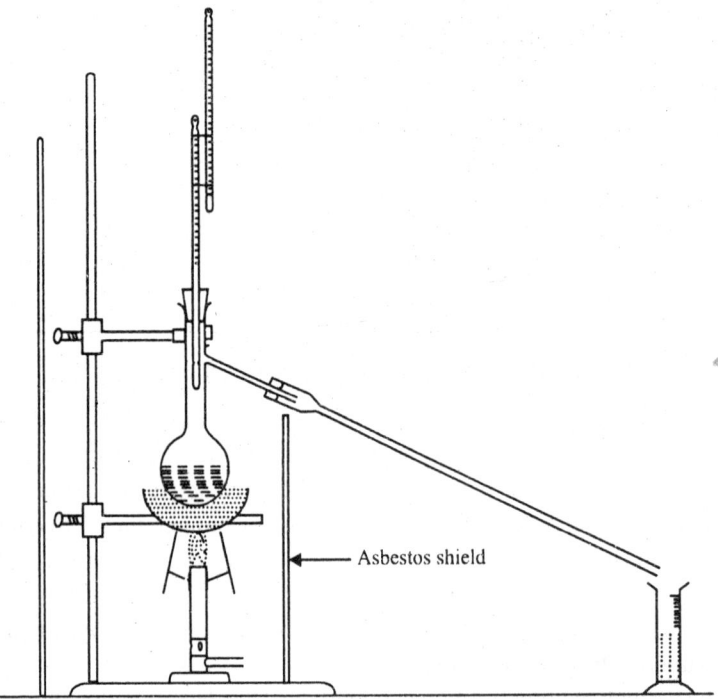

Fig. 10.4. Apparatus for the determination of boiling range.

EVAPORATION RESIDUE

An important criterion of purity is the evaporation residue; i.e. the percentage of the oil which is not volatile at 100°C. A determination of the evaporation residue is of special value in the case of the citrus oils; a low value for an expressed oil suggests the possibility of the addition of terpenes or other volatile constituents; a high value may indicate the addition of foreign material, such as, rosin, fixed oils or high boiling sesquiterpenes. In the case of rectified oils such as turpentine, a high value may indicate improper or lack of rectification or polymerisation due to age or improper storage. In the case of certain solids, such as camphor, thymol or menthol, a high evaporation residue will indicate insufficient purification.

It is important to study the odour of an oil as it volatilises during the heating. Often 'by-notes' of foreign low boiling adulterants or contaminants may be discovered.

The odour of the final residue while still hot should also be carefully studied for the addition of high boiling adulterants, such as cedarwood.

The consistency of the residue, both when hot and cool, and the colour sometimes indicates the presence of particular adulterants. For example, an orange oil, which has a brittle residue instead of the usual soft waxy residue, should be carefully investigated for rosin.

Acid numbers and saponification numbers may be determined on suspicious residues: rosin usually raises the acid number considerably; fixed oils raise the saponification number.

The fact that essential oils are complex mixtures makes an exact determination of the nonvolatile residue very difficult. 'Constant weight' cannot conveniently be attained because of the fact that waxes and other high boiling nonvolatile material tend to retain or 'fix' some of the lower boiling constituents. The constant weight can be defined as the value obtained when 'two consecutive weighings do not differ by more than 0.1 per cent, the second weighing following an additional hour of drying'. Even after 'constant weight', according to this definition, has been attained, further prolonged heating will give much lower results. Hence, a certain standardisation of technique becomes necessary.

Procedure: Weigh accurately (to the closest milligram) a well cleaned Pyrex evaporating dish that has been permitted to stand in a desiccator for 30 minutes. To this tared dish add the requisite amount of oil or solid (weighed to the closest centigram) and heat on a steam bath for the prescribed length of time. Then permit the evaporating dish to cool to room temperature in the desiccator and weigh (to the closest milligram). Calculate the nonvolatile, residue obtained, the so-called 'evaporation residue' and express as a percentage of the original oil.

	Size of sample (gram)	Period of heating (hour)
Oil bergamot	5	5
Oil grapefruit	5	6
Oil lemon	5	4½
Oil limes, expressed	5	6
Oil mace	3	8
Oil mandarin	5	5
Oil nutmeg	3	8
Oil orange	5	4½
Oil tangerine	5	5
Oil turpentine	5	4½
Oleoresin capsicum	2	4
Oleoresin ginger	2	4
Camphor	2	4
Copaiba	0.5	6
Menthol	2	2
Styrax	2	2
Thymol	2	4
Floral waters	100	After last of liquid has evaporated, heat for an additional hour.

It is well to bear in mind that the size, shape and composition of the evaporating dish employed in such a determination, as well as the size of sample and time of heating, will influence the analytical result obtained.

Flat bottom evaporating dishes of pyrex glass are very satisfactory; they offer the further advantage of more easily permitting an observation of the colour and opacity of the residue. Conventional pyrex evaporation dishes, 80 mm in diameter and 45 mm deep, are to be recommended. The use of such dishes tends to minimise the formation of polymerisation products in most cases.

Certain exceptional products will require special treatments, however; evaporation residues on such materials as diacetyl are meaningless because of the rapid formation of polymerisation products unless the determinations are carried out in vacuum with the application of little or no heat.

In evaluating oleoresins, evaporation residues should also be determined. Here it is best to express the results as 'loss of weight on heating'. The analytical results obtained will include the loss of volatile solvent as well as the loss of part of the naturally occurring essential oil. An abnormally high value often indicates the incomplete removal of the volatile solvent used in the manufacture of the oleoresin.

FLASH POINT

The flash point may prove useful in the evaluation of an essential oil. Unfortunately insufficient data exist to use this property as a criterion of quality for normal, unadulterated oils. However, the flash point has value as an indication of adulteration: additions of adulterants such as alcohol and low boiling mineral spirits will greatly lower the flash point.

Occasionally it is necessary to determine the flash point of a synthetic, solvent or a mixture because of shipping regulations. Several types of instruments are available for the determination; e.g. the Pensky-Martin closed tester (a description of the instrument and a detailed procedure for its use may be found in ASTM designation D93–42), the Tag closed tester (ASTM designation D56–36), the Cleaveland (ASTM designation D92–33) and the Tag open cup testers. The Tag open cup tester is simple, inexpensive and entirely satisfactory for use in the essential oil industry. The procedure described below is intended primarily for this instrument (Fig. 10.5).

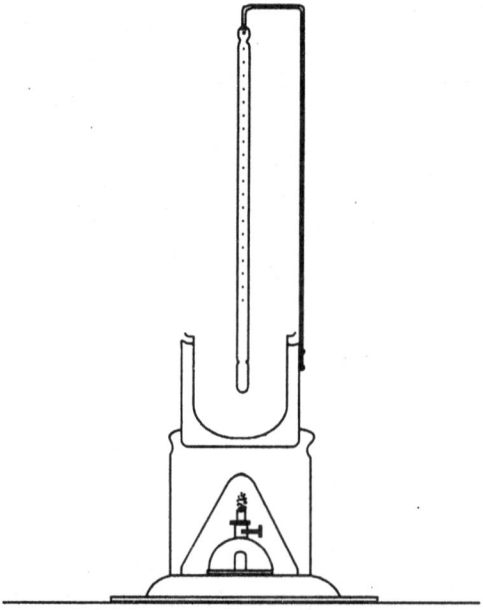

Fig. 10.5. Tag open cup tester for the determination of flash point.

Procedure: Fill the metal bath with water of about 60°F (15.6°C) temperature, leaving room for displacement by the glass oil cup which is placed in the water bath. Suspend the thermometer in a vertical position so that the bottom of the bulb is about ¼ inch from the bottom of the glass cup and so that the thermometer is suspended half way between the centre and the back of the glass cup. Fill the glass cup with the oil to be tested in such a manner that the top of the meniscus is exactly at the filling line at room temperature (i.e. ⅛ inch from the upper edge of the cup). Be sure that there is no oil on the outside of the cup or on its upper level edge; use soft paper to clean the cup in preference to a cloth. Remove any air bubbles from the surface of the oil. Adjust the horizontal flashing taper guide wire in place. The instrument should stand level and should be protected from drafts. It is desirable that the room be darkened sufficiently so that the flash may be readily discernible. Avoid breathing over the surface of the oil. Heat the water bath with a small burner so that it will raise the temperature of the oil at a rate not faster than 2°F (1.1°C) per minute without removing the burner during the whole operation.

Adjust the test flame on the flashing taper so that it is the same size as the metal bead mounted on the instrument. Apply this test flame to the oil at 5°F (2.8°C) intervals: hold the flashing taper in a horizontal position and draw it across the guide wire quickly and without pause from left to right. (The time of passage of the test flame across the cup should be approximately 1 second.)

The first or initial flash (the true initial flash should not be confused with a bluish halo that sometimes surrounds the test flame) is called the 'flash point'. Continue heating and testing the oil until the surface ignites and continues to burn until quickly blown out with a mouth-open breath. This burning point temperature is called the 'fire test' or 'fire point'. Repeat the determination and try for a flash at the proper trial temperatures indicated in Table 10.8.

Table 10.8. Trial temperature table for flash points (all temperatures in °F).

For oils expected to have a fire test of	Try for flash						
	First at			Then at			
110	85	90	95	100	105	108	110
115	90	95	100	105	110	113	115
120	95	100	105	110	115	118	120
125	100	105	110	115	120	123	125
130	100	105	110	115	120	125	130
135	105	110	115	120	125	130	135
140	110	115	120	125	130	135	140
145	115	120	125	130	135	140	145
150	120	125	130	135	140	145	150

Chapter 11

Determination of Chemical Properties of Essential Oils

INTRODUCTION

This chapter discusses the important chemcial properties of essential oils such as determination of acids, esters, alcohols, aldehydes and ketones, etc.

DETERMINATION OF ACIDS

Most essential oils contain only small amounts of free acids. Consequently the acid content is usually reported as an acid number rather than as a percentage calculated as a specific acid.

The acid number of an oil is defined as the number of milligrams of potassium hydroxide required to neutralise the free acids in 1 gram of oil. In determining the acid number, dilute alkali must be employed since many of the esters (e.g. the formates) normally present in essential oils are capable of saponification even in the cold in the presence of strong alkalies. Moreover, phenols will react with the alkali hydroxides, making it necessary to use special indicators (such as phenol red) for oils containing large amounts of phenolic bodies; this is particularly true in the case of the salicylates.

The acid number of an oil often increases as the oil ages, especially if the oil is improperly stored; processes such as oxidation of aldehydes and hydrolysis of esters increase the acid number. Oils which have been thoroughly dried and which are protected from air and light show little change in the amount of free acids.

Procedure: Weigh accurately about 2.5 grams of the oil into a 100 cc. saponification flask. Add 15 cc. of neutral 95 per cent alcohol and 3 drops of a 1 per cent phenolphthalein solution. Titrate the free acids with a standardised 0.1 N aqueous sodium hydroxide solution, adding the alkali dropwise at a uniform rate of about 30 drops per minute. The contents of the flask must be continually agitated. The first appearance of a red colouration that does not fade within 10 seconds is considered the end point.

If the determination requires more than 10 cc. of alkali, it should be repeated using 1 gram sample of the oil; if more than 10 cc. of alkali is still required, then 1 gram sample is titrated with 0.5 N aqueous sodium hydroxide solution. The acid number is calculated by means of the following formulas:

$$\text{Acid number} = \frac{5.61 \ (\text{no. of cc. of } 0.1 \ N \ \text{NaOH})}{\text{wt. of sample in gram}}$$

$$= \frac{28.05 \ (\text{no. of cc. of } 0.5 \ N \ \text{NaOH})}{\text{wt. of sample in gram}}$$

For oils containing large amounts of free acid (e.g. orris oil), the free acid content may be expressed as a percentage, calculated as a specific acid. In such cases it is well to use a 0.5 N alcoholic sodium hydroxide solution.

$$\text{Free acid content} \atop \text{(percentage)} = \frac{ma}{20w}$$

$$\text{Free acid content} \atop \text{(percentage)} = \frac{mb}{100w}$$

where, m = molecular weight of the acid
a = number of cc. of 0.5 N alkali used for neutralisation
b = number of cc. of 0.1 N alkali used for neutralisation
w = weight of sample in grams

If the acid is dibasic, the result must be divided by 2; if tribasic, by 3. In Table 11.1 are listed the molecular weights of those acids frequently encountered by the essential oil chemist.

Table 11.1. Molecular weights of acids.

Acids	Molecular wt
Monobasic acids	
Acetic	60.05
Anisic	152.14
Anthranilic	137.13
Benzoic	122.12
Butyric	88.10
Capric	172.26
Caproic	116.16
Caprylic	144.21
Cinnamic	148.15
Formic	46.03
Furoic	112.08
Lactic	90.08
Lauric	200.31
Methyl anthranilic	151.16
Myristic	228.37
Oenanthic	130.18
Oleic	282.46
Pelargonic	158.24
Phenylacetic	136.14
Phenylpropionic	150.17
Propionic	74.08
Pyruvic	88.06

(Contd...)

Acids	Molecular wt
Salicylic	138.12
Stearic	284.47
Tiglic	100.11
Undecylenic	184.27
Undecylic	186.29
Valeric	102.13
Dibasic acids	
Malonic	104.06
Phthalic	166.13
Sebacic	202.25
Succinic	118.09
Tartaric	150.09
Tribasic acids	
Citric	192.12

DETERMINATION OF ESTERS

Determination by Saponification with Heat

The determination of the ester content is of great importance in the evaluation of many essential oils. Since most esters which occur as normal constituents of essential oils are esters of monobasic acids, the process of saponification may be represented by the following reaction:

$$RCOOR' + NaOH \rightarrow RCOONa + R'OH$$

where R and R' may be an aliphatic, aromatic or alicyclic radical (R may also be a hydrogen atom).

Procedure: Into a 100 cc. alkali-resistant saponification flask weigh accurately about 1.5 gram of the oil. Add 5 cc. of neutral 95 per cent alcohol and 3 drops of a 1 per cent alcoholic solution of phenolphthalein and neutralise the free acids with standardised 0.1 N aqueous sodium hydroxide solution (this usually requires not more than 5 drops of the 0.1 N alkali). Then add 10 cc. of 0.5 N alcoholic sodium hydroxide solution, measured accurately from a pipette or a burette. Attach a glass, air-cooled condenser to the flask, 1 metre in length and about 1 cm in diameter and reflux the contents of the flask for 1 hour on a steam bath. Remove and permit to cool at room temperature for 15 minutes. Titrate the excess alkali with standardised 0.5 N aqueous hydrochloric acid. A further addition of a few drops of phenolphthalein solution may be necessary at this point.

In order to determine the amount of alkali consumed, carry out a blank determination, observing the same conditions but omitting the oil. The difference in the amounts of acid used in titrating the actual determination and the blank gives the amount of alkali used for the saponification of the esters. The blank should require an excess of about 100 per cent over the amount used in the determination. If insufficient excess is used, results will be obtained which are too low.

It is well to use saponification flasks (Fig. 11.1) made of 'jena glass' or of the special alkali resistant glass. These flasks minimise the amount of alkali consumed by the action of the sodium hydroxide on the glass itself. More accurate results are thus obtained. This is of importance when the ester determination requires more than 1 hour of refluxing, as, for example, in the case of the isovalerates.

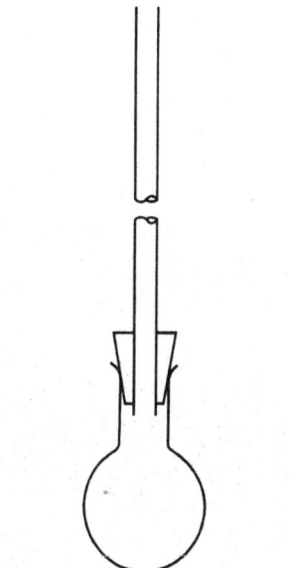

Fig. 11.1. Saponification flask.

The alcoholic 0.5 N sodium hydroxide solution is best prepared by adding 11.5 grams of metallic sodium of analytical grade to 1 litre of 95 per cent ethyl alcohol. (If larger amounts of solution are to be prepared, use 43.5 grams of sodium for each gallon of alcohol.) The sodium should be added slowly, a few small pieces at a time. After weighing out the sodium and cutting it into small pieces, it should be protected from atmospheric moisture until it is used by immersion in low boiling petroleum ether. After the required amount of sodium has been added, the solution is set aside for several days to permit any carbonate to settle; it is filtered into the reagent reservoir and permitted to stand for a few days before it is used. A clear, water white solution is thus obtained. The 0.5 N hydrochloric acid may be prepared by diluting 85 cc. of concentrated acid to 2 litres; it should then be carefully standardised.

Calculation of results

The ester content may be calculated from the following formula:

$$\text{Percentage of ester} = \frac{am}{20s}$$

where, a = number of cc. of 0.5 N sodium hydroxide used in the saponification;

m = molecular weight of the ester;

s = weight of the sample in grams.

This formula assumes that the ester is monobasic; for esters of dibasic acids (e.g. dimethyl phthalate) and dihydroxy alcohols (e.g. glycol diacetate), the ester content is divided by 2; for tribasic acids (e.g. triethyl citrate) and trihydroxy alcohols (e.g. triacetin), by 3 (this is based on the assumption that the ester is neutral in the case of di- and tribasic acids and that all alcoholic groups have been esterified in the case of esters of di- and tri-hydroxy alcohols).

The ester may also be expressed by the ester number, which is defined as the number of milligrams of potassium hydroxide required to saponify the esters present in 1 gram of oil. The use of the ester number is especially convenient when the ester present in the oil is unknown, since a knowledge of the molecular weight of the ester is not required.

$$\text{Ester number} = \frac{28.05a}{s}$$

Ester numbers are frequently used for oils which contain very small amounts of ester, e.g. oil of black pepper and oil of cubeb. A high ester number in such cases is usually indicative of adulteration.

The ester number may readily be converted to an ester content, expressed as a weight percentage, by the following formula if the acid radical of the ester is monobasic:

$$\text{Percentage of ester} = \frac{m \text{ (ester no.)}}{561.04}$$

If the acid is dibasic, the result must be divided by 2; if tribasic, by 3. Also, if the alcohol radical contains two hydroxy groups, the result (this is based on the assumption that the ester is neutral in the case of di- and tri-basic acids and that all alcoholic groups have been esterified in the case of esters of di- and tri-hydroxy alcohols) must be divided by 2; if three hydroxy groups, by 3.

In Table 11.2 are listed the molecular weights of those esters which are frequently encountered.

Modification of the general procedure

Certain esters are not completely saponified in a period of 1 hour by the procedure described above. Notable exceptions are the salicylates which should be refluxed for 2 hours; terpinyl acetate, 2 hours; menthyl acetate, 2 hours; isovalerates, 6 hours. Certain esters of sesquiterpene alcohols require 2 hours or more, e.g. cedryl acetate, 4 hours. A solution of potassium hydroxide in a high boiling solvent (such as the monoethyl ether of ethylene glycol) has been recommended for the determination of difficultly saponifiable esters. Such a solution also permits of rapid saponification (ca. 15 minutes) of other esters. Since such high temperatures may have an adverse effect upon some of the constituents of an essential oil, this method should be applied with caution.

Table 11.2. Molecular weights of esters.

Esters	Molecular wt
Esters of monobasic acids	
Allyl salicylate	178.18
Amyl acetate	130.18
Amyl anisate	222.28
Amyl benzoate	192.25
Amyl butyrate	158.24
Amyl caproate	186.29
Amyl caprylate	214.34
Amyl cinnamate	218.29
Amyl formate	116.16
Amyl furoate	182.21
Amyl heptine carbonate	210.31
Amyl laurate	270.45

(Contd...)

Esters	Molecular wt
Amyl myristate	298.50
Amyl oenanthate	200.31
Amyl phenylacetate	206.28
Amyl propionate	144.21
Amyl pyruvate	158.19
Amyl salicylate	208.25
Amyl undecylate	256.42
Amyl undecylenate	254.40
Amyl valerate	172.26
Anisyl acetate	180.20
Anisyl formate	166.17
Benzyl acetate	150.17
Benzyl benzoate	212.24
Benzyl butyrate	178.22
Benzyl cinnamate	238.27
Benzyl formate	136.14
Benzyl heptine carbonate	216.27
Benzyl phenylacetate	226.26
Benzyl propionate	164.20
Benzyl salicylate	228.24
Benzyl valerate	192.25
Bornyl acetate	196.28
Butyl acetate	116.16
Butyl benzoate	178.22
Butyl butyrate	144.21
Butyl formate	102.13
Butyl furoate	168.19
Butyl lactate	146.18
Butyl phenylacetate	192.25
Butyl propionate	130.18
Butyl salicylate	194.22
Butyl stearate	340.58
Butyl undecylenate	240.38
Butyl valerate	158.24
Cedryl acetate	264.40
Cinnamyl acetate	176.21
Cinnamyl benzoate	238.27
Cinnamyl butyrate	204.26

(Contd ...)

Esters	Molecular wt
Cinnamyl cinnamate	264.31
Cinnamyl formate	162.18
Cinnamyl propionate	190.23
Cinnamyl valerate	218.29
Citronellyl acetate	198.30
Citronellyl benzoate	260.36
Citronellyl butyrate	226.35
Citronellyl caproate	254.40
Citronellyl cinnamate	286.40
Citronellyl formate	184.27
Citronellyl propionate	212.32
Citronellyl valerate	240.38
Cresyl acetate	150.17
Cresyl butyrate	178.22
Cresyl cinnamate	238.27
Cresyl phenylacetate	226.26
Cyclohexanyl acetate	142.19
Cyclohexanyl butyrate	170.25
Decyl acetate	200.31
Decyl formate	186.29
Dimethyl benzyl carbinyl acetate	192.25
Ethyl acetate	88.10
Ethyl amyl carbinyl acetate	172.26
Ethyl anisate	180.20
Ethyl anthranilate	165.19
Ethyl benzoate	150.17
Ethyl butyrate	116.16
Ethyl caprate	200.31
Ethyl caproate	144.21
Ethyl caprylate	172.26
Ethyl cinnamate	176.21
Ethyl decine carbonate	210.31
Ethyl formate	74.08
Ethyl furoate	140.13
Ethyl heptine carbonate	168.23
Ethyl hexyl carbinyl acetate	186.29
Ethyl lactate	118.13
Ethyl methyl phenyl glycidate	206.23

(Contd...)

Esters	Molecular wt
Ethyl myristate	256.42
Ethyl octine carbonate	182.26
Ethyl oenanthate	158.24
Ethyl oleate	310.51
Ethyl pelargonate	186.29
Ethyl phenylacetate	164.20
Ethyl propionate	102.13
Ethyl pyruvate	116.11
Ethyl salicylate	166.17
Ethyl undecylate	214.34
Ethyl undecylenate	212.32
Ethyl valerate	130.18
Geranyl acetate	196.28
Geranyl benzoate	258.35
Geranyl butyrate	224.33
Geranyl formate	182.26
Geranyl phenylacetate	272.37
Geranyl propionate	210.31
Geranyl tiglate	236.34
Geranyl valerate	238.36
Guaiyl acetate	264.40
Guaiyl phenylacetate	340.49
Heptyl acetate	158.24
Heptyl caproate	214.34
Heptyl formate	144.21
Heptyl oenanthate	228.37
Heptyl propionate	172.26
Heptyl valerate	200.31
Hexyl acetate	144.21
Hexyl butyrate	172.26
Hexyl formate	130.18
Hexyl valerate	186.29
Isopulegyl acetate	196.28
Isopulegyl formate	182.26
Linalyl acetate	196.28
Linalyl anthranilate	273.36
Linalyl benzoate	258.35
Linalyl butyrate	224.33

(Contd ...)

Esters	Molecular wt
Linalyl cinnamate	284.38
Linalyl formate	182.26
Linalyl phenylacetate	272.37
Linalyl propionate	210.31
Linalyl valerate	238.36
Menthyl acetate	198.30
Menthyl salicylate	276.36
Menthyl valerate	240.38
Methyl acetate	74.08
Methyl anisate	166.17
Methyl anthranilate	151.16
Methyl benzoate	136.14
Methyl butyrate	102.13
Methyl caprate	186.29
Methyl caproate	130.18
Methyl caprylate	158.24
Methyl cinnamate	162.18
Methyl decine carbonate	196.28
Methyl formate	60.05
Methyl furoate	126.11
Methyl heptine carbonate	154.20
Methyl laurate	214.34
Methyl methyl anthranilate	165.19
Methyl myristate	242.39
Methyl octine carbonate	168.23
Methyl oenanthate	144.21
Methyl pelargonate	172.26
Methyl phenylacetate	150.17
Methyl phenylpropionate	164.20
Methyl propionate	88.10
Methyl salicylate	152.14
Methyl valerate	116.16
Neryl acetate	196.28
Neryl butyrate	224.33
Neryl formate	182.26
Neryl phenylacetate	272.37
Neryl propionate	210.31
Neryl valerate	238.36

(Contd ...)

Esters	Molecular wt
Nonyl acetate	186.29
Nonyl butyrate	214.34
Nonyl lactone	156.22
Octyl acetate	172.26
Octyl benzoate	234.33
Octyl butyrate	200.31
Octyl formate	158.24
Octyl oenanthate	242.39
Octyl propionate	186.29
Octyl valerate	214.34
Phenyl benzoate	198.21
Phenylethyl acetate	164.20
Phenylethyl anthranilate	241.28
Phenylethyl benzoate	226.26
Phenylethyl butyrate	192.25
Phenylethyl cinnamate	252.30
Phenylethyl dimethyl carbinyl acetate	206.28
Phenylethyl formate	150.17
Phenylethyl phenylacetate	240.29
Phenylethyl propionate	178.22
Phenylethyl salicylate	242.26
Phenylethyl valerate	206.28
Phenyl methyl carbinyl acetate	164.20
Phenylpropyl acetate	178.22
Phenylpropyl butyrate	206.28
Phenylpropyl cinnamate	266.33
Phenylpropyl formate	164.20
Phenylpropyl propionate	192.25
Phenylpropyl valerate	220.30
Propyl acetate	102.13
Propyl butyrate	130.18
Propyl formate	88.10
Propyl propionate	116.16
Propyl valerate	144.21
Rhodinyl acetate	198.30
Rhodinyl benzoate	260.36
Rhodinyl butyrate	226.35
Rhodinyl formate	184.27
Rhodinyl phenylacetate	274.39

(Contd ...)

Esters	Molecular wt
Rhodinyl propionate	212.32
Rhodinyl valerate	240.38
Santalyl acetate	262.38
Terpinyl acetate	196.28
Terpinyl anthranilate	273.36
Terpinyl butyrate	224.33
Terpinyl cinnamate	284.38
Terpinyl formate	182.26
Terpinyl propionate	210.31
Terpinyl valerate	238.36
Thujyl acetate	196.28
Undecalactone	184.27
Vetivenyl acetate	262.38
Vetivenyl butyrate	290.43
Vetivenyl formate	248.35
Vetivenyl propionate	276.41
Vetivenyl valerate	304.46
Esters of dibasic acids	
Diamyl phthalate	306.39
Dibenzyl succinate	298.33
Dibutyl phthalate	278.34
Dibutyl tartrate	262.30
Diethyl malonate	160.17
Diethyl phthalate	222.23
Diethyl sebacate	258.35
Diethyl succinate	174.19
Dimethyl malonate	132.11
Dimethyl phthalate	194.18
Esters of tribasic acids	
Triethyl citrate	276.28
Trimethyl citrate	234.20
Esters of trihydroxy alcohols	
Triacetin	218.20

In the case of salicylates, benzoates and phthalates, an addition of 5 cc. of water should be made before the ester is heated on the steam bath to prevent the separation of the sodium salts of the acids during the saponification.

If the oil contains large amounts of free acids, these should be determined separately by the procedure described under 'determination of acids'. The saponification number, representing the sum of the acid number and the ester number, is then determined for the oil using the general procedure described above, except that the free acids are not neutralised before the addition of the 0.5 N alkali.

In the case of oils containing large amounts of esters (e.g. oil of winter green) or esters of low molecular weight (e.g. methyl formate) or esters of dibasic or tribasic acids, it becomes necessary to vary the size of the sample and the amount of alkali employed. If 10 cc. of alkali is insufficient, 20 cc. may be used.

For synthetic esters, it is often necessary to decrease the size of the sample; usually 1 gram (of the pure synthetic) is used and 20 cc. of alkali. In the case of esters of low molecular weight or esters of polybasic acids, a 0.5 gram sample and 20 cc. of alkali may be required.

Relatively small samples are also required in the case of certain darkly coloured oils. It may also be necessary to dilute the saponified oil with alcohol in order to ascertain the end point of the titration and to use a spot-plate. The use of thymolphthalein (in place of phenolphthalein as an indicator) has been suggested for determinations involving red or brown solutions, such as result during the saponification of oleoresins. Thymolphthalein changes from a deep blue to colourless in the range pH 9.3 to pH 10.5.

The determination of the ester content by saponification will not yield satisfactory results if the oil contains appreciable amounts of aldehydes, unless the aldehydes are removed and the residual oil saponified. It has been reported that certain phenols also may interfere with the ester determination. In addition to esters, lactones may be determined quantitatively by saponification.

Determination by Saponification in the Cold

As an analytical procedure, saponification in the cold is not generally applicable. In most cases, long periods of time are necessary to complete the process; furthermore, side reactions frequently occur which give rise to inconsistent and deceptive results.

Saponification in the cold has a definite value for the determination of those esters which are very easily saponified; this is particularly true for certain formates. Thus, cold saponification is used in the analysis of geranium oils to determine the amount of 'actual formate', since the standard procedure for the determination of esters with a reflux period of 1 hour saponifies not only the geranyl formate but also other esters including geranyl tiglate.

For the determination of geranyl formate in geranium oils, the following procedure has given satisfactory results:

> *Procedure*: Into a 100 cc. saponification flask, weigh accurately about 1.5 gram of the oil. Add 5 cc. of neutral alcohol and 3 drops of a 1 per cent alcoholic solution of phenolphthalein and neutralise the free acids quickly with standardised 0.1 N aqueous sodium hydroxide solution. Add 10 cc. of 0.5 N alcoholic sodium hydroxide solution, measured accurately from a burette or pipette and titrate the excess alkali immediately with standardised 0.5 N aqueous hydrochloric acid. Calculate the ester content as geranyl formate in the usual manner.

In the case of pure synthetic formates, it is advisable to add 5 cc. of water to the flask in order to dissolve the sodium formate which otherwise may precipitate out of solution.

DETERMINATION OF ALCOHOLS

Determination by Acetylation

The alcoholic constituents of an essential oil are determined by acetylation; i.e. the oil is acetylised with acetic anhydride and the ester content of the resulting oil is determined; from this value the percentage of alcohol in the original oil may be calculated.

The basic chemical processes involved in this determination may be summarised by the following equations:

$$\left.\begin{array}{l}R1\\R2\\R3\end{array}\right\} C—OH + O \Big\langle \begin{array}{c} O{=}CCH_3 \\[4pt] O{=}CCH_3 \end{array} \longrightarrow \left.\begin{array}{l}R1\\R2\\R3\end{array}\right\} COOCCH_3 + CH_3COOH$$

$$\left.\begin{array}{l}R1\\R2\\R3\end{array}\right\} COOCCH_3 + NaOH \longrightarrow \left.\begin{array}{l}R1\\R2\\R3\end{array}\right\} COH + CH_3COONa$$

where R1, R2 and R3 may be a hydrogen atom, an aliphatic, aromatic or alicyclic radical.

For this determination, a special acetylation flask of approximately 100 cc. capacity is employed. This flask is equipped with an air-cooled condenser attached to the flask by means of a ground glass joint (Fig. 11.2). A condenser 1 metre in length is to be preferred in order to prevent the loss of volatile constituents.

Procedure: Introduce into a 100 cc. acetylation flask 10 cc. of the oil (measured from a graduated cylinder), 10 cc. of acetic anhydride (similarly measured) and 2.0 gram of anhydrous sodium acetate. Attach the air condenser and boil the contents of the flask gently for exactly 1 hour on a sand bath suitably heated by an open Bunsen flame or an electric hot-plate. Permit the flask to cool for 15 minutes and introduce 50 cc. of distilled water through the top of the condenser. Heat the flask on a steam bath for 15 minutes with frequent shaking to destroy the excess of acetic anhydride. Transfer the contents of the flask to a separatory funnel and rinse the flask with two 10 cc. portions of distilled water; add these rinsings to the separatory funnel. Shake thoroughly to assure good contact of the aqueous layer with the oil. When the liquids have separated completely, reject the aqueous layer and wash the remaining oil repeatedly with 100 cc. portions of saturated salt solution, until the washings are neutral to litmus; this usually requires three washings. Dry the resulting oil with anhydrous sodium sulphate and filter. (If the oil has been washed properly, not more than 0.2 cc. of 0.1 N aqueous sodium hydroxide solution should be required per gram of acetylised oil in order to neutralise the remaining trace of acetic acid.)

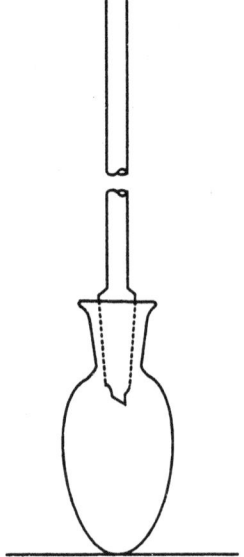

Fig. 11.2. Acetylation flask.

In order to secure accurate and reproducible results it is important to use exactly 2.0 gram of sodium acetate and to reflux the mixture for exactly 1 hour. A notable exception occurs in the case of citronella oils, which require a reflux period of 2 hours.

Calculation of Results

If the original oil contains a negligible quantity of saponifiable constituents, the free alcohol may be calculated by the following formula:

$$\text{Percentage of alcohol in the original oil} = \frac{am}{20(s - 0.021a)}$$

where, a = number of cc. of 0.5 N sodium hydroxide solution required for the saponification of the acetylised oil;

s = weight of acetylised oil in grams used in the saponification;

m = molecular weight of the alcohol.

For oils which have not been thoroughly investigated and whose alcoholic constituents are not well known, it is frequently more convenient to report the result as an ester number after acetylation.

$$\text{Ester number after acetylation} = \frac{28.05a}{s}$$

The ester number after acetylation is numerically equal to the number of milligrams of potassium hydroxide required to saponify the esters present in 1 gram of the acetylised oil.

If the original oil contains an appreciable amount of esters (as indicated by the ester number), the percentage of free alcohol may be estimated by the following formula:

$$\text{Percentage of free alcohol in the original oil} = \frac{dm}{561.04 - 0.42d}$$

where, d = (ester number after acetylation – ester number).

Although this expression is not mathematically precise, nevertheless it is sufficiently accurate for all practical work and has been used traditionally by essential oil chemists.

For the evaluation of essential oils, it is often desirable to know the percentage of total alcohol, i.e. the percentage of free alcohol plus the percentage of alcohol combined as ester present in the original unacetylised oil.

$$\text{Percentage of total alcohol in the original oil} = \left[\frac{am}{20(s - 0.021a)}\right]\left[1 - \frac{42.04e}{100(m + 42.04)}\right]$$

where, e = ester content in per cent. This formula assumes that all of the esterified alcohol present in the original oil is combined as the acetate.

All formulas in this chapter that calculate the result of an acetylation as a percentage actually refer to all constituents which are capable of acetylation under the experimental conditions, calculated as a specific alcohol. Thus for example, the 'total alcohol' in citronella oils includes not only the geraniol, free and as ester, but also all other acetylisable constituents and their esters, such as, borneol, citronellol, sesquiterpene alcohols and the aldehyde citronellal, all calculated as geraniol. These formulas further assume that the alcohol is a monohydroxy compound. Table 11.3 gives the molecular weights of alcohols frequently encountered in the analysis of essential oils.

Table 11.3. Molecular weights of alcohols.

Alcohols	Molecular wt
Amyrol	222.36
Anisyl alcohol	138.16
Benzyl alcohol	108.13
Borneol	154.25
Cedrenol	220.34
Cedrol	222.36
Cinnamyl alcohol	134.17
Citronellol	156.26
Costol	220.34
Cyclohexanol	100.16
Decyl alcohol	158.28
Duodecyl alcohol	186.33
Elemol	222.36
Farnesol	222.36
Fenchyl alcohol	154.25
Geraniol	154.25
Guaiol	222.36
Isoborneol	154.25
Isopulegol	154.25
Linaloöl	154.25
Menthol	156.26
Nerol	154.25
Nerolidol	222.36
Nonyl alcohol	144.25
Octyl alcohol	130.23
Phenylethyl alcohol	122.16
Phenylpropyl alcohol	136.19
Rhodinol	156.26
Santalol	220.34
Terpineol	154.25
Thujyl alcohol	154.25
Undecyl alcohol	172.30
Vetivenol	220.34

Limitations and modifications of the general procedure

As mentioned above, acetic anhydride employed under the experimental conditions described in the 'procedure' will react with certain compounds found in essential oils other than alcohols: phenols will be quantitatively converted into the acetates. Certain aldehydes and ketones are partially acetylated and partially destroyed or are converted to other compounds which are capable of acetylation.

Furthermore, some tertiary alcohols are not quantitatively converted to the acetate by this process of acetylation; the most important alcohols in this class are terpineol and linaloöl.

Determination of Primary Alcohols

Phthalic anhydride reacts with primary alcohols forming an acid phthalic ester.

$$
RCH_2OH + C_6H_4 \underset{\underset{O}{\overset{\parallel}{C}}}{\overset{\overset{O}{\overset{\parallel}{C}}}{\diagdown}} O \longrightarrow C_6H_4 \underset{\underset{O}{\overset{\parallel}{C}OCH_2R}}{\overset{COH}{\diagup}}
$$

Under the experimental conditions described below, this reaction takes place readily at a temperature of about 100°C in the case of primary alcohols; for secondary alcohols, the time required for reflux is greatly increased; for tertiary alcohols, no appreciable reaction occurs.

It is important that the phthalic anhydride does not contain free phthalic acid. This may be ascertained conveniently by shaking 1 gram of the anhydride with 10 cc. of benzene and warming to 40°C; a clear solution indicates the absence of appreciable amounts of phthalic acid.

Procedure: Into a 100 cc. acetylation flask introduce about 2 gram of powdered phthalic anhydride, accurately weighed and about 2 grams of the oil, accurately weighed. Add 2 cc. of benzene, measured from a graduated cylinder. Heat the flask on a steam bath with frequent shaking for 2 hours. Then permit the flask to cool for 30 minutes. Add 60 cc. of 0.5 N aqueous potassium hydroxide solution, accurately measured from a pipette or burette. Stopper the acetylation flask with a ground glass stopper and shake thoroughly for 10 minutes. Titrate the excess of alkali with standardised 0.5 N hydrochloric acid, using 3 drops of a 1 per cent phenolphthalein solution as indicator.

Run a blank determination omitting the oil, and from this calculate the amount of alkali which would be required for the weight of phthalic anhydride used in the actual determination.

Calculate the percentage of primary alcohol by the following formula:

$$
\text{Percentage of primary alcohol} = \frac{m(b-a)}{20w}
$$

where, m = the molecular weight of the primary alcohol;
b = the calculated number of cc. of 0.5 N potassium hydroxide required for the amount of phthalic anhydride used in the determination;
a = the number of cc. of 0.5 N potassium hydroxide consumed in the determination;
w = weight of oil in grams.

Determination of Tertiary Terpene Alcohols

Most tertiary alcohols suffer partial or complete breakdown and dehydration when treated with acetic anhydride. In the event that an oil contains a large percentage of such easily dehydrated alcohols, special techniques are required.

Method of Glichitch

The Glichitch method of formylation for the estimation of easily dehydrated alcohols has been successfully employed for the determination of linaloöl and terpineol.

Procedure: Introduce 15 cc. of aceto-formic acid reagent in a 125 cc. glass-stoppered Erlenmeyer flask. Cool in an ice bath and add slowly 10 cc. of the oil to be tested. Allow the mixture to stand for not less than 72 hours at room temperature. The ice in the bath should not be renewed. At the end of this interval pour the contents of the flask into a separatory funnel. Shake well with 50 cc. of ice cold water and allow to stand for 2 hours. Separate the oil and wash successively with 50 cc. of cold water, 50 cc. of a 5 per cent sodium bicarbonate solution and then with two 50 cc. portions of water. Separate the oil and dry with anhydrous sodium sulphate. Filter and saponify by refluxing with 0.5 N alcoholic sodium hydroxide. Calculate the alcohols in the usual way on the assumption that they are present as formates.

Preparation of the aceto-formic reagent: To 2 volumes of acetic anhydride, previously cooled to at least 0°, add slowly 1 volume of 100 per cent formic acid. (It is very important to use a highly purified formic acid of substantially 100 per cent strength. The usual A.R. grade of formic acid [specific gravity = 1.20; HCOOH = approximately 87 per cent] is useless for the preparation of this reagent). Mix thoroughly and then heat to 50°C for 15 minutes and immediately cool in an ice bath.

Method of Boulez

The Boulez method of acetylation makes use of a diluent in order to lessen the dehydrating effect of acetic anhydride. The period of acetylation, however, must be prolonged. This gives satisfactory results for linaloöl and terpineol if the prescribed conditions are rigidly followed. The original method suggested oil of turpentine as a diluent in the ratio of 1 part of the oil under examination to 5 parts of oil of turpentine. The chemists modified the procedure by substituting xylene as a diluent in the ratio of 1:4. The period of acetylation is very important; for terpineol 5 hours are required, longer or shorter periods give low values; for linaloöl, 7 hours. This modified procedure gives reproducible data. Great care must be exercised during this determination since any error introduced will be multiplied by 5 in the final result.

Dehydration methods

Dehydration methods are based upon the catalytic decomposition of tertiary alcohols and the splitting off of water. The amount of water obtained is determined from which the percentage of tertiary alcohol may be calculated. Such a method can be described by using zinc chloride. A very satisfactory dehydration catalyst is iodine. Additions of approximately 0.5 per cent of catalyst to the oil will prove sufficient. Such dehydration methods offer the advantage that only tertiary alcohols are determined, primary and secondary alcohol being unaffected. This is an advantage not found in the other methods described here. Hydroxy ketones and hydroxy aldehydes will interfere in this procedure, since both split off water under the experimental conditions.

A convenient method for the determination makes use of the distillation trap of Sterling and Bidwell.

Procedure: Dry the oil thoroughly by permitting it to stand overnight in contact with anhydrous sodium sulphate. Into a 1 litre, round bottom flask, introduce a sufficiently large sample, accurately weighed, to yield about 5 cc. of water upon dehydration of the tertiary alcohol. Add 0.5 per cent of solid iodine as catalyst and 500 cc. of xylene. Connect the flask to a standard Sterling and Bidwell water-trap; attach a water-cooled, straight tube condenser. Heat the flask by means of an oil bath. Measure the amount of collected water and calculate the percentage of tertiary alcohol.

This method does not yield highly accurate results, but is a convenient method for the determination of the tertiary alcohol content.

Acetyl chloride-dimethyl aniline method

This method gives exceptionally concordant and satisfactory results in the case of linaloöl and linaloöl-containing oils. It has been carefully evaluated by the members of the essential oil association of the USA. and adopted by that body. Preliminary experiments with terpineol and other tertiary terpene alcohols indicate that this may prove to be a valuable method for many tertiary alcohols. The method is described below in the final form in which it was accepted by the essential oil association for the determination of linaloöl.

Procedure: Ten cc. of linaloöl or essential oil containing linaloöl, previously dried with sodium sulphate, is introduced into a 125 cc. glass-stoppered Erlenmeyer flask cooled with ice and water. To the cooled oil is added 20 cc. dimethyl aniline (monomethyl free) and the contents thoroughly mixed, then 8 cc. acetyl chloride (reagent grade) and 5 cc. of acetic anhydride are added, the anhydride serving as a solvent to prevent crystallisation of the reaction mass. The mixture is cooled for a few minutes and permitted to stand at room temperature for one half hour after which time the flask is immersed in a water bath maintained at 40°C ± 1°C for three hours. At the end of this time the acetylated oil is washed three times with 75 cc. of ice water, then with successive washes of 25 cc. of 5 per cent sulphuric acid until the separated acid layer fails to liberate any dimethyl aniline with an excess of caustic. After removal of the dimethyl aniline, the acetylated oil is washed with 10 cc. of 10 per cent sodium carbonate solution and then finally washed neutral with water. The oil is separated, dried over anhydrous sodium sulphate and the ester number determined in the usual manner. The linaloöl content can thus be obtained directly from saponification tables or by substitution in the following formula:

$$\text{Percentage of linaloöl} = \frac{\text{cc. } N/2 \text{ KOH} \times 154.14}{20 \, (\text{wt sample} - \text{cc. } N/2 \text{ KOH} \times 0.021)}$$

As this test is further to be used for other oils containing linaloöl, besides linaloöl itself, a correction factor is necessary with oils containing significant amount of esters. For such oils, the following standard formula is recommended:

$$\text{Percentage of total linaloöl} = \frac{A \times 77.07}{B - (A \times 0.021)} \times [1(E \times 0.0021)]$$

where, A = cc. half normal alkali required for saponification

       B = weight of sample

       E = per cent of esters calculated as linalyl acetate in the original oil

Determination of Citronellol by Formylation

Most terpene alcohols are dehydrated by strong formic acid, giving rise to nonsaponifiable terpenes. A notable exception is citronellol which is converted almost quantitatively to the corresponding formate. This results in a convenient and satisfactory method for the determination of citronellol in the presence of geraniol and linaloöl.

Formylation has become a standard procedure for the determination of citronellol in rose oils. The procedure to be followed is identical to that described under 'determination by acetylation', with the exception that the 10 cc. of acetic anhydride is replaced with 20 cc. of 100 per cent formic acid and the anhydrous sodium acetate is omitted. Place in the flask short pieces of glass tubing to permit heat transfer throughout the mixture. This is particularly important if the oil contains a high percentage of geraniol, since the dehydration which results may dilute the formic acid sufficiently to cause the formation of two layers in the flask. Should this occur, there will be some danger of the lower layer becoming overheated and violently throwing out the contents of the flask through the air condenser. A small clay chip should also be placed in the flask to help prevent such overheating.

The percentage of alcohol (citronellol) in the original oil may be calculated from the amount of alkali consumed in the subsequent saponification.

$$\text{Percentage of alcohol in the original oil} = \frac{am}{20(s - 0.014a)}$$

where, a = number of cc. of 0.5 N sodium hydroxide solution required for the saponification of the formylated oil

m = molecular weight of the alcohol

s = weight of formylated oil in grams

DETERMINATION OF ALDEHYDES AND KETONES

Of the many procedures which have been suggested for the determination of aldehydes and ketones, only four general methods have attained practical significance. These are the bisulphite method, the neutral sulphite method, the phenylhydrazine method and the hydroxylamine methods.

Bisulphite Method

The bisulphite method is an absorption process based upon the general reaction (there exists some question as to the linkage of the $-SO_3Na$ group to the C atom of the carbonyl group; this linkage may occur through the S atom or possibly through the O atom):

$$RCHO + NaHSO_3 \longrightarrow RCH \begin{smallmatrix} OH \\ \\ SO_3Na \end{smallmatrix}$$

Upon shaking a measured quantity of oil with a hot aqueous solution of sodium bisulphite, an addition compound (in many cases, this addition compound is a water soluble sulphonate instead of [or in addition to] the normal bisulphite addition compound of the carbonyl group) forms which is generally water soluble and which dissolves in the hot bisulphite solution; the nonaldehyde portion of the oil separates as an oily layer which can be measured conveniently in the graduated neck of a cassia flask.

These special flasks have been known traditionally as cassia flasks because they were first used for the determination of the cinnamic aldehyde content of cassia oil. They have a large bulbous body with a long thin neck graduated in divisions of 0.1 cc. The two types (having the dimensions shown in Fig. 11.3) have proved most useful in the laboratory. The larger flask with a capacity of 150 cc. and a thin neck graduated to contain 6 cc. is very satisfactory for the determination of aldehydes and ketones. The smaller flask with a capacity of 100 cc. and a neck graduated to contain 10 cc. may also be used for such determination, although the accuracy will suffer somewhat. Furthermore, the capacity of these smaller flasks does not permit as thorough and as intimate contact of the oil and solution when the flask is shaken; if such a flask is used, the shaking should be thorough and prolonged. In general, the use of these smaller flasks is not recommended for the determination of aldehydes and ketones, unless the oil contains less than 40 per cent of reactive carbonyl compounds.

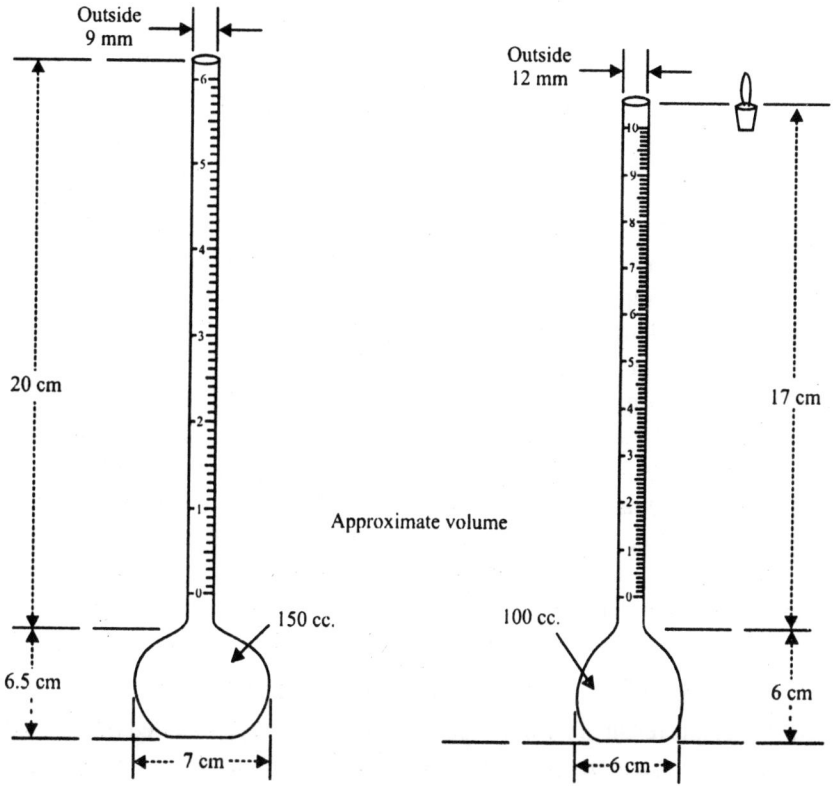

Fig. 11.3. Cassia flasks.

   The bisulphite method is perhaps the most convenient and simple of the four general methods. As such, it is frequently used in the trade because it requires no standardised solutions analytical balance or special skill. This method has proved satisfactory for the estimation of cinnamic aldehyde in cassia oil, of benzaldehyde in bitter almond oil, of citronellal in *Eucalyptus citriodora* oil; it is the commercially accepted method for the determination of citral in lemongrass oil. [The neutral sulphite method gives a more accurate value of the true citral content; in addition to citral, the bisulphite method determines other carbonyl constituents which occur as natural constituents of lemongrass oils (e.g. part of the methyl heptenone). The values obtained by the bisulphite method are generally about 4 per cent higher than those obtained by the neutral sulphite method for the normal lemongrass oils of commerce].

   The bisulphite method suffers from certain disadvantages inherent in the absorption process. Water-soluble adulterants analyse as apparent aldehyde. The time required for a determination is usually at least 1 hour. The results obtained are volume percentages. These methods are applicable only to oils containing large amounts of aldehydes or ketones. Water-soluble sulphonates may be formed from noncarbonyl compounds having double bonds; these will interfere with the accuracy of the analytical results [In this connection, only small amounts of unsaturated alcohols will dissolve if the solution of $NaHSO_3$ is stronger than molar (10.4 per cent)].

The bisulphite method suffers from further disadvantages. There is no definite indication when all of the aldehyde has completely reacted. Although satisfactory for most aldehydes, the method is not suitable for the determination of such ketones as carvone, thujone, pulegone, menthone, fenchone or camphor.

Procedure: Variations of this procedure have been suggested by other authorities. Gildemeister and Hoffmann suggest the use of a 30 per cent aqueous solution of sodium acid sulphite which does not contain too much free sulphurous acid; if necessary the solution should be neutralised with sodium carbonate. It has been the experience of the laboratories of Fritzsche Brothers, Inc., that a freshly prepared solution of $NaHSO_3$ made with Analytical Grade of reagent does not contain sufficient free H_2SO_3 to interfere with the reaction; the separation of the noncarbonyl portion of the oil is sharper and more complete if a saturated solution of $NaHSO_3$ is employed instead of a 30 per cent solution. Into a 150 cc. cassia flask, having a thin neck graduated in 0.1 cc. divisions, introduce 75 cc. of a freshly prepared, saturated, aqueous solution of sodium bisulphite [at room temperature, this will be approximately a 40 per cent (wt./vol.) solution], measured from a graduated cylinder. Pipette exactly 10 cc. of the oil into the flask. Upon thorough shaking, a semisolid mass frequently will result. Immerse the flask in a beaker of boiling water and occasionally shake until the solid addition compound has gone completely into solution. Shake the flask repeatedly to assure complete reaction of the aldehyde with the bisulphite solution. A further addition of 25 cc. of bisulphite solution is made and the flask is again repeatedly shaken. After standing undisturbed in the beaker of boiling water for 10 minutes to permit the unreacted oil to rise to the surface, add sufficient sodium bisulphite solution to force the unreacted oil into the neck of the flask. Any droplets of oil adhering to the sides are made to rise into the neck by gently tapping the flask and by rotating it rapidly between the palms of the hands. After cooling the flask to room temperature, measure the amount of unreacted oil. The aldehyde content may then be calculated by means of the following formula:

Percentage of aldehyde = 10(10 − no. of cc. of unreacted oil).

As mentioned above, this result is a volume percentage. It may be converted into a weight percentage if the specific gravity of the original oil and of the aldehyde is known:

$$\text{Percentage by weight} = (\% \text{ by volume}) \left(\frac{d_{15}^{15} \text{ of aldehyde or ketone}}{d_{15}^{15} \text{ of oil}} \right)$$

After cooling to room temperature, a small amount of the bisulphite addition compound will often precipitate out of solution, sometimes forming at the surface where the oil and aqueous layers meet; this renders an exact reading difficult. The addition of a few drops of water (added with a medicine dropper in such a way that the water runs down along the inside of the neck of the flask), which will remain temporarily on top of the bisulphite solution, gives a sharp separation of the oil and aqueous layers. If the oil contains heavy metals, these should be removed before the determination by shaking the oil thoroughly with a small amount (about 1 per cent) of powdered tartaric acid and filtering; a sharper separation of the noncarbonyl layer will then result.

The procedure described above will prove satisfactory for those aldehydes which form water-soluble sulphonates in addition to the normal bisulphite addition compound, e.g. citral, citronellal (in the determination of citronellal, the addition compound will often separate upon cooling; hence the reading should be taken as soon as the neck of the flask has cooled to room temperature), cinnamic aldehyde.

For aldehydes which form only the normal addition compound (e.g. compounds which have no double bonds other than those present in the carbonyl group or benzene ring) but which form water-soluble bisulphite addition compounds, the procedure must be modified. For the determination of phenylpropyl aldehyde (in the determination of phenylpropyl aldehyde, considerable amounts of the addition compound separate upon cooling; however, a reading is possible), benzaldehyde (use is made of the poor solubility of the benzaldehyde addition compound in saturated $NaHSO_3$ solution for the detection of benzaldehyde in cinnamic aldehyde; cinnamic aldehyde forms a sulphonate which dissolves completely in saturated $NaHSO_3$ solution. Hence, the separation of a solid addition compound upon cooling the contents of the flask to room temperature is indicative of the presence of benzaldehyde) and anisic aldehyde, use a 10 cc. sample and only 50 cc. of the saturated bisulphite solution. The normal addition compound which forms usually will not dissolve in the saturated bisulphite solution even after heating; consequently the flask should be filled by the addition of 25 cc. portions of water (Gildemeister and Hoffmann also recommend additions of water instead of $NaHSO_3$ solution for the determination of benzaldehyde, anisic aldehyde and phenylacetaldehyde) (instead of bisulphite solution). After each addition, the flask should be thoroughly shaken and then immersed in the boiling water for a period of about 5 minutes. The addition compound slowly dissolves and the nonreacting oily layer is driven into the neck of the flask and measured. Upon cooling and standing, some of the addition compound may settle out of solution. However, a reading usually may be obtained.

In general, this modified procedure will not be satisfactory for the determination of decyl aldehyde (upon cooling, the entire contents of the flask will solidify making a reading difficult), cuminic aldehyde (the addition compound formed is not sufficiently soluble even when the flask is heated), methyl heptenone (the reaction with methyl heptenone is incomplete under the condition of the determination) or phenylacetaldehyde which has polymerised. (The nonaldehyde portion settles to the bottom of the flask. Reclaire recommends the use of a special flask for this determination. The hydroxylamine method will prove entirely satisfactory.)

Neutral Sulphite Method

This is also an absorption method. Using a neutral sulphite solution, sodium hydroxide is liberated as the reaction proceeds; this must be periodically neutralised with acid to permit the reaction to go to completion.

$$RCHO + Na_2HSO_3 + H_2O \longrightarrow RCH{\overset{\displaystyle OH}{\underset{\displaystyle SO_3Na}{}}} + NaOH$$

Although this method suffers from the disadvantages of an absorption process, nevertheless it offers certain advantages over the use of the bisulphite technique. Through the use of phenolphthalein, the exact end point of the reaction may be determined. Furthermore, some ketones react with neutral sulphite completely, so that this method may be used for their determination; this is specifically of importance for the determination of carvone in spearmint, dill and caraway oils, of pulegone in pennyroyal oil and of piperitone in eucalyptus oils. Carvone reacts smoothly requiring about 1 hour for the determination. The reaction with piperitone and with pulegone is very slow: only a 5 cc. sample should be used and the flask should be heated in a bath of vigorously boiling water.

Procedure: Into a 150 cc. cassia flask, having a thin neck graduated in 0.1 cc. divisions, introduce 75 cc. of a freshly prepared, saturated, aqueous solution [at room temperature this will be approximately a 30 per cent (wt./vol.) solution] of sodium sulphite, measured from a graduated cylinder. Add a few drops of a 1 per cent alcoholic phenolphthalein solution and neutralise the free alkali with a 50 per cent (by volume) aqueous acetic acid solution. Then pipette exactly 10 cc. of the oil into the flask and shake thoroughly. Immerse the flask in a beaker of boiling water and shake repeatedly. Neutralise the mixture from time to time with the 50 per cent acetic acid ('The United States Pharmacopoeia', suggests neutralisation with a 30 per cent $NaHSO_3$ solution. However, the volume of solution frequently becomes too great to permit thorough shaking). Continue this procedure until no further pink colour appears upon the addition of a few more drops of phenolphthalein solution. Permit the flask to remain in the boiling water for an additional 15 minutes to assure complete reaction. Then add sufficient neutralised sodium sulphite solution to raise the lower limit of the oily layer within the graduated portion of the neck. Any droplets of oil adhering to the sides are made to rise into the neck by gently tapping the flask and by rotating it rapidly between the palms of the hands. After cooling the flask to room temperature, measure the amount of unreacted oil. The aldehyde content may then be calculated by means of the formula given under bisulphite method.

The neutral sulphite method is the official method of 'The United States Pharmacopoeia' for the determination of cinnamic aldehyde in cassia oil, for carvone in spearmint oil and of 'The National Formulary' for carvone in caraway oil. It proves satisfactory for the determination of citral in lemongrass oils, the reaction being very rapid.

As in the case of the bisulphite method, oils containing heavy metals should be treated with tartaric acid before a determination is attempted.

Phenylhydrazine Method

The phenylhydrazine method is seldom used today. It attained importance as the first practical method for the assay of citral in lemon oil. The official method of 'The United States Pharmacopoeia', is included here, since commercial contracts occasionally specify that aldehydes be determined by the phenylhydrazine method. An accurately measured amount of an alcoholic solution of freshly distilled phenylhydrazine is added to a weighed amount of the oil. The excess of phenylhydrazine is titrated with hydrochloric acid. A blank is run simultaneously and from the difference in the amounts of standardised hydrochloric acid required for the blank and the determination, the percentage of aldehyde is calculated.

$$RCHO + C_6H_5NNH_2 \rightarrow C_6H_5NN = CHR + H_2O$$

The method, as described, is suitable for the determination of aldehydes in the citrus oils.

Procedure: Place about 15 cc. of oil of lemon in a tared, 250 cc. Erlenmeyer flask and weigh accurately. Add 10 cc. of an alcoholic solution of phenylhydrazine (the phenylhydrazine solution should be measured accurately from a pipette or burette) (1 in 10) (not darker in colour than pale yellow) and allow it to stand for 30 minutes at room temperature. Then add 3 drops of a 0.1 per cent aqueous solution of methyl orange and neutralise the liquid by the addition of half-normal hydrochloric acid. If difficulty is experienced in determining the end point of the reaction, continue the titration until the liquid is distinctly acid, transfer it to a separatory funnel and after the layers have separated draw off the alcoholic portion. Wash the oil remaining in the funnel with distilled water, adding the washings to the alcoholic solution and titrate the latter with half-normal sodium hydroxide. Carry out a blank test identical with the foregoing, omitting the oil of lemon and note the amount of half-normal hydrochloric acid consumed. Subtract the number of cc. of half-normal sodium hydroxide from the number of cc. of half-normal hydrochloric acid consumed in the test containing the oil of lemon and this result from the number of cc. of half-normal hydrochloric acid consumed in the test without the oil of lemon. Each cc. of this difference corresponds to 0.07609 grams of aldehydes calculated as citral.

In the case of orange oils, the aldehyde is usually calculated as decyl; the factor then used is 0.07813. In the case of grapefruit oils, the aldehydes are frequently calculated as an equal mixture of octyl and decyl; the factor then used is 0.07112. The results obtained in the above method represent percentages by weight.

Hydroxylamine Methods

Two important techniques have been developed, both based upon the use of hydroxylamine for the determination of aldehydes and ketones. The first makes use of a solution of hydroxylamine hydrochloride and the subsequent neutralisation with standardised alkali of the hydrochloric acid liberated by the reaction. The second technique makes use of a solution of hydroxylamine (i.e. a solution of the hydrochloride with substantially all of the combined hydrochloric acid, previously neutralised with alkali); after the reaction with the aldehyde or ketone, the mixture is titrated with standardised acid. The latter procedure is known as the Stillman-Reed method. Both modifications are based upon the fundamental reaction:

$$RCHO + NH_2OH \cdot HCl \longrightarrow RCH{=\!=}NOH + H_2O + HCl$$

$$\begin{array}{c} R \\ \diagdown \\ C{=\!=}O + NH_2OH \cdot HCl \longrightarrow \\ \diagup \\ R' \end{array} \quad \begin{array}{c} R \\ \diagdown \\ C{=\!=}NOH + H_2O + HCl \\ \diagup \\ R' \end{array}$$

The hydroxylamine methods offer many advantages over the absorption processes. Relatively small amounts of the oil are required for a determination. The reaction of hydrolylamine with aldehydes is rapid, shortening the time required for a determination. Water-soluble adulterants which do not contain a carbonyl group do not analyse as apparent aldehyde or ketone. The methods have proved satisfactory for the determination of certain ketones (such as menthone and thujone) which cannot be determined conveniently by the absorption procedures. In fact, hydroxylamine will react with practically all aldehydes and most ketones encountered by the essential oil chemist. Furthermore, these hydroxylamine methods prove exceptionally applicable to oils which contain only small amounts of aldehydes or ketones (e.g. lemon oils) and to oils containing large amounts of free acids (e.g. orris oils). The solutions used for the standard procedure are stable and can be kept for many months; however, the Stillman-Reed solution deteriorates rapidly and is best prepared when needed.

The hydroxylamine methods have certain disadvantages not inherent in absorption techniques. It must be remembered that the calculation of results involves the molecular weight of the aldehyde or ketone, giving percentages by weight; hence adulterations with carbonyl compounds of lower molecular weight give apparent percentages which are too high. If more than one aldehyde or ketone is present in an oil, all are calculated as a specific carbonyl compound. Since the reaction of hydroxylamine is quite universal, it is difficult to determine an individual component. Nor can the carbonyl and noncarbonyl portions be separated conveniently and studied individually.

Standard procedure: Into a 100 cc. saponification flask weigh accurately the requisite amount of oil or synthetic and add 35 cc. of 0.5 N hydroxylamine hydrochloride solution, measured from a graduated cylinder. Permit the flask to stand at room temperature for the proper length of time and titrate the liberated hydrochloric acid with standardised 0.5 N alcoholic sodium hydroxide. The titration is continued until the original greenish shade of the hydroxylamine solution is obtained. A second flask containing 35 cc. of hydroxylamine hydrochloride solution may be used as a blank to assure a more accurate colour match (in the case of very darkly coloured oils, the size of sample should be greatly reduced and the end point determined with the aid of a spotplate. This is particularly important in the case of oils which have a greenish colour, e.g. wormwood oils).

$$\text{Percentage of aldehyde or ketone} = \frac{am}{20s}$$

where, a = number of cc. of 0.5 N sodium hydroxide used for neutralisation

m = molecular weight of the aldehyde or ketone

s = weight of sample in grams

Preparation of 0.5 N hydroxylamine hydrochloride solution: Dissolve 275 grams of recrystallised hydroxylamine hydrochloride in 300 cc. of distilled water; warm to a temperature of 65°C on a steam bath to yield a clear solution. Add this solution slowly to 2 gallons of 95 per cent alcohol and mix thoroughly. Then add 125 cc. of a 0.1 per cent solution of bromphenol blue indicator in 50 per cent alcohol and sufficient 0.5 N alcoholic sodium hydroxide solution to change the yellow colour of the solution to a greenish shade; this usually requires about 20 to 25 cc. of the alkali. The proper degree of neutralisation is attained when 35 cc. of the solution shows a distinct greenish shade which changes to a distinct yellow upon the addition of 1 drop of 0.5 N hydrochloric acid. A stable solution of hydroxylamine hydrochloride is thus obtained which is approximately 0.5 N; an exact adjustment is unnecessary.

For lesser quantities of solution, dissolve 34.75 grams of recrystallised hydroxylamine hydrochloride in 40 cc. of distilled water and make up to 1 litre with 95 per cent alcohol; add 15 cc. of the bromphenol blue solution and neutralise.

The proper size of sample and the proper length of time to give complete reaction and the molecular weights of the most frequently encountered aldehydes and ketones are given in Tables 11.4 and 11.5.

Stillman-Reed procedure: Proceed as directed under the standard procedure but add 75 cc. of hydroxylamine solution, measured accurately by means of a burette or pipette. At the same time run a blank determination. After standing the required length of time, titrate with standardised 0.5 N hydrochloric acid to a green-yellow end point. Care should be taken to titrate both the blank and the sample to the same end point. Calculate the percentage of aldehyde or ketone as described above.

Table 11.4. Molecular weights and reaction time of aldehydes and ketones (Part I).

Carbonyl compound	Molecular wt.	Size of sample (gram)	Reaction time
Acetaldehyde	44.05	0.5	Immediate
Acetophenone	120.14	1.0	15 min.
α-Amyl cinnamic aldehyde	202.29	1.0	24 hr
Anisic aldehyde	136.14	1.0	15 min.
Benzaldehyde	106.12	1.0	Immediate
Benzophenone†	182.21	–	–
Benzylidene acetone	146.18	1.0	15 min.
Butyraldehyde	72.10	1.0	15 min.
Camphor†	152.00	–	–
Carvone	150.21	0.5	24 hr
Cinnamic aldehyde	132.15	1.0	15 min.

(Contd ...)

Carbonyl compound	Molecular wt.	Size of sample (gram)	Reaction time
Citral	152.23	1.0	15 min.
Citronellal‡	154.25	1.0	15 min.
Cuminic aldehyde	148.20	1.0	15 min.
Decyl aldehyde	156.26	1.0	30 min.
Dodecyl aldehyde	184.31	1.0	15 min.
Ethyl amyl ketone	128.21	1.0	15 min.
Fenchone†	152.23	–	–
Furfural	96.08	1.0	15 min.
Heliotropin	150.23	1.0	15 min.
Heptyl aldehyde	114.18	1.0	15 min.
Hexyl aldehyde	100.16	1.0	15 min.
Hydrotropic aldehyde	134.17	1.0	15 min.
Ionone	192.29	0.5	24 hr
Irone	192.29	0.5	1 hr
Isovaleric aldehyde	86.13	1.0	15 min.
Menthone	154.25	0.5	24 hr
Methyl acetophenone	134.17	1.0	15 min.
Methyl amyl ketone	114.18	1.0	15 min.
Methyl heptenone	126.19	1.0	24 hr
Methyl heptyl ketone	142.24	1.0	15 min.
Methyl hexyl ketone	128.21	1.0	15 min.
Methyl nonyl ketone	170.29	1.0	15 min.
p-Methoxyacetophenone	150.17	1.0	24 hr
Nonyl aldehyde	142.24	1.0	15 min.
Octyl aldehyde	128.21	1.0	15 min.
Perillic aldehyde	150.21	1.0	15 min.
Phenylacetaldehyde	120.14	1.0	30 min.
Phenylpropyl aldehyde	134.17	1.0	15 min.
Piperitone†	152.23	–	–
Pulegone†	152.23	–	–
Salicyl aldehyde	122.12	1.0	15 min.
Thujone	152.23	0.5	24 hr
Tolyl aldehyde	152.14	1.0	15 min.
Umbellulone†	150.21	–	–
Undecyl aldehyde	152.14	1.0	15 min.
Vanillin	152.14	1.0	15 min.
Valeric aldehyde	86.13	1.0	15 min.

†Because of the slow reaction rate with hydroxylamine this method is not satisfactory for these ketones.

‡Low values are obtained for this isolate if the usual hydroxylamine hydrochloride technique is used. Fairly satisfactory results may be obtained if the solution is well cooled and the titration carried out at low temperatures (–10°C).

Table 11.5. Molecular weights and reaction time of aldehydes and ketones (Part II).

| Oil | Main carbonyl compound present | | Size of sample (gram) | Reaction time |
	Name	Molecular wt.		
Almond, bitter	Benzaldehyde	106.12	1.0	Immediate
Caraway	Carvone	150.21	1.0	24 hr
Cassia	Cinnamic aldehyde	132.15	1.0	15 min.
Cedar leaf	Thujone	152.23	1.0	24 hr
Cherry laurel	Benzaldehyde	106.12	1.0	Immediate
Cinnamon	Cinnamic aldehyde	132.15	1.0	15 min.
Citronella, Sri Lanka	Citronellal	154.25	2.5	15 min.
Citronellal, Java	Citronellal	154.25	1.0	15 min.
Cumin	Cuminic aldehyde	148.20	1.0	15 min.
Dill	Carvone	150.21	1.0	24 hr
Geranium	Menthone	154.25	0.5	24 hr
Grapefruit	Decyl aldehyde*	156.26	5.0	30 min.
Lemon	Citral	152.23	5.0	15 min.
Lemon concentrates, terpeneless and sesquiterpeneless	Citral	152.23	1.0	15 min.
Lemongrass	Citral	152.23	1.0	15 min.
Limes, distilled	Citral†	152.23	5.0	15 min.
Limes, expressed	Citral	152.23	5.0	15 min.
Mandarin	Decyl aldehyde	156.26	5.0	30 min.
Orange	Decyl aldehyde	156.26	5.0	30 min.
Orange concentrates, terpeneless and sesquiterpeneless	Decyl aldehyde	156.26	1.0	30 min.
Orris‡	Irone	192.29	1.0	1 hr
Pennyroyal§	Pulegone	152.23	0.5	about 72 hr
Peppermint	Menthone	154.25	0.5	24 hr
Rue	Methyl nonyl ketone	170.29	1.0	15 min.
Sage, Dalmatian	Thujone	152.23	1.0	24 hr
Spearmint	Carvone	150.21	1.0	24 hr
Tansy	Thujone	152.23	0.5	24 hr
Wormwood‖	Thujone	152.23	0.25	24 hr

*Occasionally the carbonyl component of grapefruit oil is reported as a mixture of equal parts of octyl and decyl aldehydes; if this is desired, use 142.24 as an average of the molecular weights.

†Very little citral is actually present in distilled lime oil. The carbonyl components consist mainly of octyl aldehyde, decyl aldehyde, dodecyl aldehyde and an unidentified aldehyde. However, it is customary to report the aldehyde content as citral.

‡It is well to titrate the reaction mixture at the end of 1 hour and then at the end of 24 hours: any appreciable difference in the two values indicates the presence of other carbonyl compounds, most likely one of the ionones. (*Contd...*)

§ Because of the slow reaction rate of hydroxylamine with pulegone, this method is not satisfactory for oil pennyroyal; use the neutral suphite method.

‖The dark colour of wormwood oils with their natural greenish tint makes the determination of thujone quite difficult. The use of a very small sample and the use of a spotplate to judge the end point is recommended. However, the accuracy of the determination suffers thereby; nevertheless an accuracy of ±5 per cent can be obtained.

Preparation of 0.5 N hydroxylamine solution: Dissolve 20 gram of recrystallised hydroxylamine hydrochloride in 40 cc. of water and dilute to 400 cc. with 95 per cent alcohol. To this solution, in a 1 litre beaker, add, with stirring, 300 cc. of 0.5 N alcoholic potassium hydroxide and 2.5 cc. of a 0.4 per cent bromphenol blue solution in 50 per cent alcohol. Permit the solution to stand for 30 minutes and filter. This solution cannot be stored for any appreciable period. A blank must always be run since the solution tends to deteriorate slowly.

In conclusion it might be well to point out that each of the general methods for the determination of aldehydes and ketones has its place in the analysis of essential oils. Thus, absorption methods permit of the easy separation of the noncarbonyl portion of the oil and of the separation of some aldehydes and ketones by regeneration from the bisulphite addition compound with strong alkali. It then becomes possible to study the odour and other properties of these individual portions and to detect more readily adulteration of the original oil. A comparison of the results from the absorption methods and from the hydroxylamine method is frequently very revealing; large differences may be indicative of adulteration with water-soluble constituents or additions of carbonyl compounds of low molecular weight.

From a consideration of the limitations of each method, it should be obvious that it is of utmost importance always to record the method used when reporting an analytical result.

DETERMINATION OF PHENOLS

Phenols react with the alkali hydroxides, giving rise to water-soluble phenolates. This is the basis of the classical method for the estimation of phenols in essential oils. Since the potassium salts of many phenols are more soluble than the corresponding sodium salts, the use of potassium hydroxide is preferred.

It must be remembered that, in addition to, the phenols, any alkali soluble material (e.g. acids) will also go into solution as well as any water-soluble constituents or water-soluble adulterants (e.g. alcohol). This will give rise to erroneous results: the apparent phenol content will be too high. Further, an aqueous solution of alkali phenolates is a much better solvent for the nonphenolic portion of an oil than is the alkali solution itself; specifically this is important in the case of terpeneless bay oils.

When the determination has been completed, it often proves of value to separate the nonphenolic portion and to study its odour. The alkaline solution of the phenolates may be freed of traces of oil by washing with ether; the phenols may then be regenerated by the addition of dilute sulphuric acid (1:3), extracted with ether, and obtained in a pure state by evaporating off the ether. (The, separated ether layer should be dried with anhydrous sodium sulphate before this final evaporation.) The presence of foreign phenolic bodies frequently may be detected by this technique. Modifications of the general procedure become necessary in the case of certain specific oils. Such modifications are noted below.

General procedure: Into a well cleaned 150 cc. cassia flask, having a long, thin neck graduated in 0.1 cc. divisions, introduce 10 cc. of the oil, measured from a pipette. Add 75 cc. of an aqueous 1 N potassium hydroxide solution, measured from a graduated cylinder. Stopper and shake thoroughly for exactly 5 minutes. Permit to stand undisturbed for 1 hour, after which the undissolved oil is forced into the neck by the addition of more potassium hydroxide solution. The alkaline solution must be added carefully to avoid disturbing the layer of separated oil. This addition may conveniently be made by clamping the flask at a slight angle on a ring stand; above the flask is placed a ring to hold a separatory funnel containing the solution of alkali which is permitted to flow down along the inside of the neck of the cassia flask very slowly. If the flow of the alkali is adjusted to about 1 drop per second, a clean separation of the oil is usually obtained (Fig. 11.4). In order to make any droplets of oil adhering to the sides of the flask rise into the neck, gently tap or revolve the flask rapidly between the palms of the hands. Measure the quantity of oil that does not dissolve in the alkali. The phenol content, expressed as a volume/volume percentage, is calculated from the following formula:

$$\text{Percentage of phenol} = 10(10 - \text{no. of cc. of undissolved oil})$$

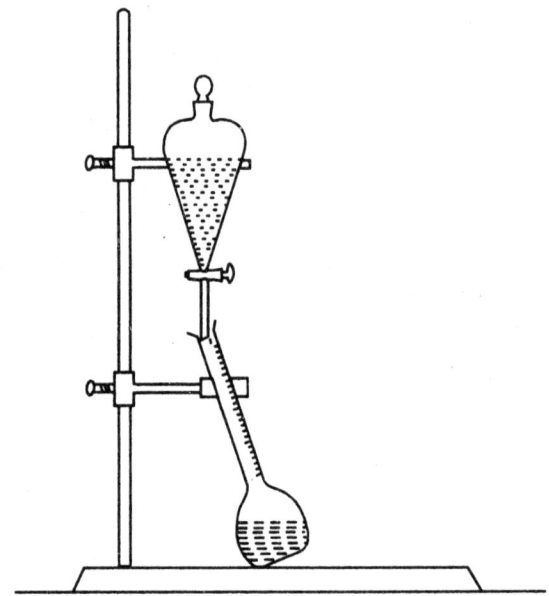

Fig. 11.4. Apparatus for phenol determination.

Oils containing large amounts of heavy metals may not give a sharp separation of the nonphenolic oily layer and the alkaline solution in the neck of the flask. Such oils should be thoroughly shaken with a small amount (about 1 per cent) of powdered tartaric acid and filtered to remove the interfering metals before the determination of phenols is attempted.

Modification of the General Procedure

Clove oils

Since clove oils contain aceteugenol in addition to free eugenol and since both constituents contribute to the value of the oil it is customary to saponify the former and report the total phenol content as eugenol. The general procedure is modified as follows:

> After thoroughly shaking the oil and alkali for 5 minutes in the cold, heat the flask on a steam bath for 10 minutes. Occasionally shake the flask during this heating to insure complete saponification. Immediately after removal of the flask from the steam bath add a further quantity of alkali in order to drive the unreacted oil into the neck of the flask. It is necessary to make this addition while the content of the flask is still hot since the nonphenolic portion may partially solidify.

Pimenta oils

The procedure described above for clove oils is also used for the determination of the phenol content of pimenta oils.

Terpeneless bay oils

Because of the solvent effect of the potassium eugenolate upon the nonphenolic constituents of a terpeneless bay oil, the whole oil will go completely into solution if a 1 N solution of potassium hydroxide is used in this determination. Therefore, it becomes necessary to reduce the strength of the alkali to 3 per cent and to use 125 cc. of this dilute alkaline solution for shaking out the phenols.

Cinnamon oils

These oils offer some difficulty to the analyst. The formation of a troublesome emulsion and a very poor separation of the oil and the aqueous layers results because of the similarity of the gravity of the oil and the gravity of the solution. It is for this reason that a 3 per cent solution cannot satisfactorily be used. Shaking for too long a period gives rise to results that are much too high. The following procedure, if followed exactly, will give results that can easily be duplicated and which represent approximately the true eugenol content:

To 50 cc. of a 1 N potassium hydroxide solution in a cassia flask add 5 cc. of the cinnamon oil. Shake well for exactly 3 minutes and let stand for 10 minutes. Fill the flask with potassium hydroxide solution, using the ring stand technique described under the general procedure. If the determination has been carried out carefully, the residual oil will rise into the neck in an unbroken column.

Thyme and origanum oils

The phenolic constituents of thyme and origanum oils consists mainly of thymol and carvacrol. The separation of the phenolic constituents is an aid in the evaluation of these oils, since oils containing predominantly thymol are generally considered of superior quality. Thymol is easily crystallised; carvacrol is a liquid at temperatures above 2°C.

The separation and examination of the phenolic portion may conveniently be carried out after the determination of the phenol content.

Pour the contents of the cassia flask (used in the assay) into a separatory funnel and permit the nonphenolic portion to separate. Filter the aqueous layer through filter paper previously wetted with water. Transfer this filtered solution to a separatory funnel and acidify with dilute hydrochloric acid (1:3) until the mixture is strongly acid to litmus. Add 50 cc. of ether and shake thoroughly. Separate the ether layer, dry with anhydrous sodium sulphate and filter. Evaporate the ether cautiously on a steam bath and pour the liberated phenols into a test tube and permit it to stand at room temperature for 30 minutes. If the phenols consist primarily of thymol, a crystalline mass results. If no crystals form after 30 minutes, cool to 5°C by means of an ice bath. Rub the side of the test tube with a thermometer or glass rod and add a small crystal of thymol to initiate crystallisation: if no crystals form after 30 minutes the absence of an appreciable amount of thymol may be assumed.

On determining phenol contents it is well to remember that water-soluble constituents may be added to increase the apparent phenol contents. Alcohol and certain glycols are such adulterants which may be occasionally encountered. If the relationship between the specific gravity and the phenol content appears abnormal, the oil should be investigated further for the presence of possible adulterants.

DETERMINATION OF CINEOLE

Of the numerous methods that have been proposed for the determination of the cineole content of essential oils, the method of Kleber and von Rechenberg, the method of Cocking and that of Scammell (modified by Baker and Smith) have proved the most valuable.

According to the Kleber and Von Rechenberg method, the congealing point of the oil itself is determined, from which the cineole content may be determined by reference to a table or graph. The presence of oxygenated constituents other than cineole has little effect upon the values obtained; an accuracy of about ±1 per cent may be obtained. 'The United States Pharmacopoeia' makes use of this method to establish a minimum of 70 per cent cineole in official eucalyptus oils. The main criticism of the Kleber and Von Rechenberg method is the inconvenience of working at greatly reduced temperatures. The exact determination of a congealing point at a temperature much below 0° often presents difficulty.

> *Procedure*: Place about 10 cc. of the oil in a heavy walled tube which is preferably equipped with an air or vacuum jacket. Immerse the tube in a mixture of ice and salt, or in a cooling bath of solid carbon dioxide in acetone. The true solidification point is determined, i.e. the temperature at which the crystals of cineole first appear as the oil is cooled and at which the crystals disappear as the temperature is permitted to rise. Several determinations of the solidifying point should be made in order to obtain an exact reading. The percentage of cineole, corresponding to this temperature can be determined directly by reference to Table 11.6.

Table 11.6. Determination of eucalyptol content by congealing point.

Temperature (°C)	Eucalyptol content (%)	Temperature (°C)	Eucalyptol content (%)
1.2	100.0	−9.0	80.3
−1.0	99.4	−10.0	78.5
0.0	97.3	−11.0	76.5
−1.0	95.3	−12.0	75.3
−2.0	93.4	−13.0	73.7
−3.0	91.5	−14.0	72.2
−4.0	89.6	−15.0	70.6
−5.0	87.5	−16.0	69.2
−6.0	85.7	−17.0	67.5
−7.0	83.7	−18.0	66.2
−8.0	82.0	−19.0	64.8

The *o*-cresol method of Cocking offers certain advantages. Since the congealing point is well above room temperature, the determination is greatly simplified. Results are easily reproducible. According to Cocking, the accuracy is approximately ±3 per cent in the case of eucalyptus and cajuput oils. The *o*-cresol method has been accepted as the official method of 'the british pharmacopoeia'. The procedure as given below is essentially the official method of 'the british pharmacopoeia'.

> *Procedure*: Into a stout walled test tube, about 15 mm in diameter and 80 mm in length, place 3 gram (accurately weighed) of the oil, previously dried with anhydrous sodium sulphate (the use of calcium chloride for drying the oil as suggested by 'the british pharmacopoeia' is not to be recommended; anhydrous sodium sulphate is much to be preferred, eliminating the possibility of

formation of addition products with primary alcohols that may be present in the oil), together with 2.1 gram of melted *o*-cresol. The *o*-cresol used must be pure and dry, with a freezing point not below 30°C. It is hygroscopic and should be stored in a small well-stoppered bottle, because the presence of moisture may lower the results. Insert a thermometer, graduated in fifths of a degree and stir the mixture well in order to induce crystallisation; note the highest reading of the thermometer. Warm the tube gently until the contents are thoroughly melted and insert the tube through a bored cork into a widemouthed bottle which is to act as an air jacket. The thermometer should be suspended from a ring stand in such a way that it does not touch the walls of the inner tube. Allow the mixture to cool slowly until crystallisation commences, or until the temperature has fallen to the point previously noted. Stir the contents of the tube vigorously with the thermometer, rubbing the latter on the sides of the tube with an up and down motion in order to induce rapid crystallisation. Continue the stirring and rubbing as long as the temperature rises. Take the highest point as the freezing point. Repeat this procedure until two readings agreeing within 0.1°C are obtained. The percentage of cineole in the oil can be computed from Table 11.7.

Table 11.7. Percentage of cineole.

Temperature	0.0	0.1	0.2	0.3	0.4	0.5	0.6	0.7	0.8	0.9
24	45.6	45.7	45.9	46.0	46.1	46.3	46.4	46.5	46.6	46.8
25	46.9	47.0	47.2	47.3	47.4	47.6	47.7	47.8	47.9	48.1
26	48.2	48.3	48.5	48.6	48.7	48.9	49.0	49.1	49.2	49.4
27	49.5	49.6	49.8	49.9	50.0	50.2	50.3	50.4	50.5	50.7
28	50.8	50.9	51.1	51.2	51.3	51.5	51.6	51.7	51.8	52.0
29	52.1	52.2	52.4	52.5	52.6	52.8	52.9	53.0	53.1	53.3
30	53.4	53.5	53.7	53.8	53.9	54.1	54.2	54.3	54.4	54.6
31	54.7	54.8	55.0	55.1	55.2	55.4	55.5	55.6	55.7	55.9
32	56.0	56.1	56.3	56.4	56.5	56.7	56.8	56.9	57.0	57.2
33	57.3	57.4	57.6	57.7	57.8	58.0	58.1	58.2	58.3	58.5
34	58.6	58.7	58.9	59.0	59.1	59.3	59.4	59.5	59.6	59.8
35	59.9	60.0	60.2	60.3	60.4	60.6	60.7	60.8	60.9	61.1
36	61.2	61.3	61.5	61.6	61.7	61.9	62.0	62.1	62.2	62.4
37	62.5	62.6	62.8	62.9	63.0	63.2	63.3	63.4	63.5	63.7
38	63.8	63.9	64.1	64.2	64.4	64.5	64.6	64.8	64.9	65.1
39	65.2	65.4	65.5	65.7	65.8	66.0	66.2	66.3	66.5	66.6
40	66.8	67.0	67.2	67.3	67.5	67.7	67.9	68.1	68.2	68.4
41	68.6	68.8	69.0	69.2	69.4	69.6	69.7	69.9	70.1	70.3
42	70.5	70.7	70.9	71.0	71.2	71.4	71.6	71.8	71.9	72.1
43	72.3	72.5	72.7	72.9	73.1	73.3	73.4	73.6	73.8	74.0
44	74.2	74.4	74.6	74.8	75.0	75.2	75.3	75.5	75.7	75.9
45	76.1	76.3	76.5	76.7	76.9	77.1	77.2	77.4	77.6	77.8
46	78.0	78.2	78.4	78.6	78.8	79.0	79.2	79.4	79.6	79.8
47	80.0	80.2	80.4	80.6	80.8	81.1	81.3	81.5	81.7	81.9
48	82.1	82.3	82.5	82.7	82.9	83.2	83.4	83.6	83.8	84.0

(Contd ...)

Temperature	0.0	0.1	0.2	0.3	0.4	0.5	0.6	0.7	0.8	0.9
49	84.2	84.4	84.6	84.8	85.0	85.3	85.5	85.7	85.9	86.1
50	86.3	86.6	86.8	87.1	87.3	87.6	87.8	88.1	88.3	88.6
51	88.8	89.1	89.3	89.6	89.8	90.1	90.3	90.6	90.8	91.1
52	91.3	91.6	91.8	92.1	92.3	92.6	92.8	93.1	93.3	93.6
53	93.8	94.1	94.3	94.6	94.8	95.1	95.3	95.6	95.8	96.1
54	96.3	96.6	96.9	97.2	97.5	97.8	98.1	98.4	98.7	99.0
55	99.3	99.7	100.0	–	–	–	–	–	–	–

It should be noted that in both methods relatively high cineole contents give more accurate analytical results. Therefore, if the cineole content of the oil is low, the determination is best carried out on a mixture of equal parts (by weight) of oil and pure cineole (melting point, 1.2°C or higher). In the Kleber and Von Rechenberg method, if the cineole content is less than 65 per cent, this modified procedure should be followed; in the o-cresol method, of Cocking, if less than 50 per cent. The cineole content of the original oil may then be calculated by means of the following formula:

Percentage of cineole in original oil = 2 × (% of cineole in mixture – 50)

The phosphoric acid method of Scammell as modified by Baker and Smith is based on the formation of a solid, loose molecular compound of cineole and phosphoric acid from which the cineole may be regenerated by the addition of water. The procedure recommended by these authors is given below:

Procedure: Place 10 cc. of the oil in a 50 cc. beaker or other suitable vessel and cool thoroughly in a bath of ice and salt. Slowly add 4 cc. of phosphoric acid (if the cineole content is below 30 per cent, add only 3 cc. of phosphoric acid), a few drops at a time, mixing the acid and oil thoroughly between each addition by careful stirring. After all of the acid has been added, permit the mixture to remain in the bath for 5 minutes to insure complete formation of the cineole-phosphoric acid addition compound. Then add 10 cc. of petroleum ether (boiling below 50°C) which, has previously been well cooled in the ice bath and incorporate well with the aid of a flat ended rod. Immediately transfer the mixture to a cooled Buchner funnel, 5 cm in diameter. Filter off the non-combined portion rapidly with the aid of a water pump. Transfer the cake from the Buchner funnel to a piece of fine calico and spread the cake with a spatula so that it covers an area of about 6 × 8 cm. Fold over the calico into a pad and place between several layers of absorbent paper. Press well for 3 minutes. Break up the cake on a glazed tile with a spatula and transfer to a cassia flask. Decompose the cineole-phosphoric acid addition compound with warm water and force the liberated cineole into the neck of the flask by the further addition of water. After the separation is complete and the contents of the flask have cooled to room temperature measure the amount of cineole.

If the cineole content is found to be above 60 per cent, repeat the determination using a sample of the oil diluted with freshly distilled pinene or turpentine oil: three volumes of oil plus one volume of pinene. Make the necessary correction in calculating the percentage of cineole.

This test gives satisfactory results with oils containing as little as 20 per cent cineole and as high as 100 per cent; in the latter case, the oil must be previously diluted as described. It is important to add the acid slowly, to have the mixture very cold and to cool the petroleum ether thoroughly before adding. Other methods for the quantitative determination of cineole have been suggested.

DETERMINATION OF ASCARIDOLE

The analysis of wormseed oils offers some difficulty because of the lack of a satisfactory method for the determination of the active principle, ascaridole.

'The United States Pharmacopoeia' based the official determination on the fact that ascaridole is soluble in dilute acetic acid. The technique consists of shaking a measured volume of the oil in a cassia flask with 60 per cent acetic acid, determining the volume of undissolved oil and calculating the ascaridole content by difference. This is a method developed by Nelson. Although this procedure represents one of the simplest determinations for ascaridole, it suffers from the fact that the analytical values are far from accurate. It has been found that normal oils containing as much as 70 to 80 per cent ascaridole (as indicated by solubility, gravity, distillation and other methods for the determination of ascaridole) often analyse as low as 55 per cent by the Nelson method. Furthermore, Reindollar has shown that 'hi-test' oils containing large amounts of ascaridole give results by this method that are too high. A further disadvantage of the Nelson method lies in the fact that the determination is by no means specific for ascaridole; additions of cineole or cineole-containing oils analyse as ascaridole. This is also true of many other oxygenated compounds, such as terpineol.

Procedure: Place 10 cc. of oil wormseed, measured from a pipette, in a 100 cc. cassia flask. Add 50 cc. of a solution of acetic acid made by diluting 60 cc. of glacial acetic acid with distilled water to measure 100 cc. Shake the mixture well for 5 minutes. Add sufficient of the acetic acid solution to raise the lower limit of the oily layer within the graduated portion of the neck and allow the liquids to separate, rotating the flask from time to time. Note the volume of the oily layer.

Percentage of ascaridole = 10 (10 – cc. of unreacted oil)

In order to overcome these difficulties, 'The United States Pharmacopoeia' later abandoned the Nelson method and then substituted the Cocking and Hymas procedure, which is give below:

Assay: Place about 2.5 gram of oil chenopodium, accurately weighed, in a 50 cc. volumetric flask, fill to the mark with 90 per cent acetic acid, mix well and transfer a portion of this freshly prepared solution to a burette, graduated in 20ths of a cc. Into a glass-stoppered Erlenmeyer flask measure, from graduated cylinders, 3 cc. of a solution of potassium iodide (prepared by dissolving 8.3 gram of potassium iodide in sufficient distilled water to make 10 cc. of solution), 5 cc. of concentrated hydrochloric acid and 10 cc. of glacial acetic acid. Immerse the flask in a freezing mixture until the temperature is reduced to –3°C, add quickly about 5 cc. of the acetic acid solution of the oil, mix it with the cooled reagent as rapidly as possible and observe the volume drawn from the burette after 2 minutes (to allow for draining). Set the stoppered flask aside at a temperature between 5° and 10°C for exactly 5 minutes; then, without diluting, titrate the liberated iodine with tenth-normal sodium thiosulphate. At the same time, conduct a blank test, but dilute the reagent with 20 cc. of distilled water before titrating the liberated iodine. The difference between the two titrations represents the iodine liberated by ascaridole. Each cc. of tenth-normal sodium thiosulphate is equivalent to 0.00665 gram of $C_{10}H_{16}O_2$.

If all conditions as outlined are rigidly followed, this method gives analytical results that are reproducible and relatively accurate for normal American oils. If, however, the ascaridole content is abnormally low, the results will not be sufficiently accurate.

Since this method is based on the oxidation of potassium iodide by the peroxide, ascaridole and the subsequent determination of the amount of free iodine, additions of oxygenated constituents should not increase the apparent ascaridole content unless the added compound is capable of oxidising the potassium iodide under the experimental conditions. Furthermore, since the liberated iodine is capable of being absorbed by unsaturates in the oil, it is very important to maintain the low temperatures as indicated in the procedure, to keep this secondary reaction at a minimum.

The tentative method for the determination of ascaridole as outlined in the methods of analysis of the association of official agricultural chemists proves too cumbersome for rapid commercial analyses and control. This method involves the reduction of ascaridole by titanium trichloride. It requires that the solution be protected from atmospheric oxygen; this entails storage of the solution under an atmosphere of hydrogen and titrations under an atmosphere of carbon dioxide. According to the experiments the results obtained by this method are fairly concordant with those obtained by the method of Cocking and Hymas. The association of official agricultural chemists' method is given below, exactly as it appears in this official work:

> *Procedure*: 'Weigh 1 ml of the oil in 100 ml volumetric flask and dilute to volume with alcohol. Place 50 ml of the $TiCl_3$ solution in Erlenmeyer flask through which current of CO_2 is passing. Fit flask with Bunsen valve, add 10 ml of diluted solution of the oil, close flask (with the Bunsen valve) and heat contents almost to boiling for 2 minutes. (Prolonged heating has no effect if contents are not boiled vigorously.) If pale violet colour of the $TiCl_3$ disappears, add more reagent to insure excess. (Formation of a white precipitate does not interfere with determination.) Add 1 ml of 5 per cent NH_4CNS solution and titrate back excess of $TiCl_3$ with the $FeNH_4(SO_4)_2$ solution in CO_2 atmosphere until faint, permanent, brownish red colour is obtained.
>
> Subtract quantity of $FeNH_4(SO_4)_2$ solution used, expressed in equivalent mg of $TiCl_3$, from number of mg of $TiCl_3$ taken. Difference is number of mg of $TiCl_3$ oxidised by oil taken. Convert mg of $TiCl_3$ oxidised into ascaridole by dividing by factor 1.1284 (1 gram of ascaridole is reduced by 1.284 gram of $TiCl_3$).

Example: 0.9600 gram of oil was made up to 100 ml and 10 ml aliquot was heated with 50 ml of the $TiCl_3$ solution (1 ml containing 0.0034 gram of $TiCl_3$). It then required 5.9 ml of the reagent, each ml equivalent to 0.01545 gram to $TiCl_3$, to back titrate. Grams of $TiCl_3$ oxidised is numerically equal to $(50 \times 0.0034) - (5.9 \times 0.01545)$, or 0.07885. Weight of oil in the aliquot was 0.0960 gram. Hence,

$$\text{Percentage of ascaridole} = \frac{0.07885 \times 100}{0.096 \times 1.284} = 72\%$$

(a) *Standard ferric ammonium sulphate solution*.: Dissolve 39.214 gram of pure, crystallised $Fe(NH_4)_2(SO_4)_2 \cdot 6H_2O$ in 200 ml of H_2O in litre flask, add 30 ml of H_2SO_4 and mix well. Weigh exactly 3.16 gram of $KMnO_4$; dissolve in 200 ml of warm H_2O and slowly add to solution in the flask, with stirring. ($KMnO_4$ solution should be just sufficient to oxidise the ferrous salt, but it is well to add the last few ml in small portions.) Cool solution and dilute to 1 litre with H_2O.

(b) *Standard titanium trichloride solution*.: Add 100 ml of commercial 15–20 per cent TiC_{13} solution to 200 ml of HCl, boil 1 minute, cool and dilute to 4500 ml with H_2O. Place solution in container with H atmosphere provision and allow to stand 2 days for adsorption of residual 0. Preserve the $TiCl_3$ solution in an atmosphere of H, taking care to have all joints air-tight and covering stoppers (preferably countersunk) with suitable wax. Standardise by titrating 20 ml of the $FeNH_4(SO_4)_2$ solution against the $TiCl_3$ solution in a protective stream of CO_2, using 1 ml of 5 per cent NH_4CNS solution as indicator. 1 ml of 0.1 N $FeNH_4(SO_4)_2 = 0.01545$ gram of $TiCl_3$.

The determination of the ascaridole content by a distillation technique is not to be recommended for routine analyses, since the ascaridole is so unstable that the oil is apt to decompose with explosive violence should the temperature not be carefully controlled.

Dodge has suggested the use of a solution of sodium bisulphite to determine the ascaridole content of wormseed oils. The difficulty of determining the exact end point and the length of time required for a determination militates against the use of this technique. In spite of its recognised deficiencies, the method of Cocking and Hymas, at the present time official in 'the national formulary' and 'the british pharmacopoeia', is probably the most useful for commercial analytical control laboratories.

DETERMINATION OF CAMPHOR

In order to determine the camphor content of essential oils (which contain no other carbonyl compounds) the gravimetric determination proposed by Aschan may be employed.

Procedure: Introduce about 1 gram of the oil, accurately weighed, into a test tube and dissolve the oil in 2 gram of glacial acetic acid. Add 1 gram of semicarbazide hydrochloride and 1.5 gram of freshly fused anhydrous potassium acetate. Triturate thoroughly with a glass rod, stopper the tube with a plug of absorbent cotton and heat three hours in a water bath at 70°C. Cool the mixture, add 10 to 15 cc. of water, stir thoroughly and transfer the precipitate quantitatively to a tared 4 to 5 cm filter. Wash with water until all water soluble matter is removed, air dry, wash with petroleum ether and dry in air to constant weight. Determine the weight of semicarbazone from the increase in the weight of the filter. Calculate the content of camphor in the original oil by means of the following formula:

$$\text{Percentage of camphor} = \frac{72.7p}{s}$$

where, p = weight of semicarbazone in grams
s = weight of oil in grams

DETERMINATION OF METHYL ANTHRANILATE

The procedure described below is based on the classical method of Hesse and Zeitschel. It depends on the actual separation of the ester from the volatile oil by the formation of the ether insoluble sulphate.

Procedure: Dissolve about 25 to 100 grams of oil in twice the volume of anhydrous ether. Cool the solution well in a freezing mixture, the temperature being reduced to at least 0°C. Add, with constant stirring, a solution of 1 volume of concentrated sulphuric acid in 5 volumes of anhydrous ether until no further precipitate forms. Collect the precipitate in a small, well-cooled Büchner funnel and wash with dry, cold ether until odourless. Dissolve this precipitate in water with the aid of alcohol if necessary and titrate with 0.5 N sodium hydroxide. Calculate the ester content by means of the following formula:

$$\text{Percentage of methyl anthranilate} = \frac{3.775a}{s}$$

where, a = cc. of alkali required
s = original weight of oil taken in grams

To this solution add an excess of 0.5 N sodium hydroxide and heat the mixture on a steam bath for 30 minutes. Titrate the free alkali which is unconsumed with 0.5 N hydrochloric acid. Calculate again the ester content by means of the following formula:

$$\text{Percentage of methyl anthranilate} = \frac{7.55b}{s}$$

where, b = cc. of alkali consumed in the saponification
s = original weight of oil taken in grams

If the ester is exclusively methyl anthranilate, *a* should be twice as large as *b*.

The procedure as described will determine all basic constituents which form ether insoluble sulphates (e.g. the methyl ester of methyl anthranilic acid) in addition to methyl anthranilate.

For the determination of methyl anthranilate in the presence of methyl N-methyl anthranilate, Erdmann has suggested a procedure based on the diazotisation of methyl anthranilate, a primary aromatic amine. The ester is washed out of the oil with dilute sulphuric or hydrochloric acid and the acid solution treated with a 5 per cent sodium nitrite solution to diazotise the amine.

The solution is then titrated with an alkaline solution of β-naphthol. (This solution is prepared by dissolving 0.5 gram β-naphthol in 0.5 cc. of sodium hydroxide, at least 30 per cent, and adding a solution of 15 gram of sodium carbonate in 150 cc. of water.)

The azo dye thereby formed is insoluble and precipitates out. The titration is continued until no further precipitation occurs.

A combination of the method of Hesse and Zeitschel and that of Erdmann can be used to determine the percentage of methyl anthranilate and of methyl N-methyl anthranilate.

DETERMINATION OF ALLYL ISOTHIOCYANATE

Several methods, both volumetric gravimetric, for the determination of allyl isothiocyanate in mustard oils have been suggested. The most satisfactory one is a modification of the official procedure of 'The United States Pharmacopoeia'. This method is based upon the reaction of the isothiocyanate radical with silver nitrate. The excess silver nitrate solution is determined by titration with standardised ammonium thiocyanate solution in the presence of ferric ion; the titration must be continued until the red colour of ferric thiocyanate is first observed.

$$C_3H_5NCS + NH_4OH + AgNO_3 \rightarrow AgNCS + C_3H_5OH + NH_4NO_3$$

Procedure: Dilute about 4 cc. of the oil, accurately weighed, with sufficient alcohol to make exactly 100 cc. of solution. Pipette 5 cc. of this solution into a 100 cc. mustard oil flask (Fig. 11.5) and add 50 cc. of 0.1 N silver nitrate solution and 5 cc. of 10 per cent ammonia solution. Connect the flask to an air-cooled reflux condenser, 1 metre long and heat on a steam bath for 1 hour. Allow the liquid to cool to room temperature and then add sufficient distilled water to fill the flask to the 100 cc. mark. Mix well and filter through a dry filter. Reject the first 10 cc. of filtrate. Transfer 50 cc. of the subsequent filtrate by means of a pipette into a 100 cc. saponification flask; add about 5 cc. of concentrated nitric acid and 2 cc. of an 8 per cent solution of ferric ammonium sulphate. Titrate the excess of silver nitrate solution with standardised 0.1 N ammonium thiocyanate. Carry out a blank determination simultaneously, using .5 cc. of alcohol and the same quantities of reagents but omitting the oil. Calculate the percentage of allyl isothiocyanate; each cc. of 0.1 N silver nitrate is equivalent to 0.004958 gram of allyl isothiocyanate.

$$\text{Percentage of allyl isothiocyanate} = \frac{19.832\ (b-a)}{w}$$

where, b = cc. of ammonium thiocyanate solution required for the blank
a = cc. of ammonium thiocyanate solution required for the determination
w = weight of oil used for the original dilution

The blank should require about 24 to 25 cc. of ammonium thiocyanate; the actual determination, about 4 to 5 cc. if a 4 grams sample of oil is employed.

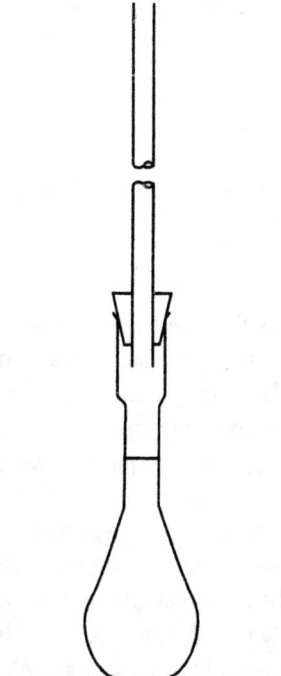

Fig. 11.5. Mustard oil flask.

DETERMINATION OF HYDROGEN CYANIDE

Hydrogen cyanide occurs in the distillates of a number of plants. It plays an important part in the medicinal value of oil of bitter almond and oil of cherry laurel. The presence of hydrogen cyanide can be ascertained qualitatively by means of the Prussian blue test.

Procedure: To 1 cc. of the oil in a test tube add 1 cc. of distilled water, a few drops of a 10 per cent aqueous sodium hydroxide solution and a few drops of a 10 per cent ferrous sulphate solution. (Such a solution of ferrous sulphate always contains a small amount of ferric salt which is necessary for this reaction.) Shake thoroughly and acidify with dilute hydrochloric acid. The precipitate of ferrous and ferric hydroxides dissolves, and in the presence of hydrogen cyanide the characteristic precipitate of Prussian blue appears.

In order to determine quantitatively the amount of hydrogen cyanide in an oil the titrimetric method of 'The United States Pharmacopoeia' has proved satisfactory. This method is based upon precipitation of the cyanide by silver nitrate solution. The end point of the reaction can be determined by the red colour of silver chromate. Part of the hydrogen cyanide found in oil of bitter almond and oil of cherry laurel is bound with benzaldehyde in the form of cyanhydrin; in order to liberate this hydrogen cyanide, a small amount of freshly precipitated magnesium hydroxide is added.

Procedure: Dissolve 0.75 gram of magnesium sulphate in 45 cc. of distilled water. Add 5 cc. of 0.5 N sodium hydroxide solution and 2 drops of a 10 per cent solution of potassium chromate and titrate the solution with 0.1 N silver nitrate solution to the production of a permanent reddish tint; this requires but a few drops of the silver nitrate solution. Pour this mixture into a 100 cc. Erlenmeyer flask containing 0.5 gram of oil of bitter almond accurately weighed. Mix well and titrate again with 0.1 N silver nitrate solution until a red tint, which does not disappear upon shaking, is produced. Conduct this titration as rapidly as possible. Calculate the hydrogen cyanide content by means of the following formula:

$$\text{Percentage of hydrogen cyanide} = \frac{0.2702a}{s}$$

where, a = number of cc. of 0.1 N silver nitrate required

s = weight of sample in grams.

DETERMINATION OF IODINE NUMBER

The iodine number of a fat or oil represents the number of grams of iodine capable of being absorbed under certain fixed conditions by 100 gram of the substance. It is an indication of the degree of unsaturation in the fatty acid radical of the glycerides. The use of iodine numbers for the evaluation of essential oils has never attained practical significance. This is due primarily to the unpredictable behaviour of such oils in the presence of iodine solutions. It has been shown frequently that the iodine numbers of many essential oils vary with the size of the sample as well as with the period of contact with the reagent. Furthermore, the results do not correspond with the theoretical values expected.

In the case of fixed oils the iodine number is an important criterion of purity. Since the essential oil chemist occasionally is faced with the evaluation of such fixed oils as persic oil, sweet almond oil, olive oil, castor oil and sesame oil, a procedure for the determination of iodine numbers is included here.

Procedure: Introduce about 0.25 gram of the oil, accurately weighed. The weight of the oil used is best determined by weighing by difference. A small bottle containing a few cc. of the oil and also a medicine dropper is accurately weighed; then about 8 or 9 drops of the oil are introduced into the Erlenmeyer flask and the bottle with the residual oil and medicine dropper is again accurately weighed. The difference represents the weight of sample used. Small 'petit cups' of glass may also be used; these cups containing the requisite amount of oil, accurately weighed are dropped into the Erlenmeyer flasks and are not removed during the determination, into a glass stoppered Erlenmeyer flask of 250 cc. capacity. Dissolve it in 10 cc. of chloroform add 25 cc. of iodobromide solution, accurately measured from a burette, stopper the vessel securely and allow it to stand for 30 minutes (in the case of castor oil, allow the mixture to stand for 60 minutes) protected from light. Then add in the order named 30 cc. of a 1 N potassium iodide solution and 100 cc. of distilled water and titrate the liberated iodine with tenth-normal sodium thiosulphate, shaking thoroughly after each addition of thiosulphate. When the iodine colour becomes quite pale, add 1 cc. of a 1 per cent starch indicator solution and continue to titration with thiosulphate until the blue colour is discharged. Carry out a blank test at the same time with the same quantities of chloroform and iodobromide solution, allowing it to stand for the same length of time and titrating as directed. The difference between the number of cc. of thiosulphate consumed by the blank test and the actual test, multiplied by 1.269 and divided by the weight of sample taken, gives the iodine number. If more than half of the iodobromide solution is absorbed by the sample of the substance taken, the determination must be repeated, using a smaller sample of the substance under examination.

The iodobromide solution may be prepared by the following method:

Dissolve 13.2 gram of reagent iodine in 1000 cc. of glacial acetic acid with the aid of gentle heat if necessary. Cool the solution to 25°C and determine the iodine content in 20 cc. by titration with tenth-normal sodium thiosulphate. Add to the remainder of the solution a quantity of bromine equivalent to that of the iodine present. Preserve in glass-stoppered bottles, protected from light.

Chapter 12

Odour Properties of Essential Oils

INTRODUCTION

An exceptionally sensitive nose is an effective aid to the survival of many animals and has undoubtedly saved many relatively defenceless species from extinction long ago. In comparison with the nose of the domestic cat or dog, the human appendage is a poor affair indeed, permitting perception of a far narrower range of odours and then only at levels of concentration much higher than is necessary for their detection by most other mammals.

We humans take little notice of smells, excepting those which arouse our curiosity, pleasure or disgust or which evoke sudden and perhaps temporarily overwhelming, yet always fleeting, recall of feelings and situations of marked pleasure or pain, long consciously forgotten, on encountering the same smell, or a very similar one many years later. It is a thought-provoking possibility that a complete record of all personal experience lies buried in the mind, awaiting just the right trigger for recall. Some people find it possible, on smelling a certain odour source, to recapture what seems to be the totality of their experience when using the same material many years ago in a learning situation of intense interest and pleasure. The instantly evocative smell on entering a school can induce a unique kind of pleasure and mental refreshment. The odour-evoked experience is usually but a flash of memory which cannot be held in the mind for contemplation, but which can be so real as to be much more than a momentary return to the past. Perhaps the infinitesimal duration of the experience concentrates its effect to the brink of reality.

The evocative property of odours may be involved, in a more general way, in the application of aromachology, the sensory aspect of aromatherapy, to the inducement of mood benefits.

At the conscious level, an odour has certain properties which we shall now discuss.

ODOUR STRENGTH

Until the recent introduction of instrumental means for the objective measurement of odours, the odour strength of a chemical, which would, of necessity, have to be highly purified, could be found only by the use of trained observers using rigorously standardised procedures of sensory estimation. Basically, these techniques involve dissolving a subject material in an odourless solvent to form a solution of known strength. This solution is then further diluted with measured quantities of the same solvent until any greater dilution of the chemical cannot be smelled at all. For a given person used as a tester, the highest dilution of the chemical which he or she can just smell is recorded as a personal 'odour threshold' for that material. From the results obtained by as large a number of other testers as reasonably possible, a figure representing an average 'minimum perceptible' concentration of the material is calculated. To obtain valid results, statistical methods have to be used to eliminate errors resulting from the subjectivity which plagues all attempts at accuracy in work of this kind.

Here are some examples of minimum perceptible values from tests using aqueous solutions of the test chemicals.

Table 12.1. Minimum perceptible values for some materials.

Test material	Odour threshold: number of grams substance dissolved in 10^{12} grams (10,00,00,00,00,000 = 1 trillion grams) water at 20°C*
Ethyl alcohol (ethanol)	10^8 = 10,00,00,000
Butyric acid (found in rancid butter)	2,40,000
Amyl acetate (odour of 'pear drops')	5000
Methyl mercaptan (CH_3SH; odour of rotting cabbage)	20
Beta-ionone (floral odour of violets)	7
2-Methoxy-3-isobutylpyrazine (intense, earthy-green odour)	2

*One gram amounts of any of the chemicals named in the above table are equivalent to approximately one-fifth of a teaspoonful. One trillion grams of water occupy, approximately, 200 million gallons—the volume of a New York skyscraper. It is not, of course, necessary to use a tank of this size for the experiments. A 'strong' solution of, say, 0.1 gram of the test substance, accurately weighed, is prepared in pure water sufficient to make 1000 grams of solution using, if necessary, an odourless co-solvent for a substance poorly soluble in water, and known dilutions of this solution are made under standardised conditions. Eventually, a dilution is reached beyond which a tester is unable to perceive any odour sensation. The tester's personal odour threshold is that previous dilution which can be just be smelled.

The odour threshold of an essential oil would depend on the odour strengths of its constituents, and the proportions in which they are present in the oil, but since these are both variable among different samples of the same oil, the property of odour threshold also is variable. Weakly odourous major constituents of essential oils, limonene in lemon oil, for example, are of odour weakening effect, whereas strongly odourous minor constituents as, for example, citral in lemon oil, together with intensely odourous trace constituents such as fatty aldehydes, contribute largely to the odour strength of the oil.

Human sensitivity to odours is weakened under cold conditions, or if the air is very dry, and so odour evaluations should be made in warm, sufficiently humid surroundings.

ODOUR CHARACTER

Until very recently, the measurement of odour character without recourse to the human nose was no more than a dream of the future for researchers working in the field of sensory perception. Today, that dream has been brought closer to realisation by the invention of detectors capable of distinguishing between certain odourous substances. These instruments do not, however, 'smell' the air dilutions of vapours presented to them, but measure the energy changes produced when the molecules of odourous vapours stick, temporarily, to specially prepared surfaces which are selective as to which molecules they will adsorb and which they will not. Adsorption differs from absorption in that it is a 'sticking to' rather than a 'soaking up' process.

It is seen on clothing when household detergents fail to remove ink stains, which only certain specially formulated stain removers will dispel, by desorption or chemical action. The minute energy changes which occur during the adsorption of odourous molecules by an 'artificial nose' are transformed into electrical energy signals, which are amplified and fed into a computer programmed to interpret them in terms of an odour profile. The advantage of a sufficiently sensitive and discriminating odour detector of this kind would be to eliminate the subjectivity inherent in odour evaluation by use of the nose.

To equal the sensitivity of the nose it would, however, have to be able to detect the almost vanishingly small concentrations of intensely odourous constituents which noticeably contribute to the odour profiles of many essential oils and perfumes and the delicate, and sometimes extremely complex, nuances that comprise the indefinable elements of 'quality' associated with fine fragrances for personal use. At the present time, odour character is mostly described in terms expressive of the distinctive odour impressions, known as odour notes, that are perceived by human observers. Just as a trained musician can name the notes of any musical chord, name the instrument sounding a note of a particular quality and even the instruments playing the different parts of an orchestral score, so a trained and experienced perfumer can name the odour notes present in a fragrance accord—the odour equivalent of a musical chord—also those of an essential oil, other raw material or finished perfume absorbed onto a smelling strip and the fragrance elements present in a finished perfume.

To describe, communicate and record information on odours some kind of code is necessary, the most obvious and commonly used being the spoken and written word. Perfumery is about feelings and emotions as much as it is about satisfying consumer needs, and for this purpose anything of a coldly scientific nature is about as useful as an electronic calculator for composing poetry. However, there is a difficulty: where odours are concerned, the English language fails us in its complete lack of a vocabulary of odour-descriptive terms.

There are, of course, words such as perfume, scent, aroma, fragrant, putrid, stink and stench, but these are colourless terms, expressive only of like or dislike.

For want of a true odour language, the odour vocabulary used in the perfume industry is made up of words referring to families of related odours, such as floral, woody, fruity and herbaceous, terms naming specific sources of odour, such as jasmine, pineapple, lavender, sandalwood and earthy, together with auxiliary expressions—sweet, dry, fresh, sharp, etc. which have been adopted from common usage in other contexts for use in reference to odours.

When smelling an essential oil or other aromatic material or perfume for the first time, it is best initially to note the relative strength of the odour perceived, then to try to identify the family of odours to which the odour of the product belongs; then, if possible, the specific odour source to which it relates. The description may then be refined by the use of auxiliary odour terms and finally presented to communicate as simple, yet complete, a description of the odour as words will permit. A touch of restraint, here, may be necessary to eliminate flatulent over-enthusiasm and promote accuracy. Like any other artistic exercise, facility in odour description improves with practice, especially if approached systematically, as it does under the imposed discipline of a training situation.

ODOUR PERSISTENCE OR LASTING POWER

The odour character of almost every essential oil changes as it evaporates from a smelling strip into the air, for the reasons that its constituents have odours that are different from one another, and because they evaporate at different speeds. This may be illustrated by means of a simple experiment in which a mixture of two aroma chemicals of different volatility and odour character, representing constituents of an essential oil, is allowed to evaporate.

In one demonstration of this kind, using smelling strips, a mixture of equal weights of benzyl acetate and eugenol was dipped to a depth of 1 cm and allowed to evaporate. For comparison, separate ½ cm dips of each of the components of the mixture were set aside to evaporate at the same time under the same conditions.

The strips were then smelled at frequent intervals until either no further odour change was observed or the odour had faded to vanishing point. The results are shown in Table 12.2.

Table 12.2. Odour persistence.

| Material | Odour | Time to disappearance of odour of | |
		Benzyl acetate (hours)	Eugenol (hours)
Mixture	Floral, spicy	7	more than 24
Benzyl acetate	Floral (jasmine-like)	3	–
Eugenol	Spicy (clove-like)	–	more than 24

The above results show that eugenol slows down the speed at which benzyl acetate evaporates. This can be explained, in part, by analogy to the relative freedom of a small crowd of people to disperse from a large, open area, contrasted with the difficulty the same people would find in attempting to disperse from the same area if the individuals were scattered among roughly the same number of other people in a crowd of twice the size.

There is, however, evidence that molecules of certain chemical classes attract one another more than can be accounted for by the forces of attraction which cause molecules of all liquids to cohere to form droplets or quantities which do not break up into smaller amounts until disturbed. This is caused mainly by a type of bonding which occurs between molecules of certain chemical families such as hydrogen bonding.

HYDROGEN BONDING AND ITS EFFECTS

The molecular weight of water, H_2O, is $(2 \times 1) + 16 = 18$; that of carbon dioxide, CO_2, is $12 + (2 \times 16) = 44$; yet carbon dioxide, with a molecule nearly two-and-a-half times heavier than a water molecule, is a gas at 20°C, and normal atmospheric pressure, while water is a liquid under these conditions. Why?

The anomalous condition of water is explained by the existence of an extra force of attraction between water molecules which is present to only a very much lesser extent between the molecules of carbon dioxide, and which is totally insufficient to maintain the coherence of carbon dioxide in the liquid state at 20°C, except under very high pressure. This attractive force is known as hydrogen bonding.

In a water molecule, there is a large difference between the electrical charge on the nucleus of the oxygen atom (eight protons give a charge of 8+) and that on the hydrogen nucleus (one proton; charge = 1+). The effect of this disparity is to displace the mean position of the pairs of electrons bonding oxygen to hydrogen in the molecule away from the hydrogen atoms and towards the oxygen atoms, electrons being negatively charged; that is, their orbitals are distorted towards the oxygen atom.

Thus, the oxygen end of the molecule gains a little extra negative charge, while the hydrogen ends lose a little of the negative charges neutralising the positive charges on the hydrogen nuclei.

This polarises the water molecule, a condition we can express by means of the following formula for water (Fig. 12.1).

The polar water molecules attract one another, forming temporary clumps which, it is deduced, continuously break up and reassemble in liquid water, effectively increasing the molecular weight of water and greatly reducing its volatility.

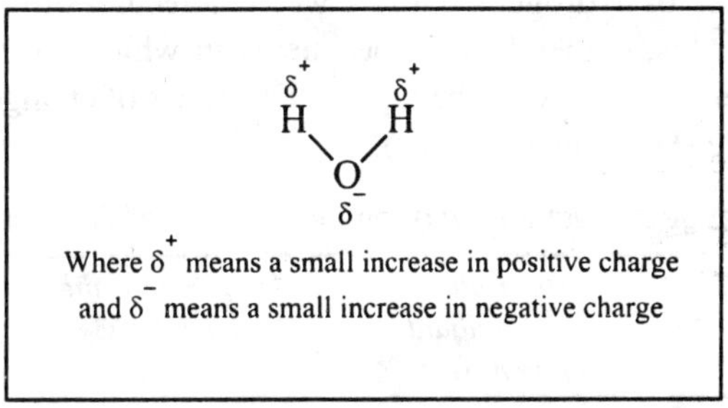

Where $\overset{+}{\delta}$ means a small increase in positive charge
and $\overset{-}{\delta}$ means a small increase in negative charge

Fig. 12.1. Polarisation of the water molecule.

A hydrogen bond is about 23 times weaker than the chemical bonds joining the oxygen atom to the two hydrogens in a water molecule, but it is about 15 times stronger than the normal forces of cohesion acting between the molecules of a liquid. This explains why water puddles evaporate without decomposition of the water. Hydrogen bonding among water molecules are shown in Fig. 12.2.

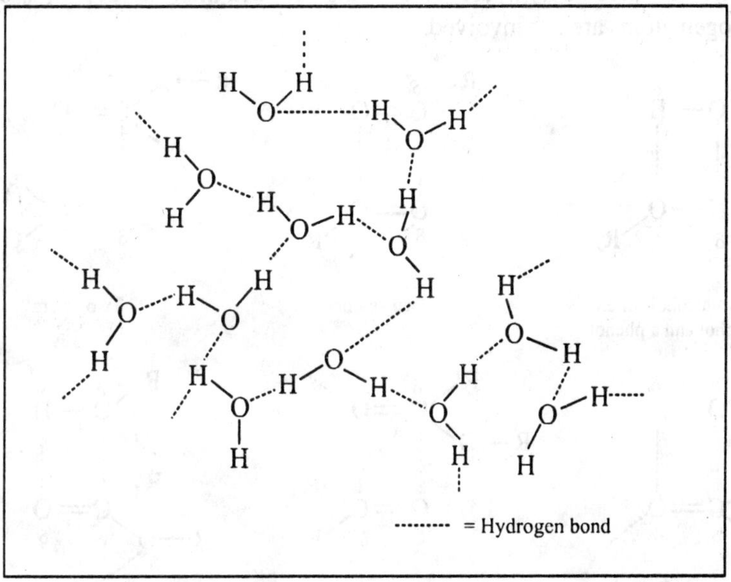

-------- = Hydrogen bond

Fig. 12.2. Hydrogen bonding among water molecules.

Without hydrogen bonding, water would be a gas as permanent as neon, and life as we know it here on earth could not exist.

Just as energy is required to break up a mechanical structure, such as a building, so energy is required at the molecular level to decompose a chemical compound. If ordinary sugar is heated it eventually melts, the molten sugar turns yellow, brown and finally black, boiling away and giving off dense, choking fumes. Ultimately, nothing remains but a black cinder of carbon and a strong, caramellic (caramel-like) kind of smell.

The sugar has decomposed into one of its elements, carbon and many odourous volatile products and this has involved the breaking of bonds. The breaking of chemical bonds requires an energy input. Conversely, when chemical bonds are formed, energy is given out, usually in the form of heat.

Evidence for the formation of hydrogen bonds between molecules of water and alcohol, and between alcohol and glycerol molecules, comes from experiments in which an increase of temperature and a decrease in volume are observed on mixing the liquids. Examples of changes of volume and temperature on mixing certain liquids are shown in Table 12.3.

Table 12.3. Examples of changes of volume and temperature on mixing certain liquids.

Composition of the mixture	Temperature of each liquid before mixing, °C	Temperature after mixing, °C	Temperature change, °C	Final volume at 22°C (cm³)
50 cm³ ethanol + 50 cm³ water	22	29	+7	93.5
50 cm³ ethanol + 50 cm³ glycerol	22	25	+3	96.0

An oxygen atom bonded to a carbon atom in a molecule is known to have a withdrawing effect on the electrons of the carbon atom, but one very much weaker than that which occurs in a water molecule (an oxygen atom has 8 protons in its nucleus; a carbon atom has 6). Aldehydes, ketones and esters in the liquid state are therefore affected by hydrogen bonding between their molecules, as shown in Fig. 12.3, even though hydrogen atoms are not involved.

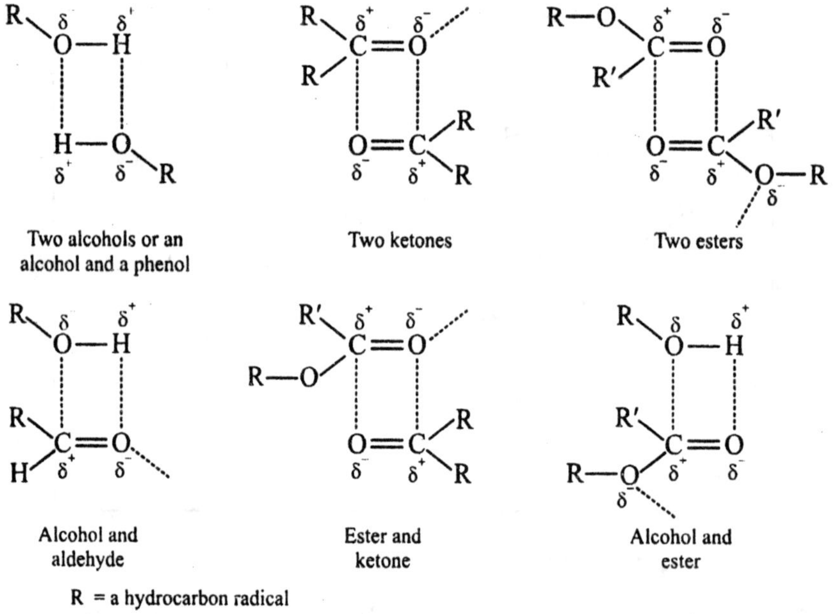

Two alcohols or an alcohol and a phenol

Two ketones

Two esters

Alcohol and aldehyde

Ester and ketone

Alcohol and ester

R = a hydrocarbon radical

R' = a hydrocarbon radical or a hydrogen atom. If a hydrogen atom, the ester would be a formate, an ester of formic acid:

Formic acid

Formate

(Note that molecules of formic acid and of all formates contain the aldehyde functional group)

Fig. 12.3. Some possibilities for hydrogen bonding among molecules of oxygenates.

The effect of hydrogen bonding among polar constituents of a liquid essential oil (i.e. the oxygenated constituents) is a tendency for smaller, faster moving molecules of relatively low molecular weight to be held back within the body of the liquid by larger, heavier molecules. We may also speculate that lighter polar molecules moving towards the surface of the liquid exert some pulling effect on heavier, polar molecules, tending to assist their movement towards the surface and so promoting their evaporation.

Hydrogen bonding undoubtedly accounts, at least in part, for the wonderfully coherent odours of flower absolutes, which are much richer in oxygenates than the corresponding distilled essential oils, if the latter exist. Lavender is a good example, here.

On carefully smelling Jasmine Absolute, occasionally, over a period of time, as it evaporates from a smelling strip, its odour is found to change, though almost imperceptibly. This absolute contains no less than 30 to 35 per cent of benzyl acetate, an ester of relatively high volatility, yet at no time during the evaporation of Jasmine Absolute is it possible to identify clearly the floral-fruity and rather coarse odour of benzyl acetate in isolation from the combined effects of the other constituents: a naturally produced blending effect for which hydrogen bonding is doubtless at least partially responsible.

The fixative effect of certain perfume ingredients in prolonging the duration of the fragrance of a perfume can, in part, be attributed to hydrogen bonding, although the presence of larger molecules in a liquid mixture of volatiles must certainly impede the evaporation of smaller ones, so exerting a purely mechanical fixative effect.

GETTING TO KNOW YOUR ESSENTIAL OILS

The range of essential oils detailed in authoritative works on aromatherapy amounts to almost a hundred different products — about one quarter of the total generally available including aromatic extracts. In the average salon perhaps no more than half this number will be in regular use, yet even a collection of forty to fifty mysterious liquids obscured behind amber glass or completely invisible within aluminium containers can present a daunting challenge to the newcomer faced with the problem of familiarisation.

Despite the ever-widening use of the computer for the storage and retrieval of information, the simple card index still has its place if systematically compiled, and can become a personal treasure to the owner, to be updated and used over and over again for many years. Such a system lends itself readily to the making of notes on essential oils and to adaptation in database form for those who prefer to work with computers.

If adopting a card index system, each card in use should be headed with the name of one of the essential oils in use, with the botanical and geographical sources and main aromatherapeutic uses recorded beneath. Following a brief, physical description of the oil, a note of its chief constituents should be entered and this should be followed by an odour profile. Beneath the odour profile, a note of the conditions under which the oil should be stored will afford a constant reminder of the delicate nature of essential oils. The reverse side of the index card may be used for other data, together with personal notes on results obtained by use of the product in aromatherapy or aromachology. Figure 12.4 shows an example of the most important items of information to record.

Most important among these entries are the odour data which, if accurate, facilitate the recognition and identification of the essential oil, and the storage directions which, if followed, ensure preservation of the properties of the oil for a considerable period of time, the length of which depends very much on the proportion of monoterpenes and aldehydes present.

It is a wise precaution to store all essential oils in a refrigerator, other than those which keep perfectly well if simply stored in a cool place and those producing crystals difficult to redissolve if refrigerated.

There is no need to worry about the essential oils of Sandalwood, Cedarwood, Patchouli or Vetivert, which if of good quality to start with will not deteriorate for many years if stored in tightly sealed containers, protected from light and stored in a cool place. Rose Otto will apparently solidify if stored in a refrigerator because it contains odourless, hydrocarbon waxes which are not too soluble in the odourous constituents of the oil and which come out of solution on cooling as a crystalline deposit, called the stearoptene, dispersed in the liquid part of the oil, the olaeoptene. Rose Otto contains about 20 per cent of stearoptene. No harm will come to Rose Otto if stored in a refrigerator, but on removal from storage for use, the crystals must be allowed to redissolve at room temperature or by the warmth of the hand; no other heat source must be used. Citrus oils, with their high content of monoterpenes, chiefly limonene, are particularly vulnerable to attack by oxygen, and suffer immediately and drastically in sunlight and if exposed to elevated temperatures.

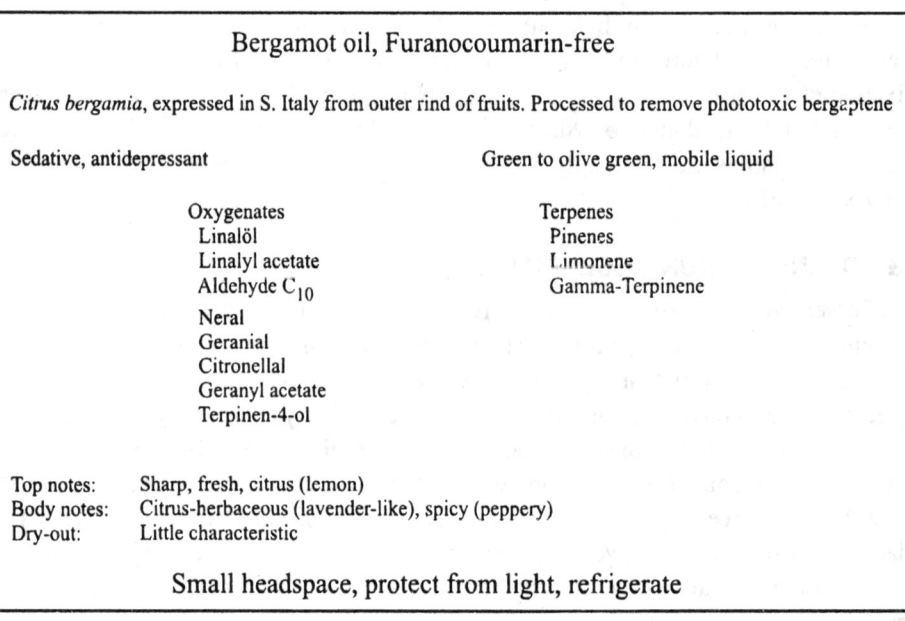

Bergamot oil, Furanocoumarin-free

Citrus bergamia, expressed in S. Italy from outer rind of fruits. Processed to remove phototoxic bergaptene

Sedative, antidepressant   Green to olive green, mobile liquid

Oxygenates	Terpenes
Linalöl	Pinenes
Linalyl acetate	Limonene
Aldehyde C_{10}	Gamma-Terpinene
Neral	
Geranial	
Citronellal	
Geranyl acetate	
Terpinen-4-ol	

Top notes: Sharp, fresh, citrus (lemon)
Body notes: Citrus-herbaceous (lavender-like), spicy (peppery)
Dry-out: Little characteristic

Small headspace, protect from light, refrigerate

Fig. 12.4. Example of index card.

Although with good storage conditions in use, the first signs of irreversible deterioration of an essential oil should never be observed, it is useful to know what these are: loss of freshness in the top note, followed by the onset of a general dullness and flatness over the entire odour profile. The odour profile of a high quality sample of each essential oil in use should be memorised, by practice in smelling, by all persons handling or using essential oils.

ODOUR PROFILING

There are very few essential oils possessing odours which do not change during the period of their evaporation from smelling strips. Exceptions to this general rule include bitter almond oil, consisting almost entirely of benzaldehyde (which, it must be admitted, undergoes oxidation on the strip, but with little odour change, to final dry-out) and wintergreen oil, composed mainly of methyl salicylate.

It is interesting that both of these constituents occur in the living plants as odourless glycosides, which are accompanied by, though separated from, the enzymes necessary for their hydrolysis. The enzymes are released by exposure of crushed bitter almond (or peach, plum, apricot or cherry) kernels, or the leaves of *Gaultheria procumbens*, respectively, to warm water, which is the treatment to which both are subjected for some time prior to distillation. The benzaldehyde released is accompanied by hydrogen cyanide, a deadly poisonous gas having an almond-like odour, most of which dissolves in the benzaldehyde. It is removed by chemical treatment of the oil before Bitter Almond Oil is offered for sale, making odour evaluation of the product less inconvenient. Benzaldehyde and methyl salicylate are shown in Fig. 12.5.

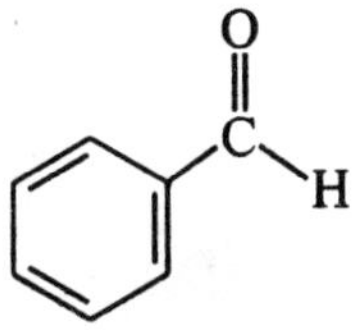

Benzaldehyde

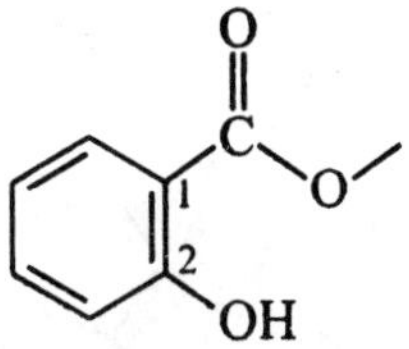

Methyl salicylate
(methyl 2-hydroxybenzoate)

Fig. 12.5. Benzaldehyde and methyl salicylate.

All other essential oils display at least some change of odour when evaporating from a smelling strip caused, as we have explained, by the different rates of evaporation and different proportions of their constituents, these changes being 'smoothed out' by the effects of intermolecular forces of attraction.

In general, with exceptions, the order of decreasing volatility of the main chemical families of constituents of an essential oil is shown in Table 12.4.

Table 12.4. Order of decreasing volatility of an essential oil's main constituents.

	Volatility	Molecular weight	Polarity	Odour
Monoterpenes	Relatively high	136	Low	Mostly weak and noncharacteristic
Oxygenates	Moderate	Most in the range 120–220	High	Mostly strong and characteristic
Sesquiterpenes	Low	204	Low	Many have characteristic odours of moderate strength

In the perfume and flavour industries it is common usage to refer to derivatives of terpenes, known chemically as terpenoids, as terpenes. In the above table the words monoterpenes and sesquiterpenes refer only to the hydrocarbons, as the figures for molecular weights indicate.

Let us look at some examples of exceptions to the data given in Table 12.4.

1. Oxygenates of low molecular weight include ethanol (mol. wt. 46) are found in Rose Otto, and methyl amyl (pentyl) ketone (mol. wt 58) in clove oils.
2. The isomeric alcohols alpha- and beta-santalol, important odourous constituents of East Indian sandalwood oil, both have a molecular weight of 220; guaiol, the main constituent of the semisolid, semicrystalline guaicwood oil of slightly smoky, rose-like odour, has mol. wt = 222 (Fig. 12.6).
3. The ketones alpha- and beta-vetivone (Fig. 12.7) make important contributions to the odour of Vetivert oil. They have mol. wt = 218.
4. The macrocyclic, musky-smelling lactone ambrettolide (Fig. 12.8), responsible for much of the odour character of ambrette seed (hibiscus seed) oil, has mol. wt = 252.

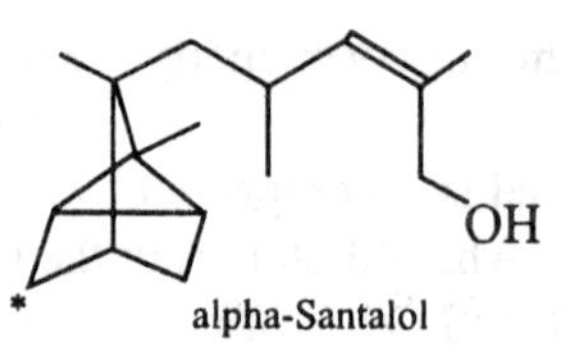

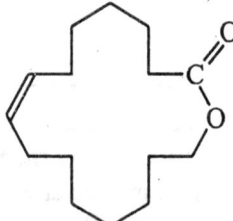

alpha-Santalol

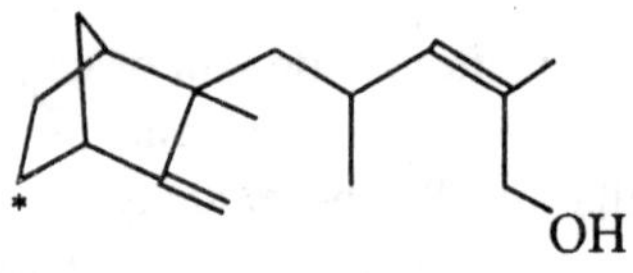

beta-Santalol

In the above diagrams the six-membered ring (indicated by *) is drawn in perspective
to make the structures clear

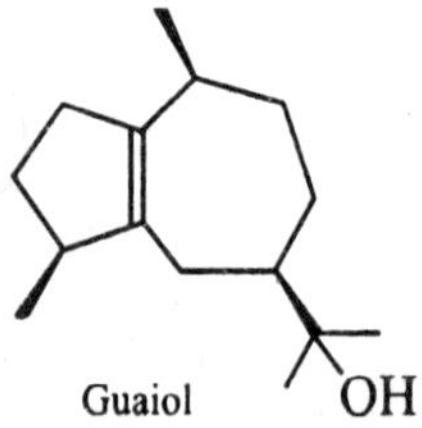

Guaiol   OH

It is worth noting the structural relationship between guaiol (colourless) and chamazulene. Three
of the bonds are shown as 'wedges', indicating that the carbon atoms at the wider ends are not in
the plane of the ring system but above it

Fig. 12.6. alpha- and beta-Santalol and Guaiol.

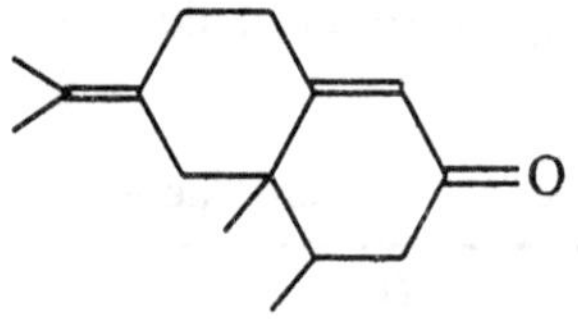

alpha-Vetivone

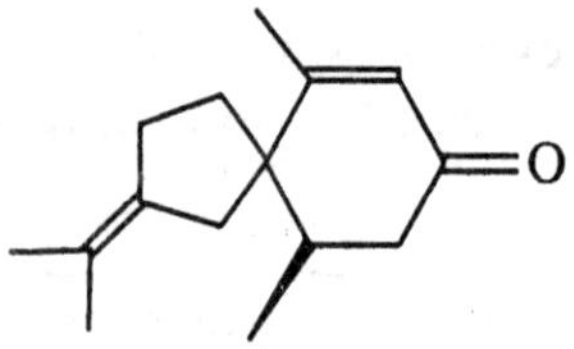

beta-Vetivone

Fig. 12.7. Vetivones.

Formula structure; the actual molecules can adopt any
shape, within the limits of their existence

Fig. 12.8. Ambrettolide.

The above structural formulae illustrate something of the molecular complexity found among the
constituents of some essential oils. This has, in some instances, resulted in difficulties of structural
elucidation which have been overcome only in very recent years with the availability of improved analytical
techniques.

With reference to the Table 12.4 and to our discussions on the effects of molecular polarity, we can
offer some further explanation of the phenomenon of odour change observed during the evaporation of an

essential oil. If the oil is totally volatile, then all of the constituents will begin to evaporate when a sample on a smelling strip is exposed to the air, but they will evaporate at different speeds. Neglecting exceptions, constituents of low polarity, low molecular weight and low odour value, that is, monoterpenes, will evaporate at the fastest rates. Molecules of most oxygenates will tend to hydrogen bond to one another, to a greater or lesser extent, prolonging the duration of the odour notes characteristic of the oil, and to some degree extending the 'life' of less volatile, oxygenated top-note constituents, such as benzyl acetate and linaloöl, if present.

Oxygenates of molecular weight around 150 to 200 evaporate quite slowly. The odour of a citrus oil, such as lemon oil, will therefore intensify on a smelling strip as the monoterpenes evaporate, because they are much more volatile and possess very weak odours in comparison with the very strong odours of the citral, fatty aldehydes, etc. comprising the oxygenates of these oils. This effect may easily be observed by taking a fresh dip of the oil after a first dip has been evaporating for about 15 minutes and comparing the odour intensities of the two samples.

Oxygenates of low molecular weight, in addition to monoterpenes, are largely responsible for the top notes of essential oils. The exception among citrus oils is bergamot oil, containing a much lower proportion of monoterpenes than the others. The odour of this oil changes, but does not intensify, on a smelling strip. Despite their generally weak odours, monoterpenes make valuable contributions to what we perceive as the 'naturalness and freshness' of the odour of an essential oil.

Oxygenates of high molecular weight evaporate only very slowly, some taking weeks, months or even years to disappear completely. Examples are guaiol, the santalols, ambrettolide and the vetivones represented in Figs. 12.6 to 12.8. The essential oils containing these constituents are extremely long-lasting on smelling strips and as perfume ingredients. Oxygenates, as indicated in Table 12.4, make the most characteristic contributions to the body notes of essential oils; in the odours of most essential oils they can be clearly smelled after much of the top note content has evaporated.

Sesquiterpenes are tenacious constituents of an essential oil, some proportions of them remaining, together with proportions of oxygenates of very low volatility, to give, as a final odour impression, the dry-out of the oil after all else has long evaporated.

It will be useful, here, to summarise some important facts concerning the evaporation of an essential oil. On first smelling a fresh dip of an essential oil, the top note, consisting of the combined odours of the most volatile constituents of the oil, is perceived. This impression is accompanied by the odours of other constituents, mainly the more volatile components of the body note complex, together with some contributions from less volatile constituents, depending on the intensities of their odours and their proportions in the oil. On smelling the same dip after an interval of time, the body notes may be observed, though always in association with lingering traces of the top note complex. With practice, these latter notes can be ignored. After a further and longer time interval the body notes will have evaporated, leaving a residual odour known as the dry-out, dry-down or end odour of the oil. Two question arise:

1. How long does it take for top notes, and body notes to evaporate?
2. What are the effects of powerful trace constituents on top notes and body notes?

These periods of time have to be estimated by smelling a genuine sample of each oil. One possible approach would be to evaluate two essential oils of different character (each providing relief from smelling the other) over 14 hours, during the course of a day when interruptions are unlikely and circumstances peaceful.

Take a dip of the essential oil and evaluate the top note complex. Allow this dip to evaporate and reevaluate briefly every 15 minutes until definite fading of the top note is observed. Allow evaporation to continue for a further 30 minutes, then compare the odour of the dip with that of a fresh dip of the same oil. By comparison, smelling the original dip first on each occasion, carefully reevaluate the top note. Finally, evaluate the body note complex. If possible, allow evaporation to continue until the body notes have completely disappeared, then evaluate the dry-out (Table 12.5).

Table 12.5. Evaluation of top and body notes and dry-out.

Time		Evaluation
hr	*min.*	
–	0	Take 1 cm dip of essential oil; label strip with name of oil, 'Dip 1' and time of dipping; smell for general impression of top note
–	15	Smell Dip 1 for general impression of any odour changes
–	30	Take second dip of the same oil; label strip with name of oil, 'Dip 2' and time of dipping. Compare odours of Dip 1 and Dip' 2, smelling Dip 1 first, now top note can be described. Carefully smell Dip 1 for provisional assessment of body notes
1	00	Smell Dip 1 for final evaluation of body notes. Compare with Dip 2 for any odour differences
1	30	Smell Dip 1, also thereafter every 30 minutes to final dry-out. Evaluate dry-out notes

All of the above evaluations should be recorded in a notebook reserved for this purpose. The body notes of some essential oils, for example, sandalwood, vetivert and patchouli, remain perceptible for days, or even weeks. If the body notes of an essential oil remain strong after 4 hours, evaluate thereafter every hour to a total of 8 hours after dipping, then every 2 hours to 14 hours after dipping. If body notes can then still be clearly smelled, it would be worth taking a fresh dip of the oil, labelled 'Dip 3' and comparing the odours of Dips 2 and 3 after a further 12 hours. A final dry-out, different in character from the body notes, may require patience, and a modicum of longevity, to reach. If the body notes simply fade, with no observable odour change, the conclusion must be that the oil exhibits no characteristic dry-out notes.

If a definite dry-out is perceived, but is found impossible to describe, the term 'nondescript' can come to the rescue. A few essential oils, of which sandalwood is a good example, possess no distinctive top notes.

The effects of powerful trace constituents depend on the character and intensities of their odours and on their volatilities. The escape of their molecules through the surface of the oil exposed to the air will be impeded by the 'crowding' effect of the much more numerous molecules of other constituents of the evaporating oil, so that whatever their polarity their effects will, to some extent, tend to persist. Trace constituents of relatively high polarity will be subject to hydrogen bonding, with the result that the notes of some of them may persist to the final dry-out of the oil. With the aromatic extracts, the absolutes and resinoids of perfumery, the persistence of body notes is extended by the presence of nonvolatile, waxy or resinous constituents. This may be caused by physical entrapment of their molecules or by hydrogen bonding, or both.

EXAMPLES OF TERMS USED IN ODOUR DESCRIPTION

The descriptive terms in the following list (Table 12.6) are those in most frequent general use for describing the odours of essential oils, aroma chemicals and perfumes. A note of the meaning of each term is followed by one or more examples of essential oils to which the term applies.

Table 12.6. Some important terms used in odour description.

Term	Explanation	Examples
Animalic	Odours associated with animals	Underlying heavy notes in jasmine and orange flower absolutes
Balsamic	Sweet and vanilla-like	Benzoin resinoid
Camphoraceous	Like camphor	Spike lavender oil
Citrus	Odours of citrus fruits	Lemon and orange oils
Coniferous	Fresh, green and resinous notes of cut, green pine cones	Rosemary oil, pine and fir oils
Earthy	The smell of rain-moistened earth	Patchouli oil
Floral	Odours of fragrant flowers	1% Rose Otto or 1% Jasmine absolute in a carrier oil
Fruity	Odours of edible fruits	Any of the citrus oils; 'Roman' chamomile oil
Green	Odours of crushed, green leaves	No common example; Violet leaf absolute is typical
Herbaceous or herbal	Odours of culinary herbs	Thyme and sage oils
Medicated	Odours suggesting medication	Wintergreen and Ylang-Ylang oils
Minty	Notes given by spearmint or peppermint leaves when stroked	Spearmint and peppermint oils
Resinous	Odours of fragrant resins	Myrrh and frankincense oils
Spicy	Odours of culinary spices	Clove, cinnamon and coriander oils
Woody	Odours of exotic woods	Sandalwood and cedar wood oils

ODOUR PROFILES OF ESSENTIAL OILS

The examples of odour profiles of essential oils completing this chapter are given for guidance and to illustrate further the use of odour-descriptive terms. The preparation of an odour profile is, of course, a subjective exercise, the outcome of which depends very much on the personal odour experience, extent of personal odour vocabulary and ability to select from it appropriate descriptive terms, of the evaluator. The given profiles are, therefore, brief and include terms referring to only the main features of the odours of 67 essential oils included in the Table 12.7. They should be studied critically and compared with personal notes on the odours of the corresponding oils.

Table 12.7. Essential oil odour profiles.

	Name of product	Top notes	Body notes	Dry-out
1.	Ambrette seed oil	Fatty, floral	Musky	Rich, sweet, floral, musky, vinous
2.	Amyris oil	Faint	Spicy	Mild, woody, pine-like, balsamic
3.	Aniseed oil	Little distinctive	Sweet, warm, anisic (characteristic of aniseed)	Warm, not distinctive
4.	Basil oil	Fresh, herbaceous, aniseed-like	Sweet, herbaceous, aniseed-like	Warm, not distinctive
5.	Benzoin, Siam, resinoid	Slightly floral, vanilla-like	Sweet, warm, vanilla-like	Balsamic-powdery

(Contd ...)

	Name of product	Top notes	Body notes	Dry-out
6.	Bergamot oil	Fresh, sharp, lemon-orangey	Herbaceous, orangey, peppery, slightly floral	Warm, like orange pith
7.	Caraway seed oil	Somewhat 'weedy', typical of caraway	Characteristic of crushed caraway 'seed'	Spicy
8.	Cedar wood oil, Virginian	Woody	Woody, somewhat oily, characteristic of cedar wood	Woody-balsamic
9.	Chamomile oil, German	Sweet, warm, herbaceous, fruity	Sweet, herbaceous, hay-like	Warm, tobacco-like
10.	Chamomile oil, Roman	Sweet, fruity, herbaceous	Warm, herbaceous, somewhat fruity	Warm, herbaceous, tea-like
11.	Cinnamon bark oil	Sweet, spicy, fruity, floral	Sweet, warm, spicy, fruity	Sweet, 'powdery'
12.	Cinnamon leaf oil	Warm, spicy, somewhat harsh	Warm, spicy, clove-like	Warm, spicy
13.	Citrus oil	Powerful, warm, ambra-like*	Rich, warm, ambra, balsamic	Dry, balsamic
14.	Clove bud oil	Fresh, spicy, warm, fruity	Warm, spicy, somewhat woody	Warm, spicy, woody
15.	Clove leaf oil	Spicy, woody	Dry, woody, spicy	Clove-like
16.	Clove stem oil	Spicy, of clove	Dry, woody, spicy	Clove-like
17.	Coriander oil	Light, peppery, woody, slightly floral	Woody, spicy, slightly floral	Warm, spicy, rather balsamic
18.	Cypress oil	Fresh, coniferous, camphoraceous	Coniferous, balsamic	Sweet, balsamic
19.	*Eucalyptus citriodora* oil	Fresh, rose-like, lemony	Rose-like, lemony	Nondescript
20.	*Eucalyptus globulus* oil	Powerful, camphoraceous	Warm, camphoraceous	Nondescript
21.	Fennel oil	Sweet, anisic, spicy	Anisic, somewhat spicy	Warm, aniseed-like
22.	Frankincense oil	Fresh, lemony, resinous	Resinous, spicy, woody	Balsamic, resinous
23.	Frankincense resinoid	Fresh, lemony, green, resinous	Resinous, balsamic	Little characteristic
24.	Galbanum oil	Powerful, fresh, sharp, green, earthy, conifer	Green, conifer, balsamic, agrestic	Dry, earthy, spicy
25.	Galbanum resinoid	Green-earth, somewhat sharp	Green, conifer, balsamic	Aldehydic, agrestic,† floral
26.	Geranium oil	Vegetable, rosey, minty	Rose-like, minty, green	Rich, rose-like
27.	Guaiacwood oil	Soft, sweet, rose-like	Sweet, rose-like, woody, slightly smoky	Nondescript
28.	Jasmine absolute	Floral, fruity, green	Heavy floral, fruity, herbaceous, animalic	Floral, fatty, heavy, animalic
29.	Juniper berry oil	Fresh, coniferous	Coniferous, woody	Sweet, warm, balsamic
30.	Labdanum resinoid	Little characteristic	Sweet, balsamic, herbaceous, ambra	Dry, woody, ambra

(Contd ...)

	Name of product	Top notes	Body notes	Dry-out
31.	Lavandin oil	Fresh, camphoraceous, herbaceous	Herbaceous, woody, lavender-like	Nondescript, warm
32.	Lavender absolute	Floral, typically lavender-like	Warm, herbaceous, lavender- and hay-like	Woody-spicy, somewhat pungent
33.	Lavender oil	Fresh, floral, slightly fruity	Herbaceous, floral, slightly woody	Nondescript
34.	Lavender spike oil	Fresh, strongly camphoraceous	Camphoraceous, herbal, lavender-like, woody	Nondescript
35.	Lemongrass oil	Fresh, citrus, slightly oily	Strong, lemony, herbal, green, tea-like ·	Herbaceous, somewhat oily
36.	Lemon oil	Fresh, light, sharp, citrus	Sweet, fresh, citrus	Warm, nondescript
37.	*Litsea cubeba* oil	Fresh, lemon-like	Sweet, fresh, lemon-like	Lemony, sharp
38.	Marjoram oil	Fresh, camphoraceous, spicy	Warm, spicy, camphoraceous, woody	Warm, spicy, woody
39.	*Mentha arvensis* oil	Fresh, minty	Rather harsh, somewhat minty, woody	Dry, herbaceous
40.	Myrrh oil	Spicy, 'medicated'	Warm, spicy, balsamic	Nondescript
41.	Myrrh Resinoid	Light, fresh, spicy	Warm, spicy, balsamic	Warm, spicy, balsamic
42.	Neroli oil	Light, fresh, floral	Light, floral, herbaceous, somewhat citrus	None
43.	Oakmoss absolute	Dry, somewhat 'seashore-like'	Mossy, woody, green, earthy, 'marine'	Warm, woody, balsamic
44.	Olibanum oil	Fresh, lemony, resinous	Resinous, spicy, woody	Balsamic, resinous
45.	Olibanum resinoid	Fresh, lemony, green, resinous	Resinous, balsamic	Little characteristic
46.	Orris oil	Floral, violet-like	Violet-like, woody, fatty	Nondescript
47.	Patchouli oil	Sweet, rich, herbaceous, balsamic	Sweet, earthy, slightly camphoraceous, spicy, woody, balsamic	Dry, woody, balsamic, spicy
48.	Petitgrain oil, Bigarade	Fresh, floral, similar to Neroli	Dry-floral, herbaceous, woody	Dry-herbaceous
49.	Pimento berry oil	Fresh, sweet, warm, spicy	Sweet, spicy, balsamic, tea-like	Fresh, sweet, spicy
50.	Pine oil, *sylvestris*	Fresh, sweet, coniferous	Coniferous, balsamic	Nondescript
51.	Rose absolute	Sweet, floral, with a beeswax note	Rich, sweet, spicy, waxy, flora	Warm, floral, honey-like
52.	Rose Otto (Rose oil)	Powerful, beeswax-like	Rich, wax, floral, spicy (clove-like)	Warm, floral, spicy
53.	Rosemary oil	Fresh, strong, camphor-aceous, resinous	Resinous, woody, herbaceous, balsamic	Dry, herbaceous
54.	Rosewood oil	Spicy, camphoraceous	Sweet, woody, floral-spicy	Woody-floral
55.	Sage oil, Clary	Sweet, light, herbaceous	Delicate, herbaceous, tobacco-like	Warm, balsamic

(Contd ...)

	Name of product	Top notes	Body notes	Dry-out
56.	Sage oil, Dalmatian	Sweet, fresh, herbal, camphoraceous	Fresh, strong, warm, camphoraceous, herbal	Little characteristic
57.	Sandalwood oil, East Indian	Little distinctive	Soft, sweet, woody, balsamic, fatty-floral	None distinctive
58.	Sandalwood oil, West Indian	Faint	Spicy	Mild, woody, pine-like, balsamic
59.	Tarragon oil (Estragon oil)	Sweet, anisic, green	Sweet, aniseed-like, spicy	None distinctive
60.	Thyme oil	Sweet, warm, 'medicated', herbal	'Medicated', herbaceous, spicy, woody	Warm, herbaceous, spicy
61.	Ti-Tree oil	Strong, camphoraceous	Warm, camphoraceous, spicy	Little characteristic
62.	Tonka absolute	Rich, sweet, warm, herbaceous	Warm, sweet, hay-like	Hay-like, coconut-like
63.	Tuberose absolute	Sweet, heavy, floral	Sweet, heavy, floral, with a caramel note	Floral, balsamic
64.	Vanilla absolute	None distinctive	Rich, sweet, balsamic	None distinctive
65.	Vetivert oil	Sweet, earthy, woody	Rich, heavy, woody, earthy, balsamic	Woody, earthy
66.	Violet leaves absolute	Green, diffusive	Green, floral, violet leaves	Woody, earthy, powdery
67.	Ylang-Ylang oil, 'extra'	Strong, sweet, 'medicated', floral	'Medicated', floral, fruity, spicy (clove)	Sweet, balsamic, floral, 'medicated'

*Resembling the odour of ambergis: musty with a note of the sea.
†An odour of the countryside.

The exchange of ideas when working with odours is most profitable for, when working with groups of students, someone very frequently suggests a feature of an odour or odour profile which he has never before considered or realised was present in a sample under evaluation. Whilst it is probably best, in the interest of concentrating contemplative thought, to work alone when first profiling an essential oil, opportunities should be sought thereafter for comparison of notes and re-examining features of profiles with colleagues. This will greatly improve your memory for odours and systematically aid familiarisation with all of the essential oils you handle or use.

Chapter 13

Special Tests and Procedures for Essential Oils

FLAVOUR TESTS

A study of the odour and flavour of an oil, isolate or synthetic is essential in judging quality and aids in the detection of adulteration. Comparison should always be made with an oil of good quality and of known purity. Organoleptic tests are unquestionably the most sensitive and satisfactory method for detecting slight spoilage in oils such as the citrus oils and in detecting burned, pyroligneous 'by-notes' resulting from improper distillation.

Procedure: Water Flavour Test: Place ½ oz. of alcohol in an 8 oz. glass. Add 1 drop of oil and then 7 oz. of cold water, the water being added slowly with-vigorous stirring. This should yield a clear or opalescent mixture, which does not separate oily droplets on the surface. The odour and flavour of these two water flavour tests should be carefully studied and evaluated.

In the case of dill oils, it is well to add 3 drops of glacial acetic acid to approximate more accurately the conditions under which this oil is usually employed. In the case of peppermint oils, it is best to add hot water; the flavour tests should be of uniform temperature and tasted while still warm.

Procedure: Sugar Syrup Test: An acidified sugar syrup is prepared by adding 1 dram of 85 per cent syrupy phosphoric acid and 7 drams (weight = DRACHM; small draught of strong drink [*drachm*]) of 50 per cent citric acid to 1 gallon of simple syrup (USP quality: approximately 65 per cent wt/wt). Dilute 2 oz. of this prepared syrup with 2 oz. of cold water. Add 1 to 3 drops of a 10 per cent alcoholic solution of the oil and mix thoroughly. The odour and flavour of these two sugar syrup tests should be carefully studied and evaluated.

These syrup tests are best prepared in widemouthed, screw-top bottles which permit of thorough mixing of the alcoholic solution and the syrup by vigorous shaking. Such syrup flavour tests are especially valuable in evaluating citrus oils, citrus concentrates, and oils and synthetics which duplicate the flavour of highly acidic fruits. In the case of sweetening agents (such as vanillin, coumarin, and heliotropin), it is well to dispense with the acidic medium and to use instead a mixture of equal parts of simple syrup and water. It should be remembered that comparison with a product of good quality is essential.

TESTS FOR HALOGENS

The presence of chlorine in a synthetic is usually indicative of insufficient purification. The detection of halogen in a reputedly natural essential oil or fraction is indicative of adulteration with a chlorine-containing synthetic. For example, cassia oils showing the presence of chlorine have probably been adulterated with impure synthetic cinnamic aldehyde.

Of the numerous procedures which have been suggested, the classical test with copper oxide (the so-called Beilstein test) proves by far the most convenient and rapid. Should this test prove inconclusive, the presence or absence of halogen should be confirmed by the combustion method, a more sensitive test.

Procedure-I. Beilstein method: Wind the end of a No. 16 gauge copper wire into a tight spiral about 6 mm long and 6 mm in diameter. Fasten the other end of this wire to a wooden handle. Heat the wire in the nonluminous flame of a Bunsen burner until it glows without colouring the flame green. Permit the wire to cool and reheat several times until a good coat of oxide has formed on the coil. Add to the cooled spiral 2 drops of the material to be tested. Ignite and permit it to burn freely in air. The wire is again cooled and 2 more drops of the material are added and burned. This process is continued until a total of 6 drops has been added and ignited. Then hold the spiral in the oxidising portion of a Bunsen flame, adjusted to about 1½ inch high. If the material is free from halogen, the flame will show no green colour. The degree of persistence of green colour is a rough indication of the amount of halogen present. A highly purified synthetic, free from halogen, will not show even a transient green colour or flash of green.

Instead of the wire spiral described above, a piece of 30 mesh copper screening (1.5 cm × 5.0 cm) may be used. The screening should be rolled tightly around a copper wire and held in position by bending back the wire and twisting securely. Such a roll of copper screening will hold about 1 cc. of oil because of surface tension.

Certain nitrogen-containing compounds may give a positive test although no halogen is present. Also, the presence of free organic acids may cause a green coloured flame since the copper salt may be sufficiently volatile; e.g. phenylacetic acid. Therefore, if a positive test is obtained, it is best to confirm such findings by the combustion method.

Procedure-II. Combustion method: A piece of filter paper about 5 × 6 cm is folded and saturated with the oil to be tested. The paper is placed in a small porcelain evaporating dish which rests in a larger watch glass. The paper is ignited and covered immediately with a 2 litre beaker, the inner surface of which has been previously moistened with water. (The watch glass should be sufficiently large to extend beyond the rim of the beaker.) After the flame has died out, the beaker is permitted to remain in position for 5 minutes. The porcelain evaporating dish is removed and the products of combustion, which have condensed on the inner surface of the beaker, are washed into the watch glass with about 10 cc. of distilled water and then poured into filter. Add to the filtrate 1 drop of nitric acid and 1 cc. of 0.1 N silver nitrate solution. If the oil is free from halogen, no turbidity should result. Since this method will detect even minute traces of chlorine, it is absolutely necessary to run a blank.

Several other tests have been described, such as the lime test, the test employing sodium peroxide, and the classical test employing molten metallic sodium. The last named test is perhaps the most sensitive, but it suffers from the inherent disadvantages of working with metallic sodium.

A special test for the detection of side chain chlorine in cinnamic aldehyde has been accepted as official in the 'national formulary', eighth edition, monograph on cinnamic aldehyde. It indicates the presence of chlorine only when it appears in the side chain. This is not intended as a general test for the detection of side chain halogen in all compounds. However, it has proven satisfactory for such synthetics as cinnamic aldehyde.

Procedure: To a 1 cc. sample of cinnamic aldehyde add 10 cc. of commercial isopropanol, 1 cc. of nitric acid (1:1) and 1 cc. of 10 per cent silver nitrate solution. Shake the mixture after the addition of each reagent. Heat to incipient boiling and permit the test tube to stand for 5 minutes. If chlorine is present in the side chain, opalescence or turbidity will result. Carry out simultaneously a blank in order to assure absence of chlorine in the reagents.

When recording the presence of halogen always designate the method employed. Also, an estimate of the relative amount of halogen present should be given; use may be made of such relative phrases as 'strongly positive', 'moderately positive', 'slightly positive', 'positive: traces' and 'negative'.

TESTS FOR HEAVY METALS

Heavy metals are often present as impurities in essential oils. It is especially important that oils be free from such impurities if they are to be used for medicinal purposes or in foodstuffs. Furthermore, the presence of heavy metals in perfume oils will often cause discolouration in such products as soaps and cosmetic creams.

A very sensitive test for heavy metals has long been official in 'The United States Pharmacopoeia' insure the absence of lead and copper. The test is based upon the fact that hydrogen sulphide will react with the chlorides of these metals to give dark coloured sulphides.

The sulphides of most metals are black or brownish black. The following represent the exceptions: the sulphides of cadmium, arsenic and tin (stannic form) are yellow; of antimony, orange; and of zinc, white. This test is especially satisfactory for the determination of small amounts of copper or lead.

Procedure: Shake 10 cc. of the oil with an, equal volume of distilled water to which 1 drop of concentrated hydrochloric acid has been added, and pass hydrogen sulphide through the mixture until it is saturated. No darkening in colour in either the oil or the water is produced in the absence of heavy metals. In order to discern any darkening if only traces of heavy metals are present, it is necessary to carry out simultaneously a blank determination to which no hydrogen sulphide is added: a comparison of the blank and the run will clearly indicate traces of heavy metals if present. Test tubes may be conveniently used for these determinations.

Often a scum will form at the surface between the oil and water layers. The formation of the scum is no indication of the presence of heavy metals, unless the scum is dark in colour.

Oils manufactured in primitive stills or oils improperly stored in metal containers (especially if the oils are not thoroughly dried) or oils containing large amounts of free acids will often contain heavy metals. Anise, bay, sweet birch, cajuput, clove, geranium, and sassafras oils usually contain heavy metals when distilled commercially. Therefore, it is well to test those oils to ascertain whether or not they have been properly treated to remove such impurities.

A metallic impurity frequently encountered in essential oils is iron. Oils distilled using iron condensers and oils stored in imperfectly lined drums frequently show the presence of this impurity. Oils rich in phenols or containing a phenol group, such as the salicylates, are often contaminated. Iron will not be precipitated by hydrogen sulphide in an acidic medium and therefore, will not give a positive heavy metals test. Ammonium sulphide or sodium polysulphide will precipitate black ferrous sulphide.

The test as described above shows a high degree of sensitivity: ten parts per million of metallic lead in oil of cloves gives a positive test; the threshold value is approximately five parts per million.

Removal of Heavy Metals

For the removal of metallic impurities from essential oils, citric or tartaric acid is frequently employed, giving rise to complex citrates and tartrates which are insoluble and which may be filtered off.

Procedure: Add to the oil a small amount of dry tartaric acid (usually ¼ to 1 per cent will prove sufficient) and shake thoroughly. Permit the acid to settle and filter the supernatant liquid. If this method should fail to remove all the metallic impurities, agitate the oil with ½ to 1 per cent of a saturated aqueous solution of tartaric acid, separate the oil, shake thoroughly with salt and filter.

The removal of heavy metals from clove, bay, pimenta and geranium oils frequently requires several treatments.

When reporting the presence of heavy metals in an oil, it is well to indicate the relative amount found by terms such as: strongly 'positive; positive; positive — small amounts; positive — traces.

TEST FOR DIMETHYL SULPHIDE IN PEPPERMINT OILS

Dimethyl sulphide occurs as a normal constituent in peppermint oils. Upon rectification of the oil obtained by steam distillation from the plant, most of this volatile compound is lost because of its low boiling point (boiling point = 37.5°–38°C). Hence, the presence of dimethyl sulphide in a peppermint oil is an indication that such an oil has not been rectified. 'The United States Pharmacopoeia' has made use of the following procedure to assure the absence of dimethyl sulphide found in nonrectified oils:

Procedure: Distil 1 cc. from 25 cc. of peppermint oil and carefully superimpose the distillate on 5 cc. of a 6.5 per cent mercuric chloride solution in a test tube. A white film does not form at the zone of contact within 1 minute.

This test is based upon the reaction of dimethyl sulphide with mercuric chloride, giving a white sulphonium compound which is insoluble in saturated mercuric chloride solution. The following modification of this official test is more sensitive and somewhat more reliable:

Dry the oil by shaking thoroughly with a small amount of anhydrous sodium sulphate in a stoppered bottle and filter. Place 25 cc. of this dried and filtered oil in a large Pyrex test tube (diameter = 22 mm, length = 200 mm) which is clamped to a ring stand at an angle of approximately 45°. Add a small piece of clay chip. Insert a tight-fitting cork equipped with a bent glass tube which extends 2 cm through the cork. The other leg of this bent tube is inserted into a second test tube which contains 5 cc. of a 6.5 per cent aqueous solution of mercuric chloride (Fig. 13.1).

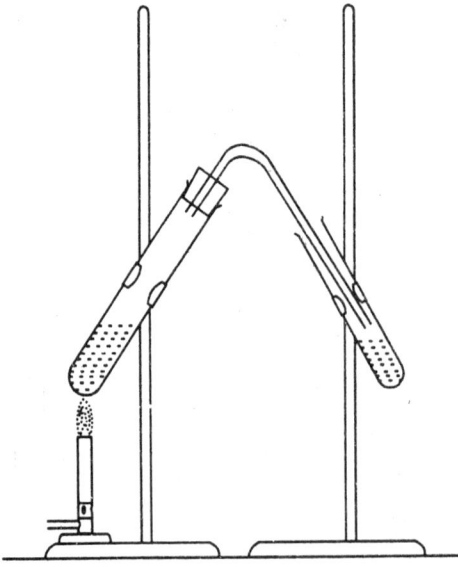

Fig. 13.1. Apparatus for the determination of dimethyl sulphide.

The tube should not dip into the solution, but should extend to within 1 cm of the surface. Apply gentle heat until the oil begins to boil. Heating is continued until the ring of condensing vapour rises to within 1 cm of the end of the glass tube. If the oil has been carefully dried and the heating has been carried out slowly, no oil will distil over into the second test tube. The formation of a white scum on the surface of the mercuric chloride solution or on the sides of this second test tube indicates the presence of dimethyl sulphide in the oil.

TESTS FOR IMPURITIES IN NITROBENZENE

Test for Thiophene

Nitrobenzene which has been manufactured from an impure grade of benzene will give a positive thiophene test, if insufficiently purified. This is due to the fact that inferior grades of benzene contain thiophene, SCH:CHCH:CH, and that all thiophene compounds give an intense blue colouration when mixed with isatin, $C_6H_4NHCOCO$, and concentrated sulphuric acid, because of the formation of indophenin, $(C_{12}H_7NOS)x$.

> *Procedure*: Shake thoroughly 5 cc. of nitrobenzene and 0.5 cc. of concentrated sulphuric acid in a test tube and add a pinch of isatin and again shake the mixture thoroughly. Permit the test tube to stand for 2 hours. No blue colouration should appear during this interval.

Soap Test

The soap test is an empirical method of testing the purity of nitrobenzene. Since a large quantity of this synthetic is used to perfume soaps, it is necessary to carry out a soap test to determine whether or not the nitrobenzene in question will cause a discolouration of the soap.

> *Procedure*: Into a large, wide Pyrex test tube of approximately 75 cc. capacity introduce 5 cc. of the nitrobenzene and 10 cc. of a 15 per cent aqueous solution of potassium hydroxide. Heat the mixture to boiling over an open flame. It is important to shake thoroughly the test tube while the mixture is heated and boiled, in order to prevent the formation of two layers. (The nitrobenzene and potassium hydroxide solution will then be thrown out of the test tube with explosive violence.) After boiling for 2 minutes, permit the test tube to stand, at room temperature, for one-half hour, and then filter the mixture through filter paper previously wetted with water. The potassium hydroxide solution passes through the wetted paper; the nitrobenzene is retained. The alkaline filtrate should be colourless or at most show only a light yellow colour. A full deep yellow indicates that the nitrobenzene has been insufficiently purified or is old. Such a product will require rectification before it is satisfactory for use in soaps.

TESTS FOR PHELLANDRENE

Phellandrene readily yields a solid nitrite which occurs as a voluminous, flocculent precipitate in the following test.

> *Procedure:* Into a test tube introduce a solution of 5 gram of sodium nitrite in 8 cc. of water. Superimpose a solution of 5 cc. of the oil in 10 cc. of petroleum ether. Add slowly 5 cc. of glacial acetic acid, shaking the tube gently with a rotatory motion. A flocculent precipitate at the junction of the two layers indicates the presence of phellandrene.

If large amounts of phellandrene are present, the petroleum ether layer will solidify to a gel-like mass. The crystals may be separated with a Büchner funnel and purified by filtering, washing with water and methyl alcohol, and finally by dissolving the crystals in chloroform and then precipitating with methyl alcohol. Since here are eight possible isomers, the melting point has little meaning unless the physical isomers are separated.

TEST FOR FURFURAL

To detect the presence of furfural in an oil, the following procedure proves satisfactory. It is based on the water solubility of furfural and on the well-known colour reaction of furfural with aniline in the presence of glacial acetic acid.

Procedure: Shake thoroughly 1 0 cc. of the oil with 25 cc. of distilled water in a separatory funnel. Permit the mixture to st. 1d until a good separation is obtained. Filter the aqueous layer through wetted paper to give a clear solution. Add 1 cc. of the filtered aqueous layer to 5 cc. of a 2 per cent solution of freshly distilled aniline in glacial acetic acid. The presence of small amounts of furfural will result in an intense deep red colour within 5 minutes. If a negative test results, extract the filtered aqueous layer with 25 cc. of ether. Cautiously evaporate the ether on a steam bath. Add 1 cc. of distilled water and then 5 cc. of the acetic acid aniline solution. The appearance of an intense deep red colour within 5 minutes indicates the presence of traces of furfural.

If a red colour is obtained, the furfural may be separated from a fresh sample of the oil (following the above procedure) and identified by the formation of a suitable derivative.

If only a small sample of the oil is available, the test may be carried out directly on the oil itself. Garratt has suggested the following method for the determination of furfural.

Procedure: To 0.1 cc. of the oil in a test tube add from a burette 5 cc. of a 2 per cent solution of freshly distilled aniline in glacial acetic acid. Protect from bright light and allow to stand for 10 minutes. Examine in a Lovibond tintometer and measure the 'red value'.

According to this authority, the test may have value for the detection of adulteration, if the adulterant has a relatively much higher furfural content than the oil to which it has been added and if the adulterant has not been treated to remove the furfural. Garratt tentatively suggests its use for the detection of light camphor oil in rosemary oils; of clove oil in bay or pimenta berry oils; of Japanese mint oil in American peppermint oil. It may also have value for the detection of added synthetic methyl salicylate to wintergreen and sweet birch oils. The 'ten-minute red values' obtained by Garratt for reputedly genuine samples of these oils are given in Table 13.1.

Table 13.1. Lovibond tintometer values for furfural-containing oils.

Oil	'Ten-minute red value'
Light camphor	1.8 to 9.2
Rosemary	0.4 to 0.8
Clove	23.0
Pimenta berry	1.1
Bay	1.4
Japanese mint	4.5 to 7.4
American peppermint	ca. 0.7
Methyl salicylate	0.0

TEST FOR PHENOL IN METHYL SALICYLATE

Methyl salicylate which has been insufficiently purified will frequently contain phenol. The presence of this impurity affects markedly the odour and flavour of the synthetic. Hence, it is well to test all samples of methyl salicylate for phenol. For routine analyses the following simple procedure has proved quite satisfactory:

Procedure I: Dissolve 5 cc. of the oil in 50 cc. of a 1 N aqueous potassium hydroxide solution. Heat on a steam bath for 2 hours, cool to room temperature, and acidify with sulphuric acid (1:3). Cautiously smell the flask for the distinct characteristic odour of phenol. If no such odour is apparent the sample may be considered free of objectionable amounts of phenol. If a phenolic 'by-note' is observed, the presence of phenol should be confirmed by the method of Dodge.

The Dodge method for the detection of phenol in methyl salicylate has proved of value as a qualitative method. Attempts have been made to convert this method to a quantitative procedure. However, these have proved unsatisfactory, particularly when applied to the natural oils of sweet birch and wintergreen.

Procedure II: Into a 100 cc. Pyrex saponification flask introduce 10 cc. of the oil in question and add 35 cc. of a 10 per cent aqueous solution of sodium hydroxide, measured from a graduated cylinder. Connect an air-cooled reflux condenser and heat the flask on a steam bath for 2½ hours. Remove the flask and allow it to cool for 15 minutes. Neutralise the saponified mixture with dilute hydrochloric acid (1:3) until the solution is distinctly acid to blue litmus paper; this requires from 3.5 to 5 cc. of acid. The hydrochloric acid should be added slowly from a burette so that no precipitation occurs. Then slowly add from a burette enough of a saturated freshly prepared sodium bicarbonate solution to just neutralise the mixture, and then an additional 0.5 cc. of the sodium bicarbonate solution. Filter into a 500 cc. distillation flask and distil with steam, using an efficient trap to prevent the mechanical carrying over of any of the solution. A 500 cc. Erlenmeyer flask may conveniently be used for this trap; the delivery tube from the side arm of the distillation flask should extend to within ½ inch of the bottom of the Erlenmeyer flask and the delivery tube from the trap to the condenser should not extend more than 1 inch below the rubber stopper into the flask (Fig. 13.2). Collect three 5 cc. portions of distillate and filter each distillate. Test for the presence of phenol by the addition of enough bromine water to give a permanent light brown colour. If phenol is present to the extent of 0.01 per cent or more, a crystalline precipitate of tribromophenol (melting point, 95°C) will form within an hour.

Procedure II is based upon the well-known fact that acids will react to form the corresponding sodium salts, but phenols will not form the corresponding phenolates when treated with sodium bicarbonate solutions. Thus the free phenol is steam distilled out of the solution in which is dissolved the nonvolatile sodium salicylate. Normal, pure wintergreen and sweet birch oils do not give a positive reaction with this procedure; certain constituents of the oils will distil which are capable of decolourising the bromine water, but which do not form crystalline derivatives under the conditions outlined. Hence, a positive test for such oils indicates adulteration with phenol-containing synthetic methyl salicylate. The test is to be considered positive only when definite crystal formation is observed within 1 hour at room temperature in the bromine treated distillates.

DETERMINATION OF ESSENTIAL OIL CONTENT OF PLANT MATERIAL AND OLEORESINS

A laboratory distillation of essential oil from plant material is often necessary in order to evaluate raw material to be used for large-scale commercial distillations. The determination of the essential oil content is also important in appraising the quality of spices and oleoresins.

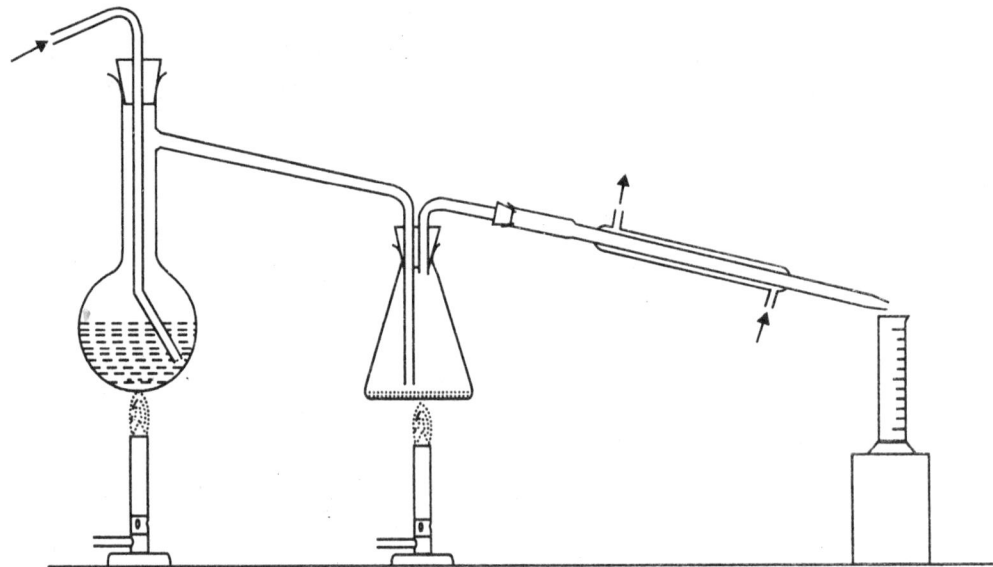

Fig. 13.2. Apparatus for the detection of phenol in methyl salicylate.

Such determinations may be conveniently carried out in a special apparatus devised by Clevenger. This apparatus offers the following advantages: compactness, cohobation of distillation waters, the actual distillation and separation of the essential oil (so that certain chemical and physical properties may be determined and so that the odour and flavour of the oil may be studied) and an accurate determination of the essential oil content using only small quantities of plant material. Furthermore, this apparatus may be used to advantage for steam rectification of small amounts of essential oils.

The apparatus consists of two specially designed oil traps and a small condenser of the 'cold-finger' type (Fig. 13.3). Two traps are supplied; one, for oils lighter than water; the other, for oils heavier than water. The diagrams are self-explanatory.

Procedure: Place a sufficient quantity of the ground or chipped material to yield 2 to 6 cc. of oil (preferably 4 cc.) in a round bottom, short-necked flask of 2-litre capacity. Add sufficient water to the flask to correspond to 3–6 times the weight of the plant material; in general, 4 times the weight is sufficient. Attach the proper essential oil trap and the condenser to the flask and add enough water to fill the trap. Place the flask in all oil bath, heated electrically or by a Bunsen burner to approximately 130°C. Adjust the temperature of the bath so that a condensate of about 1 drop per second is obtained.

Continue the distillation until no further increase of oil is observed. Usually 5 to 6 hours are sufficient, although in the case of the distillation of certain woods and roots a much longer period may be necessary. When the distillation has been completed, permit the oil to stand undisturbed so that a good separation is obtained, and so that the oil may cool to room temperature. Determine the number of cc. of oil obtained and express the yield as a volume/weight percentage; i.e. number of cc. of oil per 100 grams of plant material.

In the event that a good separation is not obtained, the oil and water may be withdrawn from the trap into a graduated cylinder; the addition of sufficient salt to saturate the aqueous layer often aids in obtaining a sharp separation. Periodic withdrawal of the oil and water into such a cylinder is sometimes necessary when the oil being distilled has a specific gravity close to that of water, or when the oil consists of two main fractions—one lighter than water, and the other heavier than water.

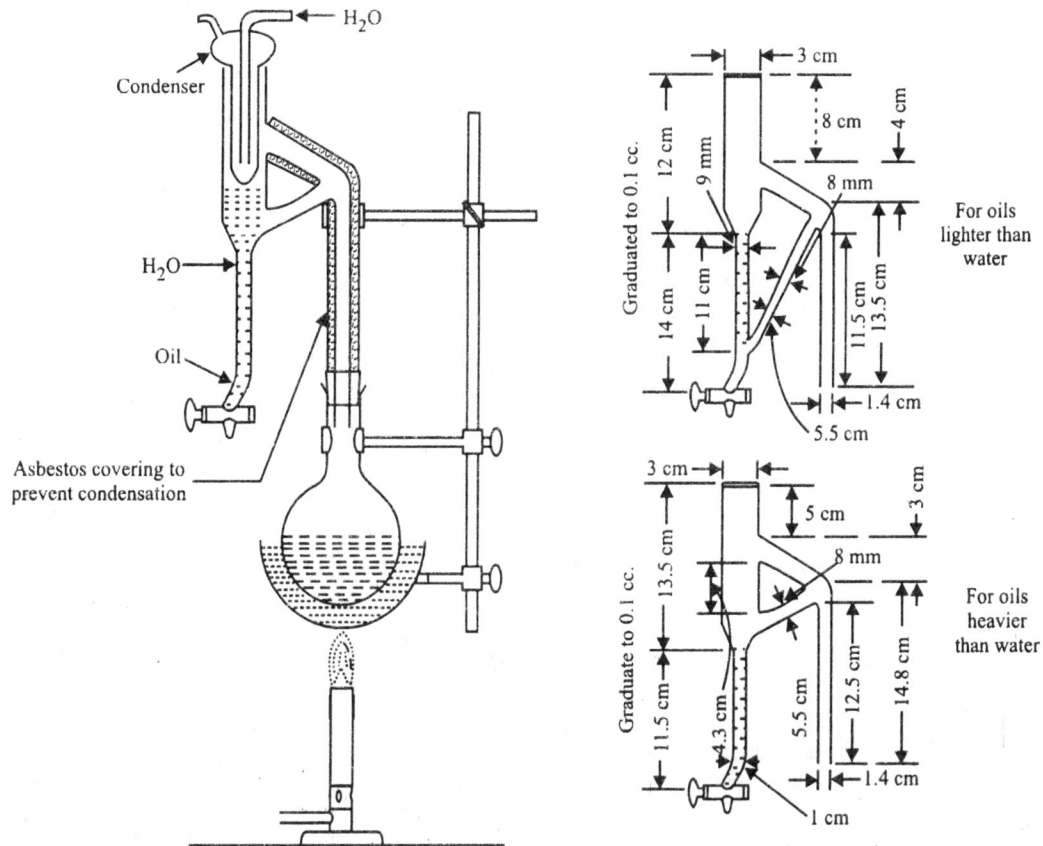

Fig. 13.3. Apparatus for the determination of the volatile oil content of plant materials.

The volume/weight may be converted into a weight/weight relationship by means of the following formula:

$$P = pD$$

where, P =   wt/wt percentage

           p =   vol./wt percentage at temperature t°C

          D =   density of oil at temperature t°C

This necessitates the determination of the specific gravity of the separated oil.

It is advisable to permit the separated oil to remain overnight in an uncorked bottle before evaluating the odour and flavour. Freshly distilled oils often have a peculiar weedy note, which soon disappears. The yield and the physico-chemical properties of the resulting oil will agree closely with the results of a commercia distillation. However, the oil from a commercial or pilot still is generally superior to that obtained in the clevenger apparatus in respect to odour and flavour.

When determining the essential oil content of oleoresins, it is best to bring the water to incipient boiling before adding the oleoresin and to distil at a faster rate. The addition of clay chips and boiling tubes will prevent undue bumping.

DETERMINATION OF ETHYL ALCOHOL CONTENT OF TINCTURES AND ESSENCES

The determination of the content of ethyl alcohol in essences, tinctures and alcoholic extracts is frequently necessary. Because of the presence of volatile esters and essential oils, a determination by distillation alone is usually impossible. Consequently these interfering substances must be removed by washing with heptane or petroleum ether before such distillation is attempted. The two procedures given below give satisfactory results:

> *Procedure—method I*: Pipette 25 cc. of the sample into a 500 cc. separatory funnel, noting the temperature. Add 100 cc. of a saturated salt solution and 100 cc. of petroleum ether. Shake thoroughly for 2 to 3 minutes and permit the mixture to stand undisturbed until a good separation is obtained (usually within 5 to 60 minutes).
>
> Draw off the salt solution into a 1 litre distilling flask. Wash the petroleum ether layer with two successive 35 cc. portions of saturated salt solution, adding both washings to the solution in the distilling flask. Discard the petroleum ether layer. Add 100 cc. water to the contents of the distilling flask; also a small amount of solid phenolphthalein and enough 10 per cent aqueous sodium hydroxide solution to make the contents alkaline to the indicator. Also add a few small clay chips and slowly distil until a distillate of about 70 cc. has been collected in a 100 cc. volumetric flask immersed in a beaker of cold water (use a straight tube water-cooled condenser). Add enough distilled water to make the volume up to about 90 cc. If the distillate remains water-white (or at most has a faint opalescence — not a turbidity), adjust the temperature to that originally observed and make up to 100 cc.

Determine the specific gravity accurately and, from this, the alcohol percentage by volume (Table 13.2). Multiply by 4 to obtain the alcohol content of the original material. If this value is above 25 per cent, determine the refractive index at 20° and compare with the value, given in Table 13.3.

Table 13.2. Alcoholometric table.

Per cent of C_2H_5OH by volume, at 15.56°C	Corresponding per cent of C_2H_5OH by weight	Specific gravity in air at 25°C	Specific gravity in air at 15.56°C
0	0.00	1.0000	1.0000
1	0.80	0.9985	0.9985
2	1.59	0.9970	0.9970
3	2.39	0.9956	0.9956
4	3.19	0.9941	0.9942
5	4.00	0.9927	0.9928
6	4.80	0.9914	0.9915
7	5.61	0.9901	0.9902
8	6.42	0.9888	0.9890
9	7.23	0.9875	0.9878
10	8.05	0.9862	0.9866
11	8.86	0.9850	0.9854
12	9.68	0.9838	0.9843
13	10.50	0.9826	0.9832

(Contd...)

Per cent of C_2H_5OH by volume, at 15.56°C	Corresponding per cent of C_2H_5OH by weight	Specific gravity in air at 25°C	Specific gravity in air at 15.56°C
14	11.32	0.9814	0.9821
15	12.14	0.9802	0.9810
16	12.96	0.9790	0.9800
17	13.79	0.9778	0.9789
18	14.61	0.9767	0.9779
19	15.44	0.9756	0.9769
20	16.27	0.9744	0.9759
21	17.10	0.9733	0.9749
22	17.93	0.9721	0.9739
23	18.77	0.9710	0.9729
24	19.60	0.9698	0.9719
25	20.44	0.9685	0.9708
26	21.29	0.9673	0.9697
27	22.13	0.9661	0.9687
28	22.97	0.9648	0.9676
29	23.82	0.9635	0.9664
30	24.67	0.9622	0.9653
31	25.52	0.9609	0.9641
32	26.38	0.9595	0.9629
33	27.24	0.9581	0.9617
34	28.10	0.9567	0.9604
35	28.97	0.9552	0.9590
36	29.84	0.9537	0.9576
37	30.72	0.9521	0.9562
38	31. 60	0.9506	0.9548
39	32.48	0.9489	0.9533
40	33.36	0.9473	0.9517
41	34.25	0.9456	0.9501
42	35.15	0.9439	0.9485
43	36.05	0.9421	0.9469
44	36.96	0.9403	0.9452
45	37.87	0.9385	0.9434
46	38.78	0.9366	0.9417
47	39.70	0.9348	0.9399
48	40.62	0.9328	0.9380
49	41.55	0.9309	0.9361
50	42.49	0.9289	0.9342

(Contd...)

Per cent of C_2H_5OH by volume, at 15.56°C	Corresponding per cent of C_2H_5OH by weight	Specific gravity in air at 25°C	Specific gravity in air at 15.56°C
51	43.43	0.9269	0.9322
52	44.37	0.9248	0.9302
53	45.33	0.9228	0.9282
54	46.28	0.9207	0.9262
55	47.25	0.9185	0.9241
56	48.21	0.9164	0.9220
57	49.19	0.9142	0.9199
58	50.17	0.9120	0.9177
59	51.15	0.9098	0.9155
60	52.15	0.9076	0.9133
61	53.15	0.9053	0.9111
62	54.15	0.9030	0.9088
63	55.17	0.9006	0.9065
64	56.18	0.8983	0.9042
65	57.21	0.8959	0.9019
66	58.24	0.8936	0.8995
67	59.28	0.8911	0.8972
68	60.33	0.8887	0.8948
69	61.38	0.8862	0.8923
70	62.44	0.8837	0.8899
71	63.51	0.8812	0.8874
72	64.59	0.8787	0.8848
73	65.67	0.8761	0.8823
74	66.77	0.8735	0.8797
75	67.87	0.8709	0.8771
76	68.98	0.8682	0.8745
77	70.10	0.8655	0.8718
78	71.23	0.8628	0.8691
79	72.38	0.8600	0.8664
80	73.53	0.8572	0.8636
81	74.69	0.8544	0.8608
82	75.86	0.8516	0.8580
83	77.04	0.8487	0.8551
84	78.23	0.8458	0.8522
85	79.44	0.8428	0.8493
86	80.66	0.8397	0.8462
87	81.90	0.8367	0.8432

(Contd...)

Per cent of C_2H_5OH by volume, at 15.56°C	Corresponding per cent of C_2H_5OH by weight	Specific gravity in air at 25°C	Specific gravity in air at 15.56°C
88	83.14	0.8335	0.8401
89	84.41	0.8303	0.8369
90	85.69	0.8271	0.8336
91	86.99	0.8237	0.8303
92	88.31	0.8202	0.8268
93	89.65	0.8167	0.8233
94	91.03	0.8130	0.8196
95	92.42	0.8092	0.8158
96	93.85	0.8053	0.8118
97	95.32	0.8011	0.8077
98	96.82	0.7968	0.8033
99	98.38	0.7921	0.7986
100	100.00	0.7871	0.7936

Table 13.3. Refractive indices of ethyl alcohol-water mixtures from 1–25 per cent.

Percentage of alcohol (by volume) at 15.56°C	Refractive index at 20°
1	1.33342
2	1.33391
3	1.33443
4	1.33495
5	1.33549
6	1.33602
7	1.33657
8	1.33711
9	1.33768
10	1.33824
11	1.33882
12	1.33940
13	1.33997
14	1.34057
15	1.34116
16	1.34176
17	1.34236
18	1.34297
19	1.34359
20	1.34420
21	1.34482

(Contd...)

Percentage of alcohol (by volume) at 15.56°C	Refractive index at 20°
22	1.34544
23	1.34606
24	1.34666
25	1.34726

The calculated index should not differ by more than 0.0002 from the experimentally determined value. A larger difference indicates the presence of some interfering substance in the alcoholic distillate. The determination should then be repeated, using the double distillation procedure.

Procedure — method II: Into a 500 cc. Erlenmeyer flask pipette 25 cc. of the sample add 50 cc. of distilled water and 25 cc. of *n*-heptane. To the 250 cc. separatory funnel add 40 cc. of *n*-heptane and connect the distilling tube and reflux condenser as shown in Fig. 13.4. Heat gently and distil slowly until 40 cc. of distillate have been collected under the heptane layer in the separatory funnel. Permit the contents of the funnel to stand undisturbed for 15 minutes to attain room temperature and drain the distillate into a 50 cc. volumetric flask. Wash the residual heptane with two 4 cc. portions of distilled water, adding these washings to the volumetric flask. Fill the flask to the mark and determine the specific gravity of the mixture and calculate the alcoholic percentage by means of Table 13.2. Multiply by 2 in order to obtain the alcohol content of the original material.

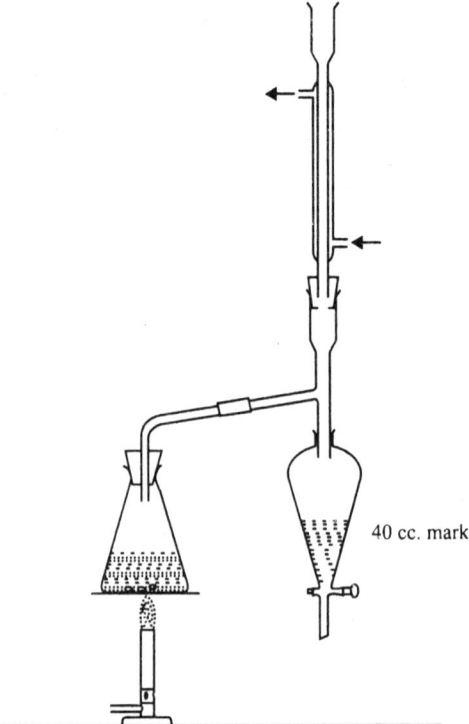

40 cc. mark

Fig. 13.4. Apparatus for the under the heptane layer in determination of alcohol.

It should be noted that certain low boiling, water-soluble constituents, such as acetic acid and acetone, will interfere in such a determination. However, most low boiling esters are readily absorbed by the heptane layer.

DETERMINATION OF WATER CONTENT

Determination by the Bidwell-Sterling Method

The most convenient method for the determination of water in essential oils, oleoresins and drugs is by the water determination apparatus of Bidwell and Sterling. The sample to be tested is distilled in this apparatus with a liquid immiscible with water, such as toluene. The special trap collects and measures the condensed water, the excess solvent overflowing and returning to the still.

Procedure: Connect the apparatus as shown in Fig. 13.5. Introduce into the 500 cc. flask, sufficient material, accurately weighed, to yield from 2 to 4 cc. of water. Add about 200 cc. of toluene to the flask and also fill the receiving trap with toluene, poured through the top of the condenser. Heat the flask gently by means of a Bunsen burner or electric hot-plate until the toluene begins to boil. Distil at a rate of about 2 drops per second until most of the water has passed over. Then increase the rate of distillation to about 4 drops per second. When no further increase in collected water is observed, continue the distillation for an additional 15 minutes. Permit the apparatus to cool. When the water and toluene have separated completely, read the volume of water and calculate the percentage present in the substance.

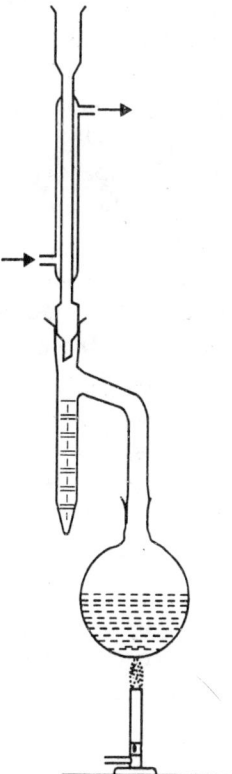

Fig. 13.5. Apparatus for the determination of water.

If the condenser and moisture trap have been thoroughly cleaned with chromic acid cleaning solution, the tendency of droplets to adhere is greatly minimised. Should such droplets of water be observed on the sides of the condenser, they may be forced down by brushing the inner tube of the condenser with a small brush previously saturated with toluene.

Determination by Karl Fischer Method

For the determination of mere traces of water, the method employing the Karl Fischer water titration reagent will prove exceptionally sensitive.

The Karl Fischer water titration reagent is a solution of iodine, sulphur dioxide and pyridine in methyl alcohol. The method depends on the oxidation of sulphur dioxide by iodine in the presence of water to form sulphuric and hydriodic acid.

$$SO_2 + 2I + 2H_2O \longrightarrow H_2SO_4 + 2HI$$

The reaction is conducted in the presence of pyridine which acts as an acid acceptor, thus enabling the reaction to go to completion. The end point is indicated by a colour change from yellow to reddish-brown, the latter being produced by the free iodine in the reagent when an excess of the reagent is added.

The method is applicable to a large number of organic and inorganic compounds, both liquid and solid. The exact limitations of the method have not been determined, but it can probably be used on all organic and inorganic compounds that do not react with the reagent and that are not naturally coloured red or brown. It is known to be applicable to organic compounds such as hydrocarbons, alcohols, esters, carboxylic acids (except formic), halogen derivatives of hydrocarbons, phenols, nitro compounds, amines and heterocyclic compounds. It is not applicable to aldehydes and ketones, nor to reducing compounds which react readily with iodine in the cold. The active hydrogen in primary and secondary amines must be blocked by solution in glacial acetic acid before titrating with the reagent.

Liquids are dissolved in a mutual solvent for both the sample and the reagent before titrating. Solids may be analysed by pulverising and dissolving or suspending in dry methyl alcohol. It is not essential that the material be soluble in methyl alcohol, as the hygroscopic nature of both methyl alcohol and the reagent will act to extract the water from the sample.

The solvent used in preparing the sample for analysis will contain some moisture, hence a blank titration must be made using the same volume of solvent and the same size flask, as the moisture in the air space is an integral part of the blank. To check the end point, breathe into the flask and the end point will disappear, but an additional drop or two of the reagent should bring back the reddish-brown colour. The choice of solvents is wide: methyl alcohol, dioxane, glacial acetic acid, chloroform, etc.

When attempting new applications of the method, i.e. with new or unknown compounds, the reactivity of the compound with the Fischer reagent must first be determined. If the compound is inert toward the reagent, the method is applicable. Also, the reagent is so avidly hygroscopic that it will dehydrate hydrated compounds. The degree of such dehydration (number of mols of water reacting with the reagent) must be determined beforehand.

All apparatus must be thoroughly dried and every precaution must be made to exclude atmospheric moisture during the titration. The titration is carried out in a small flask (125 cc. Erlenmeyer) and taken to completion rapidly. This method will detect, in general, 0.0005 gram of water, equivalent to 0.005 per cent when using a 10 gram sample.

Procedure: Pipette 10 cc. of methyl alcohol into each of three 125 cc. glass stoppered Erlenmeyer flasks, which should be kept stoppered as much as possible. Weigh accurately from a weighing pipette about 0.1 gram of distilled water into each flask. Titrate with the Karl Fischer reagent to the colour change (the colour should change from a straw yellow to a reddish-brown when the end point is reached). At the same time run a blank on the methyl alcohol. Calculate the water equivalent of the reagent by means of the following formula:

$$E = \frac{w}{A - B}$$

where, E = water equivalent of the reagent (in grams of water per cc.)
w = weight in grams of water used
A = cc. of reagent used for the determination
B = cc. of reagent used for the blank.

Into a 125 cc. Erlenmeyer flask weigh a sufficiently large sample of the material to be tested to yield approximately 0.1 gram of water. Add 10 cc. of methyl alcohol and titrate. Run a blank at the same time on the alcohol. The water content may be calculated from the following formula:

$$\text{Percentage of water} = \frac{100(A - B)\,E}{w}$$

where, A = cc. of reagent used for the determination
B = cc. of reagent used for the blank
E = water equivalent of the reagent
w = weight of sample in grams.

It is necessary to standardise the reagent daily.

The Karl Fischer water titration reagent may be purchased from chemical supply houses, or may be prepared in the following way:

Place 1 litre of dry methyl alcohol and 400 cc. of pyridine in a 2-litre reservoir of an automatic burette. Add 127 gram of iodine, stopper the bottle and swirl until the iodine is completely dissolved. Cool the bottle in a salt-ice mixture for one-half hour and then add 100 gram of sulphur dioxide, weighing by difference on a balance. The resulting solution is very hygroscopic and must be kept stoppered as much as possible. Then remove the bottle from the ice bath and insert the siphon and burette unit. Thoroughly grease the ground glass joint between the bottle and burette to give an airtight seal. Fit a calcium chloride drying tube to the opening at the top of the burette and between the bottle and hand aspirator, which is used to fill the burette. The tip of the burette is fitted with a 2-hole rubber stopper which fits the neck of the 125 cc. Erlenmeyer flask. Protect the tip of the burette when not in use.

It is best to age the solution for two to four days before using so that the variation in standardising from day-to-day will be minimised.

DETERMINATION OF STEAROPTENE CONTENT OF ROSE OILS

Oil of rose contains as a natural constituent a mixture of solid paraffinic hydrocarbons known collectively as 'stearoptene'. The highly purified stearoptene is odourless and hence contributes little to the odour value of the oil. However, for many years the quality of rose oils was judged superficially by the 'melting point' of the oil; oils with high 'melting points' were assumed to be unadulterated. As a consequence there arose the practice of adding spermaceti, tristearin, high melting paraffins and guaiac wood oil as adulterants.

'The United States Pharmacopoeia' requires a certain minimum content of stearoptene and describes a limiting test for its determination.

Procedure I: Introduce 1 cc. of oil of rose into a 25 cc. glass-stoppered, graduated cylinder and add 1 cc. of chloroform: a clear solution should result. Then add 19 cc. of 90 per cent alcohol (by volume): crystals of stearoptene should crystallise out of the solution within 24 hours, the temperature being maintained at 25°C.

A rough indication of the amount of stearoptene present in the oil can be obtained by this modified official test. Oils with high stearoptene contents will deposit an abundant amount if crystalline material immediately; oils with low stearoptene contents will sometimes separate only one or two well-formed crystals after standing 24 hours; some oils will show no separation of crystals whatsoever. The appearance of the crystals is also important; only through experience will an essential oil chemist be able to draw conclusions as to possible adulteration from the appearance of the separated material.

This test will also indicate whether or not the oil has been properly dried; a cloudy solution in one volume of chloroform is usually indicative of the presence of water in the oil.

For the determination of the amount of stearoptene, the oil is usually dissolved in dilute alcohol and chilled; the relatively insoluble paraffins separate out and can be filtered off and weighed. It is customary to use 75 per cent alcohol for this determination, although certain investigators have recommended the use of 85 per cent alcohol or acetone.

Procedure II: Dissolve 5 gram of the oil in 50 cc. of 75 per cent alcohol (by volume) with the aid of gentle heat if necessary. Cool the solution in an ice bath at 0°C for 2 hours and filter off the separated stearoptene with suction, using a well cooled Büchner funnel. Wash the stearoptene with a 50 cc. portion of 75 per cent alcohol cooled to 5°C. Remove as much of the alcohol as possible by suction, and then transfer the cake of stearoptene to a tared evaporating dish. Break up the cake with a spatula and dry in a desiccator for 24 hours. Weigh and calculate the percentage of stearoptene present in the original oil.

To be assured of the absence of adulterants, it is necessary to examine the separated stearoptene.

The naturally occurring paraffinic hydrocarbons in rose stearoptene consist of at least two components having melting points of 22° and 41°C. The mixture separated from rose oil should melt between 32° and 37°C; usually at about 33°–34°C. Additions of spermaceti, guaiac wood oil and many readily available solid paraffins will raise the melting point.

Spermaceti, tristearin or other fatty acid esters may be detected by an abnormally high ester number of the separated stearoptene. Occasionally it is possible to isolate the fatty acids from the saponified material. Guaiac wood oil consists mainly of the alcohol, guaiol; its presence will be revealed by a high ester number after acetylation of the separated stearoptene. High melting paraffins are very difficult to detect when used as adulterants for rose oils.

The appearance of the stearoptene may reveal their presence; a peculiar granular structure is frequently indicative of such additions. The appearance of the crystals which separate in the test described under Procedure I is sometimes helpful in this connection.

The congealing point of the rose oil itself is also indicative of the amount of stearoptene present in the oil. The congealing point of rose oil has been defined as that temperature at which the first crystals appear when the oil is subjected to slow cooling. (This is quite different from the true congealing point of oils such as anise.) Determine the 'congealing point' of the oil by the following technique:

Procedure III: Place 10 cc. of the oil in a test tube having a diameter of 15 mm; suspend a thermometer in the oil in such a way that it touches neither the sides nor the bottom; warm the contents of the tube to about 5°C above the point of saturation; stir well; then permit the oil to cool slowly until the first crystals appear; read the temperature. Repeat the determination.

As a general rule, good Bulgarian oils produced by the usual methods show a congealing point of 18° to 23°C.

DETERMINATION OF SAFROLE CONTENT OF SASSAFRAS OILS

The congealing point of sassafras oils gives a good estimate of the safrole content.

> *Procedure*: Determine the congealing point of the sassafras oil and estimate the safrole content from Table 13.4.

Table 13.4 will give values of the safrole content with an accuracy of about 2 per cent if the congealing point is above 2°C.

Table 13.4. Congealing point and safrole content.

Per cent safrole	Congealing point
100	11.0°C
90	7.5
80	4.6
70	1.7
60	−1.3

DETERMINATION OF CEDROL CONTENT OF CEDARWOOD OILS

For the determination of cedrol in cedarwood oils, Rabak has suggested the following method:

One hundred parts of oil are agitated vigorously with 6 parts of 65 per cent alcohol (by volume) for one to two minutes in a widemouthed, stoppered flask. Sudden and complete solidifications of the emulsion thus formed usually result if the oil contains a sufficient quantity of cedrol. If it fails to solidify add a small quantity of 'crystalline cedrol to the emulsion, and cool in a refrigerator for several hours. Filter the solidified mass with the aid of a well cooled Büchner funnel and wash the fine silky crystals with a few drops of cold 98 per cent alcohol. Weigh the dry crystals. The cedrol may be purified by dissolving it in hot alcohol, then cooling and filtering the mass.

In general, an analytical method based upon the actual separation of a constituent by physical means will not give completely accurate results. However, comparative data may be obtained provided all experimental conditions are carefully controlled.

This method appears to be of value only for obtaining comparative data when two oils are examined simultaneously; all experimental conditions should be maintained as identical as possible.

DETERMINATION OF THE COLOUR VALUE OF OLEORESIN CAPSICUM

In order to standardise the colour of oleoresin capsicum it has been found that a very close match to the natural colour can be attained with the proper mixture of solutions of potassium dichromate and cobalt chloride. The colour standard is prepared as follows:

Into a 50 cc. Nessler tube pipette 5 cc. of a 0.1 N potassium dichromate solution (4.904 gram $K_2Cr_2O_7$ per litre) and 0.5 cc. of a 0.5 N cobaltous chloride solution (5.948 gram $CoCl_2 \cdot 6H_2O$ per 100 cc.) and make up to 50 cc. with distilled water.

The colour value of the oleoresin is defined as the number of cc.'s of acetone, multiplied by 100, which are necessary to add to 1 cc. of a 1 per cent solution of the oleoresin capsicum in acetone, in order to match the colour standard as outlined above. The height of the liquid in the Nessler tube should be about 8 inches and the colour should be matched by looking down into the column and not laterally.

Procedure: Weigh accurately 1.00 gram of oleoresin and make up to 100 cc. with acetone. Pipette 1 cc. of this 1 per cent solution into a 50 cc. volumetric flask and make up to 50 cc. with acetone. Pour this dilute solution (0.02 per cent) into a burette. Introduce sufficient of this solution into an empty 50 cc. Nessler tube to approximate the colour of the standard (viewed through the length of the tube). Then add sufficient acetone to bring the volume up to about 45–47 cc. and make the final adjustment of colour by addition of small amounts of the dilute solution (0.02 per cent) from the burette.

Finally add sufficient acetone to bring the volume to exactly 50 cc. and check the colour match.

$$\text{Colour value} = 100 \left[\frac{50 - (0.02)\ (\text{number of cc. of dilute solution required})}{(0.02)\ (\text{number of cc. of dilute solution required})} \right]$$

Using this procedure, an accuracy of about ±1000 units can be obtained. The colour values will vary between 5000 and 25,000 for commercial oleoresins; a value of 14,000 is generally considered very satisfactory.

The procedure may be modified to permit the use of 100 cc. Nessler tubes and the colours of the standard and the solution of oleoresin may be accurately matched with Nesslerimeter.

Chapter 14

Detection of Adulterants in Essential Oils

INTRODUCTION

Adulterant is any substance that lessens the purity or effectiveness of a substance. It is necessary to remove the adulterants before use.

As far as adulteration is concerned, producers and distributors of essential oils are frequently painted as 'the bad guys', but it should be pointed out that their oil customers frequently demand oils below the market price while still wanting to be told that they are authentic. In this climate, the honest oil trader may find it virtually impossible to survive on the margins he is allowed to make (many have already gone bust). For example, in the late 20th Century, lavender oil (Lavandula angustifolia) was being sold almost as a loss leader by many French producers as the market was unwilling to pay a realistic price; currently, the aroma industry is dominated by a handful of large and powerful international houses whose corporate buyers often attempt to drive raw material prices to impossibly low levels, not allowing workable profits to be made. This sets the scene for unethical practices.

Essential oils should be produced by purely physical means, and be 100 per cent pure and wholly derived from the named botanical source but how are these standards to be guaranteed? No quality standards for the authentication of essential oils exist in aromatherapy, in spite of the revelations of gross adulteration of aromatherapy oils for retail sale.

DETECTION OF FOREIGN OILS IN SWEET BIRCH AND WINTERGREEN OILS

For a rapid evaluation of the quality of sweet birch and wintergreen oils, the alkali solubility test often proves of value.

> *Procedure*: Introduce 2 cc. of the oil in a 25 cc. glass-stoppered, graduated cylinder and add 23 cc. of an aqueous solution of potassium hydroxide prepared by dissolving 6.5 grams of potassium hydroxide (analytical grade) in sufficient distilled water to yield 100 cc. of solution. Shake thoroughly and permit the cylinder to stand undisturbed for 24 hours: no oily separation should result, although a separation of a solid waxy material is indicative of a normal oil.

Since the natural waxy separation melts at a relatively low temperature, care should be exercised in interpreting the results of this test in warm weather.

It is well to study the odour of the solution or any insoluble portion. Since the potassium phenolate of methyl salicylate is practically odourless, additions of foreign, odour-bearing substances may be detected.

DETECTION OF PETROLEUM AND MINERAL OIL

Oleum Test

The saturated paraffinic hydrocarbons, found in petroleum oils, are chemically very inert; they are not destroyed by fuming sulphuric acid. Other compounds are attacked, giving rise to reaction products which are soluble in sulphuric acid.

Procedure: Place 20 cc. of fuming sulphuric acid in a dry cassia flask (a narrow necked Babcock bottle may be used in place of the cassia flask; this offers the further advantage of permitting the bottle and contents to be centrifuged for better separation) of 150 cc. capacity and cool thoroughly in an ice salt mixture. Add slowly 5 cc. of the oil in question from a small burette. The oil should be added drop by drop, with frequent shaking and cooling in the ice-salt mixture, since too rapid addition of the oil is apt to cause the liberated sulphur dioxide to carry part of the acid and oil out of the flask. After the oil has been added, the flask is again shaken and permitted to stand at room temperature for 10 minutes. It is then warmed on a steam bath for 5 minutes with frequent agitation. The flask is permitted to cool to room temperature and is then filled with 95 per cent sulphuric acid. After standing overnight, the mineral oil will rise into the neck and separate as a colourless, or straw-coloured liquid. As a confirmatory test, a small amount of the separated mineral oil may be removed from the cassia flask (by means of capillary action, using a glass tube drawn out to a small tip). The refractive index of this separated oil should be less than 1.4400.

A flavour test often will prove of value for the detection of kerosene. Since petroleum fractions often contain aromatic and unsaturated compounds as well as paraffins, the separation of the paraffinic portion described above does not usually represent the total amount of added petroleum. In general, such actual separation usually is a small percentage of the adulterant. The test may be rendered more sensitive by preliminary fractionation of the oil. The addition of petroleum fractions to an oil causes a lowering of the specific gravity, index and optical rotation. The solubility of the oil usually is affected: this is the basis of the well-known Schimmel Test for citronella oils described below.

Schimmel Tests

Old Schimmel test

In order to limit the amount of adulteration of citronella oils with petroleum fractions, the chemists of Schimmel and Company introduced the well-known Schimmel test. Several modifications of this test have been proposed, but the trade accepts the following procedure in writing contracts for oils.

Procedure: Into a glass-stoppered, graduated cylinder introduce exactly 1 cc. of the oil. Add dropwise 80 per cent alcohol until a clear solution results. This should occur at 1 to 2 volumes. Add sufficient 80 per cent alcohol to bring the amount of added alcohol to 10 volumes. The solution may show a slight opalescence, but should not separate oily droplets even after standing for several hours. When adding the alcohol, violent shaking should be avoided to prevent an emulsion that will separate only after very prolonged standing.

A citronella oil meets the Schimmel test if it yields a clear solution in 1 to 2 volumes of 80 per cent alcohol and does not separate oily droplets when the amount of alcohol added is increased to 10 volumes. This test limits the amount of added petroleum fractions to about 10 per cent. If more than this amount has been added, oily droplets will form on the surface of the alcoholic solution. Additions of fatty oils will result in the formation of oily droplets which settle to the bottom.

New Schimmel test

At a later date the description of the original test was modified resulting in the so-called 'new Schimmel test'. This test is somewhat more stringent than the 'old Schimmel test' described above. A description of this test follows:

> Oil of citronella Sri Lanka must be clearly soluble in from 1 to 2 volumes of 80 per cent alcohol by volume at 20°C. Upon the further addition of alcohol of the same strength, the solution should show an opalescence at the most, but no turbidity or direct cloudiness. The alcohol must be added slowly, drop by drop; the addition being at once interrupted if a cloudiness or turbidity appears. The alcohol is then added slowly, drop by drop, until the point of highest or maximum cloudiness or turbidity is obtained. The mixture is carefully set aside and maintained at 20°C to observe if any oily constituents separate out. Ten volumes of 80 per cent alcohol at the most are added. If oil separates out immediately or after prolonged standing, the oil does not pass the 'new Schimmel test'. Strong or violent shaking must be avoided since any possible oily separation will become finely dispersed and will not separate out on standing.

Many oils will show an oily separation at the point of highest cloudiness or turbidity, but will show no oily separation if 10 volumes of 80 per cent alcohol are added.

Raised Schimmel test

In order to limit adulteration with mineral spirits to 5 per cent, the 'raised Schimmel test' was introduced. This test has never attained commercial importance.

> Oil of citronella Sri Lanka is mixed with 5 per cent of kerosene and the 'old Schimmel test' is applied, disregarding any intermediate stages of cloudiness or turbidity; i.e. simply add 80 per cent alcohol up to 10 volumes. A fresh unadulterated citronella oil will show no oily separation. Oils containing small amounts of petroleum will show an oily separation either immediately or after prolonged standing at 20°C.

This test is by far the most stringent of the three.

DETECTION OF ROSIN

In testing for rosin as an adulterant in oils, the following pertinent properties of this substance should be borne in mind. It is a nonvolatile material and consequently may be concentrated in the residue by distillation of the oil under vacuum or at atmospheric pressure; it is found also in the evaporation residue. Rosin consists primarily of complex acids and, therefore, will increase the acid number of an oil or of the evaporation residue if such residue normally consists of solid esters or paraffins; this is specifically of importance in the case of citrus oils. Rosin is soluble in most organic solvents, including petroleum ether, benzene, and xylene; since cinnamic aldehyde (the main constituent of cassia oil) is practically insoluble in petroleum ether, this permits a convenient separation of added rosin for this oil. Rosin gives a dark green copper salt when treated with cupric acetate; this salt is sufficiently soluble in petroleum ether to impart to this solvent a green colour. Rosin is a relatively high melting solid, normally a hard, noncrystalline material which fractures readily; hence the consistency of the evaporation residue is frequently altered if rosin is present.

Detection of Rosin in Balsams and Gums

Place in a small mortar 1 gram of the substance, powdered or crushed if necessary, and add 10 cc. of purified petroleum ether. Triturate well for 1 or 2 minutes. Filter into a test tube and add to the filtrate

10 cc. of a freshly prepared aqueous solution of cupric acetate (1 gram in 200 cc.). Shake well and allow the liquids to separate. The petroleum ether layer should not show a green colour.

Detection of Rosin in Cassia Oils

Shake about 2 cc. of the oil in a test tube with 10 cc. of petroleum ether. Permit the liquids to separate and decant the benzene layer into a second test tube. Add an equal volume of cupric acetate solution (1 in 1000); a green colour indicates the presence of rosin in the oil.

It is well to carry out simultaneously a test with an oil known to be free of rosin, to act as a blank. Unfortunately, tests based upon colour reactions have not proved too reliable in mixtures as complex as essential oils; nevertheless, this test will give an indication of the presence or absence of rosin.

Procedure: About 50 grams of the oil, accurately weighed, are distilled from a tared distilling flask over an open flame. Continue the distillation until decomposition is evidenced by the formation of white fumes within the flask; this usually occurs at a temperature of about 280°C. Cool the flask and weigh; calculate the percentage of residue.

This test will reveal adulteration with nonvolatile material such as rosin, if large amounts have been added. Normal oils show a distillation residue of 6 to 8 per cent or at most 10 per cent. Furthermore, the residue should be tacky, but not hard and brittle. The residue should not be higher than 5 per cent for a pure oil. Treff has pointed out that, distillation should be carried out rapidly, since the amount of residue obtained is greatly dependent upon the rate of distillation.

Procedure: Determine the acid number of the oil in the usual manner. If the oil is pure and has been properly stored, the acid number should not be greater than 15.

Detection of Rosin in Orange Oils

Determine the evaporation residue in the usual manner. In the case of pure oils this residue upon cooling should be soft and waxy, not hard, brittle or tacky. The acid number of the residue should lie between 11 and 28, the ester number between 118 and 157.

DETECTION OF TERPINYL ACETATE

It has been pointed out in the determination of esters that certain esters are not completely saponified under the standard analytical conditions if the time of reflux is limited to 1 hour. Terpinyl acetate is such an ester.

Additions of esters of this type to readily saponifiable esters (such as linalyl acetate) will be revealed by a difference in the ester numbers obtained by saponification for periods of 1 and 2 hours, respectively. Under standard conditions linalyl acetate is completely saponified in a period of 30 minutes; terpinyl acetate requires about 2 hours. Hence, an appreciable difference between the ester numbers determined after heating for 30 minutes and for 1 hour (or 2 hours) indicates the presence of certain foreign esters, such as terpinyl acetate, in oils containing only readily saponifiable esters (e.g. bergamot oil and lavender oil). If only small amounts of terpinyl acetate have been added, the difference will be too small to draw any definite conclusions. However, by modifying the experimental conditions, such small differences may be greatly magnified. The method outlined below is the classical method developed by the chemists of Schimmel and Company for the detection of terpinyl acetate as an adulterant in bergamot oils; it is also applicable to lavender oils and to synthetic linalyl acetate. With further modification, it can be used for the detection of terpinyl acetate and terpineol in numerous oils; such applications, however, should be made with discretion.

Procedure: Pipette 2 cc. of the oil into each of three tared saponification flasks and weigh accurately. To flask I add 10 cc. of 0.5 N alcoholic sodium hydroxide solution and 25 cc. of alcohol. To flask II add 20 cc. of the alkali solution, but no alcohol. To flask III add 10 cc. of the alkali solution and 5 cc. of alcohol. (The alkali solution should be measured accurately from a burette or pipette.) The contents of flask I and flask III are refluxed on a steam bath for a period of 1 hour; the contents of flask II, for 2 hours. Calculate the ester numbers for the three determinations.

In the case of pure bergamot oils, the difference between ester number I and ester number II will not be greater than 5; the usual value lies below 3. In the case of an oil adulterated with 4 per cent terpinyl acetate, the difference amounts to about 10.0; with 10 per cent terpinyl acetate, about 19.0. Furthermore, in the case of pure oils, ester number III will be approximately the arithmetical mean of ester number I and ester number II.

For oils containing larger amounts of ester, the size of the sample must be reduced; 1 cc. will often prove sufficient. In the case of synthetic linalyl acetate, a 1 cc. sample should be used and the quantities of alkali should be doubled.

Fractional saponification may also be used to detect the presence of terpineol by carrying out the determination on an acetylised oil; great discretion must be used, however, since terpineol and certain difficult saponifiable esters may be present as natural constituents or the process of acetylation may result in the formation of such esters. Recourse to fractionation of the oil or of the acetylised oil with subsequent fractional saponification of the proper fraction may frequently prove of value. Table 14.1 gives the boiling points of terpineol and terpinyl acetate at various pressures.

Table 14.1. Boiling points of terpineol and terpinyl acetate at various pressures.

	Boiling point	
Pressure in mm of Hg	*α-Terpineol*	*Terpinyl acetate*
5	92.4°C	90°–94°C
10	104.0°C	110°–115°C
760	217.5°C	220°C

DETECTION OF TURPENTINE OIL

The addition of turpentine oil as an adulterant generally reduces the specific gravity and affects the solubility and optical rotation of most essential oils. Its presence may be proved in oils which contain no pinene as a natural constituent by the separation and identification of α-pinene, the main constituent of turpentine oils.

Highly purified *d*-α-pinene has the following properties:

Boiling point	= 155°–156°C
Specific gravity at 15°C	= 0.864
Refractive index at 20°C	= 1.4656
Specific rotation at 20°C	= +48°24′
Solubility at 20°C	4 volume of 90 per cent alcohol and more

The boiling point of α-pinene lies below that of most of the terpenes and oxygenated constituents found in essential oils. Consequently, in testing for the presence of pinene it is customary to fractionate the oil, collecting the first 10 per cent or better the distillate coming over below 160°C at atmospheric pressure.

Procedure: Distil a 50 cc. sample of the oil from a three bulb, 125 cc. Ladenburg flask, collecting only the first 5 cc. Mix this distillate with 5 cc. of glacial acetic acid and cool to 0°C in a freezing bath. Add 10 cc. of amyl nitrite and then add dropwise, with constant stirring, 2 cc. of dilute hydrochloric acid (2:1). Permit the mixture to stand in the freezing bath for 15 minutes and collect the crystals which form on a Büchner funnel. Wash thoroughly with alcohol. Permit the crystals to dry at room temperature and dissolve in a small amount of chloroform. Add methyl alcohol to the chloroform solution dropwise until the nitrosochlorides precipitate out. Separate the crystals by filteration and dry at room temperature. Mount in a fixed oil (olive oil) and examine microscopically. Pinene nitrosochloride (limonene nitrosochloride, which may also be present, crystallises in needles) crystals have irregular pyramidal ends (melting point, 103°C).

DETECTION OF ACETINS

The acetic acid esters if glycerine are occasionally employed as adulterants in order to increase the apparent ester content. Since all three acetins are relatively soluble in water they may easily be washed out and tested for by the procedure described below. The least soluble of the three is triacetin; even this, however, is soluble in water to the extent of about 7 per cent. In order to insure the removal of most of the triacetin, a 5 per cent alcoholic solution is employed.

Procedure: Shake 20 cc. of the oil with 40 cc. of 5 per cent alcohol in a 125 cc. glass-stoppered, separatory funnel. When the mixture has separated completely withdraw 30 cc. of the alcoholic solution by means of a pipette and place it in a 125 cc. Erlenmeyer flask. Neutralise the solution with 0.5 N sodium hydroxide, using a 1 per cent phenolphthalein solution as indicator. Then add exactly 5 cc. of 0.5 N alcoholic sodium hydroxide and heat the mixture on a steam bath for 1 hour. Remove the flask and allow the mixture to cool. Titrate the excess of alkali with 0.5 N hydrochloric acid. At least 4.7 cc. of the acid should be used for this neutralisation.

This test is not specific for acetins; if large amounts of other water-soluble esters are present, these will appear in the dilute alcoholic layer.

DETECTION OF ETHYL ALCOHOL

Alcohol has been used frequently as an adulterant, since it is a cheap and available diluent for essential oils. The presence of ethyl alcohol as an adulterant may be readily detected by several simple tests.

Procedure I: Determine accurately the refractive index and specific gravity of the oil. Then shake thoroughly an equal volume of oil and saturated salt solution in a separatory funnel. Permit the oil to separate completely and determine the refractive index and specific gravity of this washed oil. These should not differ materially from those of the original oil. An approximation of the amount of added alcohol may be obtained from a consideration of these values.

This procedure is not specific for alcohol and will detect other water soluble adulterants.

Procedure II: Place 50 cc. of the oil (previously dried with anhydrous sodium sulphate) in a 100 cc. Ladenburg flask and distil slowly over an open flame. Collect and measure the distillate below 100°C. Since most constituents of essential oils boil much above 100°C, unadulterated oils generally show no distillate at this temperature. However, if a distillate is obtained dilute to 10 cc. with distilled water. Test a 5 cc. portion for ethyl alcohol by the iodoform test and the residual 5 cc. portion by the ethyl benzoate test.

Iodoform test: To 5 cc. of the diluted distillate add 10 drops of a 10 per cent sodium hydroxide solution and sufficient iodine potassium iodide-solution drop by drop until a faint, permanent yellow colour is obtained, indicating an excess of iodine. Allow the test tube to stand undisturbed for 5 minutes. The formation of yellow, flat, hexagonal crystals with the peculiar odour of iodoform indicates a positive reaction. If no positive result is obtained, heat the test tube to 60°C for 1 minute in a beaker of water and permit the mixture to stand for 1 hour.

The iodine-potassium iodide solution is prepared by dissolving 2 gram of potassium iodide in 8 cc. of distilled water and adding 1 gram of iodine; stir until solution is complete.

Ethyl benzoate test: To 5 cc. of the dilute distillate add 5 drops of benzoyl chloride and 2 cc. of a 10 per cent sodium hydroxide solution. Warm on a steam bath. The fruity odour of ethyl benzoate indicates the presence of ethyl alcohol.

The iodoform test will give a positive reaction with any compound containing a $CH_3\overset{\overset{\displaystyle O}{\parallel}}{C}$—group united to either a carbon or a hydrogen atom or to any chemical which is oxidised under the conditions of the test to a compound having such a structure. In particular, acetone will give a positive iodoform test. In the ethyl benzoate test, all low boiling aliphatic alcohols will give fruity odours. However, only ethyl alcohol will give positive results with both the iodoform and ethyl benzoate tests.

The presence of ethyl alcohol materially lowers the flash point of most essential oils. There exist insufficient published data on the normal limits of the flash points of the unadulterated oils to draw valid conclusions from the results of flash-point determinations.

Oils containing relatively large amounts of alcohol will form milky emulsions with water. Use of this fact may be made for a quick test.

DETECTION OF METHYL ALCOHOL

The following procedure is based upon the fact that methyl alcohol may readily be oxidised to formaldehyde by potassium permanganate in the presence of dilute phosphoric acid. The resulting formaldehyde can then be detected by means of the reaction with chromotropic acid (1,8-dihydroxynaphthalene-3,6-disulphonic acid) which gives a violet colour in the presence of sulphuric acid. The chemistry of this colour reaction is unknown.

The following compounds give no reaction with chromotropic acid: acetaldehyde, aromatic aldehydes, butyraldehyde, chloralhydrate, crotonaldehyde, glyoxal, isobutyraldehyde, isovaleraldehyde, oenanthal, propionaldehyde. Fructose, furfural, glyceraldehyde, robinose and sucrose all give yellow colours. Other sugars, acetones and carboxylic acids do not react. High concentrations of furfural give red colour.

This test is satisfactory for the detection of methyl alcohol in the presence of ethyl alcohol.

Procedure: Mix 2 drops of the alcohol in question in a test tube with 2 drops of 5 per cent phosphoric acid and 2 drops of 5 per cent potassium permanganate solution. After 1 minute, add a little solid sodium bisulphite with shaking until the mixture is decolourised. If any brown precipitate of the oxide of manganese remains undissolved, add a further drop or two of phosphoric acid and a little more sodium bisulphite. When the solution is entirely colourless, add 8 cc. of 72 per cent sulphuric acid and a small amount of finely powdered chromotropic acid. Shake the mixture well and then heat to 60°C for 10 minutes. A violet colour which deepens on cooling, indicates the presence of methyl alcohol.

The identification limit is 3.5 γ methyl alcohol; the concentration limit, 1:13600.

DETECTION OF HIGH BOILING ESTERS

Detection of Various Esters

Relatively odourless esters frequently are added to essential oils to increase the apparent ester content. Fortunately, most such esters are high boiling and permit of easy separation. The best general method for the detection of such added esters is to separate the acids and identify them. Detection of added esters of acetic and formic acid (by isolation and identification of the acids) is not practical since these acids usually occur as natural constituents of essential oils.

> *Procedure*: Saponify 10 cc. of the oil for 2 hours with 20 cc. of 0.5 N alcoholic potassium hydroxide (if the oil has a high ester number, a larger amount of alkali will be required). Add 25 cc. of water and evaporate off most of the alcohol (some chemists prefer to evaporate to dryness and then take up the residue in a small amount of water). Wash out the unsaponified oil by shaking with 3 equal portions of ether. The aqueous solution is then made distinctly acid with hydrochloric acid (1:3) and again shaken out with ether. The ethereal solution will now contain the relatively insoluble acids, such as benzoic, cinnamic, oleic, phthalic, and lauric acid. Upon evaporation of the ether these may be recovered. The aqueous solution will contain the readily water-soluble acids, such as citric, oxalic and tartaric acid. This solution should, therefore, be made just alkaline to phenolphthalein and an excess of saturated barium chloride solution added. After warming for about 10 minutes, a crystalline precipitate of the insoluble barium salts will be obtained from which the acids can be liberated and identified.

A method for the detection of esters of acids which are not readily volatile with steam, e.g. succinates, citrates, oxalates and the esters of the higher fatty acids.

> *Procedure*: Determine the saponification number of the oil in the usual manner. Then add a few drops of 0.5 N alcoholic sodium hydroxide to the contents of the saponification flask and evaporate to dryness on a steam bath. Dissolve the residue in 5 cc. of water and add 2 cc. of dilute sulphuric acid (1:3). Distil off the volatile acids with steam, using the apparatus shown in Fig. 14.1. The distillation should be carried out at such a rate that a distillate of 250 cc. is collected in the receiver at the end of 30 minutes; the volume of the liquid in the saponification flask should be kept at about 10 cc. with the aid of the small flame. Collect a further 100 cc. of distillate in a second receiver. Add few drops of 1 per cent alcoholic phenolphthalein solution to each receiver and titrate the free acids with 0.5 N potassium hydroxide solution. The first 250 cc. contain most of the volatile acids; the next 100 cc. should require only 1 or 2 drops of the alkali. From the total amount of alkali required to neutralise the acids, acid number II is calculated. A large difference between the saponification number and acid number II indicates the presence of esters of acids only slightly volatile with steam (this procedure was originally proposed for the examination of bergamot oils; pure oils showed a difference between the saponification number and acid number II of not more than 7).

The presence of the high boiling glyceryl acetates is not revealed by either of the procedures described above, since the acid liberated is acetic acid, which is volatile with steam and which occurs naturally in many oils.

Detection of Phthalates

This method is based upon a preliminary saponification of the oil, followed by a separation of phthalic acid as the lead salt. The separation is not specific since certain acids other than phthalic (e.g. oxalic, citric and phosphoric) give rise to insoluble lead salts. Therefore, it is important to regenerate the acid and determine its melting point.

Procedure: Introduce 2 grams of the oil in a 100 cc. saponification flask. Add 25 cc. of an alcoholic sodium hydroxide solution prepared by dissolving 1.25 grams of metallic sodium in 100 cc. of 95 per cent alcohol (if the oil has a very high ester number, a larger amount of alkali will be required). Saponify for 1 hour. Remove and permit the flask to cool to room temperature and then immerse it in an ice-salt mixture. After standing for 30 minutes filter off the precipitated sodium salts, using a well-cooled Büchner funnel. Wash these crystals with ice cold anhydrous alcohol. A precipitate at this point may, be indicative of any number of organic acids (phthalic, salicylic, citric or tartaric). Transfer the salt to a 250 cc. beaker and dry in an oven at 105°C for 2 hours. Cool and add 40 to 50 cc. of distilled water and 2 or 3 cc. of glacial acetic acid. Heat this solution to the boiling point and add 30 cc. of a 10 per cent lead acetate solution. Upon thoroughly cooling in an ice bath, the lead salt of phthalic acid will precipitate out almost quantitatively. The lead salts of benzoic acid, cinnamic acid and salicylic acid are soluble and remain in the filtrate. Separate the lead salt or phthalic acid by filtration. Regenerate the phthalic acid with acid, recrystallise and determine the melting point. Phthalic acid melts at about 206°C (phthalic anhydride may be formed; the anhydride melts at 131°C).

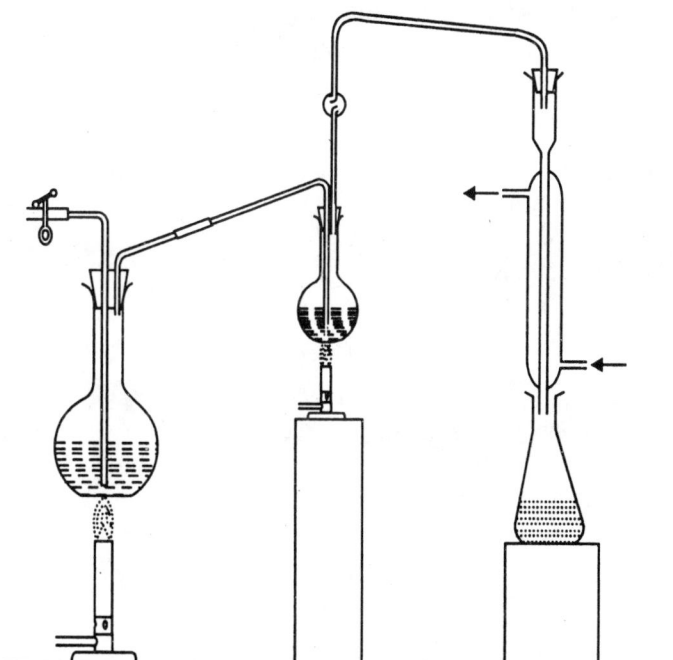

Fig. 14.1. Apparatus for the detection of high boiling esters.

DETECTION OF *MENTHA ARVENSIS* OIL

Several colour reactions have been proposed to distinguish between the oil distilled from *Mentha piperita* L. and the oil from *Mentha arvensis* L. In common with most colour reactions, these tests are not always reliable with mixtures as complex as essential oils.

The test is described below:

> *Procedure*: Mix in a dry test tube 3 drops of oil of peppermint with 5 cc. of a solution of 1 volume of nitric acid in 300 volumes of giacial acetic acid and place the tube in a beaker of boiling water. With in 1 to 5 minutes the liquid develops a blue colour which on continued heating deepens and shows a copper coloured fluorescence and then fades leaving a golden yellow solution.

The characteristic colour changes described in this procedure do not occur if an oil distilled from *Mentha arvensis* L. is examined: the acid solution then attains a light yellow colour which shows no appreciable change during the 5 minutes of heating.

It should be remembered that the colour changes described are characteristic of the oil from *Mentha piperita* L.; mixtures of this oil and *Mentha arvensis* L. give the colour changes described. Therefore, the test cannot be used to detect adulteration with *Mentha arvensis* L.

DETECTION OF VARIOUS ADULTERANTS

The physical and chemical properties of several common adulterants (which have not been thoroughly discussed previously) are briefly noted here to aid the essential oil chemist.

Cedarwood Oil

This is usually found in the last fractions owing to the high boiling points of its constituents.

d_{15}	0.951 to 0.960
α_D	−28°28′ to −35°39′
n_D^{20}	1.5030 to 1.5059
Solubility at 20°C	Often insoluble in 10 volumes 90 per cent alcohol.

Copaiba Oil

This also is found in the last fractions.

d_{15}	0.901 to 0.905
α_D	−11°18′ to −14°22′
n_D^{20}	1.4972 to 1.4990
Solubility at 20°C	Insoluble in 10 volumes 90 per cent alcohol.

Gurjun Balsam Oil

This is a high boiling oil.

d_{15}	0.918 to 0.930
α_D	−35°0′ to −130°0′
n_D^{20}	1.5010 to 1.5050
Solubility at 20°C	Insoluble in 10 volumes 90 per cent alcohol.

The following colour reaction for this oil has been recommended:

> To a mixture of 10 cc. of glacial acetic acid and 5 drops of concentrated nitric acid, add 5 drops of the oil: gurjun oil gives a purple-violet colour within 2 minutes.

A rather elaborate test describes the preparation and isolation of gurjun-ketone semicarbazone— melting point, 234°C.

Fatty Oils

Such oils greatly increase the ester number and evaporation residue of an oil. They are not volatile with steam and cannot be distilled without decomposition except at exceptionally low pressures. In general, they are very insoluble in 90 per cent alcohol and frequently insoluble in 95 per cent alcohol; castor oil proves an exception, being readily soluble in 95 per cent alcohol. The saponified oil frequently shows much foaming, owing to the formation of soaps.

PROCEDURE FOR THE INVESTIGATION OF THE CHEMICAL CONSTITUENTS OF AN ESSENTIAL OIL

Assurance of the purity of the essential oil is of primary importance in an investigation of its chemical constituents. If there is the slightest doubt as to whether or not the oil may have been contaminated or adulterated, then such an oil is worthless for the examination, because the results obtained after much labour will be open to question. Therefore, it is best for the investigator to distil the oil from the botanical, or to supervise the distillation in the producing region or factory. Such distillations should be carried out on a commercial scale in the manner in which the oil of commerce is produced; otherwise, misleading results may be obtained. If this is impossible, the oil should be obtained directly from a prime source of unquestionable repute. A representative sample of the oil to be investigated should be analysed carefully. All physical and chemical properties should be determined, including specific, gravity, optical rotation, refractive index, solubility and the percentages of esters, aldehydes, ketones, phenols, acids and alcohols. These physico-chemical properties should be compared with values given in the literature for normal pure oils. Further examination should not be attempted if these properties show any suspicious deviation from normal values. Such deviation might indicate accidental contamination, adulteration or the production of an abnormal oil.

Although an oil may have been distilled from the proper botanical material, nevertheless, it may not represent the normal article of commerce. Such factors as the degree of maturity of the botanical frequently exert an important influence on, the composition of the oil. Consider, for example, oil of coriander. If an oil is distilled from the immature and green coriander seed it will show a high decyl aldehyde content, sometimes attaining a value as high as 70 per cent. As the seed matures, the aldehyde content of the oil decreases and the linaloöl content increases, until finally an oil is obtained from mature seed which shows an aldehyde content of about 1 per cent. Needless to say, the oil having this low aldehyde content is the oil accepted in commerce as normal oil of coriander. A further difficulty exists in the proper selection of the botanical. Sometimes there are many species within a plant family but only one or more yields the desired oil or oils; the eucalypts are a good example. Occasionally there are found several varieties of the same species which may yield different oils upon distillation. The production of juniper berry oil from *Juniperus communis* L. growing in America gives rise to an oil which differs from the normal commercial product formerly obtained from *Juniperus communis* L. grown in Central Europe. This has been explained by the fact that the American oil is distilled from a variety of the true *Juniperus communis* L.; viz. *Juniperus communis* L. var. *depressa* Pursh. Physiological varieties of the same species of certain plants are also known (e.g. *Eucalyptus dives*).

The geographical location of the growing section may exert an effect upon the composition and quality of the oil. This probably results from the nature of the soil, the altitude at which the plant grows, as well as factors such as intensity of sunlight, rainfall and temperature.

Consideration should be given to the methods of distillation and production of the commercial oil and to the handling of the botanical before distillation. Some plants should be distilled as soon as cut, some after sun drying for a day, some after thorough drying in the shade, some after drying and storage for several years.

All of the above factors should be carefully considered and as much information as possible concerning the botany, geographical source, maturity, preliminary treatment of the plant material and method of production of the oil should be included in the report on the chemical constituents of the oil.

The amount of oil used for the examination is a limiting factor. The availability and the cost of the oil enter in most commercial and academic investigations. For oils that are available in relatively unlimited quantity, the difficulty of handling large amounts in a research laboratory must be considered. Such difficulty may be overcome if the manufacturing plant or factory cooperates in the investigation. It then becomes possible to fractionate large quantities of the oil. Constituents occurring in minute amounts have been identified by such a procedure. Without benefit of this preliminary fractionation, it is difficult to handle much more than 15 litres of an oil in the laboratory.

For an oil which has not been investigated previously, the first step is a general examination, followed by an investigation which endeavours to discover as many of the constituents as possible. This usually reveals those constituents which occur in substantial amounts. Frequently, indications of the occurrence of other constituents are thereby obtained, whose presence, however, cannot be established conclusively. A subsequent investigation directed solely to the isolation and identification of such individual constituents often will prove successful.

It is obvious that no comprehensive procedure can be given which will prove applicable to all essential oils. The following notes are intended merely as an aid to the chemist embarked upon such an investigation. From a study of the physico-chemical properties of the oil, a general plan for the investigation is formulated.

If the oil shows a large percentage of free acids, phenols or carbonyl compounds it is usually advisable to remove these components before fractionation. Any free acids should always be removed before further treatment of the oil. However, if phenols and carbonyl compounds are present in but small amounts, it may be better to fractionate the oil and then separate these components from the enriched fraction or fractions.

Occasionally solid constituents (such as camphor, menthol, safrole or anethole) may be separated from the whole oil by freezing, followed by filtration or centrifuging. Since such separations are never quantitative it may be advisable to freeze out these components from the enriched fraction rather than from the whole oil. If the solid constituents occur in large amounts, one may resort to a preliminary freezing, followed by fractionation of the filtrate so obtained. The enriched fractions should then be frozen and the material thus further separated added to that obtained from the original oil. The difficulty of maintaining sufficiently low temperatures during the filtration, especially for large amounts of oil, may make a separation from the whole oil impractical. In general, for the isolation and purification of the various constituents it is necessary to resort to chemical methods in addition to purely physical means.

After such preliminary treatment as indicated above, the oil or residual oil should be fractionated. This will result in a separation of the oil into a low boiling terpene fraction, and intermediate fraction, a fraction rich in oxygenated constituents, a second intermediate fraction, a fraction containing the sesquiterpene constituents and a distillation residue. The residue usually contains polymerisation products and high boiling constituents, such as azulenic compounds and the naturally occurring waxes in the case of citrus oils obtained by expression. These waxes show a tendency to 'fix' part of the volatile components. If present to any appreciable extent these waxes should be freed from the more volatile components by steam distillation or by the addition of a water-soluble glycol (e.g. diethylene glycol), followed by vacuum distillation. The latter procedure will remove most of the volatile material from the waxes, leaving a relatively inodourous residue. The glycol may then be removed from the natural constituents by washing out with water or sodium chloride solution.

Should the original analysis show a high ester content it is usually best to fractionate the oil before saponification so that the ester may be obtained in a state of relative purity for a determination of physical properties. Its components may then be identified after saponification. Since the corresponding free alcohol usually is present with the ester, saponification of the whole oil (followed by fractionation) may be preferable, especially if only small amounts of ester are present.

The treatment of an oil or fraction with reagents for the purpose of separating and purifying various constituents may cause drastic changes to occur. This may give rise to new chemical compounds not originally present as such in the oil. Intra- and intermolecular rearrangements may occur as well as degradations and dehydrations. Such possibilities must be considered in the evaluation of the final results of the investigation.

For the identification of individual constituents which have been separated and purified from the oil, two general procedures are employed: (i) the determination of physical properties including melting point (or congealing point), boiling point, specific gravity, optical rotation, refractive index and solubility in alcohol of varying strengths; and (ii) the preparation of suitable derivatives, preferably solid compounds of definite melting point capable of purification by recrystallisation. In general, the identification may be considered established if no depression is observed in the melting point when a derivative of the constituent is mixed with the corresponding derivative of a sample of known purity and constitution. In many cases compounds obtained by oxidation, reduction and condensations may be used for identification.

Other methods are often employed in establishing the identity of a constituent or derivative: combustion to determine the percentage of carbon and hydrogen and to establish the empirical formula; molecular weight determinations, especially by cryoscopic methods; molecular refraction; ignition of metallic salts, especially the silver salts of organic acids; determinations of the percentage of halogen in chlorides and bromides; and other procedures.

Chapter 15

Project Profiles for Manufacture of Essential Oils

INTRODUCTION

Essential oils for all practical purposes may be defined as odouriferous bodies of oily nature obtained almost exclusively from vegetable sources. These are generally liquid (sometimes semisolid or solid) at ordinary temperature and volatile without decomposition. Some of the essential oils are partially decomposed during distillation. Some of the project profiles of patchouli oil, eucalyptus oil, eugenol, citronella oil, perfumery compounds, palmrosa oil, chamomile oil and menthol crystals are discussed briefly. The cost estimation and profit margins are calculated on the price(s) prevailing in the year 2006.

PATCHOULI OIL

Patchouli is a herbicious plant of Libiatae family. Its botanical name is progostemon patchouli and commonly known as panadi or panch. Leaves of patchouli yield a valued oil known as patchouli oil. It is widely used in perfumery and cosmetic industry. It has property to stabilise the other oil. Hence, it is used in various perfumes as stabiliser. It has an important place in cosmetic industry because no synthetic substitutes are used in place of this oil. Sumatra and Indonesia are the main producers of patchouli oil in the world and contributes around 90 per cent share of total production. Rest 10 per cent is being produced by China, Malaysia, Brazil, and India.

The total World trade in patchouli is reported to be tune of Rs. 200 crores (1000 tons) per year most of which comes from Indonesia. (As per statistics of year 2006).

The Indian perfumery industry consumes around 70–80 tons of Patchouli oil per annum and our country is importing 80–100 tons of oil per annum.

The climatic conditions of Andhra Pradesh, Kerala, Maharashtra, Goa, Karnataka, and Orissa are found to be suitable for cultivation of patchouli plant. Hence, there is a good scope of cultivation and distillation of patchouli in our country and India can become second largest producers of patchouli oil in the world by easily producing 150 tons of oil per annum and can become self-sufficient for patchouli oil.

Market Potential

Patchouli oil is used in perfumery and cosmetic industry. Due to its unique property, it is also used as stabiliser in perfumery and cosmetic industry. In India the leaves of patchouli have been used traditionally to perfume textile such as shawls and carpets, both for its sweet smell and its insect repellent properties. The leaves are used as traditional medicine of South and South East Asia. Today world over the oil of patchouli is used in manufacture of perfumes for soaps and cosmetics.

At present there are very few industries in our country engaged in cultivation and production of patchouli and major demand is met through import.

Basis and Presumption

1. The scheme is prepared based on cultivation of patchouli and its distillation.
2. All the estimates in respect of land, building, machinery, etc. are drawn as per the prevailing prices during the preparation of scheme.
3. Land is taken on lease basis.
4. 60–70 per cent efficiency of full capacity utilisation and single shift working hours have been considered in preparation of scheme.
5. Interest rate @ 17 per cent has been considered.
6. Margin money to the extent of 25 per cent of total project cost is required by the entrepreneurs as own investment in implementing the project.
7. Minimum wages have been considered in preparation of scheme.
8. Two to three years period is considered as pay back period.

Implementation Schedule

1.	Preparation of project report	1 month
2.	Selection of site	1 month
3.	Development of land and planting of material	3½ months
4.	Registration of unit	½ month
5.	Availability of loan/finance	2 months
6.	Procurement of machinery	1 month
7.	Erection and commissioning	1 month
8.	Recruitment of staff	2 months
	Total	12 months

Technical Aspects

Cultivation/soil

The crop of patchouli grows well in humid climate with good sunlight and moderate temperature. A temperature ranges of 25°–35°C is ideal with annual rainfall of 1500–3000 mm. The plant is easily propagated by cuttings. It is recommended to use tissue cultured plants as mother plants for propagation. The crop does not tolerate water-logging and hence requires well drained soil. The land is ploughed and harrowed. At the time of planting, neem cake is preferably added into the root zone along with a first dose of fertilisers. The neem cake helps to prevent nematode attack. A luxuriant crop of patchouli utilises NPK at the rate of 150:60:60 kg. per acre per year supplemented with micronutrients. The actual requirements of fertiliser application would depend on the soil type and the method of application. This plant does not require much plant protection. However, leaf eating caterpillars and aphids are easily controlled by insecticide sprays like Diethane M-45. The affected plant should be withdrawn from the field immediately to stop the spread of disease.

The plantation of patchouli is either done through cutting or plant are made ready in nursery. The distance between the plants should be kept 60–80 cm. The crop of patchouli requires moist soil, where sufficient water is not available on soil irrigation arrangement should be made to get good yield.

The crops of patchouli are ready after 5–6 months of plantation. The plant once planted gives a good yield for about 2–3 years and can regularly be harvested every 3–4 months. Care of plants include regular irrigation and application of fertilisers. 30,000–35,000 plants per acre yield 3–4 tons of dried herbage per year. The yield is significant in drip irrigation and average 7–8 tons per year. It can also be grown as inter crop under existing coconut tree and other trees and in such case yield may be achieved around 1 to 2 tons per acre. In general complete dried leaves of patchouli yield 4 to 5 per cent of oil, while stem contains 0.5 to 0.8 per cent. Yield of oil also depends on various factors such as method of distillation, distillation time, method of drying of leaves, etc. One hectare of land yield approximately 25–30 quintals of dried leaves on three harvesting.

Distillation technology

The distillation of patchouli oil is done by hydro and steam distillation but yield and quality of oil is better in case of steam distillation. The leaves of patchouli are air dried in shade in thin layer for 3–6 days so that they lose excess moisture and can be stored without deterioration. At this stage the moisture contents of the leaves is about one per cent. The dried leaves are packed in bales and cured by ageing for few months which is essential in case of patchouli as it imparts a characteristic odour to the oil which is preferred by the perfume. The oil extracted is stored in aluminium container or galvanised iron container. The quality improves on ageing.

Quality Control/Specification

Oil of patchouli is light viscose light yellow and brown in colour. Pure oil is woody and spicy in smell. On ageing it develops sweet smell. Its specific gravity 0.963–0.974 (at 25°C).

Refractive index at 25°C	1.503–1.511
Optical rotation at 20°C	48–65°

Oil of patchouli mainly contains patchouli alcohol α-patchoulene, β-patchoulene. BIS specification No. 3398–1965 is available.

Production Capacity (per annum)

Quantity	2200 kg
Value	Rs. 29,70,000

Pollution Control

In the process of distillation of patchouli oil there is no pollution. However, wastage of spent grass, etc. should be properly disposed off. All the workers should be provided with mask and gloves.

Energy Conservation

Though there is not much scope in energy conservation in this process, however, some conservation of energy can be achieved by using insulating still which can save considerable amount of heat and thereby cutting down the cost of fuel. The most effective material for insulation is asbestos which is available in various forms. An insulation thickness of 55 mm has been found to be good enough for preventing the heat loss through surfaces.

In case of steam distillation, steam line should be made complete leak proof and insulated with suitable insulating material to prevent heat loss through leakage and radiation.

Financial Aspects

Fixed capital

Land and building

1.	Rent of land on lease for 50 hectares for 50 years @ Rs. 1200 per acre per year	Rs. 1,48,200.00
2.	Distillation shed 30′ × 80′ = 2400 sq. ft @ Rs. 100 per shift	Rs. 2,40,000.00
3.	Raw material shed 30′ × 50′ = 1500 sq. ft @ Rs. 2.80 per shift	Rs. 1,20,000.00
4.	Office-cum-store 300 sq. ft @ Rs. 80 per shift	Rs. 24,000.00
	Total	Rs. 5,32,200.00

Plant and machinery

Sr. no.	Description	No.	Value (Rs.)
1.	Distillation still and accessories (each having capacity 500 kg @ Rs. 1,00,000.00)	3	3,60,000.00
2.	Boiler	1	1,50,000.00
3.	Agricultural implements, tubewell and irrigation channel, tractor with accessories	–	1,00,000.00
4.	Laboratory equipments	–	25,000.00
5.	Installation and electrification @ 10%	–	63,500.00
6.	Office furniture and fixture	–	63,500.00
7.	Tools and equipments	–	20,000.00
	Total		7,28,500.00

Preoperative expenses	Rs. 25,000.00
Total fixed cost:	
Land and building + plant and machinery + preoperative expenses	Rs. 12,85,700.00

Working Capital

Raw material

1.	Planting material, manuring, etc.	Rs. 75,000.00
2.	Packing material (Aluminium container)	Rs. 35,000.00
	Total	Rs. 1,10,000.00

Staff and labour (PM)

Sr. No.	Designation	No.	Salary	Total salary (Rs.)
1.	Manager	1	6000	6000.00
2.	Chemist/Production Manager	1	6000	6000.00
3.	Accountant	1	4000	4000.00
4.	Operator	1	3500	3500.00
5.	Skilled workers	3	2500	7500.00
6.	Unskilled workers	5	2000	10,000.00

7.	Peon/Watchman	1	2000		2000.00
	Perquisites @ 15%				6000.00
				Total	46,000.00

Utilities (per month)

Electricity		Rs. 3000.00
Fuel (Coal)		Rs.10,000.00
Water		Rs. 1000.00
	Total	Rs.14000.00

Other contingential expenses (per month)

Stationery		Rs. 1000.00
Telephone		Rs. 2000.00
Rent		Rs. 3000.00
Travelling and transport		Rs. 7000.00
Insurance		Rs. 1000.00
Maintenance/repairing		Rs. 4000.00
Miscellaneous		Rs. 2000.00
	Total	Rs.20,000.00

Working capital (per month)

Raw material		Rs. 1,10,000.00
Salary		Rs. 46,000.00
Utilities		Rs. 14,000.00
Other contingential expenses		Rs. 20,000.00
	Total	Rs. 1,80,000.00

Working capital for 3 months   Rs. 5,40,000.00

Total capital investment

Fixed capital		Rs. 12,85,700.00
Working capital		Rs. 5,40,000.00
	Total	Rs. 18,25,700.00

Machinery Utilisation

Machinery utilisation   60 per cent

Cost of production (per annum)

1. Recurring expenses per annum		Rs. 21,60,000.00
2. Depreciation on plant and machinery @ 10%		Rs. 69,850.00
3. Depreciation on land and building @ 50%		Rs. 27,000.00
4. Depreciation on office equipment @ 20%		Rs. 2000.00
5. Depreciation on tools and equipments @ 25%		Rs. 5000.00

6. Interest on total investment @ 17%   Rs. 3,10,369.00

Total	Rs.	25,69,219.00
Say	Rs.	25,69,200.00

Turnover Per Annum

Sr. no.	Item	Quantity	Rate	Total value (Rs.)
1.	Patchouli oil	2200 kgs	1350 kg	29,70,000.00

Profitability

Profit	=	Turnover – Cost of production
		29,70,000 – 25,69,200 = 4,00,800
Net profit ratio	=	Profit × 100 = 4,00,800 × 100 = 13.49%
		Turnover Rs. 29,70,000

Rate of return

Profit × 100   =   4,00,800 × 100   = 22%

Total investment   Rs. 18,21,700

Break-even analysis

Fixed cost

1. Depreciation on plant and machinery	Rs.	69,850.00
2. Depreciation on land and building	Rs.	27,000.00
3. Rent	Rs.	36,000.00
4. Depreciation on tools and equipments	Rs.	5000.00
5. Depreciation on office equipments	Rs.	2000.00
6. Interest on total investment	Rs.	3,10,369.00
7. Insurance	Rs.	12,000.00
8. 40% annual salary	Rs.	2,20,800.00
9. 40% of other contingential expenses (except rent and insurance)	Rs.	96,000.00
	Rs.	7,79,019
Total	Rs.	8,77,79,000.00

BEP = FC × 100 = 7,79,000 × 100 = 36%

     FC + profit Rs. 11,79,800.

EUCALYPTUS OIL

Eucalyptus oil is derived from the leaves and terminal branches of 'Eucalyptus' tree by steam distillation. The oils from different species vary in composition but the oil from any one species, growing under natural conditions, maintains a comparatively constant composition.

Essential oils of eucalyptus can be grouped in following categories:

1. Pharmaceutical or medicinal oils.
2. Perfumery oils.
3. Industrial oils.

In India Eucalyptus tree was introduced into South India in 1843. The genus eucalyptus comprises over 500 species and a large number of them have been utilised for the production of essential oils. Australia is the largest producer of eucalyptus oils.

Salient Features of the Oil

The salient features of the eucalyptus oils are shown below:

1. Appearance — Colourless or pale yellow
2. Odour — Aromatic and camphoraceous
3. Taste — Spicy, pungent followed by a feeling of cold
4. Specific gravity at 15°C — 0.9065–0.9155
5. Refractive index at 25°C — 1.4580–1.4700
6. Solubility — Soluble in 1 volume of 80 per cent alcohol.

Eucalyptus oil is largely used in pharmaceuticals, mosquito and germ repellent. It also goes into perfumes and flavouring agent in dental preparation. It is an ingredient of deodourising and asepticising composition for use in theatres.

Eucalyptus oil is used locally as an antiseptic, especially in the treatment of infections of the upper respiratory tract and in certain skin diseases. It is also used in ointments for burns. Internally it used as a stimulating expectorant in chronic bronchitis and asthma. Mixed with an equal amount of olive oil it is useful as a rubefacient for rheumatism.

Cineole is the principal constituent of the medicinal oils. Cineole is of two types 1,8-Cineole and 1,4-Cineole. Their structural formula and B.P. is represented as follows:

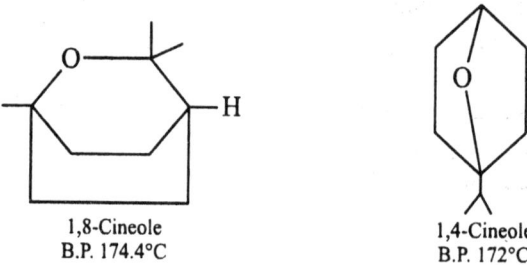

1,8-Cineole
B.P. 174.4°C

1,4-Cineole
B.P. 172°C

Markets

The world trade of eucalyptus oil is nearly 5000 tons per year. The Indian production is at the level of 275 tons. The demand in India is in increasing trend in recent years. It is good scope to set few more small scale units.

Basis and Presumptions

Efficiency and working hours considered for 80 per cent, capacity utilisation — 8 working hours/day/shift and 300 working days taken into account annually

Time period for achieving envisaged capacity utilisation — One year after trial production

Interest rate for fixed working capital — The rate of interest for term loan as well as for working capital is taken as 17 per cent which may also vary depending upon the category of entrepreneurs and the quantum of loan required

Margin money	Average
Operative period of the project	10 years
Rental value of working shed	Rs. 4000 per month
Cost of machinery and equipment	The cost of machinery and equipment, raw materials and the selling prices of the finished product are those which are existing in the market and they may vary from time to time and place to place

Implementation Schedule

Provisional SSI registration	Two weeks
No objection certificate from Pollution Control Board	Two weeks
Acquisition of land and building construction	One month
Placement of order for plant and machinery	One month
Installation and electrification	One month
Trial run	10/15 days

Technical Aspects

Process of manufacturing

Eucalyptus oil is obtained in India by the distillation of leaves and terminal branchlets of eucalyptus globules (Blue Gum tree). The leaves are collected from trees and they are dried in shade for about 3 days. The dried leaves yields upto 3 per cent of oil. The dried leaves are subjected to steam distillation. Steam distillation contains main four parts—tank, condenser, receiver, and boiler. The steam is generated in a boiler and is passed through a pipe in the tank. The tank contains a steam coil in the bottom for distribution of steam. The leaves and twigs (raw materials) is tightly packed over a case for better recovery of oil. The crude oil obtained by steam distillation is rectified after treatment with alkali. This is very necessary since the presence of valeric and other aldehydes causes coughing. Hydrogen peroxide is used for decolourising the oil.

Quality specifications

BIS-9257-1993 oil of eucalyptus citriodours (first revision) prescribes requirements and methods of sampling and test for material derived from the leaves of eucalyptus.

Annual production capacity

Quantity	30 MT
Value	Rs. 82,50,000

Approximate motive power

Approximate motive power	5 HP

Pollution control

There is small quantity of effluent which is alkaline in nature and has to be neutralised. Thus, neutralising tanks are required for this purpose before the effluent is discharged to the drain.

Energy conservation

Though there is not much requirement of power, however precautions must be taken while selecting electric motors which should be as per relevant standards.

Financial Aspects

Fixed capital

Land and building

Land 700 sq. m. @ Rs. 300 per sq. m.	Rs.	2,10,000.00
Built area, office, stores etc. 200 sq. m. @ Rs. 3000 per sq. m.	Rs.	6,00,000.00
Working shed 300 sq. m. @ Rs. 1500 per sq. m.	Rs.	4,50,000.00
Total approximate cost (land and building)	Rs.	12,60,000.00
(If rented, it will be approximately Rs. 60,000 per annum)		

Machinery and equipment

Sr. no.	Description	Indigenous/imported	Quantity	Price (Rs.)
1.	Distillation still, IMT, mild steel equipped with grid, etc.	Indigenous	1	1,00,000.00
2.	Crushing machine	Indigenous	1	30,000.00
3.	Condenser, condensing column	Indigenous	1	70,000.00
4.	Boiler	Indigenous	1	1,90,000.00
5.	Separator	Indigenous	1	35,000.00
6.	Filter press	Indigenous	1	75,000.00
7.	Rectifying column	Indigenous	1	1,50,000.00
8.	Storage tanks/vessel, etc.	Indigenous	1	50,000.00
9.	Testing equipments and glassware	Indigenous		25,000.00
				7,25,000.00
	Electrification and installation charges @ 10% of cost of machines and equipment			72,500.00
	Total cost of machinery and equipments			7,97,500.00
	Cost of office equipments/working tables, etc.			50,000.00

Pre-operative expenses

	25,000.00
Total fixed capital: (Land building + machinery and equipment + preoperative expenses)	11,32,500.00

Working capital (per month)

1. Personnel:

Sr. no.	Designation	No.	Salary	Total (Rs.)
1.	Manager-cum-manufacturing chemist	1	8000	8000.00
2.	Analytical chemist-cum-supervisor	1	7000	7000.00
3.	Accountant-cum-office assistant	1	5000	5000.00
4.	Storekeeper/Typist	1	4000	4000.00
5.	Skilled workers	1	3000	3000.00

6.	Unskilled workers	2	2500	5000.00
7.	Peon-cum-Watchman	2	2000	4000.00
				36,000.00
	15% perquisites			5400.00

2. Raw materials—per month:

Sl. no.	Particulars	Indigenous/imported	Quantity	Value (Rs.)
1.	Eucalyptus leaves	Indigenous	200 MT	4,00,000.00
2.	Aluminium/glass container of different capacities	Indigenous		40.000.00
	Total			4,40,000.00

3. Utilities:

Power	Rs.	3000.00
Coal/diesel	Rs.	25,000.00
Water	Rs.	2000.00
Total	Rs.	30,000.00

4. Other contingent expenses (per month)

Postage and stationery	Rs.	1000.00
Telephone/fax	Rs.	1500.00
Insurance	Rs.	500.00
Repair and maintenance	Rs.	2000.00
Advertisement and publicity	Rs.	2500.00
Sales expenses	Rs.	2500.00
Consumable stores	Rs.	2000.00
Transport charges	Rs.	10,000.00
Miscellaneous expenses	Rs.	3000.00
Total	Rs.	25,000.00

5. Working capital

Staff and labour	Rs.	41,400.00
Raw material	Rs.	4,40,000.00
Utilities	Rs.	30,000.00
Other contingent expenses	Rs.	25,000.00
Working capital for 3 months Rs. 5,36,000 × 3 =	Rs.	16,09,200.00

6. Total capaital investments

Fixed capital	Rs.	21,32,500.00
Working capital (for 3 montsh)	Rs.	16,09,200.00
Total	Rs.	37,41,700.00

Financial Analysis

Cost of production (per year)

Total recurring cost	Rs.	64,36,800.00
Depreciation on plant and machinery @ 10 per cent per annum	Rs.	70,750.00
Depreciation on building @ 5 per cent	Rs.	50,000.00
Depreciation on office equipments @ 20 per cent per annum	Rs.	10,000.00
Interest on total investment @ 17 per cent per annum	Rs.	6,36,089.00

| Total cost of production | | | | Rs. | 72,12,639.00 |
| Say | | | | Rs. | 72,12,600.00 |

Turnover (per year)

By sale of 3000 kgs. @ Rs. 275 per kg   Rs.   82,50,000.00

Net profit per annum

| Turnover | Cost of production | = | Net profit |
| Rs. 82,50,000.00 | Rs. 72,12,800.00 | | Rs. 10,37,400.00 |

Net profit ratio	Net profit × 100	Rs. 10,37,400 × 100		
	Turnover	Rs. 82,50,000	=	12.57%
Rate of return	Net profit × 100	Rs. 10,37,400 × 100		
	Total investment	Rs. 37,41,700	=	27.72%

Break-even point

$$BEP = \frac{\text{Fixed cost} \times 100}{\text{Fixed cost} + \text{Annual profit}}$$

Fixed cost

Depreciation on machinery and equipment @ 10% per annum	Rs.	79,750.00
Depreciation on building @ 5%	Rs.	50,000.00
Interest on total investment @ 17% per annum	Rs.	6,36,000.00
Insurance	Rs.	6000.00
40 per cent of salary and wages	Rs.	1,98,720.00
40 per cent of other contingent expenses	Rs.	1,20,000.00
Total fixed cost	Rs.	10,81,559.00
Say	Rs.	10,81,600.00

$$BEP = \frac{\text{Fixed cost} \times 100}{\text{Fixed cost} + \text{Net profit}}$$

$$= \frac{10,81,500 \times 100}{10,81,500 + 10,37,400} = 51.04\%$$

EUGENOL (FROM CLOVE OIL)

Eugenol is the characteristic constituents of the oils of cloves, cinnamon leaf, bay and pimento and is also found in numerous other essential oils. It is a liquid of powerful clove odour.

It has the following constitution:

Molecular formula: $C_{10}H_{12}O_2$

Eugenol
(Molecular mass 164.21)

Market

Eugenol is important raw material in creation of perfumes and flavours. It is used extensively in dental flavours. It is used in manufacture of vanillin. Many synthetic derivatives like methyl eugenol, eugenyl acetate, iso eugenol and its derivatives are made out of eugenol.

Basis and Presumptions

Efficiency and working hours	8 working hours/day/shift and 300 working days taken into account annually
Time period for achieving full/envisaged capacity utilisation	Within a year after trial production
Labour and wages	As per local conditions
Interest rate for fixed and working capital	The rate of interest for term loan as well as for working capital is taken as 17 per cent which may vary depending upon quantum of loan required
Margin money	Average 25 per cent
Operative period of the project	10 years
Land cost and construction cost	Rs. 5.9 lakhs
Costing of machinery and equipments	The cost of machinery and equipments, raw materials and the selling prices of the finished product are those which are existing in the market and they may vary from time to time and place to place

Implementation Schedule

Provisional registration	15 days
Sanctioning of loan	3 months
Acquisition of land and building construction	6 months
Procurement and erection of plant and machinery	2 months
Recruitment of personnel and trial run	1 month

Technical Aspects

Process outline

This scheme is based on the extraction of eugenol from essential oils such as clove oil containing 85–90 per cent eugenol. Cinnamon leaf oil (75–85 per cent), Pemento (80 per cent) and bay oil (50 per cent). The following method may be used for the extraction of eugenol from these oils:

The crude oil (clove oil) cinnamon leaf oil/pimento/bay oil, is taken in the reaction vessel fitted with agitator — 5 per cent solution of sodium hydroxide is then added into it. The mixture is agitated for about half an hour and left for separation of layer for 24 hours. The aqueous layer contains soluble sodium salt of eugenol 0:1 layer contains noneugenol. Alkaline aqueous layer is taken into neutralisation tank and acidified with 10 per cent hydrochloric acid. Liberated eugenol (0:1) is washed free of acid and then purified by fractional distillation. Distilled eugenol is packed in aluminium bottles.

Quality specifications

Bureau of Indian Standards (BIS) has laid down specification BIS: 3925–1980 for eugenol.

Annual production capacity

Sr. no.	Items	Quantity (kg)	Value (Rs.)
1.	Eugenol	25,000	93,73,000
2.	Eugenated oil (waste oil containing caryaphyllene eugenolacctate and other matter)	6000	15,00,000.00
3.	Approximate motive power	5 HP	

Pollution control

There is small quantity of effluent which is acidic/alkaline in nature and has to be neutralised. Thus, neutralising tanks are required for this purpose before the effluent is discharged to the drain. Exhaust fan is needed to keep the factory shed neat and clean.

Energy conservation

There is not much requirement of power, however, precautions must be taken while selecting electric motors which should be as per relevant standards.

Financial Aspects

Fixed capital

Land and building

Land 300 sq. m. @ Rs. 400 per sq. m.	Rs. 1,20,000.00
Built area, office stores and working shed 300 sq. m. @ Rs. 2000	Rs. 6,00,000.00
Total	Rs. 7,20,000.00

Machinery and equipments

Sl. no.	Description	Indigenous/ imported	Quantity	Price (Rs.)
1.	S.S. Reaction with stirrer 200 MS capacity	Indigenous	1	1,00,000.00
2.	S.S. settling tank 200 litres capacity	Indigenous	4	1,60,000.00
3.	S.S. Neutralisation tank 300 litres capacity	Indigenous	2	80,000.00
4.	Washing tank S.S. capacity 500 litres	Indigenous	2	1,20,000.00
5.	Distillation unit 200 litres capacity (SS)	Indigenous	1	1,75,000.00
6.	Boiler	Indigenous	1	2,00,000.00
7.	Testing equipments	Indigenous		50,000.00
8.	Electrification and installation @ 10%			88,500.00
			Total	9,73,500.00

Cost of office equipment/working tables, etc.   Rs.   30,000.00

Pre-operative expenses

Total fixed capital:

(Fixed capital + machinery and equipments + preoperative expenses)		Rs.	25,000.00
	Total	Rs.	17,48,500.00

Working capital (per month)

Personnel

Designation	No.	Salary (Rs.)	Total (Rs.)
Manager-cum-manufacturing chemist	1	8000	8000.00
Analyst-cum-Supervisor	1	6000	6000.00
Accountant-cum-office assistant	1	5000	5000.00
Typist/storekeeper	1	4000	4000.00
Skilled worker	2	3000	6000.00
Unskilled worker	2	2500	5000.00
Peon-cum-watchman	2	2000	4000.00
Total salaries			41000.00
+ Perquisite @ 15% of salary			6150.00
	Total		47,150.00
	Say		47,100.00

Raw materials (per month)

Sr. no.	Particulars	Indigenous/ imported	Quantity (kg)	Rate/ kg (Rs.)	Value (Rs.)
1.	Crude clove oil	Indigenous	2000	328	6,50,000.00
2.	Caustic soda	Indigenous	20	20	400.00
3.	Hydrochloric acid	Indigenous	30	4	120.00
4.	Laboratory chemicals indicators, reagents, etc.	Indigenous	–	–	2500.00
5.	Packaging material (Glass bottles, cartoons BOPP tapes, etc.)				20,000.00
	Total cost of raw materials				673070.00
				Say	6,73,000.00

Utilities

Power		Rs.	3000.00
Fuel		Rs.	10000.00
Water		Rs.	500.00
	Total	Rs.	13,500.00

Other contingent expenses (per month)

Postage, stationery and telephone	Rs.	2000.00
Consumable stores	Rs.	2000.00

Repair and maintenance		Rs.	2000.00
Transport charges		Rs.	5000.00
Advertisement		Rs.	2500.00
Insurance		Rs.	500.00
Miscellaneous expenses		Rs.	2000.00
	Total	Rs.	16,000.00

Total working capital

Staff and labour		Rs.	47,100.00
Raw material		Rs.	6.73,000.00
Utilities		Rs.	13,500.00
Other contingent expenses		Rs.	16,000.00
	Total	Rs.	7,49,600.00

Total capital investment

Fixed capital		Rs.	17,48,500.00
Working capital (for 3 months)		Rs.	22,48,800.00
	Total	Rs.	39,97,300.00

Financial Analysis

Cost of production (per year)

Total recurring cost		Rs.	81,95,200.00
Depreciation on plant and machinery @ 10% p.a.		Rs.	97,350.00
Depreciation on office equipment @ 20%		Rs.	6000.00
Depreciation on building @ 5%		Rs.	30000.00
Interest on total investment @ 17%		Rs.	6,79,541.00
	Total	Rs.	98,08,091.00
	Say	Rs.	98,08,100.00

Turn over (per year)

By sale of 25000 kgs. of eugenol @ Rs. 375/kg.		Rs.	93,75,000.00
Eugenated oil 6000 kgs.@ 250 per kg.		Rs.	15,00,000.00
	Total	Rs.	10,87,75,000.00

Net profit (before income tax)

Turnover	–	Cost of production	=	Net profit
1,08,75,000		98,08,100		10,66,900

Net profit ratio

Net profit ratio. $\dfrac{10,66,900 \times 100}{1,87,75,000}$ = 9.81%

Rate of return

Rate of return

$$\frac{10,66,900 \times 100}{39,97,300} = 26.69\%$$

Break-even Point (percentage of total production envisaged)

B.E.P. $\quad = \quad \dfrac{\text{Fixed cost} \times 100}{\text{Fixed cost} + \text{annual profit}}$

Fixed cost

Depreciation on machinery and equipment @ 10%	Rs.	97,350.00
Depreciation on building @ 5%	Rs.	35,000.00
Interest on total investment @ 17%	Rs.	5,79,541.00
Insurance	Rs.	6000.00
40% of salary and wages	Rs.	2,26,080.00
40% of other contingent expenses	Rs.	76,800.00
Total	Rs.	11,15,771.00
Say	Rs.	11,15,800.00

B.E.P. $\quad = \dfrac{\text{Fixed cost} \times 100}{\text{Fixed cost} + \text{Net profit}}$

$$\frac{11,15,800 \times 100}{21,82,100} = 51.13\%$$

CITRONELLA OIL

Citronella oil is obtained from two taxonomically proximal by morphologically distinguishable species. These species are chymbopogam nardus rendle, Sri Lanka variety and cymbopogan winterianus Jowitt Java citronella oil variety. Java citronella is superior than Sri Lanka citronella in terms of oil yield and quality of oil. Java citronella oil is very important essential oil widely used in perfumery and cosmetic industries. Oil is having importance due to presence of citronellal, geraniol, etc. in the oil. These aromatic chemicals can be converted to widely used perfumery product like citronellol, hydroxy citronellal, synthetic menthol, esters of gerniol and citronellol etc. Sri Lanka type of oil is used in cheap variety of perfume disinfectant and polishes.

Citronella oil is obtained from distillation of citronella grass which is a semi-perennial grass. The leaves of the grass are light green having about 1 to 2 cm broad and about 1.5 to 2 metres length.

Planting can be done through slips. Generally planting is done from onset of monsoon. But under irrigated conditions the crop can be raised throughout the year. Slips take three weeks to establish. The manure requirements is 200 kg to 300 kg of nitrogen, 100 kg of phosphate and 50 kg of potash per hectare per year. The crop provides three to four harvests per year. The first cutting is done after six months to nine months of planting and subsequent cutting are taken at an interval of 3 to 4 months. The per hectare yield of grass is 40 to 50 tons per year in first year which can go up to 60 tons per year in subsequent years. The yield of oil is 300 to 400 kg per hectare per year.

Market Potential

Citronella oil is widely used for isolation of various perfumery chemicals as well as it is used in various perfumery and cosmetic industries.

Citronella oil is also used in soap, detergents, disinfectant and polishes, etc. Due to its wide use and cheapness this oil is having export potential.

It is mainly cultivated in Assam, Tamil Nadu, Maharashtra, Karnataka, Andhra Pradesh and Orissa. In the world, China, Taiwan, Guatemala, Indonesia and Malaysia are the major producers of citronella oil. The annual world production of citronella oil is around 2500 MT. It has export potential to USA, UK, Iran, West Germany, Japan, and Hong Kong, etc.

Some parts of Orissa, where rainfall is more (2500 mm) and adequate irrigation facilities available, citronella grass is successfully cultivated.

Basis and Presumption

1. All the estimates in respect of land, building, machinery, etc. are drawn as per the prevailing prices during the preparation of scheme.
2. Land is taken on lease basis.
3. 60–70 per cent efficiency of full capacity utilisation and single shift working hours have been considered in preparation of scheme.
4. Interest rate @ 17 per cent has been considered.
5. Margin money to the extent of 25 per cent of total project cost is required by the entrepreneurs as own investment in implementing the project.
6. Minimum wages has been considered in preparation of scheme.
7. Two to three years period is considered as pay back period.

Implementation Schedule

1.	Preparation of project report	1 month
2.	Selection of site after soil testing	1 month
3.	Development of land and planting of material	3 months
4.	Registration of unit	1 month
5.	Availability of loan/finance	2 months
6.	Procurement of machinery	2 months
7.	Erection and commissioning	1 month
8.	Recruitment of staff	1 month
	Total	12 months

Technical Aspect

Cultivation/soil

Java citronella is a semi-perennial grass with reduced subsurface to surface level stem (stolen) with light green leaves, having about 1 to 2 cm broad and about 1.0 to 1.5 metres length. Though citronella requires well distributed rainfall (2000–2500 mm) persistently high relative humidity and a moderate temperature for its growth but it can also withstand drought, adjusting the harvest frequencies. Though citronella can be grown upto 900 MT above sea level, well drained alluvial, sandy loam soils are suitable for its cultivation. Hill slopes are most suitable for this crop.

Two to three times ploughed, well drained, slightly sloppy land are suitable for citronella cultivation. The citronella is propagated through slips. The slips from matured clumps are cleaned by removing dried leaves and long roots and three to four slips are planted at a spacing of 50 × 50 cm apart which can be enhanced to 90 × 90 cm in fertile areas.

Generally, citronella planting is done from onset of monsoon. But under irrigated conditions the crop can be raised throughout the year. The slips take three weeks, to establish. Weeding is essential before harvesting for good growth.

Manuring

The normal manorial requirement of citronella is 200 to 300 kg of nitrogen. 100 kg of phosphate and 50 kg of potash per hectare per year. Half of phosphate and potash are applied before planting and rest after a month of planting the crop. Nitrogen is manured in equal splits after each cutting in a year.

Field is also dusted with aldrin at the rate of 50 kg per hectare before planting to protect the slips from white ant damage. The crop mostly grow healthy except some fungal infection during rainy season. 0.3 per cent Bavistin with endrin folidol can be sprayed 15 days after harvest as a protective measure to the crop.

In well distributed rainfall areas irrigation is not required. In any regions the crop requires at least one to two irrigation per month for better growth.

Harvesting, distillation, processing and storing of oil

The crop provides three harvest per year. For better clump stability and herby) yield the first cutting is done after six months to nine months of planting and the subsequent cuttings are taken at an interval of 3 to 4 months. During first year, the herb yield varied 40 to 50 tons per hectare which can be increased upto 60 tons in subsequent years.

The herb is generally distilled immediately after harvest of the grass. The grass can be kept for a few days after cutting but it should not get damaged due to fungal growth for fermentation which will affect the oil quality. The fresh herb on hydro distillation produces 0.6 to 0.8 per cent oil in rainy season and 1.0 to 1.2 per cent oil in dry season. The oil yield varies from 300 to 400 kg per hectare per year. The distilled oil is made moisture free by adding anhydrous sodium sulphate and packed in aluminium containers and stored in dark place.

Distillation Process

Citronella oil is produced from the stem, leaves and flowers of citronella grass by hydro and steam distillation process. In the process charge is kept over a false bottom and it should be kept out of contact of boiling water. The lower part of the still is filled with water to a level just below the perforated grid or false bottom. The water is heated by direct fire at the bottom. Low pressure wet steam is generated and rises through the plant material.

The special characteristics of this method is that the steam is always saturated and never superheated. The plant materials is always in contact with the steam only and not with boiling water and thus prevents the scope of hydrolysis.

The steam carried oil with it and then passes to condenser where on cooling it is condensed in form of liquid and collected in a receiver. It takes 2 to 3 hours to distil the oil for complete distillation of one batch. The oil being lighter in weight than water can be then separated by decantation or by separating funnel. The water beneath the perforated grid should be discarded after the distillation is over and replaced with fresh water. It is necessary because soluble matter from the plant material collects in water and repeated use may cause the decomposition of the water soluble matter causing disagreeable odour.

Alternate Technology

There are various ways of distillation such as water distillation, water and steam distillation, steam distillation, distillation under reduced pressure. But water and steam distillation are most suitable and economical for Citronella oil because of simplicity. The still can be easily installed in the form thereby cutting transportation cost and avoiding disposable problems of spent up grass.

Quality control/specifications

For proper quality control of citronella oil BIS specification No. 512–1988 may be referred to.

Production capacity (per annum)

Quality	10,000 kg
Value	Rs. 27,50,000.00

Pollution control

There is not much pollution in such type of industry. Fuel should be stored preferably in a cemented floor and proper chimney height should be provided. Workers should be provided with mask and gloves. Spent grass should be properly disposed off. Spent grass is used for paper making.

Energy conservation

Though there is not much scope in energy conservation in this process. However, some conservation of energy can be achieved by using insulating material in still which can save considerable amount of heat and thereby cutting down the cost of fuel. The most effective material for insulation is asbestos which is available in various forms. An insulation thickness of 55 mm has been found to be good enough for preventing the heat loss through surfaces.

Financial Aspects

Fixed capital

Land and building

Rent of land on lease for 5 hectares for 50 years @ Rs. 1000 per acre per year		Rs.	1,28,000.00
Distillation shed 30′ × 80′ = 2400 sft @ Rs. 1 00 sq. ft		Rs.	2,40,000.00
Raw material shed 30′ × 50′ = 1500 sq. ft @ Rs. 75 per sq. ft		Rs.	1,12,500.00
Office-cum-store 500 sq. ft @ Rs. 150 sq. ft		Rs.	75,000.00
	Total	Rs.	5,55,500.00

Plant and machinery

Description	No.	Value (Rs.)
Distillation still and accessories (5 distillation units 500 kg capacity) @ Rs. 1,10,000 each	5	5,50,000.00
Ordinary furnaces	5	10,000.00
Tools and equipment	–	25,000.00
Agricultural implements tube well and irrigation channel	2	1,00,000.00

Laboratory and testing equipment	–	35,000.00
Installation and electrification	–	72,000.00
Office furniture and fixture	–	25,000.00
Total		8,17,000.00

Pre-operative expenses

Pre-operative expenses	25000.00
Total fixed capital	
(Land and building + plant and machinery + preoperative expenses)	13,97,500.00

Working Capital

Staff and labour (per month)

Designation	No.	Salary (Rs.)	Total salary (Rs.)
Manager	1	7000	7000.00
Chemist/Production manager	1	6000	6000.00
Accountant	1	4000	4000.00
Operator	3	2500	7500.00
Skilled workers	2	2500	5000.00
Unskilled workers	5	2000	10,000.00
Peon/Watchman	1	2000	2000.00
Sales man	2	4000	8000.00
			32,500.00
	Perquisites @ 15%		4875.00
		Total	37,375.00
		Say	37,400.00

Raw materials

Manuring	70,000.00
Packing materials, aluminium containers	30,000.00
Total	1,00,000.00

Utilities (per month)

Electricity	6000.00
Fuel	5000.00
Water	1000.00
Total	12,000.00

Other contingent (per month)

Stationery	1000.00
Telephone	2000.00
Rent	2500.00
Travelling and transport	5000.00
Advertisement	1500.00

Insurance		5000.00
Maintenance/repairing		3000.00
Miscellaneous expenditure		2500.00
	Total	22,500.00

Working Capital (per month)

Staff and labour		37,400.00
Raw materials		1,00,000.00
Utilities		12,000.00
Other contingent expenses		18,000.00
	Total	1,87,400.00
Working capital for 3 months		5,02,200.00

Total capital investment

Fixed capital		13,97,500.00
Working capital for 3 months		5,02,200.00
	Total	18,99,700.00

Cost of production (per annum)

Recurring cost per annum		20,08,800.00
Depreciation on plant and machinery @ 10%		79,200.00
Depreciation on land and building @ 5%		27,775.00
Depreciation on office equipments @ 20%		5000.00
Interest on total investment @ 17%		3,22,949.00
	Total	24,43,724.00
	Say	24,43,700.00

Turnover

Sr. No.	Item	Quantity	Rate	Total value (Rs.)
1.	Citronella oil	10,000 kg	@ Rs. 275 per kg	27,50,000.00

Profit	=	Turnover	−	Cost of production	=	Net profit
		27,50,000.00	−	24,43,700.00	=	3,06,300.00

Net profit ratio = $\dfrac{3,06,300 \times 100}{27,50,000}$ = 11%

Rate of return = $\dfrac{3,06,300 \times 100}{18,99,700}$ = 16.2%

Breakeven analysis

Fixed cost

Depreciation on plant and machinery	79,200.00
Rent	30,000.00
Interest on total investment	3,22,949.00

Insurance	6000.00
40% of annual salary and wages	1,79,520.00
40% of other contingent expenses (except rent and insurance)	86,400.00
Total	7,04,069.00
Say	7,04,100.00

$$\text{B.E.P.} = \frac{\text{F.C.} \times 100}{\text{F.C.} + \text{profit}} = \frac{7,04,100 \times 100}{10,10,400} = 59.83\%$$

PERFUMERY COMPOUND

A perfume may be defined as any mixture of pleasantly odourous substance incorporated in a suitable vehicle or it is a blend of two or more essence incorporated in a suitable vehicle or solvents. Originally, all the products used in perfumery were of natural origin but with the advancement in various aromatic synthetic chemical modern perfume are neither wholly synthetic nor yet completely natural. The best perfume is the art of judicious blend of two, i.e. natural as well as synthetic to balance the prices of the product and to introduce new notes of fragrance into the enhancing gamut at present available. A product made solely of synthetics tends to coarse and unnatural because of the absence of impurities in minute amounts which finish and round out the bouquets of the natural odour.

The common vehicles are modern solvent for blending perfume materials is highly refined ethyl alcohol mixed with more or less water according to solubilities of the oils employed. This solvent, with its volatile nature help to project the scent it carries is fairly inert to the solute and is not irritating to the human skin. To retain the good essence in perfume certain fixative are used which are the substances of lower volatility than the perfume oils which retard and even up the rate of evaporation of the various odourous constituents. The fixative may be animal secretion, resinous product, essential oil and synthetic chemicals. The example of different type of fixative are indicated as under.

Animal Fixative

Costor or castoreum, a brownish orange exudates of perennial glands of beaver.
    Civet — Secretion of perennial gland of civet cat.
    Musk — Secretions of perennial gland of male must deer.
Resinous: Benzoin and gums, myrrh and labdanum, balsam, etc.
Synthetic: Amyl benzoate, vanillin, phenyl ethyl alcohol, P.E. acetate, coumarin, cinamic alcohol, esters, acetophenone, musk ketone musk ambrette.

Market Potential

With the development of technology and synthetic odouriferous substances there are varieties of perfume and perfumery compound now available in the market and the demand for these odouriferous substances is also increasing very fast. The demand of such product is increasing specially due to change in life style, availability of different type of packaging materials and due to industrial development. These products are also having very good export potential.

Presently in the state of Orissa there are hardly very few units manufacturing perfumery compounds. However, it has very good scope for setting up of new units in the state.

Basis of Presumptions

1. The scheme is prepared on single shift basis and 300 working days per annum.
2. Full capacity utilisation will start from 3rd year onwards.
3. The cost of machinery, raw materials, finished product are taken as prevailing price in the market.
4. Interest rate taken @ 17 per cent per annum.
5. 25 per cent of the total investment is required as margin money.
6. Pay back period of the project will be 4 years.

Implementation Schedule

1. Preparation of project report	1 month
2. Selection of site	1 month
3. Availability of finance	2 months
4. Procurement of machineries	2 months
5. Registration of the unit	½ month
6. Recruitment of staff	½ month
7. Erection and commissioning	1 month
Total	9 months

Technical Aspect

Process outline

All the ingredients are mixed together as per required formulation in mixing tank fitted with mechanical stirrer. After completion of proper mixing the product should be packed in suitable pack. Package should contain weight batch, number, date of manufacture, expiry date, price of the product, etc. suitably printed.

Alternate technology

Manufacture of perfumery product do not require any sophisticated or various alternate technology. However, formulation of the product varies from manufacturer to manufacturer as per requirement and price of the product.

Quality Control and Standard

The product should be manufactured as per standard formulation under qualified production chemist and following specification should be followed for proper quality of the product:

BIS-2284/1988—For olfactory assessment
BIS-3261/1984(Pt.I)—Sampling and testing

Production capacity (per annum)

Quantity	150 MT
Value	Rs. 2,47,50,000.00

Pollution control

Production of perfumery compounds do not involve emission of any major pollutant in the environment. However, no objection certificate (NOC) to be obtained from state pollution control board. Workers to be provided with mask and hand gloves and processing section should be made dust free and hygienic.

Energy conservation

There is not much scope of energy conservation in perfumery compound manufacture unit. However, preventive steps should be taken to prevent unnecessary use of electric fan, light, etc.

Financial Aspects

Fixed capital

Land and building

Total covered area 200 sq. m. (rented)	Rs. 4000.00 per month

Machinery and equipment

Sr. No.	Name of machinery	No.	Value (Rs.)
1.	Mixer fitted with mechanical stirrer and 2 HP motor capacity 500 litres	1	1,25,000.00
2.	Sealing and filling machine	1	35,000.00
3.	Storage vessels (SS) 200 litres capacity	3	90,000.00
4.	Weighing machine platform type	1	10,000.00
5.	Laboratory equipments	–	25,000.00
6.	Miscellaneous apparatus	–	15,000.00
7.	Installation and electrification	–	30,000.00
8.	Office furniture, etc.	–	25,000.00
	Total		3,30,000.00

Preoperative expenses

Preoperative expenses	25,000.00
Total cost of fixed capital	3,60,000.00

Working capital (per month)

Staff and labour (per month)

Sr. No.	Designation	No.	Salary	Total salary (Rs.)
1.	Manager/production in-charge	1	7000	7000.00
2.	Chemist	1	5000	5000.00
3.	Skilled worker	2	2500	5000.00
4.	Unskilled worker	2	2000	4000.00
5.	Peon	1	2000	2000.00
6.	Salesman	1	4000	4000.00
			Total	27,000.00
			Perquisites @ 15%	4050.00
			Total	31,050.00
			Say	31,000.00

Raw material (per month)

Jasmine compound, citronella, fixative and other chemicals 12,600 kg	1,80,000.00

Utilities

Power		2000.00
Water		500.00
	Total	2500.00

Other contingential expenses (per month)

Advertisement and publicity		1500.00
Transport		2500.00
Rent		4000.00
Postage and stationery		5000.00
Packing charges		4000.00
Insurance		500.00
Miscellaneous		1500.00
	Total	15,000.00

Working Capital Requirement Per Month

Salary	31000.00
Raw materials	17,00,000.00
Utilities	25,000.00
Other contingential expenditure	15,000.00
Working capital for 3 months	55,45,500.00

Total capital investment

Working capital		55,45,500.00
Fixed capital		3,70,00.00
	Total	59,15,500.00

Cost of production (per annum)

Total recurring expenses		2,21,82,000.00
Depreciation on Machinery @ 10%		33,000.00
Depreciation on office furniture @ 20%		5000.00
Interest on total investment @ 17%		10,05,635.00
	Total	2,32,25,635.00
	Say	2,32,25,600.00

Total Sales

Sr. no.	Item	Quantity	Rate	Total value (Rs.)
1.	Perfume	150 MT	@165/kg	2,62,50,000.00

Profitability

Profit = Sales – C.P. = 2,47,50,000 – 2,32,25,600 = 15,24,400

$$\text{Net profit ratio} = \frac{\text{Profit} \times 100}{\text{Turnover}} = \frac{15,24,400 \times 100}{2,47,50,000} = 6.15\%$$

$$\text{Rate of return} - \frac{\text{Profit} \times 100}{\text{Total investment}} = \frac{15,24,400 \times 100}{59,15,800} = 25.76\%$$

Break-even analysis

Fixed cost

40% of annual salary	1,48,800.00
40% of other expenses (excluding rent and insurance)	50,000.00
Depreciation on machinery @ 10%	33,000.00
Depreciation on office furniture @ 20%	5000.00
Interest on total investment	10,05,600.00
Insurance	6000.00
Total	12,48,800.00

$$\text{B.E.P.} = \frac{\text{F.C.} \times 100}{\text{F.C.} + \text{profit}} = \frac{12,48,800 \times 100}{12,48,800 + 15,24,400} = 45\%$$

PALM ROSA OIL

If crop is harvested at full bloom or end of blooming oil yield can be achieved better. Palm rosa oil is obtained by Hydro or steam distillation.

Palm rosa oil is used in cosmetics, perfumery, soaps, detergent and flavouring tobacco. It is extensively used in India for adulterating attar or rose oil.

The Indian council of agricultural research institute (ICAR), council of scientific and industrial research (CSIR), council of aromatic plant research (CIMAP) organisations and various universities in India have worked in details on its agrotechnology. Various varieties of palm rosa have been developed by regional research laboratories (RRL), Bhubaneswar. Some of the varieties are named as:

RRL(b) 49, RRL (B) 69, RRL (B) 77, RRL (B) 77E,
IW-31245, IW-3630, Trishna, RRL-l, HR-85, etc.

Sl. No.		Growth stage oil %	Terpene	Linaloöl	Geranyl acetate	Geraniol
1.	Vegetative (75 days)	1.1%	3.8%	2.75%	20.46%	72.30%
2.	Commencement of flowering (85 days)	1.2%	5.2%	3.85%	21.36%	70.6%
3.	Full bloom stage (105–115 days)	0.4%	2.6%	2.6%	10–25%	85.30%
4.	Late seedling (125 days)	1.6%	1.6%	3.45%	6.46%	87.56%

Market Potential

Palm rosa oil is widely used in cosmetics, perfumery, soap and detergent, flavouring of tobacco and for making attar, etc. Due to its wide application, it has good demand in the country.

Presently, there are about 60 numbers of units engaged in production of palm rosa oil all over the country and about 1500 hectare of area is under palm rosa cultivation producing 200–250 MT of oil annually.

In Orissa there are 12 numbers of small scale units engaged in cultivation and processing of palm rosa oil mainly located in Ganjam, Puri and Khurda districts. These units are adopting technology supplied by RRL, Bhubaneswar. The approximate capacity of these units is about 150 MT of oil per annum. The price of the oil varies from time to time depending upon various factors, average rate of the oil is about Rs. 350–400 per kg. Palm rosa oil is not having good demand only in the country but also have good export potential. It is mainly exported to Brazil, Argentina, Indonesia and Guatemala, etc.

Keeping in view its wide use and export potential it is assumed that there is good prospect to setup some new units in the state and the country.

Basis and Presumption

1. All the estimates in respect of land, building, machinery, etc. are drawn as per the prevailing prices during the preparation of scheme.
2. Land is taken on lease basis.
3. 60–70 per cent efficiency of full capacity utilisation and single shift working hours have been considered in preparation of scheme.
4. Interest rate @ 17 per cent has been considered.
5. Margin money to the extent of 25 per cent of total project cost is required by the entrepreneurs as own investment in implementing the project.
6. Minimum wages has been considered in preparation of scheme.
7. Two to three years period is considered as pay back period.

Implementation Schedule

1. Time required for preparation of the project report — 1 month
2. Selection of site — 2 months
3. Registration of the unit — 1 month
4. Availability of loan/finance — 4 months
5. Machinery procurement — 2 months
6. Erection and commissioning — 1 month
7. Recruitment of staff — 1 month

Technical Aspect

Cultivation

Palm rosa is a perennial grass once planted, it continues to give economic yield upto 10 years. The field is well prepared before seedling or plantation. Plantation can be done in two ways:

1. Plantation through preparing nursery bed: In this method nurseries are prepared 25 cm × 25 cm size at the end of last week of May in which seeds are mixed with soil and sown by scattering. Germination starts after 4–5 days and nursery is ready within 40 to 45 days for plantation, 40–45 seedling are then transplanted in well prepared level field at a spacing of 60 × 30 cm at the set of monsoon.
2. Plantation through seeds: In this method seeds are sown in well prepared land in line of 4 cm deep at a distance of 60 cm. The dense seedling should be replaced in other places, water content

should be limited in the field till seedling grows upto 8 to 10 cm, 10 to 12 kg seeds are enough per hectare of land.

Soil and climate

Palm rosa grows well in rainfed to irrigated areas from sea level to 1000 MT. Elevation in well drained slight acidic to neutral soil, though it can be cultivated in alkali soil. Frost and winter is detrimental to its growth.

Manuring

The crop is being manured with 10 cart loads of farm yard manure at field preparation. It requires 100 kg nitrogen, 100 kg phosphate and 50 kg potash per hectare per year. P and K are provided in two equal splits, i.e. 1st as basal and 2nd after first cutting. Nitrogen is manured in three equal splits in a year, i.e. 15 days after transplanting and then after each cutting.

Disease and pest control

White ants usually attacks the dried clumps. Spreading BHC/aldrin 10 kg/ha protects the field. The minor disease and pest can be controlled by spraying Blitox and folidol once during each cutting.

Process of Manufacturing

Harvesting, distillation, processing and storing of oil: The crop is being cut 8 to 10 cm above ground and carried to distillation site.

The fresh or one to two days dried herbs are distilled by direct heating or by feeding steam. The distilled oil are made moisture free by adding common salt or sodium sulphate and packed in galvanised containers and stored in dark place.

First harvesting of grass can be done after 30 days of plantation and crop can be harvested 3–4 times in a year through which 300–350 quintals of fresh grass can be obtained per hectare of land. The leaves and stem of palm rosa contain 0.4 to 0.5 per cent of oil. Accordingly 100 kg to 125 kg of oil can be obtained per hectare of land per year.

Distillation process

Palm rosa oil is produced from the stem, leaves and flowers of palm rosa grass by hydro and steam distillation process. In the process charge is kept over a false bottom and it should be kept out of contact of boiling water. The lower part of the still is filled with water to a level just below the perforated grid or false bottom. The water is heated by direct fire at the bottom. Low pressure wet steam is generated and rises through the plant material. The special characteristics of this method is that the steam is always saturated and never superheated. The plant material is always in contact with the steam only not with boiling water and thus prevents the scope of hydrolysis.

The steam carries oil with it and then passes to condenser where on cooling, it is condensed in form of liquid and collected in a receiver. It takes to distil the oil for about 2–3 hours for complete distillation of one batch. The oil being lighter in weight than water can be then separated by decantation or by separating funnel.

The water beneath the perforated grid should be discarded after the distillation is over and replaced with fresh water. It is necessary because soluble matter from the plant material collects in water and repeated use may cause the decomposition of the water soluble matter causing disagreeable odour.

Alternate technology

There are various ways of distillation such as water distillation, water and steam distillation, steam distillation, distillation under reduced pressure but water and steam distillation is most suitable and economic for palm rosa oil because of simplicity. The still can be easily installed in the firm thereby cutting transportation cost and avoiding disposable problems of spent up grass.

Quality Control/Specification

It requires proper quality control. As per BIS-526-1968 its: (i) refractive index 1.4.69–1.4745 at 30°C, (ii) specific gravity 0.874–0.8860, (iii) optical rotation—2° to +3°, (iv) acid value—max 3.0, and (v) total alcohol calculated as geraniol – min 90 per cent.

	Production capacity (per annum)	
	Quantity	10000 kg
	Value	Rs. 27,50,000 (@ Rs. 350/kg)
Approximately motive power requirement		10 kwh

Pollution control

There is not much pollution in such type of industry. Fuel should be stored preferably in a cemented floor and proper chimney height should be provided and care should be taken for complete burning of fuel and minimising the air pollution. Worker should be provided mask and gloves and spent grass should be properly disposed of.

Energy conservation

Though there is not much scope in energy conservation in this process; however, some consideration of energy can be achieved by using insulating material in still which can save considerable amount of heat and thereby cutting down the cost of fuel. The most effective material for insulation is asbestos which is available in various forms. An insulation thickness of 55 mm has been found to be good enough for preventing the heat loss through surfaces.

Financial Aspect

Fixed capital

Land and building

Land 5000 sq. ft @ Rs. 35/sq. ft	1,75,000.00
Distillation shed (20′ × 100′) @ Rs. 100/sq. ft 2000 sq. ft	2,00,000.00
Raw material shed (20′ × 50′) @ Rs. 80/sq. ft	8000.00
Office-cum-store 800 sq. ft @ Rs. 300/sq. ft	2,40,000.00
Total	6,95,000.00

Plant and machinery

Sr. No.	Description	Nos.	Value (Rs.)
1.	Distillation still and accessories (10 distillation units 500 kg cap. @ 1,00,000 each)	10	10,00,000.00
2	Equipments, tools, etc.		25,000.00
3	Ordinary furnaces		20,000.00

4	Lab and testing equipment	35,000.00
		10,80,000.00
5	Installation and electrification	1,00,000.00
6	Office furniture and fixtures	25,000.00
	Total	12,05,000.00

Pre-operative expenses

	Preoperative expenses	
	Total fixed capital	25,000.00
	(Land and building + plant and machinery + preoperative expenses)	10,25,000.00

Working Capital

Sr. no.	Designation	No.	Salary	Total salaries (Rs.)
1.	Manager	1	7000	7000.00
2.	Chemist/Production manager	1	6000	6000.00
3.	Accountant	1	4000	4000.00
4.	Distiller	3	2500	7000.00
5.	Skilled worker	2	2500	5000.00
6.	Unskilled worker	2	2000	4000.00
7.	Peon/watchman	1	2000	2000.00
				34,000.00
	Perquisites @ 15%			5100.00
	Total			39,100.00

Raw materials (per month)

Palm rosa leaves steam		70,000.00
Packing material, aluminium containers		20,000.00
	Total	90,000.00

Utilities

Electricity	6000.00
Fuel	5000.00
Water	1000.00

Other contingent expenses (per annum)

Stationery and postage		1000.00
Telephone		2000.00
Rent		1500.00
Travelling and transport		500.00
Advertisement		2500.00
Insurance		500.00
Maintenance and repairing		3000.00
Miscellaneous expenses		3000.00
	Total	18,500.00

Working capital (per month)

Staff and labour		39,100.00
Raw materials		90,000.00
Utilities		12,000.00
Other contingent expenses		18,500.00
	Total	1,59,600.00

Working capital for 3 months		4,74,800.00
Total capital investment		
Fixed capital		19,25,000.00
Working capital		4,74,800.00
	Total	24,03,800.00

Machinery utilisation: 60 per cent

Financial Analysis

Cost of production (per annum)

Total recurring cost per month		14,22,900.00
Depreciation on plant and machinery @ 10%		1,08,000.00
Depreciation on land and building @ 5%		34,750.00
Depreciation on office equipment @ 20%		5000.00
Interest on total investment @ 17%		4,08,646.00
	Total	19,79,296.00
	Say	19,79,300.00

Turnover

Sr. no.	Item	Quantity/rate	Total value (Rs.)
1.	Palm rosa oil	10000 kg @ Rs. 275 per kg	27,50,000.00

$$\text{Profit} = \text{Turnover} - \text{cost of production}$$
$$27,50,000 - 19,79,300 = 7,70,700$$

$$\text{Net profit ratio} = \frac{\text{Net profit} \times 100}{\text{Turnover}} = \frac{7,70,700 \times 100}{27,50,000} = 28\%$$

$$\text{Rate of return} = \frac{\text{Net profit} \times 100}{\text{Total investment}} = \frac{7,70,700 \times 100}{24,03,800} = 32\%$$

Break even point analysis

Fixed cost

Depreciation on plant and machinery	1,13,000.00
Rent	18,000.00
Interest on total investment	4,08,600.00
Insurance	6000.00
50 per cent of salary and wages	1,87,700.00

40 per cent of other expenses		81,000.00
	Total	8,14,900.00

$$\text{B.E.P.} = \frac{\text{F.C.} \times 100}{\text{F.C.} + \text{profit}} = \frac{8,14,900 \times 100}{15,85,600} = 51\%$$

CHAMOMILE OIL

Essential oil obtained from the flower of German chamomile (*Matricaria chamomilla* L.) belonging to the family compositae is commercially known as 'chamomile oil'. It is also known as 'blue oil' in trade. Since it is very extensively cultivated and used in Germany, chamomile has come to be known as German Chamomile. There are two other species Roman or Egyptian chamomile and Moroccon chamomile. In India experimental cultivation of German chamomile was started in Jammu and Srinagar. The efforts to domesticate this important essential oil plant in eastern UP condition by CIMAP, Lucknow, national botanical research institute (NBRI), Lucknow have shown that not only the plant can be grown as a crop successfully but also the quality of oil is maintained to the best of standards. Chamomile oil is used in medicines, perfumes and cosmetics.

Chemical Composition

Matricaria oil (blue oil) possesses a peculiar odour and bitter aromatic flavour. The blue colour of the oil is due to the presence of Azulene (1–15 per cent). The oil also contains, matricaria ester, chamazulene, bisabolene and other terpenoids. The molecular formula of major components of matricaria oil are given as under:

Azulene

Chamazulene

Bisabolene

$$CH_3-CH=CH-C\equiv C-C\equiv C-CH=CH-COOCH_3$$

Matricaria ester

Salient features of Matricaria oil

Appearance	Deep blue viscous liquid
Odour	Strong and characteristic odour and bitter aromatic flavour
Specific gravity at 15°C	0.917 to 0.957
Acid number	5 to 50
Ester number	3 to 39
Ester number after acetylation	117 to 155
Solubility at 25°C	Even in 95 per cent alcohol soluble only with more or less pronounced separation of paraffins
Refractive index at 20°C	1.442–1.457
Optical rotation at 20°C	−1° + 3°

Market

Matricaria oil is widely used in the manufacture of pharmaceuticals and cosmetics industries. There is a great demand of matricaria oil in European countries. Since the plant has a wide range of adaptability to climate and soil, it can be grown and can be extracted on marginal soils rendered unfit for growing other economic crops.

Basis and Presumption

Working hours/shift	08 hours
Number of shift/day	One
Number of working days/annum	300
Working efficiency	75%
Time period for achieving maximum capacity	3rd year from the date of production
Labour charges	As per local conditions
Margin money	25%
Rate of interest on fixed and working capital	17%
Operative period of the project	15 years

Implementation Schedule

Preparation of project report	4 weeks
Provisional registration	1 week
Sanction of loan from bank/financial institutions	2 months
Acquisition of land and building construction	3 months
Procurement and erection of plant and machinery	2 months
Recruitment of personnel and trial run	1 month

Technical Aspects

Harvesting

The crop starts blooming from middle of February and continues till middle of April. The crop is harvested by plucking of the flowers by hand or flower scoops or strippers. When using these implements the harvesters must gather the flowers as carefully and with as little stem materials and extraneous matter as possible. The flowers are picked at the full bloom stage but not at over matured flowers stage which causes a significant decrease of oil content in the flowers. The full bloom stage is indicated by the uniformly deep yellow colour of the compound flower with the ray florets directed downwards.

Yield

From a good crop on an average 4.5 to 6.0 tons of fresh flowers can be obtained per hectare. The harvested flowers are immediately transferred to the drying shed and spread over to the ground in very thin layers and allowed to dry. Five kilograms of fresh flowers give 1 kg of air dried flowers. Shade dried flowers are steam distilled and yield about 0.8 to 2.0 per cent deep blue oil with strong smell.

Process outline

The shade dried flowers are steam distilled to obtain oil from them. The distillation must be carried out using steam of high pressure, because oil of chamomile consists chiefly of high boiling constituents, including paraffins.

Distillation of one charge requires from 7 to 13 hours. Chamomile oil may separate crystals even at 15°C, and has a tendency to form a deposit on the cool walls inside of the condenser tube. It is, therefore, necessary to stop the flow of the cooling water from time to time until the temperature of the condenser rises sufficiently for the deposit to reliquefy and flow off.

Certain constituents of the oil are soluble in large quantities of warm water, moreover the oil has a high specific gravity and tends to flow off with the distillation water in the form of a milky emulsion. For these reasons the distillation water must be cohobated, by this means as much as 30 per cent of the total oil distilled over may be recovered. On distillation of the oil the paraffins remains in the residue as a dark mass, easily soluble in other, but sparingly soluble in alcohol. The paraffin tends to retain the blue colour of the oil most tenaciously.

Quality specification

As per customer requirements, Bureau of Indian Standards has not laid down any specification so far.

Annual production capacity

Quantity	160 kg
Value	Rs. 41,60,000

Approximate motive power required

Approximate motive power required	10 HP

Pollution control

The distillation of matricalia oil from matricaria flower does not need any steps to be taken for the pollution control as no effluents to be produced are responsible for air and water pollution. However, the entrepreneurs are advised to take a no objection certificate from the State Pollution Control Board before commencement of the production.

Energy conservation

The fuel for the steam production in the boiler is coal or light diesel oil (LDO) depending upon the type of boiler. Proper care should be taken while utilising the fuel for the production of steam. It should be fed depending upon the requirement of the steam in production.

Financial Analysis

Fixed capital

Land and building

Land 400 sq. m. @ 400 value built area,		
Office, stores, etc. 150 sq. m. @ 3000		1,60,000.00
Working shed 150 sq. m. @ Rs.2500		4,50,000.00
Total cost		3,75,000.00
	Total	9,85,000.00

Machinery and equipments

Distillation still MS with pulse and discharge holes, steam pipes, etc. capacity 1 MT	1	2,00,000.00

Multitube condenser made of SS tubes with copper outer shed	2	1,50,000.00
Boiler	1	2,00,000.00
Platform weighing balance	1	50,000.00
Electrification and installation charges @ 10% on the cost of machine and equipments		61,500.00
Total cost of machinery and equipments		6,76,500.00
Furniture and fixture including office equipment		50,000.00
	Total	7,26,500.00

Pre-operative expenses

Pre-operative expenses	20,000.00
Total fixed capital (Land and building + machinery and equipments + preoperative expenses)	17,31,500.00

Working capital

Personnel

Sr. No.	Designation	No.	Salary	Total (Rs.)
1.	Manager-cum-chemist	1	7500	7500.00
2.	Storekeeper-cum-accountant	1	4500	4500.00
3.	Purchase-cum-salesman	1	5000	5000.00
4.	Clerk-cum-typist	1	3500	3500.00
5.	Boiler attendant	1	4000	4000.00
6.	Skilled workers	2	2500	5000.00
7.	Unskilled worker	2	2000	4000.00
8.	Peon	1	2000	2000.00
	Total salary and wages			35,000.00
	Perquisites @ 15% of the salary			5250.00
			Total	40,250.00
			Say	40,200.00

Raw materials (per month)

Dried flowers @ Rs.50/kg 2689 kg		1,34,900.00
Packaging materials		20,000.00
	Total	1,54,900.00

Utilities (per month)

Power		6000.00
Fuel		20,000.00
Water		1500.00
	Total	27500.00

Other contingent expenses

Postage, stationery and telephone	5000.00
Consumable stores	2000.00
Repair and maintenance	2000.00
Transport charges	8000.00
Advertisement	3000.00
Insurance	500.00
Sales expenses	8000.00
Miscellaneous expenses	2000.00
Total	**30,500.00**

Total working capital

Staff and labour	40200.00
Raw materials	1,54,900.00
Utilities	27,500.00
Other contingent expenses	30,500.00
Total	**2,53,100.00**

Total fixed investment

Fixed capital	17,31,500.00
Working capital (for 3 months)	7,59,300.00
Total	**24,90,800.00**

Financial Analysis

Cost of production (per year)

Total recurring cost	30,37,200.00
Depreciation on plant and machinery @ 10% p.a.	67,650.00
Depreciation on office equipment @ 20%	10,000.00
Depreciation on building @ 5%	41,250.00
Interest on total investment @ 17% p.a.	4,23,436.00
Total	**35,79,536.00**
Say	**35,79,500.00**

Turnover (per year)

By sale of 160 kg of matricaria oil @ Rs. 26,000/kg	41,60,000.00

Net profit/year (before income tax)

Turnover	–	Cost of production	= Net profit
41,60,000	–	35,79,500	= 5,80,500

Net profit ratio

$$\frac{\text{Net profit/year} \times 100}{\text{Turnover/year}} = \frac{5,80,500 \times 100}{41,60,000} = 13.95\%$$

Rate of return

Net profit/year × 100 = 5,80,500 × 100 = 23.30%
Total investment   24,90,800

Break even point (percent of total production envisaged)

B.E.P. =   Fixed cost × 100
                Fixed cost + Annual profit

Fixed Cost

Depreciation on machine and equipment	67,650.00
Depreciation on building	41,250.00
Interest on total investment	4,23,436.00
Insurance	6000.00
40 per cent of salary and wages	1,92,960.00
40 per cent of other contingent expenses	46,400.00
Total fixed cost	8,77,696.00
Say	8,77,700.00

B.E.P. =   8,77,700 × 100
           8,77,700 + 5,80,500 = 40%

Additional Information

This plant and machinery can be utilised for the distillation of other essential oil from flower.

MENTHOL CRYSTAL

The menthol crystals are obtained from mint oil (*Mentha oil*) which is third most important flavouring material used world over. There are several species of mint cultivated in different parts of the world. Five of them are commercially grown in India such as Japanese mint (*Mentha Arvensis*) *Mentha piperita* (Peppermint oil). *M.citrata* (Bergmot mint) *M.spieata*. Main source of method is mentha arvensis oil. The mentha oil is obtained by hydrodistillation of mentha Arvensis which is used as a source of natural menthol and dementholated oil. The main grower of mentha oil are in UP, Punjab, and Haryana. The main concentration in UP are places like Muradabad, Bareilly, Chandausi, Badaun, Sambal, and Rampur, etc. which account for around 90 per cent of country's total production of mint oil. There are around 500 numbers of small scale units in UP mainly engaged in production of mint oil with production capacity around 5000 tons annually while total production of oil in the country is reported to be 6000 tons per annum. China is the main competitor in this line.

Natural menthol has widespread use in pharmaceutical and flavouring industries due to its cooling effect and refreshing aroma. It is mainly used in toothpaste, pan masala, hair oil, chewing gum, candies and pain relieving balm, etc.

Market Potential

Due to widespread use of mentha oil and menthol crystal in different industries like cosmetics, perfumery and pharmaceutical the demand of mentha and menthol crystals is growing rapidly. The production of different type of mint oil in the country is to the tune of around 6570 MT which include Japanese Mint

6100 MT, spearmint 300 MT, peppermint 250 MT, bergmot mint 150 MT during 2004–2005. Mentha Arvensis is the best source of Menthol crystal which contain 60–75 per cent of Menthol in the oil.

Mentha oil as well as Menthol crystals have growing demand not only in national market but also have export potential and among the essential oil it has major share of export. In the world scenario India has top position in terms of production of Mint oil in the country. Other producers in the world are China, Brazil, Japan, America and Australia. In India, it is mainly produced in UP, Haryana, Himachal Pradesh, and Punjab. Total production capacity around 8500 MT per annum while demand is more than that.

In Orissa so far no unit has come up for distillation of mint oil or menthol crystals. However, there exists a very good scope for setting up of such industry in the state particularly. Menthol crystals has good demand and scope in the state which can be initially started by bringing mentha oil from UP, and other states.

Basis and Presumptions

1. The scheme is prepared for Mentha oil and Mentha crystals.
2. 300 working days 8 hours shift per day has been taken in the scheme.
3. The estimate in respect of land, building, machines, etc. are drawn as per the prevailing prices during the preparation of the scheme which may differ from place to place and time to time.
4. 60–70 per cent efficiency of full capacity utilisation has been taken into account.
5. Interest rate @ 17 per cent has also been considered.
6. Margin money to the extent of 25 per cent of total project cost is required by the entrepreneur as own investment in implementing the project.
7. Minimum wages has been taken in the scheme.
8. In the scheme the boiler has not been included as the process adopted by the unit will be based on hydrodistillation.
9. 2–3 years period is considered as a pay back period.

Implementation

1.	Preparation of project report	1 month
2.	Selection of site	1 month
3.	Development of land and planting of material	4 months
4.	Registration of unit	1 month
5.	Availability of loan finance	3 months
6.	Procurement of machinery	1 month
7.	Erection and commissioning	1 month
8.	Recruitment of staff	1 month

Technical Aspects

Distillation technology

The mentha oil is extracted by hydrodistillation process in which the raw materials like herbs is placed in perforated bottom of the distillation steel. The water is filled at the bottom of the steel. On heating over furnace the water boiled and vapour are formed which is mixed with the oil of the herbs and the oil is evaporated in form of vapour along with water which is collected with the help of condensor. On cooling, oil vapour condensed in shape of liquid which is collected in a receiver put in a water tank or water bath.

The water also condensed with the oil in the receiver which is separated through separating furnace. The oil in the receiver which is separated through separating furnace.

The oil being lighter than water comes on the top and water remains at the bottom of the receiver which is separated with the help of separating funnel. The collected oil is then stored in glass bottle or galvanised drum. To make it free from water the crystals of sodium sulphate are added.

Separation of menthol crystals from mentha oil

Mentha oil which is collected as above is used to get menthol crystal by keeping it in the deep freezer at different temperature. Mentha oil mainly contains 60–75 per cent of menthol. On deep freezing in the first step around 60 per cent of menthol crystals are formed and remaining oil is called dementholated oil which still contains 5–10 per cent of menthol which can be obtained on deep freezing. Flow diagram of menthol oil and menthol crystal is given in Fig. 15.1.

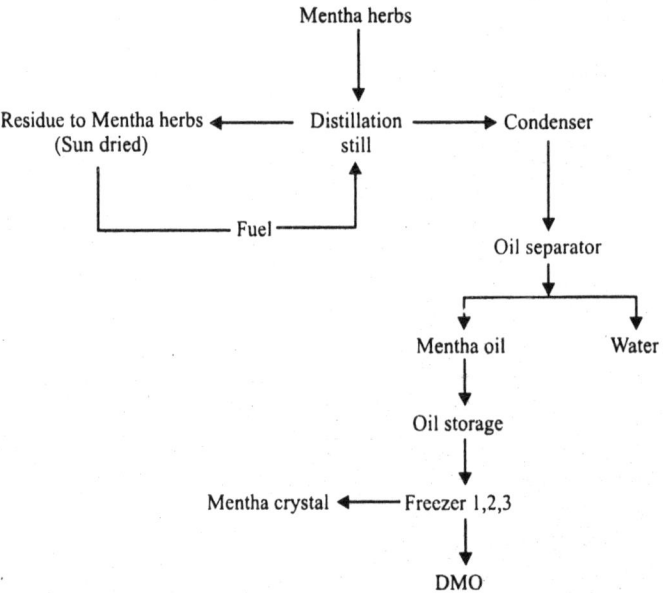

Fig. 15.1. Flow chart of menthol oil and menthol crystal.

Alternate technology

The mentha oil is also extracted by adopting steam distillation process. In the process steam is used as an extraction media which is generated through the boiler. In the process first steam is passed in the still which is filled with mentha grass. Steam carrying with oil is then condensed in form of liquid with the help of condenser. The oil is collected in a receiver through condenser and it is the separated.

Quality Control and Specifications

Menthol is white crystal solid having molecular formula $C_{10}H_{12}PH_1$, melting point 42°–43°C, boiling point 217°C. The BIS has developed specification for menthol crystal as BIS 3134–1992 which is to be followed for proper quality control of the menthol crystal.

Production capacity (per annum)

Mentha crystal	13.5 MT	54,00,000.00
Dementholated oil	9 MT	13,50,000.00

Approximately motive power

Approximately motive power	15 KW

Pollution control

There is no pollution in the process of mentha oil. However, precaution should be taken for proper maintenance of the working environment. Workers should be provided with hand gloves and mask for handling and processing of chemical.

Energy conservation

There is not much scope of energy conservation. However, proper utilisation of fuel and avoiding of unnecessary use of light and fan can save a good amount of energy. In case of steam distillation process steamline should be insulated properly to minimise radiation loss.

Financial Aspects

Land and building

Land 4000 sq. ft @ Rs. 40/sq. ft	1,60,000.00
Built up area working shed 1000 sq. ft @ Rs. 300 per sq. ft	3,00,000.00
Deep freezer rooms 20 ×15 ft = 300 sq. ft @ Rs. 1500/sq. ft	6,00,000.00
Laboratory 50 sq. ft @ Rs. 1200/sq. ft	60,000.00
Total	11,20,000.00

Plant and machinery

Sr. No.	Description	Quantity	Rate	Value (Rs.)
1.	Distillation still 1.5 ton capacity with accessories	4	1,50,000	6,00,000.00
2.	Deep freezer (one ton capacity)	3	90,000	2,70,000.00
3.	Mentha child brine basket centrifuge	1	30,000	30,000.00
4.	Storage drum for Mentha oil (galvanised 200 litres capacity)	30	–	30,000.00
5.	Aluminium condensor			20,000.00
6.	Tube well overhead tank			20,000.00
7.	Laboratory equipment			40,000.00
8.	Installation and electrification @ 10% machine cost			1,01,000.00
9.	Office furniture			2500.00
10.	Generator set			2,00,000.00
			Total	13,36,000.00

Pre-operative expenses

Pre-operative expenses	25,000.00

Total fixed capital

Total fixed capital
(Land and building + Plant and machinery + Pre-operative expenses)   24,81,000.00

Working capital

Staff and labour

Sr. No.	Designation	No.	Salary	Total salary (Rs.)
1.	Chemist manager	1	7000	7000.00
2.	Operator	1	4000	4000.00
3.	Skilled workers	3	3000	9000.00
4.	Unskilled workers	4	2500	10,000.00
5.	Clerk typist	1	4000	4000.00
6.	Peon	1	2000	2000.00
	Perquisites @ 15%			36,000.00
				5400.00
				41,400.00

Raw material (per month)

Mentha	900 MT	Rs. 900 MT	8,10,000.00
Miscellaneous item such as packaging, etc.			40,000.00
			8,50,000.00

Utilities

Electricity	10,000.00
Fuel	5000.00

Other contingential expenditure

Postage and stationery	1000.00
Telephone/Fax	2000.00
Consumables	2000.00
Maintenance and repairing	2500.00
Advertisement and publicity	2500.00
Insurance	1000.00
Transport	7000.00
Miscellaneous	2000.00
	20,000.00

Working capital (per month)

Salary	41,000.00
Raw materials	8,50,000.00
Utilities	15,000.00

Other contingential expenses	20,000.00
	9,26,400.00
Working capital for 3 months	27,79,200.00

Total Capital Investment

Fixed cost	24,81,000.00
Working capital	27,79,200.00

Cost of production (per annum)

Recurring expenses		46,32,000.00
Depreciation on plant and machinery @ 10%		1,31,100.00
Depreciation on building @ 5%		48,000.00
Depreciation on office equipment @ 20%		5000.00
Interest on total investment @ 17% p.a.		8,97,464.00
	Total	57,13,564.00
	Say	57,13,600.00

Turnover

Mentha crystal	13.5 MT	4,00,000/MT	54,00,000.00
DMO (Dementholated oil)		1,50,000/MT	13,50,000.00
			67,50,000.00

Net profit

Net profit = Turnover − Cost of production = Net profit (before tax)

67,50,000 − 57,13,600 = 10,36,400

% Net profit ratio

$$\% \text{ Net profit ratio} = \frac{\text{Net profit} \times 100}{\text{Turnover}} \quad \frac{10,36,400 \times 100}{57,13,600} = 18.13\%$$

% Rate of return

$$\% \text{ Rate of return} = \frac{\text{Net profit} \times 100}{\text{Total investment}} \quad \frac{10,36,400 \times 100}{52,60,200} = 19.70\%$$

Break-even point

Fixed cost

Depreciation on plant and machinery @ 10%	1,13,100.00
Depreciation on building @ 5%	48,000.00
Depreciation on furniture @ 20%	5000.00
Insurance	12,000.00
40 per cent annual salary	1,98,720.00
40 per cent other expenses (excluding rent and insurance)	96,000.00
	13,65,054.00
Say	13,65,000.00

$$B.E.P = \frac{\text{Fixed cost} \times 100}{\text{Fixed cost} + \text{Net profit}} \quad \frac{13,65,000 \times 100}{13,65,000 \times 10,36,400} = 56.84\%$$

ADDRESSES OF PLANT AND MACHINERY SUPPLIERS

1. M/s. Anand Engg. (P) Ltd.,
    66, MIDC, Andheri (East), Mumbai-400093.
2. M/s. National Instrument Limited,
    Jadavpur, Kolkata.
3. M/s. Kerala Engg. Works Corpn.
    National Highway, Angamali, Kerala.
4. M/s. Andhra Scientific Company.
    Mount Road, Chennai.
5. M/s. APV Engg. Company Ltd.
    7, Jessore Road, Dumdum, Calcutta.
6. M/s. Sweta Gas.
    Industrial Estate, Bareilly
    Uttar Pradesh.
7. M/s. Ganson Limited
    6, West View, Dadar, Mumbai-400014.
8. M/s. Chemical Construction Company (P) Ltd.
    57, Ring Road, Lajpat Nagar, New Delhi-110024.
9. M/s. Standard Metal Fabricators Company.
    Naraina Industrial Estate, New Delhi.

Chapter 16

Uses and Storage of Essential Oils

INTRODUCTION

Essential or as they are also called, volatile or ethereal oils, find an amazingly wide and varied application in many industries for the scenting and flavouring of all kinds of consumers finished products, some of them luxuries, most of them necessities in our advanced civilisation. Many of these products contribute directly to our health, happiness and general well-being. To underestimate their importance is to disregard entirely the physiological advantage of continuing to have available these accustomed necessities of our daily life.

Some volatile oils are more or less powerful external or internal antiseptics, others possess an analgesic, haemolytic, or antizymatic action, still others act as sedatives, stimulants and stomachics. The anthelmintic properties of certain volatile oils, especially wormseed oil, are well known.

USES OF ESSENTIAL OILS

Spices with their flavour principles, volatile oils, have been used as flavouring materials since time immemorial. Yet, not always is it sufficiently realised that they are actually indispensable to man in order to bring about proper digestion of food. The digestive juices containing digestive enzymes such as pepsin, trypsin, lipase, amylase, etc. are secreted into the stomach and intestines only when stimulated by the smell and taste of pleasantly flavoured food. The mouth 'becomes watery' and so does the stomach. As the individual digests more food with a pleasant taste, more digestive juices will be secreted, a fact equally true in the reverse.

The wide use of volatile oils in perfumes, cosmetics and the scenting of soaps hardly needs to be mentioned.

Increasingly, volatile oils and their aromatic isolates serve also for the covering of somewhat objectionable odours, as, for instance, in the case of artificial leathers. Acceptable and useful articles can now be made from raw materials that were formerly discarded or overlooked because of disagreeable odours. In most instances the incorporation of aromatics into products such as synthetic rubbers and latices has opened new and profitable fields for manufacturers.

Few people realise that in the course of a single day, from morning to night, we use or consume a great variety of volatile oils which originate from many corners of the world. All of us thereby contribute to the employment of innumerable workers and their families, often primitive peoples in distant land. Frequently these small producers depend for their income upon our continued use of these oils which have thus become really 'essential' not only to these growers for their livelihood, but also to our industries so that they may be able to manufacture their specialities, many of them marketed internationally. The essential oils industry, as such, is a small one, apt to be overlooked in the economy of a country. Its total year turnover may be estimated as amounting to only a few scores of millions of dollars, but the turnover of the consumers' finished goods, which require small additions of essential oils, reaches into many billions per year. Countless is the number of people who are involved in the developing, manufacturing, controllin advertising, marketing and selling of these products.

The following list will enumerate some of the various industries employing volatile oils, aro atic isolates or combinations. For convenience sake, they are listed alphabetically, not according to importance. While in the case of the toilet goods industry, it is possible to group the products as belonging to this one industry, such a fine distinction cannot always be made with other products. Therefore, the terms 'manufacturer' and 'industry' will have to be applied interchangeably as the groupings may require. Neither can a clear line be drawn between the products manufactured by these various industries.

Adhesives

Glues	Porcelain cements
Paper and industrial tapes	Rubber cements
Pastes	Scotch tapes, etc.

Animal feed industry

Cat foods	Dog foods, etc.
Cattle feeds	

Automobile industry

Automobile finishing supplies	Polishes
Cleaners	Soaps, etc.

Baked goods industry

Biscuits	Mince meat
Cakes	Pies
Crackers	Pretzels
Doughnuts	Puddings
Fruit cakes	Sandwich fillings, etc.
Icings	

Canning industry

Fish	Sauces
Meats	Soups, etc.

Chewing gum industry

Chewing gums	Coated gums, etc.

Condiment industry

Catsups	Pickled fish
Celery and other salts	Relishes
Chill sauces	Salad, dressings
Mayonnaises	Table sauces
Mustards	Vinegars, etc.

Confectionary industry

Chocolates	Jellies
Fondants	Mints

Gum drops
Hard candies

Panned goods
Soft centre candies, etc.

Dental preparations

Dentists' preparations
Mouth washes

Tooth pastes
Tooth powders, etc.

Exterminators and insecticide supplies

Bedbug sprays
Cattle sprays
Cockroach powders
Fly sprays
Japanese beetle attractants
Mosquito repellents

Naphthalene blocks
Paradichlorobenzene blocks
Plant sprays
Rat baits
Rodent odour eliminators, etc.

Extract industry

Commercial extracts

Home extracts, etc.

Food industry (general)

Cheeses
Cornstarch puddings
Dehydrated soups, meats and
 vegetables
Gelatine desserts
Mince meats

Pie fillers
Prepared cake mixes
Rennet desserts
Sauerkraut
Vegetable oils and fats, etc.

Household products

Bluings
Deodourants
Furniture polishes
Laundry soaps

Room sprays
Starches
Vacuum cleaner pads, etc.

Ice cream industry

Ice creams
Ices

Prepared ice cream mixes
Sherbets, etc.

Insecticide industry

Attractants
Disinfectants
Insecticides

Repellents
Sprays, etc.

Janitor's supplies

Detergents
Disinfectants
Floor polishes
Floor waxes

Scrub soaps
Sink cleaners
Sweeping compounds, etc.

Meat packing industry

Bolognas
Frankfurters

Prepared meats
Sausages, etc.

Paint industry

Bituminous paints
Casein paints

Paint diluents
Paints

Enamels
Lacquers
Paint and varnish removers

Rubber paints
Synthetic coatings
Varnishes, etc.

Paper and printing industry

Carbon papers
Crayons
Drinking cups
Industrial tapes
Inking pads
Labels

Paper bags and food wrappers
Printing and writing inks
Printing paper
Typewriter ribbons
Writing paper, etc.

Perfume and toilet industry

Baby preparations
Bath preparations
Body deodourants
Colognes
Creams
Depilatories
Eye shadows
Facial masks
Hair preparations
Handkerchief extracts
Incense

Lipsticks
Lotions
Manicure preparations
Powders
Room and theatre sprays
Rouges
Sachets
Shaving preparations
Suntan preparations
Toilet water, etc.

Petroleum and chemical industry

Bluing oils
Fuel oils
Grease deodourants
Greases
Lubricating oils
Naphtha solvents
Neoprene

Organic solvents
Petroleum distillates
Polishes
Sulphonated oils
Tar products
Waxes, etc.

Pharmaceutical industry

Antiacid tablets and powders
Cough drops
Elixirs
Germicides
Hospital sprays
Hospital supplies
Inhalants
Laxatives

Liniments
Medicinal preparations
Ointments
Patent medicines
Tonics
Vitamin flavour preparations
Wholesale druggists' supplies, etc.

Pickle packing industry

Dill pickles
Fancy cut pickles

Sour pickles
Sweet pickles, etc.

Preserve industry

Fruit butters
Jams

Jellies

Rectifying and alcoholic beverage industry

Bitters

Cordials

Rums

Vermouths

Whiskies

Wines, etc.

Rubber industry

Baby pant

Gloves

Natural and synthetic latices

Shower curtains

Surgical supplies

Synthetic rubber products of all kinds

Toys

Water proofing compounds, etc.

Soap industry

Cleaning powders

Detergents

Household soaps

Laundry soaps

Liquid hand soaps

Scrub soaps

Shampoos

Sweeping compounds

Technical soaps

Toilet soaps, etc.

Soft drink industry

Carbonated beverages

Cola drinks

Fountain syrups

Ginger ales

Root beers

Soda fountain supplies

Soft drink powders

Sundae toppings, etc.

Textlle processing products

Artificial leather and fabric coatings

Dyes

Hosiery sizing

Linoleum

Oil cloths

Sisal deodourants

Textile chemicals

Textile oils

Upholstery materials

Water proofing materials, etc.

Tobacco industry

Chewing tobaccos

Cigarettes

Cigars

Smoking tobaccos

Snuffs

Veterinary supplies

Cattle sprays

Deodourants

Dog and cat soaps

Insect powders

Mange medicines and ointments, etc.

Diversified industries

Alcohol denaturing compounds

Candles

Ceramics

Cleaners' products

Embalming fluid deodourants

Optical lenses

War gas simulants, etc.

ESSENTIAL OILS AND ISOLATES FOR CONTROLLING HOUSEHOLD INSECTS: HOUSEFLY, COCKROACH AND MOSQUITO

The use of synthetic or petroleum based insecticides for controlling household insects cause serious health hazards and environmental pollution. To overcome the problem and to search for ecofriendly insecticides, a number of essential oils and their isolates have been evaluated for use as indoor insect repellents due to their volatile nature, pleasant aroma and biodegradability. These materials have shown encouraging results for pest controlling properties with various classes of insects. The review presents the available information about the anti-insect properties of essential oils (repellency, larvicidal, ovicidal and knockdown effects) against three most common household insects, housefly, mosquito and cockroach.

The secondary metabolites produced by higher plants have relatively recently begun to be exploited for the pest control purpose. As synthetic or petroleum based insecticides pose problems of resistance, environmental pollution and serious health hazard to mankind, attempts have been made to search for new classes of insecticides, derived from plants, owing to low toxicity and less persistence in nature. Some of the plant products like alkaloids, vegetable oils, plant extracts, gums, esters, coumarin, chromenes, triterpenoids and limonoids, etc. have been evaluated for their insect-pest controlling properties. Characterisation of pyrethroids, rotenones and azadirachtin (limonoids) have led to the discovery of new molecules from botanicals as alternative pest control agents. In this conception, investigations of wide variety of essential oils and their constituents were found to possess varying degree of pest controlling properties like repellents, attractants, oviposition deterrents and antifeedants. The oils of citronella and camphor have been in commercial use as insect repellents since the first third of twentieth century, while eucalyptus oil rich in cineole (70–80 per cent) or pure cineole have also been in use as potent repellents to many insects including mosquitoes and American cockroaches. Further, the effects of constituents of oil have been observed to vary considerably between insect species, for instance three terpenoids of scot pine steam distillate were attractant to *Hylobius abietis*, a highly destructive weevil while other components were repellent to weevil. Geraniol repels houseflies but attracts honey bees.

Activities of Essential Oils and Their Isolates

Activities of essential oils and their isolates towards various insects and pests have been reviewed from time to time by many workers, but in the present review, we have concentrated on essential oils and isolates active towards household insects which are of great significance as they produce direct reflection on the civilisation, the use of mosquito lotion, moisturisers, mat, insect coils, repellent aerosols are the best example of their impact on society.

A number of household insects like cockroach, housefly, ants, mosquitoes, lice and bed bugs etc. are posing problems to mankind but the most of the work have been carried out on three insects namely housefly, mosquito and cockroach, so we have concentrated on these three insects only. Activities of essential oils and isolates against each of the three insects are presented in Table 16.1.

Table 16.1. List of essential oils producing anti-insect activity towards housefly, cockroach and mosquito.

Sr. no.	Essential oil	Anti-insect activity observed against		
		Housefly	Cockroach	Mosquito
1.	Acorus calamus	Repellent and insecticidal	–	Insecticidal
2.	Ageratum sp.	Repellent	–	–
3.	Annona squamosa	Insecticidal		
4.	Artemisia obsinthium	Insecticidal	–	–
5.	A. monosperma	Insecticidal	–	–
6.	A. vestata	Insecticidal	–	–

(Contd ...)

Sr. no.	Essential oil	Anti-insect activity observed against		
		Housefly	Cockroach	Mosquito
7.	A. vulgaris	Insecticidal	–	Repellent
8.	Allium sativum	–	–	Larvicidal and insecticidal
9.	Angelica	–	–	Insecticidal
10.	Backhousia myrstifolia	–	–	Repellent
11.	Blumea eirantho	–	–	Larvicidal
12.	Callistemon lanceolatus	Repellent	–	–
13.	Caryophyllum	–	–	Repellent Insecticidal
14.	Cedrus deodara	Insecticidal	–	Insecticidal and larvicidal
15.	Cinnamomum camphora	Repellent	Repellent	Repellent
16.	C. zeylanicum	–	Repellent	–
17.	Coriandrum sativum	Repellent	–	–
18.	Castus	–	Insecticidal	–
19.	Cuminum cyminum	–	Larvicidal	–
20.	Curcuma amada	Repellent	Repellent	–
21.	Cyathocline lyrata	Insecticidal and repellent	–	Insecticidal and repellent
22.	Cymbopogon citratus	–	Repellent	Repellent and larvicidal
23.	C. nardus	–	Repellent	Repellent
24.	C. domestica	Repellent	–	Larvicidal
25.	C. flexuosus	Repellent	–	Larvicidal
26.	C. martini var. sofia	Repellent	–	Repellent
27.	C. martini var motia	Repellent	Repellent	Repellent
28.	C. winteranisus	Repellent	–	Repellent
29.	Daucus carata	–	–	Insecticidal
30.	Daerydium franklint	–	–	Repellent
31.	Denettia tripetala	–	–	Insecticidal
32.	Eucalyptus sp	Repellent	–	Repellent
33.	Eucalyptus globules	–	–	Larvicidal
34.	E. ugenia	–	–	Larvicidal
35.	Illicium verum	Repellent	–	–
36.	Juniper berry	–	–	Insecticidal
37.	Larix decidua	–	–	Repellent, insecticidal and larvicidal

(Contd ...)

Sr. no.	Essential oil	Anti-insect activity observed against		
		Housefly	*Cockroach*	*Mosquito*
38.	*Lavendula officinale*	–	–	–
39.	*Lavendula angustifolio*	–	–	–
40.	*Linaloe*	Repellent	–	Repellent
41.	*Melaleuca bractea*	–	–	Repellent
42.	*Melia azadiracta*	–	–	Repellent and larvicidal
43.	*Mentha arvensis*	–	–	Larvicidal
44.	*Nepeta catane*	–	–	Repellent
45.	*Ocimum bacilicum*	Insecticidal	–	Insecticidal and larvicidal
46.	*Ocimum basilicum*	Insecticidal	–	–
47.	*O. gratissimum*	Repellent and insecticidal	–	–
48.	*O. kilmandscharicum*	Repellent and insecticidal	–	–
49.	*O. sanctum*	Repellent and insecticidal	–	Insecticidal and larvicidal
50.	*Onganum majorana*	–	–	Larvicidal
51.	*Pandanus odoratum*	–	Repellent	–
52.	*Pelargonium graveolens*	Repellent	–	Repellent and larvicidal
53.	Pine	Repellent	–	–
54.	*Rabdosia melissoides*	Repellent	–	–
55.	*Ricinus communis*	Repellent	–	Larvicidal
56.	Rose	Repellent	–	Repellent
57.	*Rosa damascena*	–	–	Repellent
58.	*Santalum album*	Repellent	–	–
59.	*Schinus molils*	Repellent	–	–
60.	*Syzygium aromaticum*	–	Repellent	–
61.	Terpentine	Repellent	–	–
62.	*Trachyspermum ammi*	Insecticidal and repellent	–	–
63.	*Tridax procumbens*	Insecticidal and repellent		Insecticidal and repellent
64.	*Thymus serphyllum*	Repellent	–	–
65.	*Thuja plictata*	Insecticidal	–	Repellent
66.	*Velerian*	–	–	Insecticidal
67.	*Vitex negundo*	–	–	Repellent
68.	*Zleria smithi*	–	–	–
69.	*Zingiber officinale*	–	–	Repellent

The compounds of essential oils producing anti-insect activity towards housefly, cockroach and mosquito are given in Table 16.2.

Table 16.2. List of compounds of essential oils producing anti-insect activity towards housefly, cockroach and mosquito.

Sr. no.	Compound	Anti-insect activity observed against		
		Housefly	Cockroach	Mosquito
1.	β-asarone	Insecticidal	–	Repellent
2.	Camphene	–	–	Ovicidal
3.	d-camphor	Repellent	–	–
4.	Carvacrol	Larvicidal	–	Ovicidal
5.	Carvone	Larvicidal	–	Insecticidal
6.	Carvacrone	–	–	–
7.	α-cedrene	–	–	Insecticidal
8.	8,14-cedranoxide	–	–	–
9.	Cedrol	–	–	Insecticidal
10.	Cedrene-14-al	–	–	–
11.	Cedrene-olacetal	–	–	–
12.	8, Cedrene-13-ol	–	–	Insecticidal
13.	1,8-Cineole	Larvicidal	Repellent	Ovicidal Repellent
14.	Cinneamaldehyde	Larvicidal	–	–
15.	Citral	Insecticidal Repellent and fumigant	Repellent	Ovicidal Insecticidal and insecticidal
16.	Citronellol	Insecticidal	–	Repellent and insecticidal
17.	Citronellal	Insecticidal	–	Repellent and insecticidal
18.	Chavicol	–	–	–
19.	Coumarin	–	–	Repellent
20.	Chavicol	–	–	–
21.	Eucamalol	–	–	Repellent
22.	Epi cumalol	–	–	Repellent
23.	Eugenol	Ovicidal	Repellent	Insecticidal Repellent and ovicidal
24.	Isoeugenol	–	–	Insecticidal and fumigant
25.	Farnesol	Insecticidal	–	Insecticidal
26.	Geraniol	Insecticidal	–	Ovicidal
27.	Himachelene (α, β and τ)	Insecticidal	–	–

(Contd ...)

Sr. no.	Compound	Anti-insect activity observed against		
		Housefly	*Cockroach*	*Mosquito*
28.	Himachalol	Insecticidal	–	–
29.	β-Ionone	–	–	Ovicidal
30.	*d*-limonene	Insecticidal	–	Ovicidal
31.	*l*-limonene	Insecticidal	–	Ovicidal
32.	Linaloöl	Insecticidal	–	Ovicidal
33.	Menthol	–	–	Ovicidal
34.	Menthone	–	–	Ovicidal
35.	*p*-menth-3,8-diol	–	–	Ovicidal
36.	Methyl chavicol	–	–	Insecticidal
37.	Methyl eugenol	–	Fumigant and insecticidal	–
38.	Ocimenes	–	Fumigant	Insecticidal
39.	Safrol		Insecticidal and repellent	
40.	Isosafrol	–	Fumigant Insecticidal and repellent	–
41.	β-pinene	Insecticidal	Fumigant	Ovicidal Insecticidal and repellent
42.	β-phellandrene	Insecticidal	–	Ovicidal
43.	*Trans*-piperitone	Anti-feedant	–	–
44.	Terpineole	–	–	Insecticidal
45.	Thymol	–	–	Repellent

Housefly (Musca domestica)

A number of essential oils have been reported to have repellent activity against common housefly *Musca domestica*; amongst them oils of *Cymbopogon martini* var. motia, *C. martini* var. sofia, lemongrass, Eucalyptus, sandalwood are the most effective. Kaul tested three Artemisia oils, and found maximum activity with *Artemisia vestata* oil, 10 per cent solution of this oil produced 36 per cent mortality while 20 per cent solution produced 93.3 per cent knock down effect. Salch, reported the insecticidal activity of *A. vulgaris*, *A. absinthium* and *A. monosperma* and found the insecticidal compound as 3-methyl-3-phenyl, 1-4 pentadiene. Hwang identified mosquito repellents for *A. vulgaris* oil. Pathak and Dixit reported insecticidal and repellent activity of *Tridax procumbens* and *Cyathocline lyrata* while Singh found *Cedrus deodara* oil to kill housefly at concentration less than 1 per cent. Singh and Rao tested insecticidal and repellency of thirty-one essential oils against housefly and found that essential oils of *Ocimum gratissimum* L., *Thymus serphyllum*, *Illicium verum* Hook, *Myristica fragrans* Houtt and *Curcuma amada* Roxb produced 100 per cent repellent activity whereas the oils of *Acorus calamus*, *Thymus serphyllum* and *Trachyspermum ammi* should 40 per cent insecticidal activity. Singh and Rao also found only 14 per cent mortality in adults after 24 hours, they further reported activity in the same range in other Ocimum species, viz. *O. bacilicum* (French), *O. sanctum*, *O. kilmamdscharicum* and *O. gratissimum*. Besides these, they found that the oils of *Callistemon lanceolatus, Coriandrum sativum, Cymbopogon martini, Curcuma amada, Pelargonium graveolens, Rabdasia melissoides, Santalum album* to act as repellent to housefly at various levels. Osmani prepared a cold cream containing oils of lemongrass, linaloe, rose, geranium and sandalwood which they reported to be repellent against *Musca domestica* and *Culex fatigans*. Subramanium and Raja Mohanan, evaluated fly repellent potential of terpentine, lemongrass, pine, eucalyptus and camphor oil and found that direct application of the repellent proved more effective. As for the activity of compounds are concerned against housefly many monoterpenes present in the essential oils have been evaluated, Sharma and Saxena, reported the ranges of per cent mortality rates of larva of *Musca domestica* by camphene, carvone, cineole, citral, citronellal, eugenol, farnesol, geraniol, *d*-limonene, *l*-limonens, citronellol, linaloöl, β-phellendrene and α-pinene.

Camphor has also been reported to produce knockdown effects to housefly the most active compound identified against larva is cineole which produced 62.5 per cent mortality followed by α-pipene 56.7 per cent and citronellol 43.3 per cent, while these other compounds have been reported to produce lethal action against houseflies ranging from 0–36.7 per cent in case of larva and 27.5–62.5 per cent in unclosed pupae. Sharma and Saxena, have found the inhibition to the orientation and developments of eggs of housefly by carvacrol, citral, citronellol, eugenol, farnesol and geraniol. Rani and Osmani, reported that citral as effective fumigant to act as repellent against both male and female housefly. Singh and Agarwal, reported himachalol and himachalene from *Cedrus deodara* wood oil to produce 97 per cent mortality at 0.56μ mol. concentration after 24 hours.

Yusufoflu and Hasdemir reported the oil of *Pelargonium graveolens* repellent to mosquito and housefly. Wimalartne, reported the repelling properties of essential oil of paper tree *Schinus molle* L. and identified the active ingredient responsible as *cis*-menth-2-en-1-ol and *trans*-piperitone.

Mosquito

In earlier reports by Chopra and Despanday and Tipnis, the essential oils of *Ocimum basilicum* have been found to be insecticidal and larvicidal towards mosquito. Recently Bhatnager identified methyl chavicol the major constituent of *O. basilicum* oil as more effective than eugenol are component of *O. sanctum* oil which was found to be active against three species of mosquitoes *Anapheles stephensi, Aedes aegypti* and *Culex quinquefaciatus* 0.001 ml/43 cm^2 of methyl chavicol extracted from oil of *O. bacilicum* produced 100 per cent mortality with in 10–25 minutes while the oil produced same effect with 0.003 ml/43 cm^2 concentration in 30–35 minutes. Similarly the oil of *O. sanctum* produced mortality with in 20–60 minutes with 01/43 cm^2 concentration while eugenol was effective in 10–25 minutes having 0.003 ml/43 cm^2 concentration in all the three species of mosquitoes.

Osmani and Osmani reported that the oil of *Origanum majorana* produced high mortality to the larva of *Aedes aegypti* while the oils of Geranium and *Cymbopogon citratus* were highly effective at 4th instar larval stage. Amonkar found that the oil of garlic (*Allium sativum*) is active against larva of *Aedes aegypti* while it produced knock down affects for adults, they characterised allicin a mixture of diallyl di- and tri-sulphides as the larvicidal principle. The oil was also found to be effective against *Culex fatiganes* by Kirtaniyu. Dongre and Rohlkar, found that 200 ppm solution of *Blumea eirantho* produces 100 per cent mortality to the larvae of *Culex pipens*. Singh reported that only 1 per cent concentration of *Cedrus deodara* was effective against *Anapheles stephensi*. Sharma, reported the toxic behaviour of the essential oils of angelica, calamus, carrot, cedrus, costus and valerian towards mosquitoes while oth carrot seed oil and calamus oil both were effective to filarial mosquitoes, the carrot seed oil produced significant toxicity to yellow fever mosquito and toxicity in same range toward *Culex fatigans* and

A. aegypti. Purohit, reported that 50–100 per cent solution of *Cumin cyminum* seed oil was very toxic to larva of *Aedes aegypti.* Kumar and Dutta, reported toxicity of many essential oil towards 4th instar larva of *Anopheles stephensi,* the oils are *Cedrus deodara, Cymbopogon nardus, C. flexuosus, C. martini, Lavandula officinale* (*L. angustifolia*), *Mentha arvensis, Ricinus communis, Eucalyptus globulus, Melia azadiracha, Caryptophyllus* (*Syzygium aromaticum*). Pathak and Dixit, reported the toxicity of oils of *Tridax procumbens* and *Cyathocline lyrata* against *Culex fatigans.* While Sharma, found Juniper berry oil was very toxic to *Aedes aegypti* and *Culex fatigans.* Ranweera and Dayanand, reported that the oil of *Acorus calamus* and *C. nardus* were active against larva of *Culex quinquefaciatus* while *Cymbopogon domestica* oil was lethal to larva of *Anopheles califacies.* Elemol, methyl isoeugenol are the active principle. *Larix dacidua* and *L. kaemferi* oil was reported to be repellent, insecticidal and larvicidal to *Aedes aegypti.*

A large number of essential oils have been evaluated for their repellent activity against mosquitoes. Among the earlier reports the work of Penfold and Morrison, is important as they tested forty essential oils for the repellency towards mosquitoes, the most effective oils being those of *Daerydlum franlint* (Huonpine wood), oil of leaves of *Bakhousia myrtifolia, Melaleuca bractia* and *Zieria smithi* while similar activity in the oil of *Eucalyptus* and *Caryophyllum* were reported by Mayer, after testing several essential oil against various mosquitoes, it was reported that vapours of monoterpenes nepetal acetone (Catnip), acylopentane isolated from oil of catnip plant, *Nepta catane* repell seventeen species of mosquitoes, it was also found that the thujic acid from the essential oils of wood of *Thuja plictata* is potential repellent to *Aedes aegypti.* The essential oils of *Vitex negundo* showed repellency towards *Aedes aegypti,* polar fraction of the oil protected mosquito bite for 1–3 hours. Hebbalkar and Rajdan, reported that the essential oil of *Cinnamomum camphoro, Cymbopogon martini, C. citratus, C. nardus* have repellent action against mosquitoes *Culex quinquefaciatus.* They reported complete protection against *Anopheles culifacies* and other Anopheles and 95–96 per cent protection from *Culex quinquefaciatus.*

In field trials *Cinnamomum camphora* oil protected from various *Anopheles* for about 12 hours. Essential oils of *Pelargonium graveolens* was reported to be repellent to mosquito and housefly. Trigg, has evaluated a lemon eucalyptus based insect repellent (*E. maculata, E. citriodora*) against *Anopheles gambial* and *A. funes* with *p*-menthane 3,8-idol. Tyagi evaluated repellent activity of *Cymbopogon* essential oil against mosquitoes vector of malaria, filaria and dengu fever. While Lindsay have evaluated citronella oil in the form of citronella candles, 5 per cent citronella incense for protection against field population of *Aedes* mosquitoes. Okuda reported insect repellent composition having 3–15 cinnamon oil, 4–10 parts camphor in ethanol. As for repellency of isolated compounds from essential oils Travis, reported actions of citronellal and citronellol against mosquito. Saxena and Sharma found that citral prohibited egg hatching of *Aedes aegypti* completely, while carvacrol, geraniol, eugenol prevented more than 95 per cent and others like camphene, cineole, fernesol, β-inone, pseudoinone, dselimonene, menthol, menthone, phellandrene and α-pinene produced effects at various levels, they also found that the mosquito which alighted on water surface treated with farnesol were usually unable to fly and eventually found dead. Oda reported α-cedrene, thyjoprene, 8,14-cedranoxine, cedral and 8-cedrene 13-ol produced 50 per cent mortality of *Culex pepens.* Hwary found several monoterpenes from *Artemisia* species to be excellent mosquito repellent with terpene 4-ol to be most effective. Klock reported the repellent behaviour of 1,8-cineole. Mardufa and Lubenga characterised SE ocimenone from the oil of *Tagetes minuta* toxic to *Aedes aegypti,* 40 ppm solution of the *T. minuta* oil caused 100 per cent mortality, farnesol, geraniol, citral, eugenol, terpeneal were found to exhibit toxic or and behavioural effect on mosquito, while knock down effects were found in terpenol, (–) carvone and β-citronellol by Vartak and Sharma. Naik reported β-asorone, eugenol, thymol, 1,8-cineole, coumarin as mosquito repellent *Aedes albopictus*. Watanabek isolated a new mosquito repellent compound eucamolol, epicuclamol and 4-isopropyl benzyl alcohol from *Eucalyptus camaldulensis* these are reported to be potent repellent against *Aedes aegypti, A. albopictus*. Bhatnager and Kapoor reported that methyl chavicol the major constituent of *Ocimum bacilicum* is more effective than the eugenol the major constituent of *O. sanctum* as for their insecticidal activities are concerned.

Ranweera and Dayanand reported the activity of *Acorus calamus*, *Cymbopogon nardus* against larva of *Culex quinquefaciale* and found *C. nardus* highly lethal which *C. domestica* was affective against larva of *Anapheles califacies*.

Cockroach

None of the essential oil has been reported to be insecticidal to cockroach except oil of *Denettia tripetala* by Iwabe, however few oils have been found to act as repellent. Rao recorded the repellent tendency of oil of *Annona squamosa* towards cockroaches, while Garg and Jain reported repellency of essential oil of rhizome of *Zingiber officinale* to the extent of 81 per cent. Only 1 per cent dilution of *Cymbopogon* oils. *C. nardus* and Okuda used cinnamon and camphor oils in a formulation repellent to cockroaches. *C. citratus* exhibited repellent activity against cockroaches, while pure cineole was found effective repellent by Serivenad Meloan. Essential oils of *Zingiber officinale, Pandanus odoratum, Cinnamomum zylenicum, Syzigium aromaticum* and *Cymbopogon citratus* showed dose dependent repellency to cockroaches by Ahmad. Essential oils of *Curcuma longa* and *Zingiber officinale* have been reported repellent. Regarding the insecticidal properties of isolates Vartak reported the repellency of citral and eugenol while Nagoh Shay tested nine essential oil constituents safrol, iso-safrol, methyl eugenol, α-pipene, eugenol, engenol, isoeugenol for contact and fumigant toxicity to adults female and nymphs and found that benzyne derivatives more active, more toxic and repellent to *Periplenata americana*.

Structure and activity relationship

The effect of essential oils upon insects depends on several parameters including chemical composition and species susceptibility of insects as the physiological responses of each insect species towards the same crude plant extract or essential oil was not same. Available reports reveal that lipophilic nature of compounds, alkyl side chain, free phenolic, hydroxy or methylene dioxy group (as in safarol) are significant for insecticidal activity, while aliphatic straight chain ketone and aryl ketone compound exhibit strong repelling activity, further importance of specific positions of side chain in few molecules enhance the activity. Oxygenated function (phenolic and hydroxylated) enhances the activity (e.g. citral, citronellol, eugeniol, farnesol and geraniol). The specific steriosomeric form also play an important role for the activity as is evident by the fact that sometime linalool present in different isomeric forms in various plant sources display different level of activity while the mixtures of two isomeric forms are more active. The distance of side chain, double bond from aromatic ring and substitution of methoxy group to these compounds are important for determining of their toxicity and repellency, in general benzene derivative were more active and more toxic.

APPLICATION OF ESSENTIAL OILS IN AROMATHERAPY

Aromatherapy 'Gandha cikitsa' in Sanskrit is a mode of treating a diseased condition with the help of smell. Some define this term, as a system of healing which involves the use of pure essential oils. To have remedial effect of any essential oil, the ailed person should find the smell of the oil pleasant.

If the smell doesn't appeal to the patient, it is less likely to have an enhancing effect on mood and sense of well-being. Mechanism of olfaction and psychological, metabolic and neurological effects produced by essential oil decide its healing properties. To achieve effective benefits, it is essential to have the complete oil and hence correct distillation method should be employed depending upon, source of essential oil in the plant. Before we know about essential oils and their therapeutic efficacy, it is important to know the mechanism of olfaction. Olfaction is a very complicated process, involving nose, olfactory epithelium, olfactory centre in the brain, sensory region of brain and memory. The olfactory epithelium contains olfactory cilia, connected to olfactory nerve. When a person smells any odourant molecule, it leaves an impression on sensory region and olfactory memory is established. Our olfactory system has the capacity to store more than 10000 odour memories.

Relation Between Olfaction and Moods

The molecule inhaled by nose travels to limbic region of the brain, where hypothalamus, the queen of our endocrinal system is situated. Endocrine system regulates hormonal release required for correct body functioning. Limbic system is activated with the molecule to release required hormone. Minor components of essential oils decide which hormone will be released. It is a synergic action between essential oil components and brain endocrine system and amygdala (emotional centre in the brain). Thus aromatherapy involves olfactory system and limbic system to give remedial effect.

Importance of Pure and Complete Oil for Aromatherapy

To achieve therapeutic effect using essential oil, we need to have a complete oil. Essential oil is present in various plant organs and it is distilled out from there using various methods. Most commonly used method is steam and hydro distillation. Different constituents of essential oils are distilled out depending on the system used to separate them.

Distillation of Essential Oils

Essential oils in plant are present in flowers (jasmine, rose), leaves (patchouli, geranium), stem (sandal, cinnamon), root (jatamansi, agarwood). These oils are present in oil glands and methods are used to break these oil glands to release the oil.

Hydrodistillation

Plant material and water are boiled together and along with steam, oil is separated out, which collects over water on condensation.

Steam distillation

Steam is passed through the plant material and after condensation, essential oil is recovered.

Solvent extraction

This is based on solubility of essential oil in organic material such as benzene, hexane, etc. Here, after oil is dissolved in organic solvent, under vacuum, the solvent is evaporated to obtain the oil.

Supercritical extraction

This is conducted at low temperature and high pressure. In this method there is least destruction of molecules because of low temperature. No solvent traces can remain in the oil because at room temperature it is in the gaseous form.

Importance of Natural Oils Versus Reconstituted Oils

After development of various analytical tools, it is possible to know essential oil composition and use those chemicals to have reconstituted essential oil. Most of the time, such reconstituted oil smells very much similar to the natural oil. Only expert and experienced nose could tell the difference. But when we consider aromatherapeutic efficacy, we found that synthetic oil does not perform as natural essential oil. People may think that the synthetic one makes you feel good. But then any likable fragrance can make you feel good. That does not mean that the odour has effect on central and peripheral nervous system. This was seen also when anti-microbial spectrum of synthetic and natural oil was evaluated.

Identification of Natural Oil

With the knowledge of analytical chemistry and tools, it is possible to define marker chemicals for essential oil. Thus essential oils have therapeutic values if used properly. Care needs to be taken before using it on any patient. The patient may have allergy to particular essential oil. These days, it is seen that essential oils are adulterated with cheap material. Such oil will not give any therapeutic benefit. Correct distillation methods, use of right botanical species and proper storage, is a must to have therapeutic application of essential oils. If oils are adulterated or wrong, people will not suspect the quality of oil, but the system of medicine. This needs to be taken care.

STORAGE OF ESSENTIAL OILS

From the outset it should be stated that little indeed is known about the actual processes which cause the spoilage of an essential oil. Usually it is attributed to such general reactions as oxidation, resinification, polymerisation, hydrolysis of esters and to interreaction of functional groups. These processes seem to be activated by heat, by the presence of air (oxygen), of moisture and catalysed by exposure to light and in some cases, possibly by metals. There is no doubt that oils with a high content of terpenes (all citrus oils, pine needle oils, oil of turpentine, juniper berry, etc.) are particularly prone to spoilage, due probably to oxidation and especially resinification. Being unsaturated hydrocarbons, the terpenes absorb oxygen from the air. Light seems to be of lesser importance as a factor causing deterioration, than is moisture.

Essential oils containing a high percentage of esters (oil of bergamot, lavender, etc.) turn acid after improper storage, due to partial hydrolysis of esters. The aldehyde content of certain oils (lemongrass, for example) gradually diminishes, yet much more slowly than if the isolated aldehyde (citral, in this case) were stored as such. Quite probably the essential oil contains also some natural antioxidants, yet unknown, which to a certain extent protect the aldehyde while it is contained in the oil. Fatty·oils, with a few exceptions, are very prone to oxidation, but such spoilage can be retarded or prevented altogether by the addition of suitable antioxidants, such as hydroquinone or its monomethyl ether. Certain types of essential oils, especially those containing alcohols (geranium oil, for example), are quite stable and stand prolonged storage. Still others, patchouly and vetiver, for instance, improve considerably on ageing; in fact, they should be aged for a few years before being used in perfume compounds.

As a general rule, any essential oil should first be treated to remove metallic impurities, freed from moisture and clarified and then be stored in well-filled, tightly closed containers, at low temperature and protected from light. Bottles of hard and dark coloured glass are eminently suitable for small quantities of oil, but larger quantities will have to be stored in metal drums, heavily tin lined, if possible. A layer of carbon dioxide or nitrogen gas blown into the container before it is sealed will replace the layer of air above the oil and thereby assure added protection against oxidation.

Previous to storing, as pointed out, the oil should be carefully clarified and any moisture removed as the presence of moisture seems to be one of the worst factors in the spoilage of an essential oil. The small lots can be dehydrated quite readily by the addition of anhydrous sodium sulphate, by thoroughly shaking, standing and filtration. Calcium chloride must never be used for dehydration of an essential oil, as this chemical is apt to form complex salts with certain alcohols. Larger commercial lots of oil are not always easy to clarify. Some oils, such as vetiver, give a great deal of trouble. The simplest procedure is to add a sufficient amount of common salt to the lot, to stir the mixture for a while and to let it stand until the supernatant oil has become clear and can be drawn off the tank. The lower layer will be cloudy and needs to be filtered clear. If filtration through plain filter paper does not give a clear oil, kieselguhr or specially prepared filtering clay should be placed into the filter. Care must be exercised in the selection of the filtering medium as some media, activated carbon for example, may react chemically with certain constituents of the oil and affect its quality. Large quantities of oil should be filtered through filter presses which are readily available through any supply house. Centrifuging in high-speed centrifuges is an excellent means of clarifying essential oils. Not only moisture but also waxy material depositing after a certain period of storage, if possible at low temperature in a freezing room, can thus be eliminated.

Some lots of essential oils, especially those with a high content of phenols (clove, bay, thyme, origanum, etc.) arrive from the producing fields often in a crude form and dark coloured, due to the presence of metallic impurities. Such lots must be decolourised before they can be placed at the disposal of the consumer. In many cases the dark colour may be removed by the formation of complex salts with certain organic acids. For this purpose sufficient powdered tartaric acid is added to the oil, the mixture stirred for some time and permitted to settle. The supernatant clear oil can finally be drawn off, while the lower layer has to be filtered until clear. If the treatment with solid tartaric acid does not give satisfactory results, a concentrated aqueous solution of the acid is added to the oil. After thoroughly stirring, the mixture is allowed to stand until the two liquid layers separate clearly. The upper part of the oil layer should then be sufficiently clear to be drawn off, while the lower layer and especially the intermediary layer, need further treatment by clarification and filtration. Here again high-speed centrifugings are of great help.

In cases where the colour cannot be eliminated by treatment with organic acids, the oil will have to be clarified by redistillation or rectification.

Glossary

Absolute	:	In perfumery, an aromatic extract prepared by repeated washing of a melted concrete with warm alcohol (ethanol) in a batteuse. The alcoholic solution so formed is then dewaxed by chilling to reduce its solubility in the alcohol sufficiently to precipitate the wax, which is then removed by filtration. The alcohol is recovered from the filtrate by distillation under reduced pressure. The absolute remains as a residue representing the highest concentration of, and closest approach to the quality of, the corresponding natural fragrance in general use in perfumery.
Absorption	:	A process of soaking, as water is absorbed by a sponge.
Accord	:	A harmonious blend of a small number of aromatic materials.
Acetal	:	The organic product of a chemical reaction between an alcohol and an aldehyde.
Acid	:	A compound which can donate hydrogen ions, as hydrogen chloride in contact with water donates hydrogen ions to water molecules to form oxonium ions.
Acid value	:	A measure of the proportion (or concentration) of free acid present in a product, such as an essential oil, measured as the number of milligrams of potassium hydroxide required to neutralise the free acid in one gram of the sample.
Acidic	:	Having the properties of an acid, as in the case of an aqueous solution containing a higher concentration of oxonium ions than hydroxide ions. A solution of pH less than 7.0.
Acyclic	:	Not in the form of a ring as, for example, a straight-chain or branched-chain molecular structure.
Adsorbent	:	A substance to which certain molecules will stick, as molecules of certain ink dyes stick to cotton fibres, making the stain difficult to remove.
Adsorption	:	The adherence of molecules to a surface of some kind by the formation of relatively weak intermolecular bonds.
Adulterant	:	An impurity accidentally or deliberately introduced into a product, rendering it of inferior quality.
Agarbattie	:	An Indian incense stick.
Ageing	:	The process of allowing a product to mature. In perfumery, refers to the mellowing of a perfume compound over a period of about a month, by allowing it to stand in a closed vessel in a cool place of even temperature. This allows reactive ingredients of the perfume to interact to the point of equilibrium, at which the fragrance of the perfume is at the peak of its perfection.
Aglycon	:	Any product of the hydrolysis of a glycoside other than a sugar. The hydrolysis of glycosides during the distillation of an essential oil may introduce into the oil constituents which, as such, may not occur in the oil naturally. These are volatile aglycons, which are mainly of terpenoid constitution.

477

Agrestic : Pertaining to the countryside, especially as regards odour.

Albedo : The pith, or inner rind, of a citrus fruit.

Alcohol : An organic compound characterised by the presence in its molecules of one or more hydroxy-functional groups bonded directly to a hydrocarbon structure other than a benzene ring.

Alcoholysis : A reversible reaction between an alcohol and an ester of which the result is the interchange of the hydrocarbon part of the alcohol molecules with the alcohol part of the ester molecules. Thus, in the maturing of finished, alcoholic perfumes, the ethanol used as a diluent can react, slowly and incompletely, with, for example, esters of terpenoid alcohols, such as geraniol, citronellol and nerol.

Aldehyde : An organic compound characterised by the presence in its molecules of a carbonyl group of atoms and a hydrogen atom bonded to the carbon atom of the carbonyl group. A compound of general formula R·CHO, where R represents a hydrogen atom, hydrocarbon, or substituted hydrocarbon radical.

Aldehydic : In perfumery, a fragrance note typical of fatty aldehydes: powerful, fatty or waxy and becoming pleasant only in very low concentration. Also descriptive of a perfume characterised by emphasis on aldehydic notes set within a rich, floral base.

Alkali : A compound which when dissolved in water gives rise to a higher concentration of hydroxide ions than oxonium ions. Examples are sodium, potassium and calcium hydroxides and the gas ammonia.

Alkaline : Any substance which when dissolved in water gives a solution of pH greater than 7.0.

Alkane : A saturated hydrocarbon, of the kind found in natural gas and petroleum and having the general formula C_nH_{2n+2}. The highly volatile alkane hexane, C_6H_{14}, is one of the solvents used for the extraction of aromatic botanical materials in the preparation of concretes and resinoids.

Alkene : An unsaturated hydrocarbon the molecules of which each contain one or more double covalent bonds. The simplest alkenes have the general formula C_nH_{2n}. Terpenes are alkenes of the general formula $(C_5H_8)_n$ which are important constituents of essential oils.

Alkyne : An unsaturated hydrocarbon the molecules of which each contain one or more triple covalent bonds. The simplest alkynes have the general formula C_nH_{2n-2}. Alkynes and their derivatives are uncommon as constituents of essential oils.

Allergen : A substance which causes an allergic reaction as, for example, reddening and irritation of the skin following sensitisation by contact with the same allergen. A substance to which some persons are allergic may not give rise to sensitisation in others.

Alternative medicine : Any form of medical diagnosis and treatment which is not generally regarded as orthodox, i.e. conforming to long-established principles.

Amber : A fossil resin, unrelated to ambergris. The description 'amber' is, however, commonly used in perfumery to refer to a powdery, vanilla-like note having some relationship to the odour of natural ambergris.

Ambergris : A soft black, unpleasant-smelling abdominal secretion of the sperm whale, released into the sea by the normal process of elimination or when the animal dies. The material is thought to be produced as an excretion in response to irritation by the sharp, indigestible beaks of cuttlefish, which lodge in the internal intestinal folds. On release from the animal, ambergris rises to the surface of the sea, where it may drift about for many years, becoming harder, lighter in colour and losing its unpleasant odour. Now rarely used, ambergris is said to have been the finest blending agent known to perfumery.

Ambra : A term used in perfumery to refer to an odour of ambergris as, for example, the odours of preparations of ambergris-smelling fragrance bases, labdanum and of certain aroma chemicals.

Amine : An organic compound the molecules of which are characterised by the presence of one or more amino-, NH_2, functional groups.

Amino acid : A carboxylic acid the molecules of which are characterised by the presence of one or more amino-groups, in addition to a carboxyl group. Amino acid molecules are the 'building blocks' for protein synthesis in living plant or animal cells.

Analysis : In chemistry, any process for determining the composition of a substance. Examples are the analysis of an essential oil by GLC and the subsequent determination of the composition of one of its constituents by mass spectrometry.

Animalic : A term used in perfumery to refer to an odour associated with an animal source, such as civet, or to a note of animal excreta as may be given by certain plants, such as the heavy note of indole in Jasmine absolute or orange flower absolute.

Antioxidant : An agent capable of preventing, or reducing the rate of, oxidation. The organic compounds butylated hydroxyanisole (BHA) and butylated hydroxytoluene (BHT) are antioxidants commonly used, in traces, to protect citrus oils from deterioration.

Archimedean screw : A device having the form of the shaft of a wood screw, used for transporting material through a tube in the manner of a mincing machine.

Aroma chemical : Any chemical having a useful odour and which is harmless and legal when properly used as a fragrance or flavour ingredient.

Aromachology : The study of pyschological effects of odours, particularly those of essential oils used in aromatherapy.

Aromatherapy : The use of essential oils for the treatment of human disorders. Essential oils should not be taken internally except under the supervision of a duly qualified medical practitioner.

Artefact : In reference to gas–liquid chromatography, this term refers to any product of chemical change to a constituent of a sample under analysis, brought about by the conditions of the analysis. Artefacts are revealed as peaks on a chromatogram which do not correspond to true constituents of the sample. They are frequently the result of partial decomposition of true constituents in the heating block.

Asymmetric carbon atom : A carbon atom bonded to four different atoms or groups of atoms.

Atom : The smallest particle of an element which can take part in a chemical change.

Atomic number : The number of protons in the nucleus of an atom, which is equal to the number of electrons that the atom contains.

Atomic weight : As a close approximation, the ratio of the weight of one atom of an element to the weight of a hydrogen atom taken as one atomic weight unit. For accurate scientific work, atomic masses are used, where the atomic mass of an element is the ratio of the mass of one atom of the element to 1/12 of the mass of one atom of the isotope carbon-12.

Avogadro's law   : Avogadro's law states that under the same conditions of temperature and pressure, equal volumes of all gases contain the same number of molecules (6×10^{23}, approximately). It implies that the amount of space occupied by the actual molecules of a gas is negligible as compared with the volume occupied by the gas.

Azulenes   : Members of a family of dark blue, practically odourless, volatile, unsaturated cyclic hydrocarbons occurring in essential oils obtained by distillation from certain plants, such as chamomiles, some species of artemisia and pepper.

Base   : In perfumery, a perfume ingredient specially formulated to represent a natural source or a blend of natural sources of fragrance, or an abstract fragrance concept. In chemistry, a simple definition of a base is that it is a substance which will react with an acid to form a salt and water only. More scientifically, a base may be defined as an atom, ion or molecule capable of accepting a proton.

Base line   : A horizontal line drawn on a graph (such as a chromatogram or spectrogram) by a pen recorder when receiving no signal from the instrument to which it is connected.

Basic note   : A fragrance note of extended persistence; an aromatic material of very low volatility.

Battie   : An agarbattie.

Batteuse   : A large, cylindrical vessel, standing upright and fitted with a vertical stirrer, used for breaking up a mass of a molten concrete immersed in warm ethanol. Once the concrete has been dispersed in the alcohol in the form of small globules, the alcohol can extract the essential oil it contains efficiently, forming an alcoholic extract solution ready for the next stage in the preparation of an absolute.

Benzene ring   : Term used in reference to the molecular structure of the unsaturated, cyclic hydrocarbon, benzene, C_6H_6.

Benzenoid compound   : A compound the molecules of which each contain one or more benzene rings.

Boiling point   : The temperature at which a liquid boils. Scientifically, the maximum, constant temperature at which a liquid can evaporate at a given pressure, provided it is not in the superheated condition.

Branched chain   : In chemistry, any branching arrangement of the atoms in a molecule as, for example, in the molecules of thymol and limonene.

Bridged molecular structure   : A molecular ring structure, having a skeleton usually of carbon atoms, in which one or more additional carbon atoms are bonded across the ring. Alpha- and beta-pinenes are examples of *monoterpenes* having bridged molecular structures.

Burette   : A graduated tube, commonly of 1 cm internal diameter and 50 cm^3 capacity, used in the analytical technique of titration.

Cambium   : The ring of green, living tissue situated beneath the bark of a woody stem or tree-trunk and containing vessels for transporting aqueous solutions of mineral salts from the roots to the leaves, and of elaborated nutrients from the leaves to the roots.

Capillary GLC   : A refinement of the analytical technique of gas-liquid chromatography, in which the column consists of a long (e.g. 50 metres), coiled tube of very fine internal diameter, internally coated with a thin layer of nonvolatile stationary phase material, such as a silicone oil.

Caramellic	:	Term descriptive of the odour of caramel, as given by molten sugar when heated to a high temperature.
Carbon-12	:	The isotope of the element carbon having an atomic mass of 12 precisely.
Carbonyl group	:	The divalent group of atoms consisting of a carbon atom joined to an oxygen atom by a double bond: >C=O.
Carboxyl group	:	It is monovalent group of atoms consisting of carbon atom joined to oxygen atom by a double bond and to a hydroxy-group.
Carboxylic acid	:	It is organic acid characterised by the presence in each of its molecules of one or more carboxyl functional groups.
Carrier gas	:	It is, chemically inert to all other substances involved, used to transport samples through the column of a gas–liquid chromatograph.
Carrier oil	:	It is fixed oil of a vegetable origin, such a Jojoba oil, Avocado pear oil and grapeseed oil used in aromatherapy as a solvent and diluent for essential oils.
Catalyst	:	A substance which can alter the speed (rate) of a chemical reaction and which remains unchanged in mass and composition at the end of the reaction.
Chemical properties	:	Those properties of an element or compound which are shown when the substance undergoes some change of composition as, for example, decomposition by heat, oxidation, hydrolysis or reaction with another substance.
Chemical purity	:	The extent to which a chemical, such as an aroma chemical, consists of molecules or ion-aggregates of that chemical only; usually expressed as a percentage, e.g. alpha-iso-methyl ionone, 98 per cent, the other 2 per cent consisting of acceptable impurities (which nevertheless contribute to the odour profile of the product).
Chemical reaction	:	Any rearrangement of atoms or ions in which energy, usually but not exclusively heat, is either lost or gained.
Chemical test	:	A test involving a change in the composition of the subject material, such as during determinations of the percentage of alcohols, esters, etc. in an essential oil or in a test for pH using an indicator.
Chlorophyll	:	The mixture of magnesium-containing organic pigments—chlorophyll 'a' (green) and chlorophyll 'b' (yellowish-green) found in green plants and which is necessary for photosynthesis.
Chromatogram	:	The graph of detector response against time drawn by a pen recorder in response to electrical signals originating from the detector of a gas-liquid chromatograph (see gas-liquid chromatography). It takes the form of a series of peaks corresponding to the constituents of a mixture of volatiles, such as an essential oil or perfume compound.
Chromosome	:	One of a number of microscopic, thread-like structures present in the cell nuclei of animals and plants. Chromosomes carry inherited information in the form of genes. The nature and sequence of the genes carried by the chromosomes of an organism determine the characteristics of form and constitution inherited by the organism from its parents from generation to generation.
Chypre	:	The French word for 'cyprus'. In perfumery, a type of perfume characterised by a harmony of the notes of oakmoss, sandalwood and musk in the base, floral middle notes, such as those of rose and jasmin, and a top note of bergamot and other citrus oils. The first chypre-type perfume was 'Le Chypre', launched by Coty in 1917.

Cis-trans-isomerism	:	The occurrence of two different geometrical forms of molecules of the same unsaturated compound. In the *cis-*, or (Z-) form, identical atoms or groups of atoms are on the same side of a double bond. In the *trans-*, or (E-) form, the same groups of atoms are on opposite sides of the double bond.
Citrus oil	:	An essential oil obtained from the oil glands of the flavedo of a citrus fruit.
Civet	:	In perfumery, the glandular secretion obtained from the civet, *Viverra civetta*, and other species of *Viverra*, animals related to the weasel.
Classic perfume	:	A perfume accorded the distinction of representing the highest level of fragrance creation. A supreme example of the perfumer's art.
Coeur	:	The French word for 'heart'. The heart or main fragrance theme of a perfume, particularly in reference to a perfume for personal use.
Cohobation	:	A process of redistillation of distillation waters in order to recover dissolved essential oil.
Colation	:	The removal of contaminating, insoluble particles from a liquid by straining through muslin, cotton wool, tow, etc. A process of coarse filtration.
Colloidal solution (or Colloidal sol)	:	A dispersion of ultra-fine particles in a continuous medium as, for example, of solubilised *micelles* of an oil in water. Colloidal particles, though invisible, will scatter light, so that a beam of light, itself invisible in a dust-free room, can be seen if passed through a colloidal solution.
Column	:	In GLC, the long tube, containing the stationary phase, through which the carrier gas transports the vapourised sample for separation of constituents.
Compound	:	In chemistry, a substance composed of atoms of two or more elements bonded together in fixed and definite proportions by mass. In perfumery, a finished perfume composition in concentrated form.
Concentration	:	A process of increasing the proportion of a required substance present in a mixture, or the weight per unit volume of a substance present in a mixture as, for example, the concentration in grams per litre of an alkali or acid in a standard solution.
Concrete	:	In perfumery, an aromatic, waxy or fatty extract prepared by washing a natural, aromatic source material with a pure, volatile hydrocarbon solvent, such as hexane, followed by recovery of the solvent. Most concretes are amorphous, solid or semi-solid masses containing essential oil, natural wax and pigments from the source.
Condensation	:	The change of state of a substance from gas or vapour to liquid or solid. As used in organic chemistry, condensation is a term of indefinite meaning, usually referring to a process of synthesis between two reactants, in which a covalent bond is formed between a carbon atom of one reactant and a carbon atom of the other, with the elimination of a small molecule of some kind, such as water.
Condenser	:	In distillation, a cooling device for removing sufficient heat from the distillation vapour to enable it to change to the liquid state (or to the solid state if, as in the case of Orris oil, the product is solid at room temperature).
Coppiced	:	The regrowth of a tree in the form of thin stems after felling to leave a stump.
Corps	:	A prepared fat, such as a mixture of purified suet or lard, as used in the enfleurage process.
Correction factor	:	A figure by which the recorded percentage of a constituent of a mixture of volatiles, as given by GLC analysis, has to be multiplied to find its true percentage in the mixture.

Cosolvent	:	A solvent which increases the solubility of a solute in the principal solvent of a solution. Water, for example, dissolves about 9 per cent of its weight of phenyl ethyl alcohol at ordinary room temperature. The addition of increasing amounts of ethanol to water progressively increases the solubility of the aroma chemical.
Covalent bond	:	A bond between two atoms consisting of a shared pair of electrons. See also double bond.
Covalent compound	:	A compound consisting of atoms of two or more elements joined by covalent bonds.
Creativity	:	In perfumery, the artistic composition of an original perfume from aromatic raw materials.
Croton oil	:	A fixed oil obtained from the seeds of *Crotum tiglium*, a tree cultivated in Southeast Asia, and once used in medicine in minute doses as a powerful cathartic and counterirritant. Not suitable as a carrier oil for aromatherapeutic purposes.
Cyclic	:	In chemistry, descriptive of a molecule containing one or more rings of atoms, such as the molecules of benzene and cyclohexane.
Defleurage	:	The removal of spent flowers from the chassis in the enfleurage process.
Depart	:	Abbreviation for the French expression '*note de départ*', meaning '*top note*'.
Derivative	:	In perfumery, a single constituent or a mixture of constituents, separated from an essential oil or aromatic extract. Linaloöl, isolated from rosewood oil, terpeneless petitgrain oil and petitgrain terpenes are examples of derivatives.
Dermatology	:	The study of the histology, physiology and pathology of the skin and the treatment of skin diseases.
Desorption	:	The detachment of adsorbed atoms or molecules (see Adsorption) from an adsorbent as, for example, following the headspace capture of a flower fragrance for analysis of the desorbed vapour by capillary GLC.
Detector	:	A device which responds to a change of some kind in its environment as, for example, a change of temperature, pressure, electrical conductivity (as with the flame ionisation detector used in GLC) or radiation of some kind. Electrical signals from a detector of an analytical instrument, such as a gas-liquid chromatograph, are transmitted, after amplification, to a computer and pen recorder for the purposes of visual display and permanent recording of the analytical results.
Determination	:	In chemistry, any process of analysis leading to a quantitative result.
Dextrorotatory	:	The property of a material, such as d-limonene, to rotate the plane of polarised light in a clockwise direction.
Diffusion	:	The spontaneous spreading out of a gas or vapour, or of a solute placed in a solvent in which it is soluble, to become evenly distributed throughout the whole of the available space.
Dissociation	:	A chemical process in which molecules split into smaller groups of atoms or molecules or into ions. An example is the dissociation of water molecules into hydrogen ions and hydroxide ions; another is the dissociation of molecules of acids into ions on contact with water.
Distillate	:	Any product of distillation collected in the receiver of a still.
Distillation	:	The process of vapourising a substance in a distillation vessel and collecting the product of cooling the vapour in a separate vessel or in the case of reflux distillation, in the same vessel.

Double bond	:	A linkage between two atoms, consisting of two bonding pairs of electrons.
Dry down	:	The final residue of odour remaining after the almost total evaporation of an aromatic material or perfume.
(E-)	:	Abbreviation, used in chemistry, for the German word *entgegen*, meaning 'opposed to', in reference to the *trans-* form of a pair of geometrical isomers [see *cis- trans-* isomerism and also (Z-)].
Electron	:	A negatively charged particle, of mass approximately 1/2000 of that of a proton.
Electronic nose	:	An electronic instrument for the characterisation of odours independently of the human nose.
Electron shell	:	A region of space around the nucleus of an atom containing one or more electron orbitals.
Electrovalency	:	The combining power of an atom, numerically equal to the number of electrons that it can lose or gain to form an ion.
Element	:	A substance composed of atoms, the nuclei of all of which contain the same number of protons. It follows that the atoms of an element will all contain the same number of electrons, external to the nucleus, equal to the number of protons. This number is unaffected by the presence of neutrons in the nuclei of the atoms. Isotopes of the same element therefore have identical chemical properties.
Emollient	:	A material capable of restoring the flexibility and elasticity of the skin.
Empatage	:	In enfleurage, the process of spreading the *graisse* on the glass plate of a chassis.
Empirical formula	:	The simplest formula expressing the composition of a chemical compound. For example, the molecular formula for ethanol is C_2H_5OH, corresponding to the empirical formula C_2H_6O.
Enantiomer (or Enantiomorph)	:	An optical isomer.
Enantiomorphism	:	The existence of optical isomers of the same chemical compound.
End point	:	The point during a titration at which neither of the reactants is in excess, as at the point of neutrality when an alkali is titrated with an acid.
Enfleurage	:	The process of absorbing the fragrance (as essential oil) from living flowers of the same kind into specially purified, preserved fat over a period of many hours.
Enzyme	:	A biochemical catalyst, such as the zymase of yeast used in fermenting certain natural sugars to ethanol and carbon dioxide in the brewing industry.
Essential oil	:	The term 'essential oil' is frequently used quite loosely, to refer to any fragrant product from a natural source, whether distilled, extracted or expressed. Most commercial essential oils do not, in fact, conform to a strict definition, which may be stated as follows: 'An essential oil is a totally volatile product, obtained from a natural source of a single species, which corresponds to that species in chemical composition and odour.'
Ester	:	The organic product of a reaction between an alcohol or phenol and a carboxylic acid.
Esterification	:	The type of reaction by which an ester is synthesised from an alcohol or phenol and a carboxylic acid.
Ester value	:	The percentage of an ester in an essential oil.
Ether	:	An organic compound the molecules of which are characterised by the presence of an oxygen atom bonded to two hydrocarbon chains, ring systems or other hydrocarbon molecular structures.

Evaporation	:	The physical change of a liquid or solid to the vapour state.
Extending	:	The practice of increasing the quantity of an aromatic material by the addition of a cheaper material without altering the properties, in particular the odour and appearance, of the material to a generally perceptible extent.
Extract	·	The soluble matter obtained from a natural source, such as jasmin flowers, by washing with a pure, volatile solvent and subsequent recovery of the solvent by distillation, usually under reduced pressure. The concretes, absolutes and resinoids of perfumery are examples of extracts.
Expression process	:	A mechanical process of scarification or compression for obtaining the essential oils from citrus fruits.
Exudate	:	A resinous product, such as benzoin, frankincense or myrrh, produced by the cambium of a woody plant, either naturally or in response to wounding or removal of bark.
Fatty aldehyde	:	A straight chain or branched chain aldehyde having the general formula $C_nH_{2n+1} \cdot CHO$. Molecules of the fatty aldehydes commonly used in perfumery contain from 7 to 14 carbon atoms.
Fermentation	:	A process of the partial decomposition of organic matter, catalysed by enzymes as in the fermentation of grape sugar (dextrose) by the zymase of yeast in the making of wine. Useful perfume ingredients can be produced by the bacterial fermentation of certain terpenes.
Fine fragrance	:	A fragrance of the highest quality.
Fixation	:	The technique of prolonging the lasting power of the main fragrance theme of a perfume.
Fixative	:	A material, such as sandalwood oil, capable of prolonging the effects of the main fragrance theme of a perfume. Resinoids are excellent fixatives by virtue of their content of odourless resin.
Fixed oil	:	An oil, such as a vegetable oil, which is nonvolatile at ordinary temperatures and atmospheric pressure.
Flame ionisation detector (FID)	:	A device for detecting the vapours of constituents of mixtures of volatiles, such as essential oils or perfumes, which have been separated by a GLC column. The separated vapours pass through a small flame of burning hydrogen, wherein they burn, causing changes of electrical conductivity between two electrodes at high potential difference placed near to the flame. These changes are approximately proportional to the relative amounts of the constituents in the original sample.
Flavedo	:	The coloured part of the rind of a citrus fruit.
Floret	:	A small flower, usually one of a cluster, such as the florets of hyacinth or lilac blossom which together form complete flowers.
Floriental	:	An oriental type perfume displaying emphasis on floral notes, such as those of exotic flowers—jasmine, tuberose, gardenia, plumeria, etc.
Fond	:	The French word for 'base' or 'foundation', used in reference to the base of a perfume.
Formulation	:	The process of composing a formula for a product of some kind, such as a perfume.
Fougère	:	French word meaning 'fern'. A type of perfume based on a combination of oakmoss or treemoss and the aroma chemical coumarin, and displaying emphasis on lavender in the top note.

Fraction	:	In chemical and perfume technology, a separately collected portion of the distillate from the distillation of an essential oil or crude aroma chemical.
Fractional distillation	:	A distillation process in which portions of the distillate having different boiling points or ranges of boiling point, are collected in separate receivers.
Fractionating column	:	A hollow, vertical column, made of glass, stainless steel or other nonreactive, nonabsorbent material, used for separating fractions from the vapours rising up the column from a distillation vessel beneath.
Fragmentation pattern	:	The displayed results of the separation of fragments of the molecules of a chemical compound bombarded by high-energy electrons in a mass-spectrograph.
Frankincense	:	A resinous exudate from the trunk of the tree *Boswellia carterii* and other species of *Boswellia*. Known also as *olibanum*.
Frequency	:	Number of complete vibrations (cycles) per second. Measured in Hertz (Hz).
Functional group	:	A group of bonded atoms or a single atom, which is the most chemically reactive part of a molecule.
Furanocoumarins	:	Derivatives of coumarin, certain of which are phototoxic, found as constituents of citrus oils and some other essential oils also known also as bergaptenes.
Gas–liquid chromatography	:	In analytical technique for separating the constituents of a minute sample of a mixture of volatiles, such as a natural aromatic material or a perfume, and recording the results of the analysis. The sample is vapourised and the constituents separated by virtue of differences in their solubilities in a nonvolatile absorbent coating the inner walls of a long capillary tube (the chromatography column) through which they pass. The vapourised sample is carried through the column in a low stream of helium or nitrogen and all constituents are kept in the vapour state by means of hot air circulating round the column. The results of the analysis are recorded as a series of peaks, drawn by a pen recorder, each one of which corresponds, with respect to its position, to a constituent of the sample.
Gel	:	Colloidal solution in which the colloidal particles are combined with the solvents to form a semi-solid, such as a jelly.
Gene	:	A unit of the molecular genetic code, located on a chromosome. Sequences of genes provide the programme whereby specific anatomical and physiological features of an organism are passed on from one generation to the next.
Genetic	:	Pertaining to the means whereby inherited characteristics of a living organism are transmitted from one generation to the next.
Genetic code	:	The sequence of information, in the form of units of three organic, nitrogen-containing bases called codons, which, as present in genes, determines the composition of all proteinaceous matter in a plant or animal cell. Each codon codes for the biosynthesis of one specific amino acid of the molecular chain of a protein.
Genotype	:	The genetic constitution of an organism, as determined by its genetic code.
GLC match	:	A mixture of aromatic materials prepared to conform to the results of analysis by GLC of a perfume compound or complex aromatic material such as a fragrance base.
GLC trace	:	A chromatogram.
Glycoside	:	A member of a family of plant cell constituents which on hydrolysis undergo partial decomposition to a sugar and another compound, called an aglycon.

Some aglycons are volatile and if formed during the distillation of an essential oil, appear as constituents of the oil.

Graisse	:	A French word, meaning 'grease', formerly used in perfumery in reference to the mixture of purified fats used in the enfleurage process.
Halo effect	:	A perceived impression that the functional performance of a perfumed product is better than that of the same product which is either unperfumed or perfumed with a less suitable fragrance.
Harmony	:	In perfumery, a pleasing blend of fragrance notes having a smooth, unified effect.
Headspace	:	The space bounded by the walls of a container, the closure and the surface of its contents.
Headspace analysis	:	Analysis, by gas–liquid chromatography, of the gas or vapour present in a headspace.
Heartwood	:	The internal, nonliving part of a woody stem, branch or tree-trunk.
Heating block	:	The part of a gas–liquid chromatograph, situated at the entrance to the column, where injected samples for analysis are quickly vapourised by heat.
Hedonic	:	Pertaining to pleasant and unpleasant sensations, or sensual pleasure.
Herbivore	:	A plant-eating animal.
Hertz	:	Unit of frequency in cycles per second.
Histology	:	The study of the fine structure of animal and plant tissues.
Holistic medicine	:	Any form of medicine in which treatment is decided after consideration of the conditions of the entire organism to be treated, rather than by deduction from the symptoms of the disorder.
Homologous series	:	A series of organic compounds in which successive molecules differ only by a $-CH_2-$, or methylene, group of atoms.
Humectant	:	A hygroscopic substance, such as glycerol (glycerine), which can moisturise the skin by absorbing water vapour from the air and possibly also by promoting the upward movement of water to the skin from subcutaneous tissues.
Hydrocarbon	:	A compound composed of molecules consisting of atoms of carbon and hydrogen only.
Hydrogen bond	:	A weak, electrostatic bond formed between oppositely charged parts of polar molecules, such as the oxygen atom of an alcohol molecule and the hydroxy-hydrogen atom of another molecule of the same or a different alcohol.
Hydrogen ion	:	A hydrogen ion is a proton as produced, for example, by the dissociation of a molecule of an acid. In aqueous solution, a hydrogen ion combines immediately with a water molecule to form an oxonium ion.
Hydrolysis	:	The decomposition of a compound by water. Esters, for example, may under suitable conditions be hydrolysed to the alcohols and carboxylic acids from which they are derived.
Hydroxide ion	:	The negatively charged ion OH^-, produced by the ionisation of water molecules and characteristic of alkalis.
Hydroxy-group	:	The functional group $-OH$, present in water molecules and molecules of alcohols, and distinguished from the hydroxide ion by its electronic configuration and lack of negative charge.
IFA	:	International fragrance association. The voluntary body, based in Switzerland, which advises the perfume industry on the safety of fragrance ingredients.

Imine	:	An organic compound characterised by the presence in its molecules of an imino, >NH, functional group, as present in the indole molecule.
Indicator	:	A substance used, usually in very small amounts, to test for the presence or absence of another substance, to estimate the extent to which a reaction has taken place, to determine the concentration of a substance or to measure the pH of a solution.
Inflorescence	:	A collection of florets, together forming a complete flower, as found in the blossoms of hyacinths and members of the botanical family of Compositae, e.g., dandelions and daisies.
Infrared	:	An instrumental technique for measurement of the absorption of infrared radiation spectrophotometry (heat rays) over a range of frequencies by the molecules of a material, such as an (IRS) aroma chemical, essential oil or perfume compound. The infrared spectrogram, which is the analytical result of the IRS of a material, is extremely useful for purposes of identification as, like a fingerprint, it is unique to that material under standardised conditions of analysis.
Injection port	:	The fine hole through which samples, of the order of less than one microlitre, are injected into a gas–liquid chromatograph.
Inorganic chemistry	:	The study of the chemical behaviour of elements and of compounds of elements, other than carbon, but including ionic compounds such as carbonates and simple molecular compounds such as carbon dioxide.
Instrumental analysis	:	Analysis of any kind performed by an advanced analytical instrument, such as a chromatograph.
Integrator	:	A dedicated computer of the kind used to calculate the results of analysis performed by gas–liquid chromatography.
Interface	:	The boundary between two immiscible liquids or solids, or between a liquid and a solid.
Ion	:	An electrically charged atom or group of atoms, such as the sodium ion, Na^+.
Ionic association	:	The association (NB not combination) of ions to form an ionic compound, such as sodium chloride: $Na^+ + Cl^- \rightarrow Na^+Cl^-$.
Ionic combination	:	The chemical interaction of a metallic element with a non-metallic element to form an ionic compound. The reaction involves ionisation of atoms of the metal by electron loss to form positively charged metal ions, and of atoms of the nonmetal by gain of electrons lost by the metal atoms to form negatively charged nonmetal ions. The oppositely charged ions then associate to form ion-aggregates comprising the compound formed.
Ionisation	:	Any process of the formation of ions.
Isolate	:	A term usually employed to refer to a single constituent separated from a mixture of volatiles such as an essential oil. Typical examples are citral from lemongrass oil and linaloöl from rosewood oil.
Isomer	:	One of two or more chemical compounds, of which the molecules contain the same number of atoms of the same elements, but in which these atoms are combined or arranged in different ways. Examples of pairs of isomers are ethanol and dimethyl ether (C_2H_5OH and CH_3OCH_3, respectively), alpha- and beta-pinenes, in which the only difference is that of the position of the double bond in the molecules, the *cis-/trans-*isomers geraniol and nerol and the optical isomers *d-* and *l-*limonene.

Isomerism	:	The existence of isomers. See isomer.
Isotopes	:	Atoms of the same element containing different numbers of neutrons. The isotopes of a given element have the same chemical properties, but different physical properties, such as relative atomic mass and (hence) density.
Juice	:	Anglicised version of the French word *jus*, meaning 'juice', used colloquially in reference to a perfume compound.
Ketone	:	An organic compound characterised by the presence in its molecules of a carbonyl functional group bonded to two hydrocarbon radicals: $R \cdot CO \cdot R'$.
Key base	:	In perfumery, a mixture consisting of all the ingredients of a perfume compound which are essential to the specific character of the fragrance.
Key ingredient	:	In perfumery, an ingredient of a perfume essential to the specific character of its fragrance.
Lactone	:	An organic compound characterised by the presence in its molecules of an ester functional group as part of a ring system.
Laevorotatory	:	The property of a material, such as an essential oil, to rotate the plane of polarised light anticlockwise.
Latent heat of fusion	:	The quantity of heat required to melt a given mass of a solid to liquid at the melting point. This same quantity of heat is given out by the same weight of the liquid when it solidifies at the melting point. The melting point of a solid may therefore be defined as that temperature at which the liquid and solid states of a substance can coexist: an equilibrium temperature when the rate at which melting is taking place is equal to the rate of solidification.
Latent heat of a vapourisation	:	The heat required to vapourise a given mass of a liquid at the boiling point. This same quantity of heat is given out by the same weight of the vapour when it condenses, at the boiling point. The boiling point of a liquid may therefore be defined as the temperature at which the liquid and vapour states of a substance can coexist: an equilibrium temperature when the rate at which vapourisation is taking place is equal to the rate of condensation of the vapour.
Lift	:	The property of certain aromatic materials, such as ylang-ylang oil, extra, to render middle notes of a perfume perceptible in the top note.
Longitudinal waves	:	Alternate regions of compression and rarefaction propagated from a source through a medium of some kind, such as air or water in the case of sound waves.
Maceration	:	The process of allowing a definite weight of extractable matter to soak, in a closed vessel for several days, in a definite weight of alcohol of given strength to produce a crude tincture. The tincture is filtered and adjusted to standard strength with respect to its odour or content of an active ingredient, allowed to mature and finally filtered bright ready for use. Tinctures are today almost obsolete in both perfumery and pharmacy.
Marine	:	In perfumery, a note of the sea or seashore. The term 'oceanic' is an alternative and more expressive term having a similar meaning.
Mass number	:	The sum of the numbers of protons and neutrons in the nucleus of an atom.
Mass spectrometry	:	An instrumental analytical technique for determining the composition of a compound, usually an organic compound.
Matching	:	The copying of a perfume or complex perfume ingredient for the purpose of duplicating its fragrance and other properties.

Maturation	:	The ageing of a finished alcoholic perfume until fully mellowed.
Membrane	:	In biology, a thin, flexible sheet of tissue, such as the epidermis of the skin or of a leaf.
Meta-	:	In chemistry, a prefix referring to positions in a benzene ring which are separated by one carbon atom of the ring as, for example, the 1,3-positions.
Metastable	:	A transient condition of a system or part of a system, such as exists in a supercooled liquid. A liquid in this condition remains liquid at temperatures below the melting point, and is an example of a substance in a metastable state. Certain aroma chemicals, having melting points a few degrees above normal room temperature, such as diphenyl oxide, $C_6H_5OC_6H_5$, melting point 26.5°C, frequently show this phenomenon. Solidification occurs on sufficiently disturbing the supercooled liquid or on adding to it a crystal of the solid.
Micelles	:	Colloidal particles consisting of droplets of oil surrounded by molecules or ions of a surfactant which prevent the droplets from coalescing. Soap and soapless detergents are surfactants which form micelles with oily dirt ready for washing away.
Microlitre	:	One millionth of a litre.
Middle note	:	A fragrant note of intermediate volatility and lasting power.
Miscible	:	Capable of complete mutual dispersion in another substance. Liquid aromatic materials are in most cases mutually miscible in all proportions.
Molar	:	In chemistry, a molar solution is a solution containing one mole of a dissolved solute per litre of solution.
Molarity	:	The number of moles of a solute dissolved in one litre of a solution.
Mole	:	In chemistry, the quantity of an element or compound contained in its formula weight.
Molecular formula	:	The formula expressing the true numbers of atoms of the different elements present in a molecule of a compound.
Molecular geometry	:	The patterns of arrangement of the atoms in a molecule.
Molecular structure	:	Term used in reference to the shape of a molecule, as determined by the nature and direction of the bonds holding its atoms together.
Molecular weight	:	To a close approximation, the molecular weight of an element or compound is the ratio of the weight of one molecule of the substance to the weight of one atom of hydrogen taken as one atomic weight unit.
Molecule	:	The smallest particle of an element or compound which can exist on its own.
Monomer	:	A chemical compound capable of undergoing polymerisation.
Monoterpene	:	A terpene of molecular formula $C_{10}H_{16}$.
Mossy	:	An odour recalling Oakmoss or Treemoss absolute: woody, green, earthy and 'marine' in character.
Moving phase	:	In gas–liquid chromatography, the carrier gas.
MS	:	Mass spectrometry.
Mucus	:	The glairy, colloidal solution produced by mucous cells (goblet cells) which covers a mucous membrane, keeping it moist.
Musk	:	Natural musk is the dried, glandular secretion of the male musk deer, formerly used in perfumery as a fixative.
Naphthenic	:	An odour recalling that of naphthalene, the organic compound from which old-fashioned moth balls are made. Pure indole has a naphthenic odour.

Nature identical	:	Term designating a synthetic organic compound of the same composition and molecular structure as the same compound as it occurs in nature.
Nervous impulse	:	A wave of electrical negativity which flows over a nerve fibre from the point of stimulation to a synapse.
Neutron	:	An electrically neutral particle of unit mass present in the nuclei of the atoms of all elements other than hydrogen of unit atomic mass. The effect of the presence of neutrons in an atomic nucleus containing more than one proton is to bind the protons together.
Nitrile	:	An organic compound characterised by the presence of a cyano, functional group: $-C\equiv N$.
Nanometer(s) (nm)	:	A nanometer is one thousand millionth (10^{-9}) of a meter; a millionth of a millimeter.
Noodles	:	In soap technology, noodles are small, rounded masses of unperfumed soap base.
Nucleus	:	In chemistry, the positively charged, central body of an atom. In biology, a dense, organised, proteinaceous body found in the protoplasm of a plant or animal cell, containing hereditary material and controlling the metabolic activities of the cell.
Odourant	:	Any substance having an odour.
Odour balance	:	The odour effect of a blend of aromatic materials in which none of the constituent fragrance notes is more prominent than any of the others.
Odour masking	:	Rendering an unwanted odour imperceptible by means of a stronger odour, the effect of which is acceptable.
Odour note	:	A distinctive odour impression, i.e. one which can be recognised and identified.
Odour profile	:	A complete description of an odour in written, diagrammatic or graphical form, resulting from olfactory evaluation or instrumental measurement.
Odour purity	:	The extent to which the odour of a test sample of an aromatic material or perfume conforms to the odour of a standard sample of the same product.
Odour threshold	:	The least concentration or highest dilution, at which the odour of an odourant can be detected under standardised conditions.
Oleo-gum resin	:	A plant exudate consisting of a mixture of an essential oil, water-soluble gum and resin. Several of these natural products are purified by solvent extraction for use as resinoids in perfumery.
Oleoptene	:	The oily, odourous part of an essential oil, such as Rose Otto, which also contains volatile, odourless matter in solution or as a crystalline deposit.
Oleo-resin	:	A plant exudate consisting of a mixture of essential oil and resin. A small number of these products find use in perfumery as resinoids after purification by solvent extraction or other means.
Olfactory	:	Pertaining to the sense of smell.
Olfactory fatigue	:	Temporary loss of sensitivity to the odour of an odourant continuously smelled over a period of time. Fatigue to a certain odour leaves the nose fully sensitive to all other odours which it is able to detect. Recovery from olfactory fatigue is rapid and complete when the responsible odourant is no longer smelled.
Olfactory hairs	:	The submicroscopic, thread-like projections of primary olfactory nerve fibres of the olfactory organ which support odour-sensitive sites for detecting the presence of odourous molecules.

Olfactory organ	:	The twin, odour-detecting membranes of the nose situated on either side of the nasal septum (the partition between the two nostrils) within the nasal cavity.
Optical isomers	:	These are different optically active forms of the same chemical compound, in which the molecule of one form is the mirror-image of that of the other form. One of a pair of optical isomers, the *d-* form, rotates the plane of polarised light in a clockwise direction, while the other isomer, the *l-* form, rotates it in an anticlockwise direction. Interesting examples are *d-* and *l-* carvones, occurring as the chief odourous constituents of caraway oil and spearmint oil, respectively, and possessing the odours characteristic of the parent oils. This example illustrates the fact that optical isomerism can give rise to odour differences between stereoisomers.
Optical rotation	:	Rotation of the plane of polarised light by transmission through an optically active substance. Almost all essential oils show optical activity at least to some degree, arising from their content of optically active constituents.
Orbital	:	A region of space around the nucleus of an atom where an unpaired electron or an electron pair is most likely to be found.
Organ	:	The traditional arrangement of shelving holding a perfumer's palette of aromatic materials, so named for its resemblance to the console of a cinema organ. Now almost totally replaced by arrangements less conducive to creative thought.
Organic chemistry	:	The study of the chemical behaviour of compounds of carbon, other than carbon-containing ionic compounds such as carbonates and similar molecular compounds such as carbon dioxide.
Organic compound	:	A carbon compound other than a simple, ionic compound containing carbon, such as a carbonate or similar molecular compound such as carbon dioxide.
Oriental	:	A type of perfume characterised by a heavy and very long-lasting fragrance.
Ortho-	:	In chemistry, the prefix ortho- refers to adjacent positions in a benzene ring as, for example, the 1,2-positions.
Oxidation	:	A chemical reaction in which oxygen combines with an element or compound, or in which hydrogen is removed from a compound. A more fundamental concept is that oxidation is the loss of one or more electrons by an atom, ion or molecule.
Oxonium ion	:	The ion H_3O^+, formed by loss of a proton, H^+ (a hydrogen ion) from an acid molecule and its combination with a water molecule.
Oxygenated constituent	:	A constituent of an essential oil or aromatic extract containing combined oxygen.
Ozonic	:	A fresh odour note, similar to the odour of ozone (O_3) often found in the fragrances of modern consumer products, such as domestic laundry detergents.
Palette	:	By analogy with the palette of colours of an artist, the range of aromatic materials available to a perfumer.
Para-	:	In chemistry, the prefix para- refers to two positions in a benzene ring which are opposite to one another, i.e. separated by two carbon atoms as, for example, the 1,4-positions.
Partition	:	In physical chemistry, the distribution of a solute between two immiscible solvents in contact with one another. Thus if an essential oil is shaken with the solvents pentane and 50 per cent aqueous methanol, both oxygenates and terpenes will become partitioned between both solvents, with most of the terpene content dissolved in the pentane and most of the oxygenate content in the weak methanol. The phenomenon of partition affords a means for the preparation of terpeneless essential oils.

Patage	:	In the process of enfleurage patage is the inversion of the *chassis*, following defleurage so that the lower layer of graisse is now the upper layer, ready for a fresh charge of flowers.
Pathogenic	:	Disease-producing.
Peak area	:	The area of a peak on a chromatogram, which is approximately proportional to the amount of the constituent that it represents in the product subjected to analysis.
Peak height	:	The vertical distance from the base line of a chromatogram to the apex of a peak and which is proportional to the peak area.
pH	:	A measure of the acidity or alkalinity of an aqueous solution, expressed as a numerical value on a scale from 0 (extremely acidic) to 14.0 (extremely alkaline). A pH value of 7.0 expresses neutrality. (Scientifically, the pH of a solution is measured as the logarithm to base 10 of the reciprocal of the hydrogen ion concentration in moles per litre.)
Permanent gas	:	A gas, such as oxygen, nitrogen or hydrogen, which is difficult to liquefy.
Phenol	:	The organic benzenoid compound C_6H_5OH or any other compound of which the molecules each have one or more hydroxy groups bonded directly to a benzene ring.
Photocatalysis	:	A changing of the rate of a chemical reaction by the incidence of light. Essential oils deteriorate very much faster when exposed to sunlight than they do in darkness.
Photosynthesis	:	The manufacture of the sugar glucose in the leaves of a green plant from carbon dioxide and water in the presence of chlorophyll, using sunlight as a source of energy and with the evolution of oxygen.
Phototoxic	:	This term describes the property of a substance to exert a toxic effect in the presence of light, particularly sunlight as, for example, bergaptene in bergamot and some other essential oils.
Physical properties	:	Those properties of a substance which do not involve chemical change, such as melting point, boiling point, specific gravity or refractive index.
Physical test	:	A test, such as the determination of melting point or measurement of specific gravity, which does not involve a chemical change (change of composition).
Pilot-scale process	:	A process using apparatus of size intermediate between laboratory scale and industrial large scale, designed to facilitate determination of the conditions required for safe and efficient full-scale operation. Pilot-scale equipment is used, for example, for development of the full-scale manufacture of new aroma chemicals.
Plane of polarisation	:	The set of parallel planes in which rays of light travel following polarisation.
Polarisation	:	The filtration of rays of light orientated in all planes at right angles to their direction of travel, to allow only those rays orientated in a single set of parallel planes to pass through.
Polariscope (or polarimeter)	:	An instrument for measuring the optical rotation of a transparent liquid or solid.
Polariser	:	An optical filter for polarising light rays.
Polar molecule	:	A molecule on which there is an uneven distribution of electrical charge, such as a water molecule and molecules of alcohols, aldehydes and carboxylic acids.

Polyfunctional	:	A term used in reference to a molecule, such as that of vanillin, which contains functional groups of more than one kind.
Polymer	:	A larger molecule formed by the bonding together of small molecules, or parts of smaller molecules, of one or more monomers; a compound of high molecular weight formed by the bonding of molecules of one or two compounds of low molecular weight.
Pommade	:	The type of product resulting from enfleurage; it consists of graisse which has become saturated with essential oil exhaled by fragrant flowers.
Position isomerism	:	Isomerism in which the isomers differ in respect of the position of the functional group(s) in their molecules.
Pot	:	A distillation or reaction vessel.
Potential difference	:	A difference of electrical charge between two points, such as the poles of an electrical cell or other source of current.
Protein	:	A natural polymer of very high molecular weight, present in all living matter. A protein is formed by the linking together of amino acid molecules, with the elimination of water molecules.
Proton	:	A positively charged particle of unit atomic mass, which occurs in the nuclei of all atoms.
Protoplasm	:	The complex, organised, colloidal contents of all living cells.
Qualitative	:	A term descriptive of a test for identifying the atoms, ions or molecules present in a chemical compound or the components of a mixture.
Quantitative	:	A term descriptive of a test for determining the percentages of the elements combined in a compound or of the components of a mixture.
Radical	:	An atom or group of atoms having one or more unpaired electrons; symbol R.
Raschig rings	:	Rings made of glass, ceramic or other nonreactive material used in a fractionating column to increase the internal surface area available for condensing vapours rising up the column.
Reaction pathway	:	A succession of chemical reaction steps in which the product of one reaction is caused to undergo a further reaction to give an intermediate product until a required product is finally formed.
Reactive	:	In chemistry, a term applied to a substance which readily undergoes chemical change.
Reagent	:	Any substance which can undergo a chemical reaction. Applied mostly to chemicals used for testing purposes.
Receiver	:	In distillation, a vessel placed at the outlet of the condenser to collect the distillate.
Receptor	:	In biology, a cell or collection of cells capable of responding to a particular kind of stimulus, such as odourous molecules.
Reconstitution	:	In perfumery, the synthetic or largely synthetic reproduction of an aromatic material of natural origin. The term is also used to refer to the product of an exercise of this kind.
Reduction	:	In chemistry, the opposite of oxidation: a chemical reaction in which oxygen is removed from a compound or in which hydrogen combines with an element or compound. More fundamentally reduction is any reaction in which electrons combine with an atom, ion or molecule.

Reflux distillation	:	A process of distillation in which the distillation vapours are condensed by a vertical condenser and are continuously allowed to run back into the distillation vessel beneath. Used in chemical synthesis when a reaction mixture has to be heated for a time without loss of volatile material by evaporation, as in the manufacture of aroma chemicals.
Refractive index	:	In practical terms, a measure of the bending of parallel rays of light of a given frequency when passed from a less dense medium into a denser medium. In more precise, scientific terms, it is the ratio of the speed of light of given frequency in a vacuum to the speed of light in a medium of some kind at a specified temperature.
Refractometer	:	An instrument for measuring refractive index.
Relative atomic mass	:	The ratio of the mass of one atom of an element to $\frac{1}{12}$ of the mass of an atom of the isotope carbon-12 taken as 12 atomic mass units precisely.
Relative molecular mass	:	The ratio of the mass of one molecule of an element or compound to $\frac{1}{12}$ of the mass of an atom of the isotope carbon-12, taken as 12 atomic mass units precisely.
Resinoid	:	A purified, resinous plant exudate, such as an oleo-resin or oleo-gum resin.
Resolving power	:	In gas–liquid chromatography, the least amount of a volatile compound that a chromatograph can measure.
Respiration	:	The production of energy in an animal or plant cell by the enzyme-catalysed combustion of foodstuffs, chiefly glucose.
Retention time	:	In gas-liquid chromatography, the time which a vapourised compound takes to pass through the column.
Reversible reaction	:	A chemical reaction which can proceed in either direction according to prevailing conditions, such as the concentrations of the reactants and products of the reaction.
Reworking	:	In perfumery, the production of a close match of an original perfume, usually for the purpose of replacing ingredients which have become unavailable or too costly by equivalent materials likely to remain available for the foreseeable future.
Research institute for fragrance materials (RIFM)	:	A voluntary organisation, based in the United States, for testing the safety of perfume ingredients.
Rose alcohols	:	The rose-smelling alcohols citronellol, geraniol, nerol and phenylethyl alcohol, which occur in Rose Otto.
Saturated compound	:	An organic compound the molecules of which contain no multiple bonds.
Saturated solution	:	A solution containing as much of a solute as the solvent can hold at a stated temperature.
Scarification	:	A process of scraping as used, for example, in the mechanical expression of Bergamot oil from the peel of the fruit.
Sensory	:	In general, pertaining to the senses. In perfumery the term refers specifically to the sense of smell as, for example, in the expression 'sensory perception', meaning the process of smelling.
Septum	:	In gas–liquid chromatography, a small thin, flexible partition sealing off the injection port, through which samples for analysis are injected into the heating block for vapourisation.
Sesquiterpene	:	A terpene of molecular formula $C_{15}H_{24}$ ($1\frac{1}{2} \times C_{10}H_{16}$).

Shelf life	:	The period of time following manufacture during which a product remains fit for use.
Shoulder	:	In gas-liquid chromatography, the appearance of the apex of a smaller peak merged with the side of a larger peak due to imperfect separation of the corresponding volatiles.
Side chain	:	A chain of atoms joined to a ring or straight-chain molecular structure.
Side reaction	:	An unwanted chemical reaction, yielding an impurity, which takes place during a reaction for producing a required product.
Silicone	:	An organic, silicon-containing, linear or cyclic polymer of general formula $(R_2SiO)_n$, where R is a hydrocarbon radical. Depending on the value of n and on molecular structure, silicones take the form of oils, greases, rubbers, etc. which use for many different purposes, e.g. as water repellents, foam suppressants, lubricants, surfactants, flexible tubing, electrical insulators, etc.
Skeletal formula	:	A formula for an organic compound in which bonds between the carbon atoms are represented, but symbols for carbon atoms and for hydrogen atoms bonded to carbon atoms are generally omitted on the understanding that they are present. The conventional symbols are used to represent atoms of other elements present.
Snell's law	:	The natural law upon which measurements of refractive index are based. When a ray of light passes from a less dense medium to a denser medium the ratio of the sine of the angle of incidence to the angle of refraction is constant for a given pair of media at constant temperature. This relationship was discovered by the Dutch physicist Willebrord Snell.
Solubiliser	:	A water soluble surfactant capable of mediating the formation of a colloidal solution in water of water-immiscible liquids such as perfume compounds by the formation of micelles.
Solute	:	The dissolved substance in a solution.
Solvent extraction	:	The separation of soluble matter from a natural source material by a pure, volatile solvent, as in the preparation of extracts from aromatic sources, also of absolutes from concretes.
Specification	:	A statement of important properties of a product, to which all other samples or batches of the same product must conform to be acceptable.
Specific gravity	:	The ratio of the weight of a substance to the weight of an equal volume of water measured at a stated temperature.
Spectrogram	:	A graph or diagram of a spectrum, such as a spectrum resulting from the infrared spectrophotometric examination of an essential oil, showing the degrees of absorption of infrared rays over a range of different wavelengths under standardised conditions. In infrared spectrophotometric transmittance, the reciprocal of absorption, is recorded by the spectrometer.
Standard sample	:	A sample of a product which conforms to a specification for the product, and which is kept for purposes of comparison with batch samples for purposes of quality evaluation.
Standard solution	:	A solution containing a known weight of a given reagent in a known volume of solution.
Stationary phase	:	In gas-liquid chromatography, the general name give to the nonvolatile absorbent with which the interior of a capillary column is coated. The stationary phase, in conjunction with the carrier gas, effects separation of the vapourised constituents of a sample subjected to analysis.

Steam distillation	:	A process of distillation in which steam under pressure is used to heat the charge and release and vapourise the volatiles that it contains.
Stearoptene	:	Any volatile solid material from an essential oil following distillation, such as the mixture of colourless, waxy, odourless, crystalline hydrocarbons which separates from a genuine sample of Rose Otto on cooling in a refrigerator.
Stereospecific	:	Term used to designate a pure, synthetic stereoisomer, or to refer to a type of synthetic process which yields a pure stereoisomer.
Still	:	Any form of distillation equipment, usually excepting that used for reflux distillation.
Still head	:	The removable top part of a distillation vessel leading to and in many cases continuous with the vapour pipe.
Still note	:	An unpleasant, vegetable-like or cabbagey note commonly found in freshly distilled essential oils, caused by the presence of traces of very highly odourous organic sulphides, such as dimethyl sulphide, $CH_3 \cdot S \cdot CH_3$, formed by the partial hydrolysis of proteinaceous matter. Still notes can be eliminated by brief aeration of an essential oil so affected. The presence of 'burnt' or 'smoky' notes in an essential oil which should not display them is indicative of scorching of the charge and hence of a poor quality product. 'Burnt' notes are not true still notes cannot be eliminated. Birch tar oil and cade oil are produced by the destructive distillation of birch bark and juniper twigs, respectively. Both possess highly 'smoky' or 'burnt' odours but are not true essential oils. Guaiacwood oil and Chinese cedarwood oil are examples of essential oils possessing characteristically slightly 'smoky' or 'burnt' notes when of completely acceptable quality.
Straight chain	:	In organic chemistry, this term refers to a series of carbon atoms bonded together in succession.
Stretching	:	A form of adulteration of a costly aromatic material with cheaper material with the object of increasing the quantity without noticeably altering the odour character or strength. It should be noted that certain products so 'stretched' are perfectly usable as ingredients of consumer product perfumes, where the genuine counterparts would be too expensive to use or simply not available in sufficient quantities for bulk usage.
Striage	:	The making of furrows in enfleurage graisse following empatage to increase the surface area for absoprtion of flower fragrances (the natural essential oils of fragrant flowers).
Subjectivity	:	Dependence on human judgement and opinion.
Sublimation	:	In chemistry, the vapourisation of a solid or the solidification of a gas or vapour, without the appearance of the intermediate liquid phase.
Substantivity	:	In perfumery, the property of certain aromatic materials and perfumes to adhere to a surface, from which they are slowly released, yielding odour over very long periods of time. The term is used particularly in reference to lingering fragrance notes of a perfume in a product under in-use conditions. Examples are the 'fresh air', 'ozonic' or 'marine'-type notes found in certain domestic laundry product fragrances and in some fabric softeners, which survive the washing, rinsing, drying and airing sequence to render the linen clean-smelling.
Substituent	:	An atom or group of atoms replacing a hydrogen atom in a molecular structure, such as a hydroxy-functional group substituting for a hydrogen atom of a benzene ring in a molecule of a phenol.

Surfactant	:	A surface-active agent such as soap or a household detergent.
Surface active agent	:	A substance which can reduce surface tension; a surfactant.
Surface tension	:	The stretching force acting at the surface of a liquid. The existence of surface tension at the surface of water is shown by the rapid bursting of bubbles formed by vigorous agitation of the water. The addition of a surfactant reduces the stretching forces which break the bubbles, rendering them more permanent.
Synapse	:	A narrow gap between the endings of two nerve fibres in close association, across which nervous impulses are transmitted chemically.
Synthesis	:	The building up of a more complex chemical compound from elements or from simpler compounds.
Synthetic oil	:	A term sometimes loosely applied to refer to an aroma chemical, a perfume compound of synthetic composition or to an oily, odourless chemical, such as isopropyl palmitate or isopropyl stearate, which is nonvolatile under ordinary conditions of temperature and atmospheric pressure.
Temperature programming	:	In GLC, the computer-controlled increasing of temperature of the column at a predetermined rate to ensure that all components of a sample pass completely through it, and are not left behind to emerge during the next analysis.
Terpene	:	An unsaturated hydrocarbon of empirical formula $(C_5H_8)_n$, where $n = 1$ (hemiterpenes), 2 (monoterpenes), 3 (sesquiterpenes), 4 (diterpenes), 5 (sesterterpenes) or 6 (triterpenes). Terpenes occurring in distilled essential oils have $n = 2$ or 3, rarely 4. Higher, non-volatile, terpenes occur in plant extracts.
Terpeneless essential oil	:	An essential oil from which all or part of the terpene content has been removed by vacuum fractionation or solvent extraction, or a combination of both processes.
Terpenoid	:	A derivative of a terpene, such as citral, terpineol, linalyl acetate, etc. In industry, terpenoids are commonly referred to as terpenes.
Tête	:	A French word meaning 'head', used in perfumery to refer to the top note of an essential oil or perfume.
Thermal decomposition	:	A process of molecular fragmentation which occurs to a compound heated to a temperature high enough to break bonds. The higher the temperature to which a compound is heated, the more violent are the vibrations of its molecules until a temperature is reached when their structures begin to come apart.
Thermal stress	:	A condition of molecular vibration, brought about by heating a compound, which tends to strain certain of the bonds in their molecules to the point of structural breakdown.
Thermostatic control	:	The automatic control of temperature within narrow limits by means of a thermostat. This form of control is applied to the column of a gas–liquid chromatograph, which is contained in an oven fitted with a computer controlled thermostat and a fan to distribute heated air evenly throughout the length of the column. The oven temperature is usually set to increase progressively to a predetermined maximum during an analysis.
Thurible (or censer)	:	A container for glowing charcoal and incense used for purposes of religious ceremony. The thurible is supported by chains, usually held by hand, although there are certain places of worship where very large thuribles are suspended from the ceiling. The charcoal heats the incense, causing vapourisation and some thermal decomposition of its constituents, so producing fragrant smoke.

Swinging or looping of the thurible improves the air supply to the charcoal so that it does not burn out. A small door set in the body of the thurible provides for replenishment of the incense from time to time.

Tincture : In perfumery, an odour-standardised alcoholic solution of extractable matter from a source of aroma, prepared by maceration. Tinctures of musk, civet, ambergris and castoreum were once in regular use as perfume ingredients.

Titration : Measurement of the concentration of the solute in a solution. The following are the essential steps:

(a) A burette is filled to the zero mark with the required standard solution.

(b) An accurately measured volume of the solution whose concentration is to be found (the test solution) is transferred to a small flask.

(c) The standard solution is slowly added from the burette to the test solution in the flask, with constant gentle mixing of the contents of the flask until, at the end point, a colour change or a sharp change of electrical resistance occurs, whereupon the volume of the standard solution added is measured. From this measurement, and knowing the concentration of the standard solution, the concentration (or titre) of the test solution may be calculated. Modem equipment for titration is automatic and computer-controlled; it performs all the required calculations and displays the results.

Toilet water : A fragrant product consisting of a weak solution (not more than about 8 per cent) of a perfume compound dissolved in aqueous alcohol, intended for liberal application to the skin after bathing as a means of physical and mental refreshment. As the product rapidly evaporates, it loses its most energetic molecules (molecules of the alcohol-and-water base). The energy required for this evaporation is heat, which is withdrawn from the skin. The skin thus quickly cools, and at the same time the refreshing fragrance of the perfume is perceived. The heat transferred to the evaporating product is known as latent heat of vapourisation.

Top note : The first sensory impression perceived on smelling an aromatic material, perfume or perfumed product. It consists of the vapours of the most volatile together with some proportion of the lesser volatile ingredients of the perfume.

Total quality management (TQM) : A system of quality management aimed at the total elimination of product rejects by making all employees of a manufacturing company personally responsible for the quality of their work. TQM, if correctly applied, extends to every single employee, from the chief executive to the trainee. It should be noted that systems of TQM can be applied with advantage to all areas of human activity.

Transpiration : The evaporation of water from the leaves of a green plant. This process eliminates excess water from the plant, cools the leaves for maximum efficiency of photosynthesis and assists the transport of water and dissolved nutrients from the root system to all other living parts of the plant.

Transverse waves : Waves, such as those of the sea or of radiant energy, which travel in planes perpendicular to their direction of movement.

Triangle test : A form of sensory test designed to reveal differences in the odours of standard and test samples of an aromatic material, perfume or flavour compound which may be very small yet important. Two smelling-strip dips of equal depth are taken from the test material and one of the same depth from the standard, using strips inscribed with identification marks. The object of the test is to identify the strip smelling differently from the other two. The test is conducted with the reference marks of the strips unseen, so that the tester is unaware of their identity. Since any given triangle test is highly subjective, it should be carried out by more than one person independently and the result discussed.

Trickle down effect : The diffusion of fragrance ideas originating in the fine-fragrance sector of perfumery to the area of general perfumery and their appearance in mass-market products for domestic or personal care. Fragrance ideas may also 'trickle across' from one highly popular fragranced product to new products of the same or of a different kind. Very occasionally they even 'trickle up' as, for example, in the instance of a well-known fragrance initially appearing in a bath-time product being later refined and reintroduced as a fine fragrance for personal use.

Triple bond : A linkage between two atoms consisting of three bonding pairs of electrons.

Unsaturated compound : A compound of which the molecules each contain one or more double or triple bonds.

Vacuum fractionation : Fractional distillation carried out in a vacuum to reduce the boiling point of the charge to a temperature at which thermal stress will not occur.

Vacuum stripping : Removal of the last traces of a volatile substance, such as a solvent, from a product by evaporation in a vacuum.

Valency : The combining power of an atom, ion or radical.

Vapour : As usually employed, this term refers to a gas under such conditions that a small increase of pressure or decrease of temperature will cause it to condense, as water vapour condenses at the dew point.

Vapour pipe : The pipe leading from the still head to the condenser of a still.

Vegetable oil : A nonvolatile oil, consisting largely of esters of higher alcohols and higher carboxylic acids, from a vegetable source such as sweet almonds, jojoba seeds or wheat germ. Most purified vegetable oils are faintly odourous from traces of volatiles they contain.

Vibrational theory : A theory of odour detection, recently advanced by Luca Turin, which suggests that odourous molecules stimulate odour-sensitive sites on the olfactory hairs by their vibrations. This theory is subject to confirmation by further research as an alternative to the site-fitting theory of Amoore.

Viscosity : The internal friction experienced by a liquid which opposes its tendency to flow freely.

Vital force : The hypothetical force which was held to exist only in living matter and which was believed to be necessary for the synthesis of organic compounds. The idea of a 'vital force' was overthrown in 1845 by the German chemist Hermann Kolbe, who performed a total synthesis of acetic acid from its elements.

Volatile : Descriptive of a substance which evaporates when exposed to the air. Used also as a generic name for low boiling-point constituents of a natural source of aroma or flavour.

Volatility : The speed or rate at which a substance evaporates. In perfumery, the concept of volatility leads to the classification of aromatic materials as top, middle or basic notes.

Water distillation : A slow process of distillation in which aromatic plant material is kept in contact with boiling water for the purposes of volatilising its essential oil for subsequent condensation and collection. Only essential oils which resist thermal decomposition and the hydrolysis of their constituents, such as clove bud oil, can be produced successfully by water distillation.

Wavelength	:	The distance between two successive crests or two successive troughs of a train of transverse waves, or between two successive points of maximum compression or of maximum rarefaction in a train of longitudinal waves.
Worm	:	The coiled part of the vapour pipe of a still which is immersed in the cold water of the condenser.
X-ray diffraction	:	The scattering of X-rays by the atoms or ions of a crystalline solid to form a pattern of luminous spots on a screen, from which the arrangement of the particles forming the crystal may be deduced.
Ylang-Ylang	:	An expression in the Tagalog language of the Philippine Islands referring to something which nods and waves in the breeze, in the manner of the flowers of the Ylang-Ylang tree.
(Z-)	:	Abbreviation for the German word *zusammen*, meaning 'together' and referring to the *cis-* form of a pair of geometrical isomers.

References

Bayer, S., *Estimation of Essential Oils in Drugs and Plant Material*, Chem. Abstracts 30, 570.

Beckly, V.A., *Essential Oils and Their Methods of Production in Kenya*, Kenya Colony Department of Agricuture.

Braverman, J.B., *Citrus Products,* Interscience Publishers, Inc., New York.

Budyko, M.I., *Identification of Essential Oils,* Progress Publishers, Moscow.

Cash, L.S. and Fawsitt, C.E., *Estimation of Cineole in Essential Oils by the Cocking Process*, Chem. Abstracts 18, 1730.

Chopra, R.N., Nayar, S.L., *Glossary of Indian Medicinal Plants*, Council of Scintific and Industrial Research, New Delhi, India.

Cocking, T.T., *Estimation of Cineole in Camphor Oils*, Chem. Abstracts 21, 3252.

Dugan, L. Jr. and Haendler, H., *Benzylideneaminomorpholine Compounds*, Chem. Abstracts 37, 130.

Dugan, P.R., *Terpeneless Oils*, Plenum Publishing Corporation, London.

Eaton, J.L., *Essential Oil Industry of Seychelles*, Colony of Seychelles, Department of Agriculture.

Ernest Guenther, *Essential Oils*, D. van Nostrand Reinhold Company, New York.

Francis, D., *Notes on Analysis of Essential Oils*, Chem. Abstracts 34, 4862.

Ginzberg, A.S., *Simplified Determination of Essential Oils in Plants*, Chem. Abstracts 27, 372.

Greene, L.W., *Chemical Microscopy of Essential Oils*, D. van Nostrand, New York.

Hidy, G.M., *Species and Oleoresins,* Heinemann, London.

Hufenuessler, R.M., *Preparation of Terpeneless Oils*, Gordon and Breach Publishers, New York.

Pino, J.A., *Composition of the Essential Oil from Leaves and Flowers*, D. van Nostrand, New York.

Reclaire, A. and Frank, R., *Perfumery Essential Oil Record*, Chem. Abstracts 32, 8302.

Rosenberg, H.R., *Chemistry of Terpenes*, Interscience Publishers Inc., New York.

Sabetay, S., *Simplified Procedure for the Analytical Oximation of Aldehydes and Ketones*, Chem. Abstracts 33, 1268.

Scott, W.W., *Determination of Solubility of Oils and Fats*, Standard Methods of Sampling, D. van Nostrand, New York.

Wasicky, R. and Rottar, G., *Estimation of Essential Oils in Drugs and Plant Material*, Chem. Abstracts 27, 3557.

Whiestler, R.L., *Industrial Oils*, Academic Press, New York.

Zimmermann, *Analytical Methods for Perfumery Essential Oil*, Gordon and Breach Publishers, New York.

Index